Healthy Ageing

The Role of Nutrition and Lifestyle

Healthy Ageing
The Role of Nutrition and Lifestyle

The Report of a British Nutrition Foundation Task Force

Chaired by
Professor John C. Mathers

Edited by
Sara Stanner
Dr Rachel Thompson
Professor Judith L. Buttriss

(W)WILEY-BLACKWELL

A John Wiley & Sons, Ltd., Publication

Published by Wiley-Blackwell
for the British Nutrition Foundation

This edition first published 2009
© 2009 British Nutrition Foundation

Blackwell Publishing was acquired by John Wiley & Sons in February 2007. Blackwell's publishing programme has been merged with Wiley's global Scientific, Technical, and Medical business to form Wiley-Blackwell.

Registered office
John Wiley & Sons Ltd, The Atrium, Southern Gate, Chichester, West Sussex, PO19 8SQ, United Kingdom

Editorial offices
9600 Garsington Road, Oxford, OX4 2DQ, United Kingdom
2121 State Avenue, Ames, Iowa 50014-8300, USA

For details of our global editorial offices, for customer services and for information about how to apply for permission to reuse the copyright material in this book please see our website at www.wiley.com/wiley-blackwell.

Library of Congress Cataloging-in-Publication Data

Healthy ageing : the role of nutrition and lifestyle : the report of a British Nutrition Foundation task force / chaired by John C. Mathers; edited by Sara Stanner, Rachel Thompson, Judith L. Buttriss.
　　　　 p.　;　cm.
　　Includes bibliographical references and index.
　　ISBN 978-1-4051-7877-8 (pbk. : alk. paper)　1. Older people—Health and hygiene.　2. Older people—Nutrition.　3. Aging—Nutritional aspects.　4. Health behavior.　5. Lifestyles—Health aspects.　I. Mathers, John C.　II. Stanner, Sara.　III. Thompson, Rachel, Dr.　IV. Buttriss, Judith.　V. British Nutrition Foundation.
　　[DNLM: 1. Aging.　2. Aged.　3. Health Behavior.　4. Life Style.　5. Nutrition Physiology. WT 104 H434803 2009]
　RA564.8.H456 2009
　613′.0438—dc22
　　　　　　　　　　　　　　　　　　　　　　　　　　　　　　　　　　　　2008031224

A catalogue record for this book is available from the British Library.

Set in 9.5/11.5 pt Times by SNP Best-set Typesetter Ltd., Hong Kong
Printed in Singapore by C.O.S. Printers Pte Ltd

1　2009

Contents

This report is the collective work of all the members of the Task Force.
Authors of the final draft of each chapter are given below.

Foreword

Over the past couple of centuries, one of the most remarkable human achievements has been the apparently inexorable increase in life expectancy observed in most countries. For example, life expectancy of Japanese women has increased by about 40 years in the last 160 years and one in four Japanese girls born in the millennium year 2000 can expect to celebrate their 100th birthday. Sadly, in most cases the greater number of life years has brought with it more years of chronic morbidity so that much of humankind's experience of ill health and expenditure on medical and social care (especially in Western countries) are concentrated in the later years of life. Indeed, for a large proportion of common chronic medical conditions, age is the single greatest risk factor.

This worldwide increase in lifespan is evidence of considerable malleability in the ageing process and the challenge is to understand the factors influencing ageing so that strategies which facilitate healthy ageing (maintenance of the healthy ageing phenotype) can be maximised. Emerging evidence suggests that nutrition and lifestyle may be key environmental determinants of ageing because they have profound effects on the genomic and cellular damage which appears to be the fundamental cause of reduced function and increasing frailty which characterise physiological ageing. With this background, it was very timely for the British Nutrition Foundation to set up a Task Force to assess the role of nutrition and, to a lesser extent, physical activity in ageing. After an overview of the basic biology of ageing, we opted to take a systems approach and reviewed the evidence that nutrition influenced ageing of several of the major body organs and tissues including brain, gastrointestinal tract, musculoskeletal tissues, eyes, cardiovasculature and skin as well as the immune and endocrine systems. As far as possible, we focused attention on evidence from studies in humans rather than in experimental animals. Each chapter was drafted by one or two Task Force members and then critiqued by the rest of the Task Force.

It soon became clear that we need to take a life-course approach to nutrition and ageing and that, whilst there is encouraging epidemiological evidence that dietary choices influence ageing, there is a paucity of intervention studies which have tested the impact of particular nutrients, foods or dietary patterns on ageing in general or ageing of particular body systems. The significant gaps in knowledge are highlighted as priorities for future research and we hope that these recommendations will be useful to funding agencies, as well as to researchers, as increasing attention is focused on addressing the biological, medical and social aspects of the almost universal demographic shift in the age profiles of populations. In addition, as is now usual, this Task Force Report summarises the key points of each chapter in a question and answer format and considers the practical implications for public health.

In preparation of this Task Force Report, I have been privileged to work with a very talented and enthusiastic group of experts to whom I offer my grateful thanks. In addition, on behalf of the external Task Force members, I thank the BNF scientists who, in addition to authoring a number of chapters, provided a very efficient secretariat. Their support has been invaluable.

Professor John C. Mathers
Chair of the Task Force

Terms of Reference

The Task Force was invited by the Council of the British Nutrition Foundation to:

(1) Review the present state of knowledge of the link between dietary and lifestyle factors and the ageing process.

(2) Prepare a report and, should it see fit, draw conclusions, make recommendations and identify areas for future research.

British Nutrition Foundation
Healthy Ageing: The Role of Nutrition and Lifestyle
Task Force Membership

Chair:

Professor John C. Mathers, Professor of Human Nutrition, Human Nutrition Research Centre, School of Clinical Medical Sciences, University of Newcastle, Newcastle upon Tyne NE2 4HH

Members:

Professor Judith L. Buttriss
Director General
British Nutrition Foundation
High Holborn House
52–54 High Holborn
London WC1V 6RQ

Dr Robert Clarke
Reader in Epidemiology and
    Public Health Medicine
Clinical Trial Service Unit and
    Epidemiological Studies Unit
University of Oxford
Richard Doll Building, Old Road
    Campus
Roosevelt Drive
Oxford OX3 7LF

Professor Paul Dieppe
MRC Senior Scientist and
    Professor of Musculoskeletal
    Sciences
Nuffield Department of
    Orthopaedic Surgery
University of Oxford
Windmill Road
Oxford OX3 7LD

Professor Astrid E. Fletcher
Professor
Department of Epidemiology
    and Population Health
London School of Hygiene &
    Tropical Medicine
Keppel Street
London WC1E 7HT

Professor Thomas B.L. Kirkwood
Director, Institute for Ageing
    and Health and Centre for
    Integrated Systems Biology of
    Ageing and Nutrition
Henry Wellcome Laboratory for
    Biogerontology Research
Newcastle University
Campus for Ageing and Vitality
Newcastle upon Tyne NE4 SPL

Dr Susan A. Lanham-New
Reader in Nutrition
Nutritional Sciences Division
Faculty of Health and Medical
    Sciences
University of Surrey
Guildford GU2 7XH

Dr Nigel Loveridge
Senior Scientist, Bone Research
   Group (Medical Research
   Council)
Department of Medicine
University of Cambridge Clinical
   School
Addenbrooke's Hospital (Box
   157)
Cambridge CB2 2QQ

Dr Jonathan R. Powell
Unilever Corporate Research
Colworth Park
Sharnbrook
Bedford MK44 1LQ

Professor Michael J. Rennie
Professor of Clinical Physiology
University of Nottingham
School of Graduate Entry
   Medicine and Health
Derby City Hospital
Uttoxeter Road
Derby DE22 3DT

Professor Ian R. Rowland
Head of the Hugh Sinclair Unit
   of Human Nutrition
University of Reading
Whiteknights
Reading
Berkshire RG6 6AS

Ms Sara Stanner
Senior Nutrition Scientist
British Nutrition Foundation
High Holborn House
52–54 High Holborn
London WC1V 6RQ

Professor Angus Walls
Professor of Restorative
   Dentistry
Newcastle University
School of Dental Sciences
Framlington Place
Newcastle upon Tyne NE2 4BW

Dr Emilie A. Wilkes
Clinical Research Fellow
Graduate Entry Medical School
University of Nottingham
Derby City Hospital
Uttoxeter Road
Derby DE22 3DT

Observer:

Dr Alison Tedstone
Food Standards Agency
Aviation House
125 Kingsway
London WC2B 6NH (observer
   from January 2003)

Contributors:

Ms Julie M. Thompson
Unilever Corporate Research
  (*at time of writing*)
Colworth Park
Sharnbrook
Bedford MK44 1LQ

Mologic Ltd (*current address*)
Colworth Park
Sharnbrook
Bedford MK44 1LQ

Ms Brigid McKevith
Senior Nutrition Scientist (until
  2006)
British Nutrition Foundation
High Holborn House
52–54 High Holborn
London WC1V 6RQ

Dr Linda J. Wainwright
Unilever Research and
  Development
Colworth Park
Sharnbrook
Bedford MK44 1LQ

Dr Martin R. Green
Unilever Research and
  Development
Colworth Park
Sharnbrook
Bedford MK44 1LQ

Dr Gail Jenkins
Unilever Reseach and
  Development
Colworth Park
Sharnbrook
Bedford MK44 1LQ

Dr Rosalyn J. Forsey
Unilever Corporate Research
  (*at time of writing*)
Colworth Park
Sharnbrook
Bedford MK44 1LQ

LCG Bioscience (*current address*)
Bourn Hall Ltd
Bourn
Cambridge CB3 7TR

Dr Graham Pawelec
Tübingen Ageing and Tumour
  Immunology Group
Centre for Medical Research,
  ZMF
University of Tübingen Medical
  School
Waldhornlestrasse 22
D-72072 Tübingen
Germany

External reviewer:

Professor Stuart Milligan
Professor of Reproductive
  Biology
Room 2.11N Hodgkin Building
King's College London
Guy's Campus
London Bridge
London SE1 1UL

Editors:

Ms Sara Stanner
Senior Nutrition Scientist
British Nutrition Foundation
High Holborn House
52–54 High Holborn
London WC1V 6RQ

Dr Rachel Thompson
Senior Nutrition Scientist
British Nutrition Foundation
High Holborn House
52–54 High Holborn
London WC1V 6RQ

Professor Judith L. Buttriss
Director General
British Nutrition Foundation
High Holborn House
52–54 High Holborn
London WC1V 6RQ

Secretariat:

Ms Brigid McKevith
Senior Nutrition Scientist (until
  2006)
British Nutrition Foundation
High Holborn House
52–54 High Holborn
London WC1V 6RQ

Ms Heather Caswell
Research Assistant
British Nutrition Foundation
High Holborn House
52–54 High Holborn
London WC1V 6RQ

1
Diet and Nutrition Issues Relevant to Older Adults

1.1 Introduction

This Task Force Report aims to identify steps that can be taken from a nutritional perspective to help the older adults of tomorrow to lead healthier lives. Subsequent chapters will discuss:

- the basic biology of ageing;
- the effect of ageing on a range of different organ systems and how a life-course food and nutrition approach, together with regular physical activity, may minimise or delay these effects; and
- public health recommendations and approaches that should be undertaken to improve the health of future older adults.

This first chapter sets the scene. It provides some details of the demographics of ageing and describes current patterns of ageing and health. It highlights some of the diet and nutrition issues relevant to today's older adults, many of which will be expanded in subsequent chapters.

Within this Task Force Report, definitions from the World Health Organization (WHO) are used; that is 'older' refers to a person aged 65 years or over and the 'oldest old' refers to those aged 80 years or over. However, it is important to recognise that definitive categorisation of older people is difficult, as 'old' is an individual-, culture-, country- and gender-specific term. For example, in developing countries many people are functionally 'old' in their forties and fifties (World Health Organization 2001). This means that older adults are a very heterogeneous group.

1.1.1 Demographics

Over the past hundred years many changes have impacted on people's lives. In some parts of the world during this time, life expectancy has almost doubled, at the same time fertility rates have declined, leading to changes in the demographics of the population.

Population ageing (characterised by a decline in the proportion of children and young people and an increase in the proportion of older people) has, until recently, been associated with the more developed regions of the world. For example, nine out of the ten countries with more than 10 million inhabitants, and with the largest proportion of older people, are in Europe (World Health Organization 2002a). However, the number of older people living in less developed regions is expected to increase from ~400 million.

1.1.1.1 Worldwide

The number of older people is set to increase (Figure 1.1), although it is important to note that the proportion of older people within the total population varies widely among countries *e.g.* from about 4% in Cambodia to around 14% in Japan in 2004 (World Health Organization Regional Office for the Western Pacific Region). From 1970 to 2025, a 223% growth in older adults is expected worldwide, so by 2025 there will be ~1.2 billion people over the age of 60. Decreasing fertility rates and increasing longevity will ensure the continued 'greying' of the world's

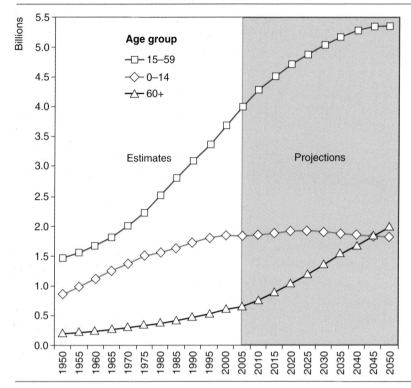

Figure 1.1: World population by age groups, 1950–2050. Source: United Nations Population Division, *World Population Prospects: The 2006 Revision.* Fact Sheet. Series A. New York: United Nations Department of Economic and Social Affairs, March 2007.

population, despite setbacks in life expectancies in some African countries (due to AIDS) and in some newly independent states (due, for example, to increased deaths caused by cardiovascular disease and by violence).

Over half the world's older people live in Asia and it is expected that Asia's share of the world's oldest people will continue to increase by the greatest amount. For example, it is projected that, by 2025, the proportion of older adults in Japan will increase to 26% of the population, and in China from 6.5% to 12% (World Health Organization Regional Office for the Western Pacific Region).

In 2002, globally, people over the age of 80 numbered ~69 million, the majority of whom lived in more developed regions of the world. This age group is the fastest growing segment of the older population (World Health Organization 2002a), owing to increased longevity, and is expected to increase with the post-Second World War baby-boom generation approaching their sixties (Ministry of Health 2002).

1.1.1.2 The UK

As in many other developed countries, life expectancy in the UK has continued to rise (Figure 1.2). In 1901, life expectancy at birth for females was 49 years and for males 45 years, whereas by 2002 life expectancy had risen to 81 and 76 years respectively. Consequently, the number of older people in the UK is increasing. The proportion of people aged 50 years or over has increased from 16 million in 1961 to 19.8 million people in 2002, a 24% increase. It is estimated that this number will continue to increase, with an estimated 27 million people aged 50 years or over by 2031 (National Statistics Online 2004) (see also Chapter 14, Section 14.1).

The proportion of people aged 85 and over will increase too. In 2001, this subgroup accounted for only 1.9% of the population; by 2031 it is estimated that it will make up 3.8% of the population. Currently, a very small proportion of older people in Great Britain are from non-white minority ethnic

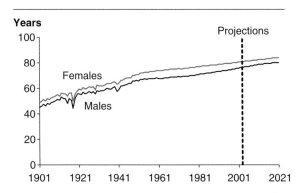

Figure 1.2: Life expectancy at birth in the UK. Source: Government Actuary's Department (www.gad.gov.uk); Babb *et al.* (2006).

groups (1%) but this will increase in the coming years.

1.1.1.3   Europe

Similar changes in demographics have been seen across Europe. Between 1960 and 2002 the proportion of older people in the EU-15 rose from 11% to 16%. Data for the EU-25 show a similar trend, although there is some variation between countries (*e.g.* 17.5% of Germany's population are aged 65 or over, while in Ireland and Liechtenstein it is closer to 11%). It is estimated that by 2010 there will be twice as many older people as in 1960 (69 million vs. 34 million), although as a proportion of the global population of older adults, Europe's share will decrease the most over the next two decades (World Health Organization 2002a).

Growth among those aged 80 or over is even more pronounced and it is estimated that between 2000 and 2010 the numbers of people in this age group will rise by 35%. Belgium, France, Italy and Luxembourg are expected to experience the largest increases (43–49%), while in Denmark and Sweden, growth of this age group will be negligible (Eurostat 2004).

1.1.1.4   The United States

In 2002 the older population of the US numbered 35.6 million, representing about 12.3% of the total population. It is expected that by 2030 the older population will have more than doubled to about 71.5 million; that the proportion of older people

from ethnic minorities will increase (from 16% in 2000 to 26% in 2030) and that the 'oldest old' will increase (from 4.6 million in 2002 to 9.6 million in 2030) (Administration on Aging 2003).

1.1.1.5   Other regions and countries

Africa: It is projected that Africa will experience an increase in absolute numbers of older people. For example, in western and northern Africa the number of older adults is expected to increase nearly five-fold between 1980 and 2025. A feature of ageing in Africa is the number of older people who live and work in rural areas (World Health Organization Regional Office for Africa).

China: According to 2003 estimates, 7.5% of the Chinese population are 65 years old and over. With continuing ageing of the population, the proportion of the people who are over 65 is projected to increase to 8.3% by 2010, 12% in 2020 and 22.6% by 2040. In 1990, about 30% of the people over 65 years of age were above the age of 75 years; this proportion is projected to rise to 35% by 2020, and 50% by 2050.

New Zealand: As in other developed countries, the proportion of older adults in the New Zealand population has increased (Figure 1.3). It is estimated that from 2001 to 2051 it will increase from 12% of the total population to 26%. The number of people aged 85 and over is projected to increase by 485% between 2001 and 2051. In comparison, the total population aged 65 and over is estimated to increase by 158% and the New Zealand population by only 20% (Ministry of Health 2002).

1.2   Ageing and health

Although data increasingly indicate that old age itself may not necessarily be associated with increased health service expenditure, the number of people reporting long-standing illness increases with age. For example:

- Baseline data from the Survey in Europe on Nutrition and the Elderly, a Concerted Action (SENECA) study of ~2,500 men and women from 17 towns in 11 countries across Europe, found the percentage of people suffering from a chronic

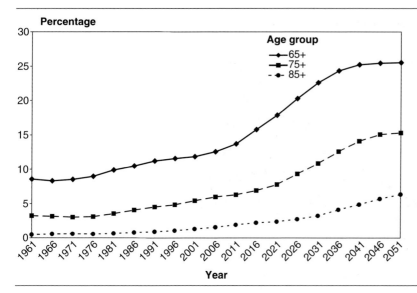

Figure 1.3: Changes in older adults – New Zealand population 65+, 75+ and 85+ as a percentage of the total population: 1961–2051. Source: Statistics New Zealand, *Census of Population and Dwellings 1961–1996 and Population Projections* (1999 base).

disease ranged from 59% (Yverdon, Switzerland) to 92% (Vila Franca de Xira, Portugal) (Schroll *et al.* 1991).

- Follow-up data from SENECA found that on average 68% of participating men and 78% of women aged 75–80 years had at least one chronic disease, with large variations between countries (*e.g.* 40% of Spanish men compared to 100% of Portuguese women have at least one chronic disease) (M. Schroll *et al.* 1996).
- In the US, 50% of older people had chronic diseases or some other form of disability (Blanc *et al.* 2004). The most frequently occurring conditions in 2000–1 were hypertension (49.2%), arthritic symptoms (36.1%), heart disease (31.4%), sinusitis (15%) and diabetes (15%) (Administration on Aging 2003).
- In Australia, survey data found that the prevalence of most conditions increased with age, to the extent that at least one long-term condition was reported for almost all (99%) of those aged 75 years and over. Among those aged 55 years or older, the most common long-term conditions included sight problems, arthritis, back and disc problems, hypertension and hearing loss (Australian Bureau of Statistics 2002).

Detailed statistics for the UK can be found in Chapter 14, Section 14.5.

Chronic or non-communicable diseases become the leading causes of morbidity, disability and mortality in all regions of the world as people age. A life-course approach to chronic disease has arisen against a background of increasing evidence that the risk of many chronic diseases is not just determined by risk factors in mid-adult life but begins in childhood or adolescence and potentially earlier during fetal development (Aboderin *et al.* 2002) (Figure 1.4).

The proportion of people reporting a disability tends to increase with age; additionally, the severity of disability increases with age. For example, data from New Zealand show that while 14% of women and 12% of men aged 15–44 years reported a disability; in those aged 75 years and above the proportion increased to 69% of women and 64% of men (Ministry of Health 2002). Similarly, the Health Survey for England 2001 indicates that while 66% of men and 68% of women aged 65–74 years reported no disability, less than a third of those aged 85 or older were disability-free. Among these age groups, prevalence of serious disability increases from 9% to 33% in men and from 9% to 42% in women (Figure 1.5) (Bajekal and Prescott 2003) (see Chapter 14, Section 14.5).

Older adults are disproportionately affected by sensory impairments (Desai *et al.* 2001). For example, in the US, although older people make up

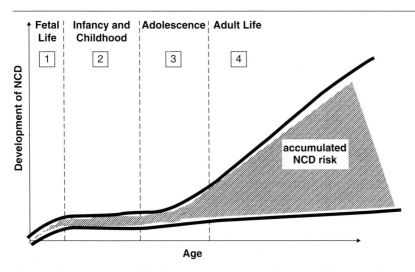

The risk of non-communicable diseases accumulates with age and is influenced by factors acting at all stages of the life span. The main factors at different stages of life include the following:

1 Fetal Life
fetal growth, maternal nutritional status, socioeconomic position at birth

2 Infancy and Childhood
growth rate, breastfeeding, infectious diseases, unhealthy diet, lack of physical activity, obesity, socioeconomic position

3 Adolescence
unhealthy diet, lack of physical activity, obesity, tobacco and alcohol use

4 Adult Life
known adult behavioural and biological risk factors

NCD: Non-communicable disease.

Figure 1.4: Life-course approach to non-communicable disease prevention.
Source: Aboderin *et al.* (2002).

only 12.8% of the population, they account for approximately 37% of hearing-impaired individuals and 30% of all visually-impaired individuals. It is estimated that worldwide about 4% of persons aged 60 and over are blind (60% of whom live in Sub-Saharan Africa, China and India). The major age-related causes of blindness and visual disability include cataracts (nearly 50% of all blindness), glaucoma, macular degeneration and diabetic retinopathy (World Health Organization 2002a) (see Chapter 9, Section 9.1). The Health Survey for England 2001 found 3%, 7% and 21% of men aged 65–74, 75–84 and 85+ years and 4%, 10% and 19% of women aged 65–74, 75–84 and 85+ years had moderate or serious sight disability, defined as not being able to recog-

nise a friend at a distance of 4 metres when wearing their glasses or contact lenses (Bajekal and Prescott 2003), and 62% of those aged 75 years and over reported more general eye complaints (see Chapter 14, Section 14.7). While globally over 50% of older people may have some degree of hearing loss (World Health Organization 2002a), in England lower levels have been found – 28% of men and 30% of women aged 85 years or older in the Health Survey for England had moderate or serious hearing disability (Bajekal and Prescott 2003). Both visual and hearing impairments can cause difficulties with communication; this can lead to frustration, low self-esteem, withdrawal and social isolation, increase vulnerability and limit quality of life (World Health Orga-

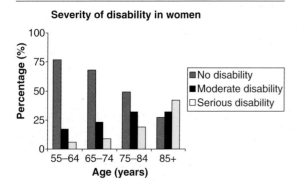

Figure 1.5: Severity of disability in women and men in England.
Source: Bajekal and Prescott (2003). Reproduced under the terms of the Click-Use Licence.

nization 2002a). Problems with locomotion (*e.g.* walking and climbing stairs), personal care (*e.g.* dressing and feeding oneself) and communication affect older adults more than younger adults (Bajekal and Prescott 2003).

Across Europe the number of older people free of any health problems, illness or disability has been shown to decrease with increasing age (Figure 1.6).

1.2.1 Causes of death

The main cause of death varies with age. For example, in 2002 the most common cause of death for people aged 50–65 years in the UK was cancer, while over the age of 65 circulatory diseases were the most common cause, with heart disease as a cause of death decreasing with increasing age and stroke increasing (National Statistics Online 2004).

Table 1.1 shows the leading causes of death in older people in a number of countries. However, the major causes of death can vary according to gender and race. For example, US data from 1997 show that diabetes was the third leading cause of death among older American Indian and Alaskan Native men and women, it was the fourth leading cause of death among older Hispanic men and women and ranked sixth among white men and women and older Asian and Pacific Islander men (Federal Inter-agency Forum on Ageing-Related Statistics 2004).

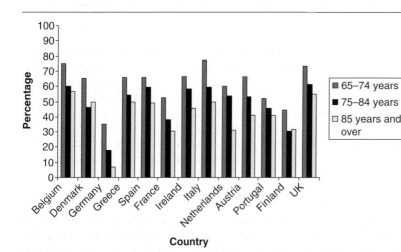

Figure 1.6: Percentage of older people free of any physical or mental health problem, illness or disability.
Source: ECHP UDB, EUROSTAT (06/2003).
© European Communities, 1995–2007.

Table 1.1: Leading causes of death among older people in selected countries

Country	Year	Leading causes of death (% of total deaths in older adults)	Reference
Australia	1999	Circulatory system (46%) Cancer (25%) Respiratory system (9%)	World Health Organization statistics
America	2001	Heart disease (32.4%) Cancer (21.7%) Cerebrovascular diseases (8.0%)	National Center for Health Statistics
Chile	1999	Circulatory system (34%) Cancer (22%) Respiratory system (17%)	World Health Organization Statistics
England and Wales	2002	Circulatory system (42%) Cancer (24%) Respiratory system (15%)	National Statistics Online (2004)
France	1999	Circulatory system (35%) Cancer (24%) Respiratory system (9%)	World Health Organization statistics
Germany	1999	Circulatory system (58%) Cancer (22%) Respiratory system (7%)	World Health Organization statistics
Ireland	1999	Circulatory system (45%) Cancer (21%) Respiratory system (19%)	World Health Organization statistics
Japan	1999	Circulatory system (34%) Cancer (27%) Respiratory system (16%)	World Health Organization statistics
New Zealand	1996–98 combined	Ischaemic heart disease (25.8%) Cancers (19.55%) Other circulatory disease (13.5%) Respiratory diseases (13.98%) Stroke (10%)	Ministry of Health 2002

1.2.2 Quality of life

Quality of life (QoL) issues in ageing also need to be recognised and addressed because the term 'health' encompasses more than just the absence of disease. For example, the WHO (2001) defines health as the state of complete physical, mental and social wellbeing.

The factors important in QoL may differ from person to person, but independence, self-esteem and socio-economic security are typically key factors. It is important to recognise that, as some foods have symbolic meaning and particular food habits are influenced by religious, cultural, social and emo-tional experiences, some dietary interventions may not lessen disability or extend life expectancy but may still be worthwhile if they enhance the individual's QoL (Wahlqvist and Saviage 2000). Equally, in some older adults, traditional food will be preferred even if it is known that these foods are not nutritionally ideal. Control of food choice and/or preparation may improve self-esteem in some older adults.

1.3 Ageing, gender and ethnicity

As mentioned above, there are gender differences with respect to ageing. Women outlive men in virtually all societies, so that there are more older women than men (World Health Organization 2002a). Men are more likely to engage in behaviours known to lead to health problems and premature mortality such as poor diet, smoking and excessive consumption of alcohol and other substances harmful to health. This means that women generally have a longer life expectancy and in developed countries men's life expectancy is at least five years lower than women's (Payne 2004). But it appears that this gender inequality is slowly changing, in some countries at least. For example, in Great Britain, death rates for men have fallen faster than for women over the last 30 years and are expected to continue. There were 28% more women than men aged 50 and over in 1961 but only 18% more in 2002, and by 2031 the number is expected to have reduced further, to 14% (National Statistics Online 2004).

Health inequalities have been noted among people of different ethnic groups, for example life expectancy varies by race. In New Zealand, the life expectancy of Maori and Pacific people is lower than that of the general population due to higher mortality rates, particularly for circulatory diseases and cancers, at earlier ages. In the 65–74 age group, the Maori mortality rate is 104% higher than that of European/other New Zealanders. The mortality rate for Pacific peoples aged 65 and over is also much higher than for European and other groups of the same age (77% higher) (Ministry of Health 2002).

Some ethnic groups are more susceptible to certain chronic diseases. In the UK the risk of stroke is higher among men from African-Caribbean and South Asian communities (Department of Health 2001). *The Health Survey for England 1999 – The Health of Minority Ethnic Groups* found higher rates of cardiovascular disease among South Asian groups compared with the general population, and Black Caribbean men and women had a higher prevalence of diabetes (Erens *et al.* 2001).

Nationally representative data from the US have also shown differences in nutritional intakes and status between different ethnic groups. The Third National Health and Nutritional Examination Survey (NHANES III, 1988–94) found that, compared to non-Hispanic whites, older non-Hispanic blacks and Mexican Americans generally had lower mean dietary intakes and a higher prevalence of inadequate iron and zinc intakes, or intakes below the recommendation for calcium (Ervin and Kennedy-Stephenson 2002).

The British National Diet and Nutrition Survey (NDNS) for older people does not provide information according to ethnic group. However, the *Health Survey for England 1999 – The Health of Minority Ethnic Groups* specifically focused on ethnicity and found differences in eating habits among minority ethnic groups (Erens *et al.* 2001). For example, the proportion of Chinese men and women who consumed fruit and vegetables six or more times a week (46% and 53% of men and 60% and 69% of women, for fruit and vegetables respectively) was higher than corresponding proportions of all other minority ethnic groups, and a higher proportion of Bangladeshi men (13%) and women (11%) than of other minority ethnic groups consumed red meat six or more times a week (Erens *et al.* 2001).The participants (adults over 16 years) in this survey were not segmented by age and no comparisons were made with the general population (also see Chapter 14, Section 14.5.1).

A series of smaller studies have also noted differences in nutrient intakes between ethnic groups:

- A study of 2655 older adults found that, compared to whites, African-Americans were more likely to have inadequate intakes for most nutrients (American Dietetic Association 2000).
- The San Luis Valley Health and Aging Study found Hispanic participants were more likely than non-Hispanic whites to report inadequate intakes of vegetables, problems with teeth or dentures, difficulty preparing meals and lack of money to buy food (Marshall *et al.* 1999).
- An American study found that Hispanic older adults consumed fewer saturates and simple sugars and more complex carbohydrates than did non-Hispanic whites, although those Hispanics who had been living in the US for a longer period of time tended to have macronutrient profiles more like those of the non-Hispanic whites (Bermudez *et al.* 2000).
- A UK study of men and women aged 25–79 years from Pakistani, European and African-Caribbean communities found iron intakes were low among the African-Caribbean group (Table 1.2).

As the proportion of older people from ethnic minorities is projected to increase in many countries, and because of the health inequalities described above, it is important that robust data are collected on these groups of older adults.

Table 1.2: Nutrient intake per day (means)

Nutrient	Men			Women		
	White European (n = 38)	African-Caribbean (n = 99)	Pakistani (n = 34)	White European (n = 48)	African-Caribbean (n = 147)	Pakistani (n = 50)
Iron (mg)*	15.5	12.1	14.8	14.8	10.1	14.1
Calcium (mg)*	1133	939	605	1063	828	601

*Reference nutrient intake (RNI): iron 8.7 mg/day for men and 14.7 mg/day for women; calcium 700 mg/day for adults.
Source: Vyas *et al.* (2003).

1.4 Costs of an ageing population

A large proportion of public health funds are spent on older adults, that is to say, although older people account for only 16% of the UK population, just over a third of hospital and community health service spending can be attributed to them (Wanless 2004). Additionally, in England almost two-thirds of general and acute hospital beds are occupied by people over 65 (Department of Health 2001).

As well as impacting on health care spending, an increase in the average age of the population has consequences in relation to the workforce and pensions. The changing age composition of the population will reduce the proportion of workers and increase the number of dependent older adults, but several factors may influence these changes. For example, the increase in experience associated with an older workforce will typically raise average earnings and productivity per worker (Rogers *et al.* 2000). 'Savings' may be made from the decreased per capita expenditure on school education as the proportion of the population of school age will be reduced.

1.5 Nutritional requirements of older people and current recommendations

1.5.1 Energy

Energy is needed by the body for a number of different functions (FAO/WHO/UNU 2004). The largest component of energy expenditure is that required to maintain physiological equilibrium and is referred to as basal metabolic rate (BMR). BMR is influenced by fat-free mass, age, sex, thyroid hormones and protein turnover. Energy is also required to digest and absorb food and for the regulation of body temperature (thermogenesis), as well as for physical activity. In addition, energy is required for growth, pregnancy and lactation. Energy requirements are estimated from measures of energy expenditure and revised values for the UK population are expected to be published in 2008. Recommendations are also being reviewed from a European perspective by the European Food Safety Authority (EFSA).

There is much interest in how the components of total energy expenditure (TEE) change with age. Generally, among healthy people living in developed countries, TEE decreases with age (Elia *et al.* 2000). A decrease in BMR with age has been reported by the Food and Agriculture Organization (FAO), with estimates of decreases of 2.9% and 2% per decade for normal weight men and women, respectively (FAO/WHO/UNU 2004). However, this decrease is not linear. Ageing is associated with quantitative changes in body composition, with body mass tending to increase from adulthood to 70–75 years (and thereafter decrease), while fat-free mass increases (Kendrick *et al.* 1994; Ritz 2001). This means that, for a given bodyweight, older people tend to have less muscle and more fat, leading to a decrease in the BMR.

The effect of ageing on thermogenesis is not clear. Several studies have investigated the effect of ageing on the diet-induced thermogenesis (DIT) component of energy expenditure (summarised by Elia *et al.* 2000) but results are inconsistent, with some studies showing no difference in DIT between young and older adults, and others reporting a greater DIT in younger individuals compared to older ones. However, as DIT is affected by a number of factors including the composition and consistency of food intake, body composition, visceral fat accumulation in women, physical activity level and heredity factors, more studies controlling for these factors are required to better understand the contribution of DIT to TEE in older adults.

As people age they often become more sedentary, leading to a decrease in energy expenditure (National Academy of Sciences 2002). But this is not always the case. For example, a prospective study in the US found that on retirement people tended to increase their sport and physical activity participation (Evenson *et al.* 2002). In the UK, energy requirements in older people are based on assumed physical activity levels (PALs) relative to basal metabolic rate (*i.e.* 1.5 × BMR). However, the number of older adults used in formulating these predictive equations is usually small (*e.g.* 50 men and 38 women in Scholfield 1985) and typically they include small numbers of people from ethnic minorities, limiting the generalisability of the equations. A recent study of ~280 older adults found that metabolic requirements were overestimated by predictive equations, while physical activity levels were underestimated compared to empirical measurements (Blanc *et al.* 2004). Several smaller studies have found energy requirements to be underestimated in older men and older women (Roberts *et al.* 1992; Reilly *et al.* 1993). Another small study by Fuller *et al.* found that although the mean daily energy requirement equalled 1.5 times the BMR, there was substantial variation between a random sample of 23 older men (standard deviation 0.2 times the BMR), with significant differences between those living in their own home and those in sheltered accommodation (Fuller *et al.* 1996).

In the UK (as in other countries) the estimated average requirements (EAR) for energy for older adults have been set at lower levels than for younger adults (see Table 1.3). This lower value is to take into account the changes described above. The FAO/WHO/UNU Report concluded that energy requirements for older adults should be calculated based on physical activity levels, placing great importance on accurately estimating the BMR of older adults. Although the FAO/WHO/UNU Report continued to use Scholfield's (1985) equations for estimating BMR from bodyweight (FAO/WHO/UNU 2004), as more information becomes available on the BMR of older adults with differing lifestyles, ethnicity and body composition, the predictive equations may need to be revised. As noted, expert committees are in the process of con-

Table 1.3: Estimated average requirements (EAR) for energy

Age	EAR	
	MJ/d	Kcal/d
Men		
19–50	10.60	2550
51–59	10.60	2550
60–64	9.93	2380
65–74	9.71	2330
75+	8.77	2100
Women		
19–50	8.10	1940
51–59	8.00	1900
60–64	7.99	1900
65–74	7.96	1900
75+	7.61	1810

Source: Department of Health (1991).

sidering whether current energy recommendations for people in the UK and also across the EU are appropriate.

Chronic diseases can affect energy balance in many different ways. BMR can be increased (*e.g.* during metabolic stress and with fever) or decreased (*e.g.* because of reduced body mass). With many diseases energy expenditure due to physical activity is decreased, but in some instances may be increased (*e.g.* in patients with severe muscular spasms) (Elia *et al.* 2000). Medication may also change energy expenditure (Ritz 2001). Elia *et al.* (2000) detailed a limited number of studies of TEE in older adults with disease but concluded from the available information that a significant rise in TEE is generally not observed in chronic disease because increases in BMR are balanced by reductions in physical activity (Table 1.4).

1.5.2 Bodyweight

Recommendations to maintain a healthy bodyweight are relevant to all sections of the population, including older adults. Malnutrition predisposes to disease, delays recovery from illness and adversely affects body function, wellbeing and clinical outcome (Malnutrition Advisory Group 2003), while being obese increases the risk of many chronic diseases (British Nutrition Foundation 1999). Body mass index (BMI, a measure of weight and height) is used to identify individuals who are underweight (BMI <18.5 kg/m^2), and those who are overweight (25–

Table 1.4: Energy expenditure in free-living, 'healthy' subjects and patients with selected diseases

	No. of subjects (gender)	Age (y) and SD	BMR measured (MJ/day) and SD	TEE (MJ/day) and SD	Physical activity energy expended	
					(MJ/day) and SD	(MJ/kg/day) and SD
Healthy subjects	150 (M)	72 ± 8	6.44 ± 0.89	10.79 ± 2.09	3.27 ± 1.61	0.044 ± 0.021
	100 (F)	68 ± 6	5.53 ± 0.08	8.85 ± 1.49	2.22 ± 1.2	0.033 ± 0.019
Parkinson's disease	16 (M)	62 ± 8	6.92 ± 1.18	9.26 ± 1.95	1.42 ± 1.53	0.018
Alzheimer's disease	30 (13 M/17 F)	73 ± 8	5.38 ± 0.95	7.95 ± 2.16	1.78 ± 1.32	0.028
Lung cancer	8 (5 M/13 F)	68 ± 12	6.39 ± 1.04	8.73 ± 2.38	1.34 ± 1.35	0.019

BMR: basal metabolic rate; F: female; M: male; SD: standard deviation; TEE: total energy expenditure.
Source: *European Journal of Clinical Nutrition*, **54 (Suppl 3)**, S92–S103; Elia *et al.* (2000).

29.9 kg/m^2) or obese (>30 kg/m^2). While BMI is an important component of many malnutrition screening tools (*e.g.* the UK malnutrition universal nutrition tool; MUST), it has been suggested that BMI is not a good marker of body composition in older people because height and lean body mass decrease with ageing (Beck and Ovesen 1998; Visscher *et al.* 2001) (see also Chapter 10, Section 10.6.2). There may also be difficulties in obtaining accurate height measurements in some older adults (*e.g.* some may be unable to stand straight or may be unsteady on their feet). Surrogate measures such as using demi-span (the distance from the middle of the sternal notch to the tip of the middle finger when the arm is stretched out laterally) can and have been used. For example, the British National Diet and Nutrition Survey obtained reliable measures of demi-span for around 1000 free-living older people and around 200 older people in institutions. The ratio of height to demi-span was 2.11 for free-living men and 2.15 for free-living women. There was no significant association between this measure and age, which suggests that any height differences observed in the survey were cohort effects rather than age-related spinal shrinkage.

As highlighted by the American Dietetic Association (2000), the appropriate range of healthy BMIs for older adults is controversial. For example, the US Longitudinal Study of Ageing, a prospective cohort study of over 7000 people, found that a relatively high BMI (30–35 kg/m^2 for women and 27–30 kg/m^2 for men) was associated with minimal risk for mortality in adults older than 70 years of age (Allison *et al.* 1997). Similarly, the Cardiovascular Health Study (a cohort study of over 4000 non-

smoking men and women aged 65–100 years) found that the association seen between higher BMI and mortality in middle age did not appear to be a risk factor for five-year mortality in older American adults (American Dietetic Association 2000). In their review, Beck and Ovesen (1998) concluded that different cut-off points should be used for older adults, *i.e.* BMI < 24 kg/m^2 in older adults may be associated with health problems in some older adults, while a BMI of 24–29 is a healthy weight for most older adults.

There are also questions about the applicability of reference data for a range of anthropometric measurements for older adults, including BMI (Chumlea and Sun 2004), with Bannerman *et al.* (1997) identifying a need for contemporary reference data.

1.5.3 Macronutrients

In the UK, dietary recommendations for fat, carbohydrate and dietary fibre are the same for older people as for the rest of the adult population (Department of Health 1991). A similar situation exists in many other countries although, in the US and Canada, recommendations for fibre vary with age and gender to take into account the median energy intake of the different groups (National Academy of Sciences 2002. See Lunn and Buttriss 2007).

Protein recommendations for adults in some countries change with age. In the UK, the reference nutrient intake (RNI) for protein was set in 1991 and was based on the 1985 recommendations from the FAO/WHO/UNU (Department of Health 1991). It assumed that older people had the same

Table 1.5: Reference nutrient intake (RNI) for vitamins and minerals for adults (50+ years)

Nutrient	RNI
Calcium (mg/d)	700
Phosphorus (mg/d)	550
Magnesium (mg/d)	270 women, 300 men
Sodium (mg/d)	1600
Potassium (mg/d)	3500
Chloride (mg/d)	2500
Iron (mg/d)	8.7
Zinc (mg/d)	7.0 women, 9.5 men
Copper (mg/d)	1.2
Selenium (μg/d)	60 women, 75 men
Iodine (μg/d)	140
Thiamin (mg/d)	0.8 women, 0.9 men
Riboflavin (mg/d)	1.1 women, 1.3 men
Niacin (mg/d)	12 women, 16 men
Vitamin B_6 (mg/d)	1.2 women, 1.4 men
Vitamin B_{12} (μg/d)	1.5
Folate (μg/d)	200
Vitamin C (mg/d)	40
Vitamin A (μg/d)	600 women, 700 men
Vitamin D (μg/d)	(10 μg/d after age of 65 years)

Source: Department of Health (1991).

requirements for protein as younger adults (0.75 g protein/kg/day). As older adults have less lean body mass per kg bodyweight, the RNI for younger adults is slightly higher (see Section 1.6.2 for details of protein intakes in Great Britain). In a report by the Committee on Medical Aspects of Foods (COMA), guidance was given for the UK population as a whole to avoid high protein intakes (defined as intakes of more than twice the RNI; *i.e.* over 1.5 g protein/kg/day) (Department of Health 1991). This may be of particular importance to older adults, as the report suggested that high intake of dietary protein increases glomerular filtration rate, which may be related to the age-related decline in renal function. In the US and Canada recommendations exist regarding the amount of amino acids that should be consumed (reported as mg/g protein for the different amino acids), but recommendations for older adults in these countries are the same as for other age groups (National Academy of Sciences 2002).

There are ongoing discussions about the validity of protein requirements based on the FAO/WHO/UNU report, with various researchers concluding that protein requirements may be higher in older adults. For example, an American study found net nitrogen balance was negative among older adults

consuming 0.8 g protein/kg/day and positive for those consuming 1.62 g protein/kg/day (more than twice the UK RNI) (Campbell *et al.* 1994). The authors estimated that the intake required for nitrogen balance was 1 g/kg/day. Similarly, Evans and Cyr-Campbell (1997) suggested a safe protein intake for older adults of 1.25 g/kg/day and that the recommendations should be set at 1–1.25 g/kg/day. A review on protein requirements by Millward and Jackson (2004) highlighted some of the problems encountered when establishing protein recommendations, for example the lack of consideration given to the potential influence of metabolic adaptation on dietary requirements. The authors calculated protein requirements in relation to energy requirements (predicted for different physical activity levels), to generate reference ratios for protein energy/total energy (reference P/E ratio) as a function of age, bodyweight, gender and physical activity level. Reference P/E ratios were adjusted using the proposed values for amino acid requirements and from these calculations the authors concluded that a number of sub-groups could be at risk of inadequate protein intakes, including large, older sedentary women. This conclusion is in contrast to those reached by other researchers (see Chapter 6, Section 6.8).

Protein requirements may be increased by illness, surgery, infection, trauma and pressure ulcers, and long-term inadequate protein intake may result in further loss of muscle mass, impaired immune function and poor wound healing (Chicago Dietetic Association 2000).

1.5.4 Micronutrients

Recommendations for intakes of micronutrients among UK adults aged 50 years or older are shown in Table 1.5. As can be seen, the only change in recommendations for older adults is for vitamin D. It is assumed that individuals aged 4–64 years will obtain adequate amounts of vitamin D through the action of sunlight; however, this conclusion has been challenged recently (see Chapter 4, Section 4.2.3 and Chapter 14, Section 14.3.2). Older adults typically go out of doors less than younger age groups and are less efficient at producing vitamin D from sunlight. Therefore, an RNI of 10 mg/day for older adults was set, with the expectation that the majority of older people would need vitamin D supplementation to achieve this level (Department of Health

1998a). Micronutrient intakes among older adults are discussed in Section 1.6.3.

In the US, Dietary Reference Intakes (DRIs) are provided for older adults in two life-stage brackets: 51–70 years and older than 70 years. To date, recommendations are the same for both groups, with the exception of vitamin D, which is higher in the older group, and sodium, which is lower in the older age group (National Academy of Sciences 2004; www. iom.edu/Object.File/Master/21/372/0.pdf, accessed 13 April 2007).

1.5.5 Fluid

Fluid requirements in adults are about 1 ml/kcal (30 ml/kg bodyweight), *i.e.* approximately 6–8 cups, mugs or glasses of fluid per day, although this intake level may not be sufficient to meet the fluid needs of underweight adults (World Health Organization 2002b). In the US, adequate intakes of fluids from drinks are estimated to be 3 L/day, in addition to water provided by food, which is estimated as just under 900 ml/d on average (National Academy of Sciences 2004) (see Chapter 14, Section 14.5.4). Fluid needs increase with environmental temperature, fever, vomiting, diarrhoea and drug- and caffeine-induced fluid losses (Chicago Dietetic Association 2000).

The prevalence of dehydration is controversial but it is thought to be a potential problem in older adults, especially in the oldest old and those living in institutions. According to the WHO (2002b), increased risk of dehydration in older adults is due to:

1. Reduced fluid intake, with evidence that even healthy older adults feel less thirst in response to water deprivation. Other factors such as delirium, dementia, diuretic use, swallowing problems, laxative abuse, incontinence (with urinary incontinence reportedly affecting about half of older adults living in institutions and 15–30% of those living in the community; Williams and Pannill, 1982; Resnick 1996) and problems with dexterity or mobility can also increase the tendency towards dehydration in some older adults.
2. Increased fluid loss. A reduction in renal concentrating capacity in response to dehydration and decreases in plasma rennin activity and aldosterone secretion mean that older adults are less able

to concentrate urine compared to younger individuals and therefore have a higher minimum urine output.

1.5.6 Physical activity

Physical activity has been demonstrated to benefit all people regardless of age, stage of life, gender or socio-economic status. The benefits of physical activity for older adults in relation to specific organ systems are covered in subsequent chapters (see Chapter 4, Section 4.2.4.1; Chapter 8, Sections 8.2.2 and 8.3.8; Chapter 10, Section 10.8; Chapter 12, Section 12.5.2.1; Chapter 13, Section 13.4.1 and Chapter 14, Section 14.4 for a summary). However, more generally, strength training can increase muscle size (see Chapter 6, Section 6.10), which may stimulate more aerobic activity. It may also have an important impact on energy balance because of an increased resting metabolic rate and an increase in energy expenditure (Evans and Cyr-Campbell 1997). Additionally, depending on the type of physical activity, participation may provide social interaction which can have a positive impact on quality of life.

Recommendations for physical activity among adults in the UK (Department of Health 2004a) (at least 30 minutes' moderate activity at least five times a week) are applicable to older adults. In addition, older people should aim to maintain mobility through daily activity; activities that promote and improve balance, strength and coordination are encouraged. The importance of physical activity in the prevention and treatment of diabetes and coronary heart disease has been highlighted in the Department of Health's National Service Framework (NSF) reports. For example, the NSF for diabetes highlights that physical activity and weight loss should be the first intervention for people with newly diagnosed type 2 diabetes (Department of Health 2001), while the NSF on coronary heart disease highlights the role that regular physical activity plays in reducing the risk of developing cardiovascular disease (Department of Health 2000b) (see Chapter 14, Section 14.6).

The American Agency for Healthcare, Research and Quality suggests at least 30 minutes of physical activity on most days of the week for older people, but *The Guidelines for Americans* recommend approximately 60 minutes of moderate to vigorous intensity activity on most days of the week to obtain greater health benefits (Department of Health and Human Services). These guidelines also recommend at least 60–90 minutes of daily moderate-intensity physical activity to sustain weight loss in adulthood.

The WHO's (2003a) global strategy on diet, physical activity and health recommends that all people should engage in adequate levels throughout their lives, and recognises that different types and amounts of physical activity are required for different health outcomes: at least 30 minutes of regular, moderate-intensity physical activity on most days reduces the risk of cardiovascular disease and diabetes, colon cancer and breast cancer. More activity may be required for weight control. Evidence exists that it is never too late to start and that all age groups can benefit (Buttriss and Hardman 2005; Blair 2007) (see Chapter 14, Section 14.6).

1.6 Food patterns, nutrient intakes and nutritional status of older people

1.6.1 Food patterns

Differences in food patterns have been observed among people of different ages. National cross-sectional survey data suggest that the diets of older UK adults (50–64 years) are typically closer to the dietary recommendations than those of younger adults (under 35 years) (see Chapter 14, Section 14.5).

Older adults consume more fruit and vegetables than younger adults, *e.g.* the average daily intake for men aged 19–24 years was 1.3 portions compared with 3.6 portions in men aged 50–64 years. Similarly, women in the youngest age group consumed considerably less fruit and vegetables than those women in the oldest age group on average (1.8 portions vs. 3.8 portions). For nearly half of the types of fruits and vegetables, a significantly lower proportion of men and women aged 19–24 years consumed the item compared with the oldest age group, *e.g.* 30% of men and 43% of women in the youngest age group ate leafy green vegetables compared with 64% of men and 70% of women in the oldest age group. Other foods less likely to have been consumed by the youngest group of men and women compared with the oldest group are shown in Table 1.6 (see also Chapter 14, Section 14.5.5).

Results from the British survey for older adults (65+ years) indicated that men generally ate larger quantities than women (Finch *et al.* 1998). No significant differences in the types of food eaten were observed between men and women in institutions, but in the free-living group men were more likely than women to consume meat and meat products, eggs, table sugar and alcoholic drinks, while women were more likely to consume cottage cheese, yogurt and fromage frais. A more traditional eating pattern was observed in the group resident in institutions and for older free-living participants, *e.g.* these groups were more likely than younger free-living age groups (aged 65+) to eat cereal-based milk puddings (Finch *et al.* 1998). Using data from this survey, Pryer *et al.* (2001) divided the free-living older adults into clusters (traditional, mixed diet and healthy diet), based on consumption of different foods, and found that men and women in the traditional and mixed-diet groups were more likely to be smokers and from the manual social class; they were more likely to be in receipt of a state benefit and to be on a lower income compared to those individuals in the healthy diet group. An age effect was seen, with a higher proportion of younger individuals being categorised in the healthy diet group and more of the oldest old group in the traditional or mixed diet groups.

Much effort has been directed towards identifying food patterns associated with health in older populations. Trichopoulou *et al.* (1995) found that among a sample of older Greek adults, a one unit increase in diet score (based on eight component characteristics of the traditional diet common in the Mediterranean region) was associated with a 17% reduction in overall mortality (9% confidence interval, 1% to 31%). Similarly, The Healthy Ageing: a Longitudinal Study in Europe (HALE) reported that individuals aged 70–90 years following a Mediterranean-type diet and lifestyle had a more than 50% lower rate of all-cause and cause-specific mortality (Knoops *et al.* 2004). The benefit of a Mediterranean-type diet has been demonstrated in other settings. Kouris-Blazos *et al.* (1999) found mortality reduction increased with diet score among Greek-Australians and Anglo-Celts living in Melbourne, Australia. A cross-sectional analysis of food patterns of participants of the SENECA follow-up study found that north and south European eating patterns emerged (Schroll *et al.* 1996). The southern food pattern seemed more in line with guidelines for healthy eating, being rich in grains, vegetables, fruit, lean meat and olive oil.

Table 1.6: Main differences in the eating behaviour of British respondents by age group*

Men aged 19–24 years more likely to eat	Men aged 50–64 years more likely to eat
Pasta	Wholemeal bread
Pizza	Whole-grain and high-fibre breakfast cereals
Coated chicken and turkey	Fruit pies
Burgers and kebabs	Other cereal-based puddings
Potato chips	Whole milk
Savoury snacks	Skimmed milk
Carbonated soft drinks (not low calorie)	Cottage cheese
Alcopops	Eggs
	Pork and dishes
	Liver, liver products and dishes
	Oily fish
	Raw carrots
	Peas
	Green beans
	Leafy green vegetables
	Tomatoes – not raw
	Other potatoes and potato dishes
	Apples and pears
	Citrus fruits
	Bananas
	Canned fruit in juice
	Other fruit
	Preserves
	Wine
	Low alcohol and alcohol-free beer and lager
	Coffee

Women aged 19–24 years more likely to eat	Women aged 50–64 years more likely to eat
Coated chicken and turkey	Wholemeal bread
Burgers and kebabs	Whole-grain and high-fibre breakfast cereals
Savoury snacks	Fruit pies
Carbonated drinks (not low calorie)	Buns, cakes and pastries
Concentrated soft drinks (not low calorie)	Cream
Concentrated soft drinks (low calorie)	Eggs
Beer and lager	Egg dishes
Alcopops	Coated and/or fried white fish
	Other white fish dishes
	Oily fish
	Raw tomatoes
	Peas
	Leafy green vegetables
	Carrots – not raw
	Tomatoes – not raw
	Apples and pears
	Citrus fruits
	Bananas
	Canned fruit in juice
	Canned fruit in syrup
	Other fruit
	Preserves
	Fortified wine
	Low alcohol and alcohol-free beer and lager
	Coffee
	Soup

*Dietary patterns change with age.
Source: Finch *et al.* (1998).

1.6.2 Nutrient intakes

A number of dietary surveys and studies have been undertaken in older adults in a range of different locations. Examples of some of these studies are shown in Table 1.7, along with average values. While these studies show that older people are generally well-nourished, they have highlighted low intakes of fibre and a range of micronutrients, especially in some sub-groups of older adults (see Chapter 14, Section 14.5).

1.6.2.1 Great Britain

The most recent NDNS of older adults was published in 1998. Two nationally representative samples

Table 1.7: Selected dietary surveys and studies showing low intakes of various nutrients in older populations

Country	Nutrients and proportion of study population with low* intake (%)	Age range of subjects	Reference
Australia	Vitamin A Magnesium Potassium Calcium (12–24% men and 14–61% women)	>65 years	Bannerman *et al.* (2001)
Germany	Fibre (38%) Vitamin D (75%) Folate (37%) Calcium (35%)	≥65 years	Volkert *et al.* (2004)
Great Britain	(Results given for free-living men, free-living-women, men and women living in institutions, respectively) Vitamin A (5, 4, 1, 1%) Riboflavin (5, 10, 3, 3%) Vitamin B6 (2, 3, 1, 2%) Folate (1, 6, 4, 5%) Vitamin C (2, 2, 0, 0%) Iron (1, 6, 5, 6%) Calcium (5, 9, 1 >0.5%) Magnesium (21, 23, 39, 22%) Potassium (17, 39, 28, 42%) Zinc (8, 5, 13, 4%)	≥65 years	Finch *et al.* (1998)
Spain**	Vitamin A (14–65%) Vitamin D (47–97%) Vitamin E (54–95%) Thiamin (0–50%) Riboflavin (0–53%) Vitamin B6 (12–89%) Vitamin B12 (1–23%) Folate (2–88%) Vitamin C (0–48%) (At blood levels, deficiencies of vitamins B_{12}, A and E were infrequent, but for all other vitamins prevalence of deficiency varied within a wide range)	All ages included in analysis	Ortega *et al.* (2001)
US**	Calcium (males 70–75%, females 87%) Zinc (males 35–41%, females 36–45%) Vitamin D (up to 90%)	≥60 years	Ervin and Kennedy-Stephenson (2002) C. Moore *et al.* (2004)

*Low has been defined differently in various countries.
**Details on a limited number of nutrients available.

Table 1.8: UK dietary reference values (DRVs) for fat and carbohydrate as a percentage of food energy, and intakes of older adults (aged 65 years and above)

% of food energy unless otherwise stated	Population average	Free-living		Living in institutions	
		Men	Women	Men	Women
Saturated fatty acids	11				
Cis polyunsaturated fatty acids	6.5				
Cis monounsaturated fatty acids	13	11.0	11.0	10.5	10.5
Trans fatty acids	2	1.5	1.5	1.8	1.8
Total fat	35	35.7	36.1	35.1	34.8
Non-milk extrinsic sugars	11	13.2	11.5	17.9	18.5
Intrinsic and milk sugars and starch	39	35	36	32.9	32.8
Total carbohydrate	50				
Non-starch polysaccharide (g/d)	18	13.5	11.0	11.0	9.5

Source: Finch *et al.* (1998).

were drawn from older adults: one of free-living individuals and one of individuals living in institutions (Finch *et al.* 1998). The free-living sample generally had 230 people for each category (age groups 65–74, 75–84 and 85 and over), but there were low numbers of men in the oldest age group so it was agreed that the target for this group would be 100. The survey included an interview to provide general information; a four-day weighed dietary record of food and drinks consumed; physical measurements and requests for blood and urine, and an interview to provide information on oral health (see Section 1.6.1 for information on dietary patterns).

Average daily energy intakes in the free-living population were 8.02 MJ (1909 kcal) for men and 5.98 MJ (1422 kcal) for women aged 65–74 years, while for those men and women living in institutions the mean daily intake was 8.14 MJ (1935 kcal) and 6.94 MJ (1650 kcal) respectively. These intakes were below the estimated average requirements (EAR) of 9.71 MJ and 7.96 MJ, for men and women respectively. The largest contribution to recorded energy

intake was made by cereals and cereal products (providing 34% of energy intake in the free-living group and 38% in the institution group).

Average intakes of macronutrients and fibre are shown in Table 1.8. Briefly, protein intakes were above the estimated requirements, but there was a large variation in intakes (from 33.7 g in men and 30.8 g in women up to 96.7 g in men and 85.2 g in women) and a decrease was seen with age. The main sources of protein were meat and meat products (32% of average daily intake for free-living participants and 26% for those in institutions), cereals and cereal products (24% for the free-living and 29% in institutions) and milk and milk products (19% for the free-living and 22% in institutions).

The average daily intake of total carbohydrate was slightly lower than the current UK DRV. Cereals and cereal products were the main source of carbohydrates, followed by vegetables, including potatoes. The average daily intake of non-milk extrinsic sugars (NEMS) was above the DRV of 11%, particularly in those older adults living in institutions where there was a high intake of NMES and a relatively low intake of other carbohydrates.

With regard to fat, intakes for all groups were close to the DRV of 35% of food energy, while average intakes of saturated fatty acids were above the recommended 11% of food energy in all older adults (with average intakes representing ~15% of food energy), with milk, fat spreads, meat and cereal products being the main sources. Intakes of *trans* fatty acids were below the recommended upper limit of 2% of energy (1.5% of food energy in free-living older adults and 1.8% in those living in institutions) (see Chapter 14, Section 14.5.2).

Average fibre intakes (measured in the UK as non-starch polysaccharides, NSP) among older adults were well below the 18 g recommendation in all groups. Intakes of fibre were found to decrease with age among the free-living participants, but not within institutions.

More free-living older adults consumed alcohol than those participants in institutions (85% of free-living men and 70% of women vs. 30% of those living in institutions). Free-living men had a higher average daily intake than women; a similar pattern was seen among those in the institution group, although intakes were far lower.

Table 1.9 shows the average intake of a range of vitamins and minerals as a proportion of the RNIs, the amounts believed to cover the needs of 97.5% of the population. Vitamin D intakes were particularly low, and average folate intake (in women living in institutions) was close to the RNI. For the minerals, average intakes of potassium and magnesium were well below the RNIs, zinc was close to the RNI and the average iron intakes of both groups of women were also close to the RNI, as were average calcium intakes in free-living women. It is interesting to note that, with one or two exceptions, the intakes of vitamins and minerals in the participants living in institutions were lower than those of free-living participants (though they were generally above the RNI). However, for several nutrients, namely calcium, riboflavin and vitamin A, those in institutions fared better. These three nutrients are provided by milk, and milk intake was higher than in the free-living subjects.

Although the average intakes of most nutrients were well above the RNI, a small proportion of subjects had intakes below the lower reference nutrient intake (LRNI) (the quantity sufficient for

Table 1.9: Intakes of vitamins and minerals from food in older people (% RNI)

	Free-living		Living in institutions	
	Men	Women	Men	Women
Vitamin A	168	161	151	160
Thiamin	166	148	149	142
Riboflavin	134	130	138	147
Niacin	200	206	170	194
Vitamin B$_6$	168	160	154	158
Vitamin B$_{12}$	404	298	329	304
Folate	135	103	117	99
Vitamin C	167	152	124	119
Vitamin D	41	29	38	33
Iron	127	99	111	94
Calcium	119	99	136	123
Phosphorous	225	180	218	192
Magnesium	85	73	72	70
Sodium	168	128	170	138
Potassium	78	63	69	61
Zinc	93	98	88	101
Iodine	134	106	138	125

Source: Finch *et al.* (1998).

only 2.5% of the population). There is no LRNI for vitamin D; however, virtually all the subjects had intakes below the RNI (Table 1.10). A substantial proportion of subjects had intakes of magnesium and potassium below the LRNI. There was evidence that the situation worsened in the older age group for some micronutrients (riboflavin, vitamin B$_6$, vitamin C, iron, magnesium, potassium and zinc).

1.6.3 Nutritional status

1.6.3.1 Bodyweight

Involuntary weight loss predicts morbidity and mortality. It is estimated that, in the general population, one in seven older adults has a medium or high risk of malnutrition. The prevalence is higher in subjects who are living in institutions (Malnutrition Advisory Group 2003). The NDNS identified more older adults with a BMI ≤20 within institutions than free-living (16% of men and 15% of women living in institutions vs. 3% free-living men and 6% women). Risks to health are associated with excess bodyweight, and although there is some uncertainty

Table 1.10: Proportion of older people with micronutrient intakes from food below the LRNI (%)

	Free-living (%)		Living in institutions (%)	
	Men	Women	Men	Women
Vitamin A	5	4	1	1
Thiamin	>0.5	>0.5	1	>0.5
Riboflavin*	5	10	3	3
Niacin	>0.5	>0.5	>0.5	>0.5
Vitamin B$_6$*	2	3	1	2
Vitamin B$_{12}$	>0.5	1	nil	Nil
Folate*	1	6	4	5
Vitamin C*	2	2	1	Nil
Vitamin D	97% below RNI		99% below RNI	
Iron*	1	6	5	6
Calcium	5	9	1	>0.5
Magnesium*	21	23	39	22
Sodium	nil	nil	nil	Nil
Potassium*	17	39	28	42
Zinc*	8	5	13	4
Iodine	2	6	1	1

*Proportion increases with age.
LRNI: lower reference nutrient intake; RNI: reference nutrient intake.
Source: Finch *et al.* (1998).

about whether the cut-offs used are appropriate for all older adults (see Section 1.5.2 and Chapter 10, Section 10.6.2), a large proportion of older adults in the NDNS were found to be obese or overweight when using these cut-offs (67% of free-living men and 63% of free-living women; 46% of men and 47% of women living in institutions).

1.6.3.2 Micronutrient status

In contrast to the NDNS findings regarding micro-nutrient intakes, the results on nutritional status highlighted larger proportions of older British adults with low status (Table 1.11). The situation was typically worse among those in institutions; additionally those in institutions had lower vitamin E, beta-carotene and retinol indices (not shown). Indices of magnesium and potassium were not included but may have also been low on the basis of the intake data. Vitamin C status was particularly low in those living in institutions without their own teeth (Table 1.12) and the data suggested that half the subjects had an intake below the level regarded as signifying biochemical depletion.

Of particular concern is the number of older adults with low status of vitamin D (see below), and

Table 1.11: Proportion with a low status of selected nutrients

	Free-living (%)		Living in institutions (%)	
	Men	Women	Men	Women
Iron (Hb)*	11	9	52	39
Vitamin C*	14	13	44	38
Folate	15	15	39	39
Vitamin B$_{12}$	6	6	9	9
Thiamin	8	9	11	15
Riboflavin	41	41	41	32
Vitamin D*	6	10	38	37

*Proportion increases with age.
Source: Finch *et al.* (1998).

Table 1.12: Mean vitamin C status

	Plasma vitamin C* (µmol/L)
Free-living, own teeth	49.1
Free-living, without teeth	39.4
Institutional care, own teeth	24.6
Institutional care, without teeth	21.1 (median 11.4)

*Below 11 µmol/L indicates biochemical depletion.
Source: Steele *et al.* (1998).

Table 1.13: Prevalence of iron deficiency anaemia (%) among older adults

	SENECA baseline (Lesourd *et al.* 1996) (excluding those in psychogeriatric nursing homes)		SENECA follow-up (Lesourd *et al.* 1996) (excluding those in psychogeriatric nursing homes)		NHANES II (Looker *et al.* 2002) (free-living)		NDNS (Finch *et al.* 1998) (free-living/living in institutions)	
	Men (n = 975)	Women (n = 946)	Men (n = 570)	Women (n = 594)	Men	Women	Men	Women
WHO criteria*	4.6	5.5	6.0	5.0	4.5	3.5	11/52	9/39
NHANES II criteria**	4.1	4.2	4.0	3.5	4.5	3.5	–	–

*Men Hb < 130 g/L; women Hb < 120 g/L.
**Men Hb < 126 g/L; women Hb < 117 g/L.
NDNS: National Diet and Nutrition Study; NHANES: National Health and Nutritional Examination Survey, SENECA: Survey in Europe on Nutrition and Elderly, a Concerted Action; WHO: World Health Organization.

of iron, folate and vitamin B_{12}. In the US NHANES III, there was evidence of anaemia due to nutrient deficiency in one third of older adults (Guralnik *et al.* 2004). Table 1.13 shows the prevalence of iron deficiency anaemia in several studies, including the NDNS, where the highest prevalence in the free-living group of low haemoglobin concentrations was among those aged 85 years and over, although among those in institutions there was little variation with age (Finch *et al.* 1998).

Plasma 25 hydroxyvitamin D (25 OHD) is used as a measure of vitamin D status, with the lower level of the normal range for plasma 25 OHD usually considered to be 25 nmol/L (see Chapter 4). As can be seen from Table 1.11, a proportion of older adults had low vitamin D status and this was considerably greater in those living in institutions (Finch *et al.* 1998) (see Chapter 4, Section 4.2.3 and Chapter 14, Section 14.3.2).

It is worth highlighting that many of the reference values used for determining micronutrient status were not determined for use specifically with older adults. So while these figures are useful, it is likely that a limited number of older adults were used in setting such values, making their relevance for older adults questionable (Brachet *et al.* 2004). It may be useful to identify specific reference values for older adults.

1.6.3.3 *Physical activity*

Although the NDNS of older adults did not collect data on physical activity levels, there is some information on self-reported levels of physical activity

among older adults living in England from the 2003 Health Survey for England report, which highlighted an increase in the proportion of men and women meeting the physical activity target in all age groups, except for those aged 75 and over (Sproston and Primatesta 2004).

An earlier report found that the majority of older adults in care homes were classed as inactive, with significantly more women (86%) than men (78%) in this category. Inactivity levels were highest in nursing homes, with about nine in ten residents not having done a continuous walk of 15 minutes or more in the past month, and lowest in private residential homes (seven in ten men; eight in ten women) (Bajekal 2002) (see Chapter 14, Section 14.6).

1.7 Determinants of food and nutrient intake and status in older people

Many factors influence food and nutrient intake and therefore status. A sufficient energy intake may be important for an adequate nutrient intake because those older adults with a low energy intake may not compensate for the low micronutrient intake by eating foods with a higher nutrient density (K. Schroll *et al.* 1996; Bannerman *et al.* 2001). However, a high energy intake does not guarantee an adequate nutrient intake (De Groot *et al.* 2000). Several nutritional surveys have shown a gradual decrease in energy intake as people progress into old age, along with increasing numbers with low micronutrient intakes and/or status amongst the oldest (*e.g.* Finch *et al.* 1998).

1.7.1 Ill health, disease and disability

Physical and mental health problems, illness and disability can affect people of different ages. However, as people get older their daily activities are more likely to be hampered by such problems, so that within Europe among those aged 85 or over, from 43% (Belgium) to 93% (Germany) of the population may be affected (Figure 1.6).

Ill health and disease may affect nutrient intake/status in various ways. For example, periods of ill health can lead to weight loss because of decreased intakes (*e.g.* loss of appetite) and/or increased requirements (*e.g.* metabolic stress and fever increase energy requirements) (De Groot *et al.* 2000; Ritz 2001). Depression (see Chapter 8, Section 8.4) has been shown to be a major cause of weight loss, and this may be an important factor for some older adults: the SENECA study (1996) found 12% of men and 28% of women were depressed. More recently, it was found among a sample of 1800 older adults that depression severity made a larger independent contribution to three out of four general health indicators (mental functional status, disability and quality of life) than medical co-morbidities, highlighting the importance of recognising and treating depression (Noel *et al.* 2004).

Disability can affect the activities of daily life, such as shopping, preparing and cooking food and eating. Researchers in Italy found that from a sample of ~1500 older adults, those reporting difficulties in three or more nutrition-related activities had a significantly increased risk of an inadequate intake of energy and vitamin C (Bartali *et al.* 2003). Similarly, a smaller American study of housebound older adults (n = 123) found better calcium, vitamin D, magnesium and phosphorus intake among those with less disability. Greater BMI was directly associated with worse lower extremity performance and indirectly with greater severity of disability (Sharkey *et al.* 2004).

Those older adults who took part in the NDNS and were unwell were, on average, found to have lower intakes of protein, total carbohydrate and starch, although there was no significant effect on energy intake. Free-living men who were unwell and whose eating was affected had lower intakes of vitamins A, D, pantothetic acid and riboflavin, and lower intakes per unit energy of retinol, vitamin B_{12}

and vitamin D. These differences were not seen in free-living women and there were few differences among older adults living in institutions (Finch *et al.* 1998).

1.7.2 Poor dentition

Although few relationships have been observed between dentition and macronutrient intake (De Groot *et al.* 2000), data do suggest that poor dentition may impact on micronutrient intake. For example, the NDNS found an association between oral function and nutrient intake. Those older adults with no or few natural teeth ate a more restricted range of foods, influenced by their perceived inability to chew. For example, they were less likely to choose foods that need chewing, such as apples, raw carrots, toast, nuts and oranges. An association was also found between oral function and status (iron, vitamin C, vitamin E and retinol status was lower in those without teeth or with few teeth) (Steele *et al.* 1998). For more on the NDNS and dental status, see Chapter 3, Section 3.3. Similarly, the American NHANES III survey found that among adults aged 50 years or over, those with impaired dentition had consistently lower healthy eating scores (a measure of dietary quality), consumed fewer servings of fruit and had lower serum values of β-carotene and ascorbic acid (Sahyoun *et al.* 2003).

1.7.3 Living in institutions

There is wide variation between countries in the proportion of older adults living in a care home or institution. Table 1.14 shows the use of residential and home care services across a selected number of European countries. In England and Wales, 2.6% of men and 5.9% of women live in a residential or nursing home (National Statistics Online 2004), while in the US and New Zealand, about 4% and 5% of older men and women, respectively, live in a nursing home (Ministry of Health 2002; National Center for Health Statistics 2005).

The Health Survey for England 2000 found that the proportion of men and women in care homes eating fruit and red meat six or more times a week was about half that in private households (Bajekal *et al.* 2003) and, as highlighted in Section 1.6.2, although there were few differences in macronutri-

Table 1.14: Use of residential and home care services across a selected
number of European countries

Country	Estimated % of older adults		Reference
	Living in institutions	Receiving formal help at home	
France	6.5	6.1	Jacobzone (1999)
Greece	1.0	N/A	Mestheneos and Triantafillou (1999)
Italy	3.9	2.8	Jacobzone (1999)
Poland	0.7	1.0	Bień *et al.* (1999)
Sweden	8.7	11.2	Jacobzone (1999)
UK	5.1	5.5	

Table 1.15: Intakes of selected nutrients by social class,
free-living subjects

	Non-manual		Manual		RNI
	Men	Women	Men	Women	
Riboflavin, mg	1.96	2.17	1.68	1.46	1.3/1.1*
Folate, µg	295	239	266	209	200
Vitamin C, mg	85.6	85.2	60.3	54.2	40
Vitamin E, mg	11.8	11.9	8.8	7.0	–
Iron, mg	12.4	9.5	10.9	8.4	8.7
Magnesium, mg	278	217	237	184	300/270*
Potassium, mg	2933	2409	2550	2076	3500
Zinc, mg	9.3	7.5	8.5	6.6	9.5/7.0*

*RNIs for men and women.
RNI: reference nutrient intake.
Source: Finch *et al.* (1998).

ent intake, data from Great Britain generally found lower micronutrient intakes among those older adults living in institutions compared to those free-living individuals. Similarly, biochemical and haematological indices of nutritional status were generally poorer among those in institutions (Table 1.14). This may be in part due to ill health and drug–nutrient interactions, which may be higher in those in care homes compared to the free-living population (see Sections 1.7.1 and 1.7.5).

1.7.4 Socio-economic status, poverty and economic uncertainty

The NDNS found lower intakes of a range of nutrients among those free-living subjects from manual households compared with those in non-manual households. In some cases (*e.g.* magnesium and potassium), intakes were quite low in comparison with the RNI, particularly among women (Table 1.15). Additionally, associations between socio-economic status (SES) and low nutrient status among older British adults have been seen, *e.g.* lower plasma selenium among those receiving state benefits (Bates *et al.* 2002) and variations in methylmalonic acid concentrations (a measure of vitamin B_{12} status) and receipt of state income benefits, social class of head of household and education (Bates *et al.* 2003). Data from the US found that older adults from food-insufficient families were more likely to have diets that might compromise their health, *e.g.* lower intakes of energy, vitamin B_6, magnesium, iron and zinc and lower serum concentrations of vitamin A and vitamin E (Dixon *et al.* 2001).

Poverty can be a barrier to adequate food intake and therefore can influence nutritional status. Data from the US show that a substantial proportion of older people live in poverty or near poverty (~17% in 1998), with older women experiencing twice the rate of poverty of men. In addition, those older adults living alone or with non-relatives are also more at risk of poverty than those living with families (American Dietetic Association 2000). Data for Great Britain show that over 30% of those classified as living on a persistent low income were pensioners, and were less likely to move out of poverty (Babb *et al.* 2006).

Even if older people are not living in poverty, most live on a fixed income. As expenses increase (*e.g.* cost of utilities), they may result in reduced food intake, thereby increasing the risk of malnutrition.

1.7.5 Drug–nutrient interactions

It is estimated that over 30% of all prescription drugs are taken by older adults, and older adults are the highest users of over-the-counter drugs too (McCabe 2004). It is not surprising, therefore, that older adults are at high risk of experiencing drug–nutrient interactions (Chan 2002).

In England, older adults living in care homes are more likely to be on prescribed medication (92% of men and 97% of women) than those living in private households (77% of men and 80% of women) (Bajekal 2002). Polypharmacy (taking four or more prescribed medicines) was also more common in care homes, where 71% of both men and women were on four or more drugs compared with about a third of men and women in private households (Bajekal 2002).

Four types of drug–nutrient interactions have been defined (Chan 2002):

- *ex-vivo* bio-inactivation (interaction through biochemical or physical reaction);
- interactions affecting absorption;
- interactions affecting systemic/physiologic disposition; and
- interactions affecting the elimination or clearance of drugs or nutrients.

In particular, a healthy gut is important for the metabolism of many drugs (McCabe 2004) (see Chapter 12).

While interactions may be quickly recognised when a food or a nutrient interferes with the action of a drug in a hospital setting, it is less likely that a drug interfering with nutritional status will be recognised, monitored or diagnosed elsewhere, particularly in outpatient or nursing home settings.

Herbal medicines and dietary supplements are commonly used by older people – the NDNS found 19% and 26% of free-living men and women, respectively, took supplements. Among men and women living in institutions 18% and 19% respectively took supplements (Finch *et al.* 1998). As some of these supplements can interact with drugs (*e.g.* gingko biloba and aspirin interact), doctors and health professionals need to be aware of these interactions and monitor their patients accordingly (Dergal *et al.* 2002).

1.7.6 Taste and smell

Chemosensory impairment in older people has been indicated in a number of laboratory studies (*e.g.* Schiffman *et al.* 1994; Nordin *et al.* 2003). A number of medical conditions (Table 1.16), as well as a range of medications including drugs to lower cholesterol and blood lipids, drugs for arthritis and pain, drugs

Table 1.16: Examples of medical conditions that may alter taste or smell

Nervous	Alzheimer's disease
	Bell's palsy
	Multiple sclerosis
	Parkinson's disease
Nutritional	Cancer
	Chronic renal failure
	Liver disease
	Niacin, vitamin B_{12} and zinc deficiency
Endocrine	Adrenal cortical insufficiency
	Diabetes mellitus
	Hypothyroidism
Local	Allergic rhinitis, atopy and bronchial asthma
	Sinusitis and polyposis
Viral infections	Acute viral hepatitis
	Influenza-like infections

Source: *European Journal of Clinical Nutrition,* **50 (Suppl 3)**, S54–S63; Schiffman and Graham (2000).

for hypertension and heart disease and antihista-mines, can alter taste or smell (Schiffman and Graham 2000). However, according to Mattes (2002), data on the prevalence of chemosensory shifts over the lifecycle are rare (see Chapter 3).

1.8 Conclusions

As people are now generally living longer, the number of older adults is increasing. Unfortunately, these extra years are not always spent in good health as there tends to be an increase in the presence and number of chronic conditions with older age. This provides a number of challenges, including economic ones especially with regard to health care

costs, pensions and the workforce. Compared to other life-stages, comparatively little is known about nutritional requirements of older adults. Food patterns and nutritional intake and therefore nutritional status are influenced by a range of factors which need to be considered with all sub-groups, but especially the older age group. While older adults have generally been found to be well nourished, low intakes of fibre and a range of micronutrients have been found, especially among some sub-groups. Considering the important role diet plays in health and disease prevention as well as treatment, it is important that the diets of older adults as well as younger adults are improved to reduce the burden of disease and increase quality of life.

1.9 Key points

- The trend of an increasing proportion of older adults and a decreasing proportion of children will continue in developed countries while spreading to less developed countries. The fastest growing segment of the older population is among the oldest old – those aged 80 years and older – and in Great Britain there will be a growing proportion of older adults from non-white minority ethnic groups in this segment.
- While old age *per se* is not necessarily associated with poor health, the number of people reporting long-term illness and disability increases with age. Older adults are also disproportionately affected by sensory impairments.
- Women tend to have a longer life expectancy than men, although in some countries this is changing. Life expectancy also varies by race; some ethnic groups are more susceptible to some chronic diseases.
- An ageing population impacts on health care spending and also has consequences in relation to the workforce and pensions.

- The energy, macronutrient and micronutrient requirements of older adults are not yet fully understood. The relevance of using a range of anthropometrical and biochemical measurements for older adults is unclear; much of the reference data for these measurements included few older adults.
- A number of surveys and studies in a range of countries have found that while older adults are generally well nourished, low intakes of fibre and a range of micronutrients have been found, especially in some sub-groups. Of particular concern is the number of older adults with low status of vitamin D, and of iron, folate and vitamin B_{12}.
- Food and nutritional intake (and therefore status) is influenced by a range of factors, including ill health, disease and disability, poor dentition, institutionalisation, socio-economic status, poverty and economic uncertainty.

1.10 Recommendations for future research

- Most of the reference data used to establish energy and other nutrient requirements have used limited numbers of healthy older adults and very little representation from different ethnic groups. The UK DRVs for older adults could be reviewed taking into account the research findings accumulated since the early 1990s.

- More work could be undertaken to increase understanding of the particular nutritional needs of the oldest old, the fastest growing age group of the population, and those with disabilities and diseases, which are common among older adults.

1.11 Key references

Finch, S., Doyle, W., Lowe, C., *et al.* (1998) *National Diet and Nutrition Survey: People Aged 65 Years and Over. Volume 1: Report of the Diet and Nutrition Survey.* London, The Stationery Office.

SENECA investigators (1996a) Food patterns of elderly Europeans. *European Journal of Clinical Nutrition,* **50 (Suppl 2)**, S86–S100.

SENECA investigators (1996b) Health and physical performances of elderly Europeans. *European Journal of Clinical Nutrition,* **50 (Suppl 2)**, S105–11.

SENECA investigators (1996c) Mental health: minimal state examination and geriatric depression score of elderly Europeans in the SENECA study of 1993. *European Journal of Clinical Nutrition,* **50 (Suppl 2)**, S112–16.

World Health Organization (2002a) *Active Ageing. A Policy Framework.* Geneva, World Health Organization.

2
The Basic Biology of Ageing

2.1 Definitions

Although the ageing process is familiar to us all, it is important to be precise about what we mean by key terms such as 'ageing', 'lifespan' and 'longevity'. There are no universally agreed definitions of these terms and so we begin by explaining the sense in which we shall use them here.

'Ageing' is the most difficult of the terms about which to be precise. It can mean simply the property of becoming chronologically older and, when used in this sense, it does not necessarily carry any association of decline. It can, for example, describe the growing up of an infant to a child. However, it is often used to refer principally to the changes that occur during later life when it is characterised by a progressive, generalised impairment of function, leading to increasing frailty, likelihood of disease and eventually death. For this reason, it is common to apply an actuarial definition which says that ageing is defined by an accelerating increase in the age-specific death rate. This definition is useful, for example, to distinguish between animal species in which ageing occurs and those, such as *Hydra*, in which it does not. The human increase in age-specific death rate is well described by an exponential increase in age-specific mortality. Interestingly, this increase is apparent from puberty onwards, with mortality rate doubling every eight years. This almost lifelong pattern reveals that ageing, even when defined in terms of intrinsic deterioration, does not begin in middle life but is part of a much more extensive continuum.

'Lifespan' will usually be taken to mean the specific measure of an individual's length of life, as with an individual measure of height or weight. Average or maximum lifespan thus refers to statistics measured on populations. 'Longevity' will be used in the more general sense of referring to length of life as an attribute, without necessarily specifying whether this describes an individual, a population or a species.

A rather more difficult, but potentially useful, concept is 'biological age', as opposed to the chronological age measured strictly by a clock or calendar. An individual who ages more slowly than the average, in terms of the phenotypic changes associated with increasing frailty, will have a biological age less than his or her chronological age, and vice versa. Although this concept is attractive in the context of interventions that might potentially alter the rate of ageing, its utility is limited so far by a shortage of good biomarkers of ageing to provide the necessary scale by which biological age might be measured.

2.2 Current understanding of ageing and its genetic basis

A common misconception about the ageing process is that organisms such as humans are programmed to die, perhaps because this is necessary to get rid of older generations and make space for the new. The fallacies in this view have been thoroughly described (Kirkwood and Cremer 1982; Kirkwood 2005) and will be summarised only briefly here. The main objection is that there is little evidence that ageing serves as a major contributor to mortality in natural populations (Medawar 1952), which means that ageing apparently does not serve the role suggested for it. The theory also embodies the questionable supposition that selection for advantage at the species level will be more effective than selection among individuals for the advantages of a longer life. Ageing is clearly a disadvantage to the individual, so any mutation that inactivated any hypothetical 'ageing genes' would confer a fitness advantage, and therefore the non-ageing mutation should spread through the population.

If ageing is not actively programmed, how can it be accounted for in terms of natural selection? The key comes from looking more closely at the observation that ageing makes negligible contribution to mortality in wild populations of animals. For example, 90% of wild mice are dead by age 10 months, although the same animals might live for three years if protected (Austad 1997). This has an important bearing on how far the mouse genome should invest in mechanisms for the long-term maintenance and repair of its somatic (non-reproductive) cells. If 90% of wild mice are dead by 10 months, any investment in maintenance to keep the body in good condition much beyond this point can benefit at most 10% of the population. This immediately suggests that there will be little evolutionary advantage in building long-term survival capacity into a mouse. The argument is further strengthened when we observe that nearly all of the survival mechanisms required by the mouse to combat intrinsic deterioration (DNA damage, protein oxidation *etc.*) require metabolic resources. These are scarce, as is evidenced by the fact that the major cause of mortality for wild mice is cold, due to insufficient energy to maintain body temperature (Berry and Bronson 1992). From a Darwinian point of view, the mouse will benefit more from investing any spare resource into thermogenesis or reproduction than into better DNA repair capacity that it needs to ensure adequate function for a limited time period.

This concept, with its explicit focus on evolution of optimal levels of cell maintenance, is termed the disposable soma theory (Kirkwood 1977, 1997). In essence, the investments in durability and maintenance of somatic tissues are predicted to be sufficient to keep the body in good repair through the normal expectation of life in the wild environment, with some measure of reserve capacity. Thus, it makes sense that mice (with 90% mortality by 10 months) have an intrinsic lifespan of around three

years, while humans (who probably experienced something like 90% mortality by age 50 in our ancestral environment) have an intrinsic lifespan limited to about 100 years. The distinction between somatic and reproductive tissues is important because the reproductive cell lineage, or germ line, must be maintained at a level that preserves viability across the generations, whereas the soma needs only to support the survival of a single generation. As far as is known, all species that have a clear distinction between soma and germ line undergo somatic senescence, while animals that do not show senescence, such as the freshwater *Hydra* (Martinez 1998), have germ cells distributed throughout their body.

The disposable soma theory leads to a number of clear predictions about the nature of the underlying mechanisms that result in age-related frailty, disability and disease. In essence, ageing is neither more nor less than the progressive accumulation through life of a variety of random molecular defects that build up within cells and tissues. These defects start to arise very early in life, probably *in utero*, but in the early years both the fraction of affected cells and the average burden of damage per affected cell are low. However, over time the faults increase, resulting eventually in age-related functional impairment of tissues and organs, which can be seen as a progressively reduced ability to cope with physiological challenges.

This view also helps us examine the sometimes controversial relationship between 'normal ageing' and age-related disease. At one extreme, the term 'normal ageing' is reserved for individuals in whom identifiable pathology is absent. An obvious difficulty that arises, however, when any attempt is made to draw a line between normal ageing and age-related disease is that as a cohort ages, the fraction of individuals who can be said to be ageing 'normally' declines to very low levels. Whether the word 'normal' can usefully be applied to such an atypical subset is debatable. The majority of chronic, degenerative conditions, such as dementia, osteoporosis and osteoarthritis, involve the progressive accumulation of specific types of cellular and molecular lesions. Since the ageing process, as we have seen, is likely to be caused by the general accumulation of such lesions, there may be much greater overlap between the causative pathways leading to normal ageing and age-related diseases than has hitherto

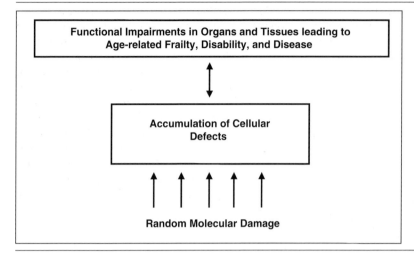

Figure 2.1: Schema of the ageing process.
The ageing process is driven by a lifelong accumulation of molecular damage, resulting in gradual increase in the fraction of cells carrying defects. After sufficient time has passed, the increasing levels of these defects interfere with both the performance and functional reserves of tissues and organs, resulting in age-related frailty, disability and disease.
Source: Kirkwood (2005).
Reprinted with permission from Elsevier.

been recognised (see Figure 2.1). In the case of Alzheimer's disease, most people above 70 years of age have extensive cortical amyloid plaques and neurofibrillary tangles (the so-called 'hallmarks' of classic Alzheimer's disease) even though they may show no evidence of major cognitive decline (Neuropathology Group. Medical Research Council Cognitive Function and Aging 2001).

2.3 Mechanisms of cellular damage

Ageing is highly complex, involving multiple mechanisms at different levels. Much recent evidence suggests that an important theme linking several different kinds of damage is the action of reactive oxygen species (ROS; also known as free radicals) which are generated as by-products of the body's essential use of oxygen to produce cellular energy (Martin *et al.* 1996; von Zglinicki *et al.* 2001). Of particular significance are the contributions of ROS-induced damage to cellular DNA through (i) damage to the chromosomal DNA of the cell nucleus resulting in impaired gene function, (ii) damage to telomeres – the protective DNA structures that appear to 'cap' the ends of chromosomes (analogous to the plastic tips of shoelaces), and (iii) damage to the DNA that exists within the cell's energy-generating organelles, the mitochondria, resulting in impaired energy production. In addition, it is becoming apparent that, with age, there are progressive changes to epigenetic markings (see Section 2.3.4) of the genome (principally changes in DNA methylation) which may have profound effects on gene expression and cell function.

2.3.1 DNA damage and repair

Damage to DNA is particularly likely to play a role in the lifelong accumulation of molecular damage within cells, since damage to DNA can readily result in permanent alteration of the cell's DNA sequence. Cells are subject to mutation all the time, both through errors that may become fixed when cells divide and as a result of ROS-induced damage which can occur at any time. Numerous studies have reported age-related increases in somatic mutation and other forms of DNA damage, suggesting that an important determinant of the rate of ageing at the cell and molecular level is the capacity for DNA repair (Promislow 1994; Bürkle *et al.* 2002).

Although DNA damage may take many forms, it is estimated that oxidative damage is among the most important, accounting for large numbers of oxidative hits per cell per day. A key player in the immediate cellular response to ROS-induced DNA damage is the enzyme poly(ADP-ribose) polymerase-1 (PARP-1), which recognises DNA lesions and flags them for repair. Grube and Bürkle (1992) discovered a strong, positive correlation of PARP activity with the species lifespan; cells from long-lived species having higher levels of PARP activity than cells from short-lived species. In a similar vein, it was found that human centenarians, who have often maintained remarkably good general health, have a significantly greater poly(ADP-ribosyl)ation capacity than the general population (Muiras *et al.* 1998).

2.3.2 Telomeres

In many human somatic tissues a decline in cellular division capacity with age appears to be linked to the fact that the telomeres, which protect the ends of chromosomes, get progressively shorter as cells divide (S.-H. Kim *et al.* 2002). This is due to the absence of the enzyme telomerase, which is normally expressed only in germ cells (testis and ovary) and in certain adult stem cells. Some have suggested that in dividing somatic cells telomeres act as an intrinsic 'division counter', perhaps to protect us against runaway cell division as happens in cancer but causing ageing as the price for this protection (Campisi 1997). Erosion of telomere length below a critical value appears to trigger activation of the same kinds of cell cycle checkpoint as are involved in the more general cellular response to DNA damage, especially the p53/p21/pRb system which responds to DNA damage by inducing cell cycle arrest.

While the loss of telomeric DNA is often attributed mainly to the so-called 'end-replication' problem – the inability of the normal DNA copying machinery to copy right to the very end of the strand in the absence of telomerase – it has been found that stress, especially oxidative stress, has an even bigger effect on the rate of telomere loss (von Zglinicki 2002). Telomere shortening is greatly accelerated (or slowed) in cells with increased (or reduced) levels of stress. The clinical relevance of understanding telomere maintenance and its interaction with stress is considerable. A growing body of evidence suggests that telomere length is linked with ageing and mortality (*e.g.* Cawthon *et al.* 2003). Not only do telomeres shorten with normal ageing in several tissues (*e.g.* lymphocytes, vascular endothelial cells, kidney, liver), but also their reduction is more marked in certain disease states. For example, there appears to be a 100-fold higher incidence of vascular dementia in people with prematurely short telomeres (von Zglinicki *et al.* 2000). Viewed together with the observation that oxidative stress accelerates telomere loss, the intriguing possibility arises that prematurely short telomeres *in vivo* are an indicator of previous exposure to stress and may, therefore, serve as a prognostic indicator for disease conditions in which oxidative stress plays a causative role (von Zglinicki 2002). A recent cross-sectional study in women has shown that telomere length decreased steadily by 27 base pairs (bp) per year of age. However, telomeres were 240 bp shorter in obese than in lean women, *i.e.* in terms of telomere length, the obese women were nine years older than their lean counterparts. In addition, there was a significant dose-dependent reduction in telomere length with amount and duration of cigarette smoking (Valdes *et al.* 2005).

2.3.3 Mitochondria

An important connection between oxidative stress and ageing is suggested by the accumulation of mitochondrial DNA (mtDNA) deletions and point mutations with age (Wallace 1992). Mitochondria are intracellular organelles, each carrying its own small DNA genome, which are responsible for generating cellular energy. As a by-product of energy generation, mitochondria are also the major source of ROS within the cell, and they are, therefore, both responsible for, and a major target of, oxidative stress. Any age-related increase in mutation of mtDNA is likely to contribute to a progressive decline in the cell and tissue capacity for energy production. Age-related increases in frequency of cytochrome c oxidase (COX)-deficient cells have been reported in human muscle (Muller-Hocker 1989; Muller-Hocker *et al.* 1993; Brierley *et al.* 1998) and brain (Cottrell *et al.* 2001), associated with increased frequency of mutated mtDNA.

Until recently, the evidence for age-related accumulation of mtDNA mutations came mainly from tissues such as brain and muscle where cell division in the adult, if it occurs at all, is rare. This led to the idea that accumulation of mtDNA mutation was driven mainly by the dynamics of mitochondrial multiplication and turnover within non-dividing cells (Kowald and Kirkwood 2000). However, recent work has revealed a strongly age-dependent accumulation of mtDNA mutations in human gut epithelium, which has the highest cell division rate of any tissue in the body (Taylor *et al.* 2003). Thus, it appears that mtDNA mutation accumulation may be a widespread phenomenon.

2.3.4 Epigenetic changes

Epigenetics describes modifications to the genome which are copied from one cell generation to the next but which do not involve changes to the primary DNA sequence (Egger *et al.* 2004). Such modifications include DNA methylation and post-translational modifications of histone 'tails' which protrude from the globular protein core of nucleosomes (these are the structural units of chromatin consisting of DNA wrapped around octets of histone proteins). It is possible that these two types of modification occur together, perhaps even acting cooperatively, but, in the context of ageing, most of the available data relate to changes in DNA methylation.

Ageing is associated with a simultaneous reduction in the total methyl content of the nuclear genome and hypermethylation (increased [abnormal] methylation) of a subset of cytosine-rich regions known as CpG islands in the promoters (regulatory regions of DNA upstream of the coding sequence) of certain genes. Similar changes (although, probably, in different genes and in other DNA domains) occur during tumorigenesis (tumour development) and Holliday (1987) suggested that these altered epigenetic markings may be responsible for abnormalities in gene expression during both oncogenesis (the process of developing tumours) and ageing. It has since been demonstrated clearly that CpG island hypermethylation results in silencing of the associated gene. For example, Issa *et al.* (1994) observed that ageing was accompanied by increased methylation of the CpG island in the promoter region of the oestrogen receptor (ESR1) gene and was associated with loss of expression of the protein. Promoter hypermethylation of several genes with increasing age has now been reported for several tissues including colorectal epithelium (Issa *et al.* 1994), cells of the immune system (Issa 2003), and the gastric mucosa (G.H. Kang *et al.* 2003). In addition to aberrant (abnormal) gene expression, loss of normal methylation patterns in tumours and in ageing tissues may be causal for genetic instability (Lengauer *et al.* 1997). These losses of epigenetic control may have adverse effects on the ability of the cell to maintain homeostasis.

2.3.5 Proteins

So far, we have concentrated on damage to DNA. However, damage can also affect any of the macromolecules that make up the cell, as well as those that form extra-cellular structures such as cartilage and bone. In particular, damage to protein molecules occurs to a considerable extent, and accumulation of faulty proteins contributes to important age-related disorders such as cataract, Parkinson's disease and Alzheimer's disease (see Chapter 8). In some ways, the accumulation of defective proteins is harder to explain than the accumulation of DNA damage, since individual protein molecules are subject to a continual cycle of synthesis and breakdown. Thus, damage to any individual protein molecule should be cleared as soon as that molecule is degraded. The exceptions occur when the defective protein molecules become resistant to breakdown, for example, because they form aggregates large enough to withstand the normal removal systems. It is the build-up of such aggregates that is commonly linked with cell and tissue pathology.

2.3.6 Interactions between mechanisms

We have so far considered a number of distinct mechanisms that can contribute to cellular ageing. For each of these, there is evidence supporting the hypothesis that it is indeed an agent of senescence. However, the extent of the contribution to senescence almost invariably appears too small for the mechanism to be a sufficient explanation of age-related degeneration. The obvious solution to this conundrum is that cellular ageing is multi-causal and that the various mechanisms all play their part. For example, a build-up of mitochondrial DNA mutations will lead to a decline in the cell's energy production, and this will reduce the capacity to carry out energy-dependent protein clearance. Mitochondrial mutations may also interfere with signalling pathways for cell death by apoptosis (programmed cell death) (Mathers 2003) and so allow the survival of cells carrying damaged genomes. In recent years, novel methods based on computer modelling of interactions and synergism between different ageing mechanisms have begun to build a better, more integrated picture of how cells break down with age (Kirkwood *et al.* 2003).

2.4 Metabolic factors affecting ageing

Of particular significance in terms of metabolic factors influencing ageing rates has been the discovery that insulin signalling pathways appear to have effects on ageing that may be strongly conserved across the species range (Gems and Partridge 2001). Insulin signalling regulates responses to varying nutrient levels and so the discovery of the major role for these pathways in ageing fits well with the central concept of the disposable soma theory, namely that ageing results from and is controlled by the metabolic allocation of the organism's metabolic resources to maintenance and repair.

One of the clearest examples of how metabolic signalling affects ageing and longevity, comes from a study on genes of the insulin signalling pathway in *C. elegans* (Murphy *et al.* 2003). When threatened with overcrowding, which the larval worm detects by the increasing concentration of a pheromone, it diverts its development from the normal succession of larval moults into a long-lived, dispersal form called the dauer larva (Larsen *et al.* 1995). Dauers show increased resistance to stress and can survive very much longer than the normal form, reverting to complete their development into adults should more favourable conditions be detected. An insulin/IGF (insulin-like growth factor)-1-like gene, *daf-2*, heads the gene regulatory pathway that controls the switch into the dauer form, and mutations in *daf-2* produce animals that develop into adults with substantially increased lifespans (Kenyon *et al.* 1993). In common with other members of the evolutionarily conserved insulin/IGF-1 signalling pathway, *daf-2* also regulates lipid metabolism and reproduction. The *daf-2* gene product exerts its effects by influencing 'downstream' gene expression, in particular via the actions of another gene belonging to the dauer-formation gene family, *daf-16*, which it inhibits (Kimura *et al.* 1997). It was shown by Murphy *et al.* (2003) that more than 300 genes appeared to have their expression levels altered by *daf-16* regulation. These genes turned out to be a heterogeneous group in which three major categories could be discerned. The first category comprised a variety of stress-response genes, including antioxidant enzymes. A second group encoded antimicrobial proteins, important for survival in this organism because its death is commonly caused by proliferation of bacteria in the gut. A third group included genes involved in protein turnover, which is an important cellular maintenance system. Thus the metabolic regulation of the rate of ageing in *C. elegans* is mediated through genetic effects on a diverse array of survival mechanisms, in line with the predictions of the disposable soma theory.

2.5 Energy (calorie) restriction in rodents

The effect of food restriction (calorie restriction) on lifespan in laboratory rats was first described by McCay *et al.* (1935). Many studies have confirmed this result and extended it to mice (Weindruch and Walford 1988; Sprott 1997). Long-term food restriction results in a small, lean rodent with impaired fertility, but which is otherwise healthy and active and lives as much as 40% longer, on average, than an *ad-libitum* fed control. Rodents kept on restricted diets have less body fat and smaller major organs (Weindruch and Sohal 1997).

One of the curious features of food-restricted rodents is that they appear to have a general up-regulation of mechanisms protecting against accumulation of somatic damage. Protein turnover (Lewis *et al.* 1985; Ward and Shibatani 1994), serum corticosteroids (Masoro 1995), DNA repair activity (Haley-Zitlin and Richardson 1993), cystolic antioxidants (Yu 1994) and the expression of heat shock proteins (factors which recognise molecules altered by stress and mark them for renaturation or destruction) (Heydari *et al.* 1996) all remain at youthful levels for longer. This enhanced somatic protection and repair is associated with a delay in many aspects of age-related pathology. Incidence rates of spontaneous and chemically induced tumours are greatly reduced (Weindruch and Walford 1982; Klurfeld *et al.* 1987; Schwartz and Pashko 1994). The age-related decline in efficiency of wound healing is also delayed (Reed *et al.* 1996). Also, calorie restriction virtually eliminates the development of autoimmune diseases in susceptible strains of mice (Weindruch and Sohal 1997).

The fact that animals which are severely short of food *increase* their investment in cellular maintenance functions is at first sight puzzling, particularly since one of the leading physiological explanations of ageing, the disposable soma theory (Kirkwood 1977; Kirkwood and Holliday 1979; Kirkwood and Rose 1991), suggests that ageing occurs because natural selection favours a strategy in which investments in somatic maintenance are limited in order to spare precious resources for growth and reproduction (see Section 2.2). Thus, the fact that food-restricted rodents up-regulate their maintenance seems at first sight counterintuitive. A suggestion to resolve this paradox is that the primary role of the food-restriction response is to shift resources away from reproduction during periods of famine, when the likelihood of reproductive success is small, and to invest as much of the resultant saving as possible into increased somatic maintenance. The potential benefit is that the animal gains an increased chance of survival with a reduced intrinsic rate of senescence, thereby permitting reproductive value to be preserved for when the famine is over (Harrison and Archer 1989; Holliday 1989; Phelan and Austad 1989). A detailed quantitative development of this hypothesis using a dynamic resource allocation model revealed that the effect could be the result of the suggested evolutionary process provided that the following conditions were satisfied: (i) there is a substantial initial cost to reproduction; and (ii) juveniles are at a disadvantage during periods of food shortage (Shanley and Kirkwood 2000).

2.6 Early life effects

The possibility that adaptive plasticity of ageing and lifespan, *i.e.* an evolved capacity to alter the course of the life history in response to adverse circum-

stances, occurs also in humans has been raised by the discovery that the fetal nutritional environment can affect the risk of developing age-related diseases in the adult (O'Brien *et al.* 1999; Barker *et al.* 2002; Bateson *et al.* 2004; Gluckman and Hanson 2004). Whether these effects are mediated by adaptive plasticity affecting the allocation of metabolic resources to somatic maintenance remains to be discovered.

It is clear, however, that in terms of underlying mechanisms of ageing there is a continuum between early and late life, which is played out through the accumulation of molecular and cellular defects and which can be influenced by nutrition and other life-style factors as illustrated in Figure 2.2.

Early life effects can also be important in creating variability in the ageing process through the impacts of damage on processes of development. The overall process of morphogenesis is remarkably reliable. Nevertheless, small early perturbations can result in large effects, and there is evidence of significant organ size variations among genetically identical organisms (Finch and Kirkwood 2000). In addition to variations in the endpoints of development, such

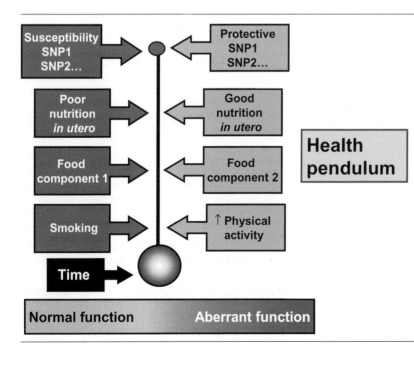

Figure 2.2: The health pendulum.
Conceptual model of major factors influencing cellular function during the life-course with implications for modulation of the ageing trajectory.
SNP: Single nucleotide polymorphism.
Source: Modified from: Mathers (2002).

as adult organ size, there can be significant variations in the timing of key developmental events, such as puberty (vom Saal *et al.* 1990).

2.7 Nutrition and antioxidants

Nutrition appears be an important determinant of life expectancy. For example, observational studies have shown that those who adhere to a Mediterranean diet have reduced overall mortality (Trichopoulou *et al.* 2003, 2005). Whilst nutrition may be an important modulator of the ageing trajectory, there is as yet no proof of the role played by any specific food component in influencing longevity. However, recent research has suggested that dietary factors may play an important role in influencing the rate at which the genome (and probably other cell macromolecules) sustains damage that is fundamental to the ageing process.

We have hypothesised that aberrant gene expression, resulting from unrepaired damage to the genome, is causal for the loss of capacity for homeostasis which is characteristic of ageing. Therefore, dietary factors which limit damage or which enhance repair would be expected to modify the rate of biological ageing. The most extensively studied aspect of DNA damage, modifiable by dietary factors, is oxidative damage by reactive oxygen species. Trace metals (including zinc and selenium), vitamins (including A, C and E) and non-nutrients (such as lycopene and polyphenols) all play a role in scavenging free radicals and so preventing oxidative damage to DNA as well as to cellular lipids and proteins. Whilst the role of dietary antioxidants in prevention of DNA damage is now well established, recent research has shown that certain antioxidants may have an additional role in enhancing DNA repair (Brash and Havre 2002).

Humans and other mammals have evolved a range of DNA repair mechanisms (including one-step repair, base excision repair, nucleotide excision repair and DNA mismatch repair) which detect and repair different kinds of DNA damage. Selenium was the first of the antioxidant nutrients for which evidence emerged for a role in enhancing DNA repair. Addition of extra selenium (in the form of selenomethionine) induced base excision repair via P53 activation in normal human fibroblasts *in vitro* (Seo *et al.* 2002). It is possible that higher intakes of zinc in older individuals may help ensure optimal function of both base excision and nucleotide excision repair since several of the proteins involved in these repair systems are zinc finger (which enable the proteins to interact with DNA and to regulate gene expression) or zinc-associated proteins (Ho 2004). Importantly, there is now evidence that nutrition may enhance DNA repair in humans *in vivo*. Collins *et al.* supplemented the diets of healthy volunteers (26–54 years) with one or more kiwi fruit (rich in vitamin C and other phytochemicals with antioxidant activity) for three-week periods (Collins *et al.* 2003). In addition to the expected increases in antioxidant status of plasma and of lymphocytes, Collins *et al.* observed that the extra fruit reduced endogenous oxidation of purines and pyrimidines in lymphocytic DNA and significantly enhanced ($P < 0.001$) base excision repair in lymphocytes. Interestingly, the kiwi fruit supplementation had no detectable effect on expression (at the mRNA level) of two key genes, *OGG1* and *APE1*, responsible for DNA repair, so further work is needed to ascertain the mechanisms underlying the enhanced DNA repair and to determine which components of the fruit delivered this protection. Recently, tentative evidence has emerged from a human epidemiological study that low folate status may limit the cell's ability to carry out nucleotide excision repair (Q. Wei *et al.* 2003). Given the age-related decline in folate status manifested as a rise in plasma homocysteine concentration, this is a potentially important observation which should stimulate further investigation.

2.8 Nutrition and inflammation

Finch and Crimmins (2004) have argued that lifetime exposure to infectious diseases and other sources of inflammation are important determinants of longevity. Ageing is associated with a greater risk of dysfunction of the immune system and with development of a chronic inflammatory state. Inflammation may be a key factor in the impaired immune function and progressive loss of lean tissue during ageing (Grimble 2003) and appears to accelerate age-related changes in CpG island methylation (Issa *et al.* 2001; G.H. Kang *et al.* 2003) (see Chapter 11). These adverse effects, which decrease the capacity for homeostasis, may be attributable, at least in part, to impaired nutrition so that interventions using nutrients with anti-inflammatory properties such as vitamin E and *n*-3 polyunsaturated fatty acids may reduce levels of inflammation and improve cell and tissue function (Grimble 2003). During ageing, lean tissue tends to be lost and be replaced by fat so that for a given BMI, older persons will tend to have higher body fat content. Since obesity is characterised by mild chronic inflammation (Trayhurn 2005), the increase in prevalence of overweight and obesity (until about age 75 years) is likely to exacerbate any age-related increase in inflammation.

2.9 Nutrigenomics

The application of high throughput genomics tools (nutrigenomics) (van Ommen and Stierum 2002; Muller and Kersten 2003; Oommen *et al.* 2005), especially when a systems biology approach is adopted, offers a powerful new way of investigating the role of diet in influencing the biology of ageing. Systems biology describes an approach to investigating biological complexity which involves the integrated work of several disciplines including biologists, mathematicians and computer scientists. To date, much of the work in this area has been restricted to studies of global changes in gene expression (using genome-wide micro-array expression analysis) in tissues from animals subjected to calorie restriction but, together with applications of proteomics and metabolomics, these nutrigenomics approaches are likely to yield important novel data not only on the process of ageing, but also on the mechanisms by which food components modify ageing.

C.K. Lee *et al.* (1999) were the first to publish data on global gene expression during ageing and on the impact of calorie restriction on these changes. In mouse muscle, ageing resulted in a differential pattern of gene expression characteristic of increased stress response with reduced expression of biosyn-thetic and metabolic genes. Calorie restriction partially or completely reversed these alterations in both muscle (C.K. Lee *et al.* 1999) and in liver (Cao *et al.* 2001). Age-associated induction of genes encoding inflammatory and stress responses in the mouse brain were also attenuated by calorie restriction (Lee *et al.* 2000). Even relatively short periods (2–8 weeks) of calorie restriction produced a rapid and progressive shift in hepatic gene expression patterns towards those seen in rodents exposed to long-term calorie restriction (Dhahbi *et al.* 2004).

2.10 Conclusions

1. Ageing is a process of cumulative cell and tissue dysfunction that is driven by faults in the synthesis, modification and clearance of macromolecules.
2. Genes that influence longevity act through their effects on setting the levels of activity of key molecular and cellular maintenance systems. The genetic contribution to human ageing thus determines the likely trajectory that an individual will follow in terms of maintenance and ultimate erosion of the systems supporting survival.
3. Although genes set the individual expected rate of accumulation of damage, many environmental factors may impact on the rate of damage accumulation, for better or for worse.
4. Nutrition in particular may have an important effect since, on the one hand, a poor diet will contain factors that are intrinsically damaging, either at low levels or when consumed to excess; and on the other, nutrition can have important beneficial effects on the rate of ageing, not only because cell maintenance functions depend on an adequate supply of energy, but also because some nutritional ingredients can aid in the protection against damage, *e.g.* dietary antioxidants.

2.11 Key points

- The process of ageing is *not* genetically programmed. It appears to result from the accumulation of damage to cells and to the macromolecules – especially DNA – within cells.

- External factors that enhance cellular damage, such as stress and poor nutrition, are likely to speed up the ageing process. Both obesity and smoking are associated with a reduction in telomere length – a

Continued

potential biological marker of the ageing process.

- As yet there is limited understanding of the molecular mechanisms by which individual nutrients or other food constituents could affect

the accumulation of the cellular and molecular damage responsible for ageing. However, anti-oxidant food components are likely to be protective and there is some evidence that nutrients, *e.g.* selenium, may enhance DNA repair.

2.12 Recommendations for future research

- Further research is needed to develop robust biomarkers of the ageing process in humans which can be applied in both observational studies and in intervention studies designed to reduce the rate of biological ageing.

- Further work should examine in detail how nutrition can impact, in particular in beneficial ways, on the networks for cell maintenance and repair. To gain the necessary level of understanding is likely to require a systems-biology approach.

2.13 Key references

Bateson P, Barker D, *et al.* (2004) Developmental plasticity and human health. *Nature*, **430**, 419–21.

Finch CE and Crimmins EM (2004) Inflammatory exposure and historical changes in human life-spans. *Science*, **305**, 1736–9.

Gluckman PD and Hanson MA (2004b) The developmental origins of the metabolic syndrome. *Trends in Endocrinology & Metabolism*, **15**, 183–7.

Kang GH, Lee HJ, *et al.* (2003) Aberrant CpG island hypermethylation of chronic gastritis, in relation to aging, gender, intestinal metaplasia, and chronic inflammation. *American Journal of Pathology*, **163**, 1551–6.

Kirkwood TBL (2005) Understanding the odd science of aging. *Cell*, **120**, 437–47.

3
Healthy Ageing: Teeth and the Oral Cavity

3.1 Changing oral health status with age

The historical view of the oral health status of older people is characterised by large numbers of people with no natural teeth (edentulous) who rely on removable prostheses for adequate oral function. This pattern is currently changing rapidly throughout the world. Whilst there are still high levels of edentulism among the oldest old today, there is a progressive trend for retention of teeth among younger people, which will gradually spread into old age over the next 20–30 years. This pattern is exemplified for the adult population in Figure 3.1 for the UK, but is also seen in many other countries for which such data are available (Table 3.1). Those countries in which there is no projected decline in edentulism already show such low levels that it is not realistic to expect any further reduction. Implicit in this is an understanding that there will always be some people who have no natural teeth, either because of their susceptibility to oral disease, notably periodontal disease, or because they do not regard oral health as a particular benefit and opt for tooth extraction rather than retention when attending the dentist. In some countries this decision may also be an economic one, as extraction is usually much cheaper than attempts to maintain or restore a broken down tooth.

In all countries there are also significant variations in oral health status both in different regions and with social class, with higher levels of tooth retention in the higher social groups and more affluent areas of a country. This is illustrated using UK data in Table 3.2.

This change is occurring because of altered patterns of dental care, which used to be dominated by tooth extraction and is now more focused on restoration and retention of teeth. There is also a greater social awareness of the benefits of retaining some natural teeth for both aesthetic and functional reasons. This will result in more teeth being present and susceptible to dental diseases, in particular dental caries and periodontal disease, in older people at the same time that the size of the older population is also increasing.

3.2 Impact of nutrition on oral disease

3.2.1 Dental caries (tooth decay)

Dental caries is an environmental disease that is a product of the interactions between bacteria on the surface of teeth and fermentable sugars in food. Bacterial plaque begins to form on the surface of teeth immediately after they are cleaned, but does not reach maturity until it is about four days old. Mature plaque which has a characteristic microbial flora is capable of metabolising sugars to produce acid. Once the pH of the plaque falls below the critical pH for demineralisation of tooth tissue the surface and sub-surface tissue begin to dissolve. This process can be reversed by the mouth's defence mechanisms, which include dilution and buffering of the plaque acids and active remineralisation of any demineralised surfaces by saliva. Dental caries occurs when the balance of influences causing demineralisation and remineralisation lies in favour of the demineralisation process (Figure 3.2). This balance may be affected in four ways during ageing; exposure of dentine, presence of fluoride, oral hygiene and saliva flow.

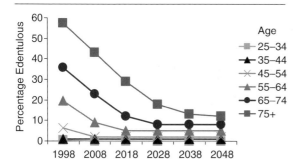

Figure 3.1: Projected changes in the proportion of the population edentulous over the next 40 years. The data are based on national epidemiological data gathered on a decennial over the last 40 years. The greatest changes are in the oldest age groups over this period.
Source: Kelly *et al.* (2000). Reproduced under the terms of the Click-Use Licence.

Table 3.1: Prevalence of edentulousness for people aged 60 and over

		1980s	1990s	2000s
Denmark	65–74	51	40	27
France	65–74		16.3	15.5
Netherlands	65–74	65.4	61	
US	Over 60s	31	25	
UK	Over 65s	67	46	

Source: www.whocollab.od.mah.se/euro/denmark/denmark.html; Bratthall (2006).

3.2.1.1 Mineralised tissues

The tooth comprises two mineralised tissues. The enamel covers the crown of the tooth and is the tissue that is normally exposed in the oral environment. It is highly mineralised (98%) and has a relatively low critical pH for dissolution (about pH 5.5). The enamel covers a less mineralised tissue dentine which is the vital core of the tooth. Dentine not only forms the core of the crown but also the whole of the structure of the root of the tooth. With age there is an increased tendency for the root tissue to become exposed close to the gum margin as a consequence of periodontal disease and gum recession. This exposed dentine is more susceptible to demineralisation than enamel, with a critical pH closer to 6. An individual may be caries-free for many years until dentine starts to become exposed. This change in the

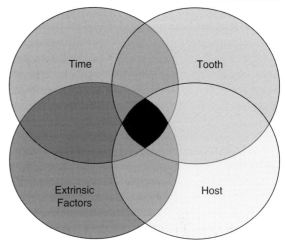

Figure 3.2: The multifactorial origin of dental caries. Dental caries is a multifactorial disease of infectious origin. Decay occurs when the extent and severity of the demineralising challenge in the mouth is greater than the ability of the natural defence mechanisms in the oral environment to repair the damage. This will be affected by variables such as the individual's ability to produce an adequate volume of saliva, the quantity and particularly the frequency of intakes of sugars and the susceptibility of the host.

threshold for progressive demineralisation can result in decay occurring in a previously stable oral environment when enamel alone was exposed.

Furthermore, both enamel and dentine undergo surface change with time of exposure in the oral environment. This occurs as a consequence of the dynamic demineralisation/remineralisation balance which occurs throughout normal oral function. With each remineralisation cycle, the mineral content of the surface of the tooth becomes ionically more complex and chemically more stable, with the incorporation of trace elements such as strontium, magnesium, zinc and fluoride into the crystal structure. These trace elements come from the diet, including the water supply. It takes up to six months of exposure in the oral environment for a *new* enamel or dentine surface to become modified in this way. Such new surfaces can either occur through loss of tissue attachment at the gum margin, with periodontal disease exposing root dentine, or through a dentist removing the surface layer (which is very shallow) when providing a filling for a tooth.

Table 3.2: Variations in the rates of edentulism with age, gender and social background from the National Diet and Nutrition Survey for people aged 65 years and over

Socio-demographic variables	Base	% Edentate	% 1–20 teeth	% ≥21 teeth	Mean no. of teeth
Gender					
Men	391 (52%)	37	46	17	9.6
Women	362 (48%)	56	33	11	6.4
Age group					
65–74	325 (43%)	32	46	22	11.1
75–84	285 (38%)	50	39	11	7.2
85+	143 (19%)	70	29	1	3.1
Social class					
Non-manual	362 (48%)	38	43	19	9.8
Manual	347 (46%)	53	38	9	6.3
Region					
Scotland	69 (9%)	51	39	10	7.3
Northern	172 (23%)	62	27	11	5.6
Central, South-west England and Wales	314 (42%)	44	43	13	8.5
London and South-east	198 (26%)	34	47	19	9.9
Education attainment					
High	75 (10%)	31	39	31	12.1
Low	677 (90%)	48	40	12	7.6

1–20 teeth: compromised dentition; >21 teeth: intact dentition.
Source: Steele *et al.* (1998). Reproduced under the terms of the Click-Use Licence.

3.2.1.2 *The role of fluoride*

Fluoride has a number of important roles in helping to prevent tooth decay. The relative balance of these roles depends on the nature of exposure to fluoride, that is whether it is present in an all-pervasive sense (usually as a consequence of either naturally occurring fluoride in the water supply or artificial supplementation of the water supply), or episodically through the use of fluoride containing toothpastes and mouth rinses.

Enamel and dentine that develop in people who have lifelong exposure through water fluoridation contain significant quantities of fluorapatite as opposed to hydroxyapatite. Fluorapatite is more resistant to demineralisation and hence imparts resistance to decay to such teeth; the benefits of this resistance are greatest for exposed smooth surfaces of the teeth like the root surface.

Fluoride is also critical to the surface maturation process described above. In the presence of small quantities of fluoride (which can come from toothpaste, the water supply or food sources such as tea) the remineralisation process is enhanced and fluoride becomes incorporated into the mineral matrix

of the surface of the tooth converting the original mineral hydroxyapatite into fluorapatite.

Until recently the relative importance of these two mechanisms was unclear, particularly for the adult. It has been established that lifelong residence in a community with natural or artificial fluoridation of the water supply or early-life exposure to such water imparts some defence against caries (Burt *et al.* 1986; Stamm *et al.* 1990). One of the arguments used against community water fluoridation programmes has been that there is no established benefit for adults of drinking fluoridated water. However, there is now compelling evidence from both the US and Ireland that the incorporation of fluoride at optimum levels in the water supply has a benefit in preventing dental caries over and above that that is derived from incorporation of fluoride in teeth during their development in childhood through this mechanism. The Irish data contrast the root caries experience of older adults living in cities which have benefited from water fluoridation to the level of 1 mg/L for 25 years with that for rural communities over the same period where the water is not fluoridated. The comparison showed a 7 percentage point reduction in root caries in people from the fluoridated communities (18.9%

of exposed surfaces with caries compared with 11.7%) (Whelton *et al.* 1993). The two American studies likewise contrast root caries experience of individuals who have been exposed to fluoridated water in adulthood with those who have not, in Iowa and New York. They both show reductions in decay either in terms of prevalence (Brustman 1986) or incidence of new lesions (Hunt *et al.* 1989). The impact of this benefit varies with length of exposure to fluoridated water but reductions in both the prevalence and severity of root caries have been shown with long-term exposure to fluoridated water as adults.

As little as 10% of the domestic water supply in the UK has either natural or added fluoride to the perceived optimum of 1 mg/L. There have been concerns that at this level there is an increased risk of excess intakes and hence toxicity from fluoride through a combination of water and foods. This concern was addressed by the UK Committee on Toxicology and was shown to be unfounded (COT 2003).

Finally, fluoride plays an important part in the arrest and reversal of decay. Again, this is mediated by its action in enhancing the rate and effectiveness of the remineralisation process of demineralised tooth tissue. Fluoride preparations, in the form of gels or mouthwash, form an important part of a dentist's armamentarium in helping to manage decay in older people.

3.2.1.3 Oral hygiene

There is a tendency for the quality of an individual's personal oral hygiene to deteriorate with age. This is likely to be due in part to increasing difficulty for the individual in undertaking intricate tasks like cleaning teeth and in part due to alterations in the shape of the gum as a consequence of periodontal disease and gum recession. As the gum architecture becomes more complex, intricate techniques are required to clean the surfaces of teeth close to the gum margin making the process more difficult for older people. Furthermore, as the gum recedes the shape of the teeth changes with grooves and hollows on the root surfaces becoming exposed into the mouth. Again these are more difficult to clean than the smooth convex surfaces people usually cope with well. This is compounded by relatively low rates of attendance at the dentist among older people and consequently there are limited opportunities for education about the required techniques. Poor oral

hygiene is the shared aetiological variable that is responsible for the link between unmanaged periodontal disease and root caries.

3.2.1.4 Saliva

There are profound alterations in the structure of salivary glands with increasing age. Youthful salivary tissue is densely packed with the secretory elements for saliva (the salivary acini). With ageing, these acini are replaced progressively with fatty and fibrous tissue. Current evidence would suggest that salivary flow under stimulated conditions is unaffected by these changes in healthy older people. There is some evidence that resting flow rates from the minor salivary glands and the sub-mandibular glands may be reduced by these changes. It is thought that this apparent dichotomy between marked change in structure and apparently minor change in function is brought about by increases in stimuli for salivary secretion (this pattern is also seen for gut motility which is maintained in increasing age by increased rates of stimulation). However, the reserve capacity of the salivary glands (the difference in secretory capacity between that which is used routinely to maintain normal rates of flow and the maximum potential flow for the gland) is markedly reduced. As a consequence, challenges to that reserve capacity brought about by drugs or disease result in reduced rates of flow which may extend to overt dry mouth or xerostomia (Figure 3.3) (Baum *et al.* 1992; Ghezzi and Ship 2003). Such challenges are common in older people, particularly as a consequence of polypharmacy (Figure 3.4) (Närhi *et al.* 1992).

Saliva has many roles in the mouth but is critical to the defence mechanisms against dental caries by acting as a buffer for plaque acids, a diluent and a remineralising solution. Levels of demineralisation that do not cause problems in subjects with normal salivary flow cause problems with decay in people with xerostomia as oral homeostasis is impaired.

3.2.2 Sugars consumption

Sugars are an important component of all diets and yet they are also responsible for being the source of acids that result in tooth decay. There is a considerable body of evidence linking caries to sugars intake in younger people, including national epidemiological studies (Figure 3.5). However, there are fewer

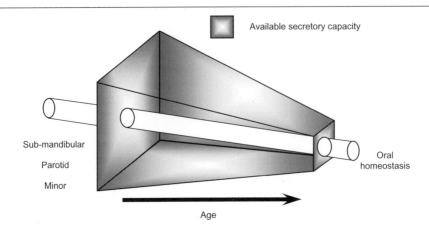

Available secretory capacity

Sub-mandibular

Parotid

Minor

Oral homeostasis

Age

Figure 3.3: The ability of salivary glands to produce saliva decreases with increasing age as a consequence of pathological changes within salivary gland tissue.
There is some reduction in salivary flow rate with increasing age, but the magnitude of the change is small and probably not of clinical significance. Of much greater impact is the effect of drugs on salivary flow and other causes of dry mouth. Any challenge to salivary output has a greater impact in older people as a consequence of their lower salivary reserve (*i.e.* the difference between the available secretory capacity and the amount of saliva needed for normal function).
Source: Baum *et al.* (1992). Reproduced with permission from the Copyright Clearance Centre.

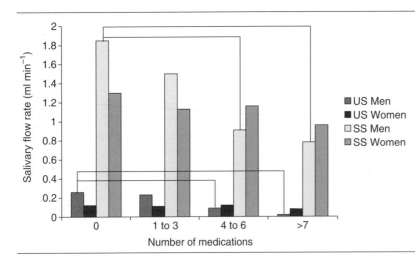

Figure 3.4: The effect of taking multiple medications on salivary flow in a population of older Finnish people. The groups linked by the bars were significantly different from each other, as were the flow rates for men and women. SS: stimulated salivary flow; US: unstimulated salivary flow. Source: Närhi *et al.* (1992). Reproduced by permission of the International and American Associations for Dental Research.

data which link decay in older adults to sugars consumption. Vehkalahti was able to demonstrate a link between the use of sugars in tea and coffee and root caries in a Finnish population (Vehkalahti and Paunio 1988) and Steele *et al.* (2001) found a twofold increase in risk of root caries in subjects with high frequency of sugars intake in their analysis of the UK National Diet and Nutrition Survey for people aged 65 and over. One particular area of concern is the high level of untreated dental caries in institutionalised populations. This is the result of a combination of poor access to dental care and also a

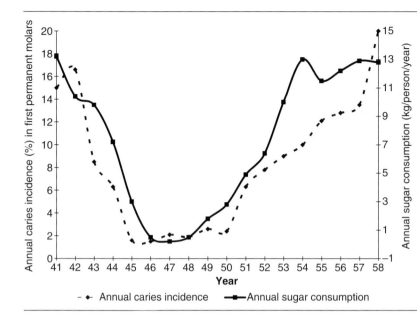

Figure 3.5: The relationship between caries in first permanent molars in Japanese schoolchildren and annual sugar intake between 1941 and 1958. The relationship between dietary intake of sugars and caries activity is striking in this example.
Source: Takahashi (1961). Reproduced by permission of the Tokyo Dental College.

relatively cariogenic diet with a high frequency of sugars intake daily.

There are three variables that determine the impact of dietary sugars on the teeth: age, frequency and quantity.

3.2.2.1 *Which sugars are important?*

It is clear that the most cariogenic sugars are highly refined carbohydrates, particularly sucrose, but also glucose. Natural fruit sugars, like fructose and those in milk (lactose), can also be metabolised by plaque bacteria to produce acids but are more difficult for the bacteria to metabolise and hence are less acidogenic. It is also relatively unusual for people to have diets that include high frequency of intake of such sugars. Finely ground starch can also be metabolised to produce acids by oral bacteria, but again at lower levels than seen with sucrose.

Refined sugars are widely used in the food industry as sweetening agents and as preservatives. In this latter role they are often described as hidden sugars as many savoury foods contain substantial quantities of added sugar (prime examples are tomato ketchup, chutney and baked beans, but there are many others). High-starch snack foods can also contribute to the development of caries lesions.

3.2.2.2 *Is frequency or quantity important?*

When sugars are taken into the oral environment they are metabolised by plaque bacteria, which produce acids as a by-product. This results in a reduction in oral plaque pH with a characteristic pattern of a rapid fall to a pH of about 5.3 followed by a progressive rise back to normal levels of oral pH (about 6.8). Demineralisation occurs during the period when the plaque pH lies below the threshold level for the tissue concerned. Hence for each episode of pH fall, dentine will be exposed to a longer period of demineralisation than enamel (Figure 3.6). Remineralisation and repair occur during times when plaque pH is above the demineralising threshold. Evidence would suggest that the frequency of sugars intake is more important than the overall quantity of sugars ingested in predicting the severity of caries seen. With relatively low frequency of intake the natural defence/repair mechanisms have an opportunity to be effective, however when frequencies are high demineralisation dominates, tipping the process away from repair towards decay. There is no evidence on what frequency of sugars intakes might be regarded as safe for root caries; the evidence that is available relates to enamel caries in younger subjects where dentists would normally recommend no more

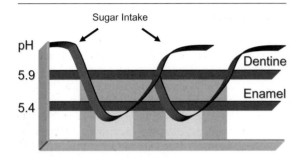

Figure 3.6: A schematic diagram of the effect of intake of sugars on the pH of mature dental plaque. There is an immediate reduction in plaque pH followed by a slow rise back to baseline levels. This has a greater impact in terms of the length of time the plaque is below the critical pH for demineralisation of the tooth surface for dentine compared with enamel. The higher pH of demineralisation for dentine may also allow bacteria which cannot initiate demineralisation of enamel because they do not produce sufficient acid to lower the pH to 5.4 to cause this for dentine at a pH of 5.9.
Source: Reproduced by permission of Ageing Clinical & Experimental Research.

than four episodes of sugar-containing foods or drinks intake per day. This would include sugar used to sweeten tea and coffee. It is of note that the mean number of sugars intakes daily for the free-living 65 and over population in the UK was 5.1, rising to 7.9 for the institution sample in the 65 and over NDNS programme (Steele *et al.* 1998).

One specific problem that relates to older infirm individuals is the use of energy supplements as part of their diet to try to maintain an adequate calorific intake. These supplements are often in liquid or syrup form and are drunk over extended periods of time by their users, resulting in long periods during which demineralisation can occur. The syrupy nature of these preparations is of particular relevance as their rate of oral clearance will be low, especially in individuals with impaired salivary flow.

3.2.2.3 Sugars in medicines

Sugars are used in medicines as preservatives in syrups and mixtures, and to mask the bitter flavour of drugs. There has been a long and successful cam-paign for the replacement of sugars in medicines for children with artificial sweeteners and other agents. Drugs delivered to adults are commonly taken in tablet or capsule form, but there is increasing use of liquid preparations in older adults and also drugs which have prolonged oral clearance (tablets that are sucked or chewed, for example, rather than swallowed). Currently, most of these drugs retain sugars as sweeteners or preservatives, which can pose a problem in relation to decay in susceptible individuals. Similarly, chewable preparations that have an intrinsically low pH (for example, vitamin C preparations) will add to the overall acid burden of the oral environment.

3.2.2.4 Caries prevention

There are three strategies that can assist with caries prevention in relation to sugars intake: reducing frequency, sugars replacement and use of chewing gum.

1. *Reducing frequency:* If the frequency of sugars consumption can be reduced to 3–4 times daily then the normal remineralising capacity of the mouth should be able to cope with resulting acid challenge. Within limits, the overall quantity of sugars taken on each occasion is irrelevant.
2. *Sugars replacement:* One factor that can assist with reducing the frequency of sugars intake is sugars replacement with other sweetening agents that cannot be fermented by oral bacteria to produce acids. Such sweeteners come in two forms:
   - intense sweeteners (*e.g.* saccharine, sucralose and acesulfame K), which are commonly used to sweeten drinks and are widely available for consumer use through products such as Sweetex®, Splenda® and Hermesetas®, along with a variety of proprietary brands.
   - bulk sweeteners (*e.g.* isomalt, sorbitol, xylitol), which are used in prepared foods to replace the bulking effect of sugars. One complication of their use is that they are not absorbed across the gut wall and hence remain in the gut, then pass through the large bowel. They remain osmotically active in the large bowel, reducing the capacity for water uptake from the stool. If taken in large quantities, this can result in osmotic diarrhoea. Xylitol is of particular

benefit as it both replaces sugar as a sweetener but also has the additional property of inhibiting the metabolic pathway that results in acid production by *strep mutans* in dental plaque.

The quantity of such sweeteners that can be added to foods is carefully regulated (FSA 2002).

3. *Chewing gum:* Chewing has the effect of stimulating salivary output. Saliva has a number of roles in caries prevention: it dilutes and buffers plaque acids and it is a potent remineralising agent for demineralised tooth tissue. The fall in pH associated with sugars intake is dramatically modified if it is followed by a period of chewing gum (Figure 3.7). This effect occurs with both sugar-containing and sugar-free gums, but obviously the latter are preferable, particularly those that contain xylitol (Dodds *et al.* 1991). One trial of a gum chewing programme in an institutional setting in the UK showed dramatic reductions in the development of new carious lesions using a gum containing xylitol, fluoride and a topical antimicrobial chlorhexidine gluconate (Simons *et al.* 2002).

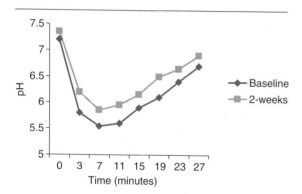

Figure 3.7: The influence of chewing gum on both the fall in salivary pH for a given acidogenic challenge and the rate of recovery from the fall in pH.
The subjects were all individuals who had not been previous habitual gum chewers and were encouraged to chew gum regularly after and between meals for a two-week period.
Source: Dodds *et al.* (1991). Reproduced by permission of the International and American Associations for Dental Research.

3.2.3 Erosion

Erosion is acid-mediated dissolution of tooth tissue, where the acid is not produced as a consequence of the metabolism of sugars by bacteria. The acids involved can be intrinsic (regurgitated gastric acid) or extrinsic (from foods/drinks or occasionally industrial sources) in origin. Whilst there is no evidence of a link between loss of tooth structure in older adults and dietary acids on an epidemiological basis, there is compelling evidence from the national surveys of children's and adults' dental health for the UK of high levels of erosive pattern tooth tissue loss (the pattern of loss of mineralised tooth tissue from the surfaces of teeth associated with acid dissolution has specific characteristics that enable the dentist to differentiate between this and other forms of tooth wear). The inability to relate this to dietary patterns in a cross-sectional study of older people simply reflects the complexity of the aetiology of tooth wear. The extent and severity of tissue destruction is of particular concern in the young, as the loss of significant quantities of enamel is irreversible and is likely to pose a significant risk to future oral health status (Table 3.3).

3.2.4 Antioxidants and periodontal disease

Periodontal disease is the single most common chronic inflammatory disease in man (see Chapter 10, Section 10.6.6 for the suggested link with cardiovascular disease). It results in very limited morbidity until the loss of bony attachment is sufficiently severe to cause mobility of the teeth and ultimately tooth loss. This can occur simply through shedding or as a consequence of a dentist extracting teeth.

The disease is susceptible to all of the normal influences on chronic inflammatory pathways, which will include the effects of nutritional antioxidants in moderating inflammatory change. There have been some attempts to moderate the severity of this disease with both locally and systemically delivered antioxidant supplements, however these have shown little benefit in any age group of the population.

3.2.5 Nutrients and oral mucosal health

The evidence for alterations in the oral mucosae with age is equivocal. There is some evidence for mucosal atrophy with reductions in the attachment

Table 3.3: Proportion of children aged 12 and 15 with tooth surface loss on the surfaces of permanent incisors and first permanent molars

		Age			
		12 years		15 years	
		1993	2003	1993	2003
		Percentage of children			
Incisors	Buccal				
	Any	9	12	12	14
	Into pulp/dentine	*	*	*	*
	Lingual				
	Any	27	30	27	33
	Into pulp/dentine	1	3	3	5
Molars					
	Any		19		22
	Into pulp/dentine		2		4

*Denotes proportions <1%.
The buccal surface of a tooth is the surface closest to the lips or cheek; the lingual surface of a tooth is the surface closest to the tongue.
Source: United Kingdom (1993, 2003); Chadwick and Pendry (2004).
Reproduced under the terms of the Click-Use Licence.

apparatus between the mucosa and the dermis (the rete pegs) from specific areas of the mouth (*e.g.* the lateral border of the tongue). The impact of these changes on the susceptibility of the mucosa to nutritional deficiencies is unclear. The oral mucosal lining has a very rapid rate of turnover like many other mucosal surfaces within the gastrointestinal tract. Consequently, reductions in micronutrients that are critical for mucosal turnover and integrity will manifest themselves with oral mucosal lesions at a relatively early stage.

3.2.5.1 Iron, vitamin B₁₂ and folate

These micronutrients are critical for maintenance of oral mucosal integrity; deficiency states will result in mucosal change affecting both the tongue and the oral mucosal lining. The tongue tends to lose the irregularity on its surface, producing a smooth surface that is often also bright red in appearance rather than the pink of keratinised oral mucosa. Oral ulceration is more common, particularly minor oral ulcers, as are red lesions (erythroplasias) of the oral mucosae. The latter are regarded as pre-malignant lesions. Iron deficiency is also associated with burning mouth syndrome in older people (a condi-

tion where sufferers complain of a painful burning mouth particularly when eating some foods), angular cheilitis (sores at the corners of the mouth which may also be infected with either candida or staphylococci), and a mucosal stomatitis associated with the area beneath the plate of an upper denture, again candida are commonly involved.

3.2.6 Alcohol

Oral health is reduced in subjects with relatively high alcohol intake. The oral health changes include:

- Erosive pattern tooth wear in people who are professional wine tasters due to the acidity of many wines, and also in alcoholics due to a combination of pH of the drink itself plus chronic regurgitation of stomach contents into the oral environment as a consequence of alcohol-induced gastric mucosal irritation.
- Increased levels of dental caries through the sugars and acid contents of drinks, as well as through generalised neglect in individuals who become addicted to alcohol. This is a particular problem currently in young people who drink alcopops, which contain high levels of sugar as well as acids as flavouring agents.

- Increased risk of oral cancer, with some variation in risk associated with both the patterns of alcohol consumption and the type of alcohol consumed. It is thought that the concentration of some cancer-preventing compounds like polyphenols in some forms of alcoholic beverage may moderate the interaction between the intake of alcoholic drinks and cancer risk (Petti and Scully 2005).

3.2.7 Oral cancer

There are some nutritional links to oral cancer, through the pre-malignant lesions associated with iron deficiency as well as high levels of alcohol intake, and specific problems associated with tobacco (either when smoked or in smokeless forms), betel quid and areca nut. The estimated relative risk of developing oral cancer in individuals who chew areca nut alone is 58.4 (95% CI: 7.6–447.6) (Lu *et al.* 1996). Chewing betel quid is endemic in the Indian subcontinent and increasing among Indian ex-patriots in the UK. This combination of tobacco leaf and slaked lime is particularly harmful, resulting initially in sub-mucous fibrosis and subsequently in overt squamous carcinoma (Zain *et al.* 1999; Warnakulasuriya 2004).

3.2.8 Smoking

Smoking tobacco products has a number of adverse effects on oral health.

3.2.8.1 Dental caries

Smokers have a higher incidence of carious lesions than non-smokers, on both the crowns and roots of teeth. The mechanism for this interaction is unclear; if anything smokers show greater levels of salivary output than non-smokers. However, it has been reported that smokers are more likely to consume sugars-containing drinks and snacks than non-smokers and generally their oral hygiene is poorer. These effects influence both coronal and root surfaces of teeth (Axelsson *et al.* 1998; Fure 2004).

3.2.8.2 Periodontal disease

There are strong links between smoking and periodontal disease. These have been reviewed recently by Palmer and co-workers (2005). Fundamentally,

smoking not only influences the development and flora of bacterial plaque on the surfaces of teeth, it also exerts direct effects on the gingival and periodontal tissues by modifying the rate of blood flow through these tissues. It also affects both the humoral and cell-mediated immune responses, which are key to defence against periodontal disease. There are also thought to be some local effects on the fibroblasts of the gingival tissues. These effects also occur with smokeless tobacco use (Fisher *et al.* 2005) and cessation of smoking is associated with better outcomes to care in dental patients (Preshaw *et al.* 2005).

3.3 Impact of the oral environment on nutrition

3.3.1 Chewing efficiency, digestion and foods choice

Food is ingested through the mouth, and chewing, along with salivary enzymes, is an important component of the initiation of digestion of foods. Chewing also serves to comminute foods so that a bolus can be formed and swallowed. This process of breaking up food and converting it into a bolus to be swallowed is associated with the release of tasteants from the food enhancing our enjoyment of the things we eat.

Hence, it would be reasonable to assume that the health status of the mouth might influence diet and nutrition. The numbers and distribution of teeth are going to influence the ease of chewing, as is the presence of complete dentures. Chewing with conventionally retained dentures can be likened to an oral juggling act, where the prostheses are controlled by the actions of the oral musculature and the forces of adhesion and cohesion holding them in place against the edentulous mucosa. Food acts as a profound destabilising influence in this process as forces are applied eccentrically to the dentures, unless the bolus can be manipulated such that chewing occurs simultaneously on the right and left sides.

3.3.1.1 Masticatory efficiency

The ability to break down foods into controlled lumps by chewing to permit swallowing is usually assessed by measuring the size of test food samples that have been chewed for a specific number of chewing cycles by study participants. The test food is expectorated and the residue analysed using a sieving method or, more recently, using image analysis techniques.

This test methodology has consistently demonstrated reduced efficiency in chewing with reducing numbers of teeth, with teeth and removable partial dentures compared with a similar number of natural teeth, and with complete dentures compared with a natural dentition (Feldman *et al.* 1980; Gunne 1985; Akeel *et al.* 1992; van der Bilt *et al.* 1993; Mowlana *et al.* 1994). Ageing alone has little effect on chewing efficiency, although there is some suggestion in the literature of reduced oral motor function in older people, probably relating to altered muscle bulk (Baum and Bodner 1983; Newton *et al.* 1993).

Masticatory efficiency and digestion: In the 1950s Farrell showed that the ability to chew does not influence our ability to digest food with a modern diet. Muslin bags containing samples of unchewed, partially chewed and fully chewed foods were swallowed by young, healthy volunteers. The bags were retrieved after passage through the bowel and analysed for the extent of digestion of the foods within the bag. He showed that the quality of digestion was independent of the extent by which the food had been chewed but was dependent on the food type (Farrell 1956; 1957).

This work was informative, but its relevance in an older population is unclear. There are profound changes in the bowel with ageing, including reductions in the rate of gastric motility and atrophy of the villi on the walls of the bowel (see Chapter 12). These changes influence the ability of an older person to digest and absorb foods, but Farrell's work has not been repeated in an older population. There has been very little further work in this area, but a more recent paper demonstrates altered availability of sugars from food if foods are swallowed whole rather than having been chewed (Read *et al.* 1986), while Pera and co-workers (2002) have shown that gastric emptying times are reduced for foods that are masticated more thoroughly compared with those that are chewed less well.

Masticatory efficiency and food choice: Whilst it may be the case that digestion *per se* is not influenced by mastication, there is compelling evidence that food choice is affected by our ability to chew.

As masticatory efficiency reduces, people report increasing difficulty chewing foods and individuals thus affected choose not to eat foods that are difficult to chew. This is of particular importance for those foods that could be regarded as more difficult to chew, for example raw carrot, nuts, fibrous vegetables and some fruits. In addition, green leafy vegetables are a particular problem for individuals who use dentures. The leaf can become stuck to the surface of the denture making the individual uncomfortable. The leaf can often not be removed without taking the denture out of the mouth; something that is socially unacceptable. People become handicapped by their dentition and as a consequence suffer impaired intakes of fruit and vegetables and some key nutrients (Moynihan *et al.* 2000). One area of particular concern is the level of non-starch polysaccharides (dietary fibre) intake that is markedly reduced in older people compared with dietary reference values (Yurkstas and Emerson 1964; Feldman *et al.* 1980; Chauncey *et al.* 1984; Moynihan *et al.* 1994; Joshipura *et al.* 1996; Krall *et al.* 1998).

In addition to these areas of reduction in nutrient intake, there are also reports of increases in intakes of saturated fatty acids, cholesterol and energy in older people with reducing numbers of teeth (Krall *et al.* 1998).

Recent data from the UK and the US have confirmed these associations between edentulism and food selection (Krall *et al.* 1998; Sheiham *et al.* 2001a; Nowjack-Raymer and Sheiham 2003) (Table 3.4). Further and more detailed analysis of the dental, nutritional and biochemical data from three large studies (the longitudinal Veterans Administration Aging Study in Boston and the cross-sectional National Diet and Nutrition Survey for adults aged over 65 years in the UK and NHANES III survey in the US) have clarified these relationships, demonstrating clear associations between oral health status, nutrient intake and biochemical markers of nutritional status. Summaries of these data are given in Table 3.5 for nutrient intake and biochemical markers of nutritional status. These outcomes are independent of the effects of age, gender, regional variation within a country and socio-economic group (Sheiham *et al.* 2001a; Nowjack-Raymer and Sheiham 2003).

The impact of the effect of masticatory efficiency on food selection is liable to be compounded by

Table 3.4: Comparative data from the UK National Diet and Nutrition Survey and the US Veterans Administration Longitudinal Study of Aging for dietary intake, divided into individuals with an intact dentition (with 21 or more teeth), a compromised dentition (fewer than 20 teeth) or edentulous (no natural teeth)

Nutrient and UK dietary reference value for comparison	Intact		Compromised		Edentulous	
	UK	US	UK	US	UK	US
Protein, g/day (63 g/day)	72.3	80	66.6	74	60.1	68
NSP, g/day (25 g/day)	16.2	21	12.9	19	11.0	16
Calcium, mg/day (800 mg/day)	883	773	812	677	722	689
Niacin, mg/day (15 mg/day)	33.8	32	31.0	28	27.0	34
Vitamin C, mg/day (60 mg/day)	82	156	73	146	60	127

NSP: non-starch polysaccharide.
Source: Krall *et al.* (1998); Sheiham *et al.* (2001b). Reproduced by permission of the International and American Associations for Dental Research.

Table 3.5: Relationships between oral health status and biochemical markers of micronutrient status

		NDNS (UK)		NHANES III (US)	
		Dentate Adjusted Mean	Edentate Adjusted Mean	Dentate Adjusted Mean (SE)	Edentate Adjusted Mean (SE)
Ascorbate	μmol/L	49.1	39.4		
Retinol	μmol/L	2.30	2.09		
α tocopherol	μmol/L	38.6	37.0		
Vitamin C	mg/dL			0.95 (0.06)	0.87 (0.09)
Folate	ng/dL			6.1 (0.6)	4.7 (0.9)
β-carotene	μg/dL			16.6 (2.4)	9.8 (3.6)

Figures in parentheses are the standard error of the adjusted mean of the values.
Original data amalgamated from referenced sources.
Source: Sheiham *et al.* (2001b); Nowjack-Raymer and Sheiham (2003). Reproduced by permission of the International and American Associations for Dental Research.

food preparation. There would be an increased likelihood of fresh foods being over-prepared (*e.g.* removal of the skin from fruits and vegetables) or over-cooked by a person with reduced chewing efficiency in an effort to make their consumption practical. A broad range of nutrients are affected by these phenomena, including foodstuffs that are thought to be important for cancer prevention (*e.g.* non-starch polysaccharides or dietary fibre) and for cellular defence and potentially combating the effects of ageing (*e.g.* the antioxidant micronutrients vitamins C and E). Hung and co-workers (2003) examined the effect of tooth loss on dietary patterns during eight years of follow-up in the US health professional ageing study. They showed that over that period there was a general trend for dietary quality to improve for all subjects. However, the magnitude of the improvement was lower in people who had had five or more teeth extracted during that period. Those who had had more teeth extracted were more likely to have stopped eating apples, pears and raw carrots and showed smaller reductions in intake of cholesterol, greater reductions in consumption of polyunsaturated fat, and smaller increases in consumption of dietary fibre and whole fruit than those who had no teeth extracted during the same period.

Oral health interventions alone to increase the functionality of the mouth, either by making dentures or fixed prostheses for patients, have little impact on dietary patterns. However, when an oral health intervention is paired with tailored dietary advice aimed at the 'stage of awareness of need to change' of the individual concerned, significant improvements in fruit and vegetable consumption can be achieved (Bradbury *et al.* 2006).

3.3.2 Salivary changes with age and disease

Historically, salivary flow was thought to reduce with increasing age. Contemporary studies are less clear in their outcomes. Some have shown no changes with increasing age, whereas others have tended to show changes, particularly among women (Yeh *et al.* 1998; Ghezzi, Wagner-Lange *et al.* 2000). The age-associated change in women is also related to menopausal status, however these are closely correlated, so identification of a casual relationship is difficult. It is of note that the most profound changes in

unstimulated salivary output were seen around the time of the menopause in the study by Yeh *et al.* (Figure 3.8). However, the magnitude of the change is relatively small and may not be of clinical significance, particularly relative to the changes seen with medication use in the same age groups (Ghezzi, Lange and Ship *et al.* 2000). Alterations are seen in salivary composition, with some variation in the mineral balance of saliva along with alterations in the mucins (Table 3.6) (Dodds *et al.* 2005). The clinical significance of these changes is unclear, however the alterations in ionic content may be related to variations in taste perception seen in older subjects and the reduction in histatin output may result in altered susceptibility to candidal infection. (Histatins are part of the *non-specific* immune defence mechanisms contained within saliva and are thought to have a particular role in protecting the mucosa from fungal infection.)

There are significant alterations in minor salivary gland output with age (the minor glands lie immediately beneath the oral mucosa and empty directly onto the mucosal surface). These glands have a highly mucous secretion, as well as being responsible for much of the secretory immunologloglobulin A (IgA) and immunoglobulin G (IgG) in the oral environment. Again, the clinical significance of these changes is unclear, however there will be reduced mucosal immunity as a consequence of this change.

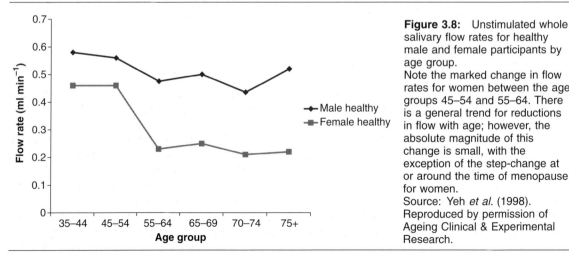

Figure 3.8: Unstimulated whole salivary flow rates for healthy male and female participants by age group.
Note the marked change in flow rates for women between the age groups 45–54 and 55–64. There is a general trend for reductions in flow with age; however, the absolute magnitude of this change is small, with the exception of the step-change at or around the time of menopause for women.
Source: Yeh *et al.* (1998). Reproduced by permission of Ageing Clinical & Experimental Research.

Table 3.6: Age-related changes in salivary composition and output

	Stimulated parotid saliva	Unstimulated sub-mandibular saliva	Stimulated sub-mandibular saliva
Concentration			
Protein (mg/ml)	⇑	⇑	⇓
Na (mEq/L)	⇓	⇓	⇓
K (mEq/L)	⇑	⇑	⇑
Cl (mEq/L)	⇓	⇑	⇓
Ca (mEq/L)	⇑	⇑	⇑
Lactoferrin	⇑		⇑
Lysozyme	=		⇓
SIgA	⇑		=
Albumin	⇑		=
Cystatin	nd		=
MG1	nd		⇓
MG2	nd		⇓
HRP1	=		⇓
HRP3	⇓		⇓
HRP5	⇓		⇓
Output			
Protein (mg/ml)	=	⇓	⇓
Na (mEq/L)	⇓	⇓	⇓
K (mEq/L)	=	=	⇓
Cl (mEq/L)	⇓	⇓	⇓
Ca (mEq/L)	=	⇓	⇓

MG1 and MG2 are two distinct groups of salivary mucins with molecular weights of 103 and 130–50 kDa, respectively.
HRP1, 3 and 5 are salivary histatins (histidine rich proteins) which have potent anti-candidal effects.
Cystatin and salivary mucins are not present in parotid saliva.
Source: Dodds *et al.* (2005). Reproduced by permission of Elsevier.

3.3.2.1 *Pathological change in gland function*

The most common cause of dry mouth (xerostomia) in older people is as a side-effect of drugs used to manage other medical problems. The secretory control of saliva is complex, but involves α and β adrenergic receptors, muscarinic cholinergic receptors, as well as intracellular calcium channel signalling (Figure 3.9). It is also influenced by the hydration state of the individual concerned. Any drugs which impact on these receptors have the potential to reduce salivary output. These drugs are commonly given in combination and their effects are synergistic in relation to salivary output (Sreebny and Schwartz 1997).

Other causes of xerostomia are Sjögren's syndrome and either surgical removal of gland tissue or destruction of the gland as a secondary effect of radiotherapy used in managing head and neck malignancy.

Dry mouth is a significant cause of morbidity for sufferers and results in difficulties in speech, chewing and swallowing, and derangement of taste. All of these effects can result in altered patterns of foods consumption and food choice.

3.4 Taste and smell

Alterations in chemosensory perception are relatively common with ageing. Adjusted national estimates from the US National Health Information Survey of 1984 showed 1.4% of the population with disorders of smell and 0.6% with disorders of taste (Finkelstein and Schiffman 1999). The prevalence of these conditions increased exponentially with age, with 40% of individuals with chemosensory problems being aged 65 or older. Using multivariate analysis, general health status, other sensory impairment, functional problems and a variety of other

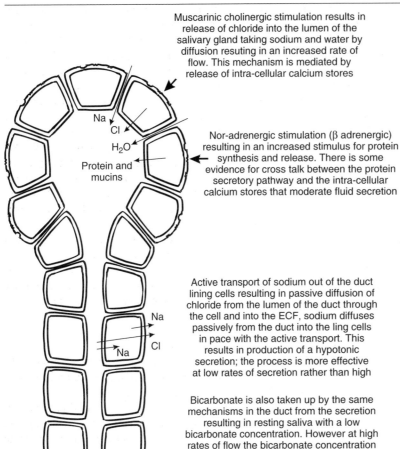

Muscarinic cholinergic stimulation results in release of chloride into the lumen of the salivary gland taking sodium and water by diffusion resuting in an increased rate of flow. This mechanism is mediated by release of intra-cellular calcium stores

Na
Cl
H_2O
Protein and mucins

Nor-adrenergic stimulation (β adrenergic) resulting in an increased stimulus for protein synthesis and release. There is some evidence for cross talk between the protein secretory pathway and the intra-cellular calcium stores that moderate fluid secretion

Active transport of sodium out of the duct lining cells resulting in passive diffusion of chloride from the lumen of the duct through the cell and into the ECF, sodium diffuses passively from the duct into the ling cells in pace with the active transport. This results in production of a hypotonic secretion; the process is more effective at low rates of secretion rather than high

Na
Cl
Na

Bicarbonate is also taken up by the same mechanisms in the duct from the secretion resulting in resting saliva with a low bicarbonate concentration. However at high rates of flow the bicarbonate concentration increases to levels above those of plasma (about 60mM). The mechanism for this is unclear but may be linked to the active transport of chloride which drives the production of the fluid in saliva

Figure 3.9: A schematic diagram illustrating the major influences on saliva formation within the salivary gland. ECF: extracellular fluid. Source: Dodds *et al.* (1991). Permission granted by the International and American Associations for Dental Research.

health-related characteristics were also associated with chemosensory difficulties.

3.4.1 Alterations in taste perception with age

The sensations of taste are derived from sensory taste buds located on the dorsum of the tongue, the soft palate, the pharynx, larynx, epiglottis and the upper third of the oesophagus. There is little evidence of loss of taste cells in normal, healthy adults with increasing age.

Tasteants must be dissolved in saliva to pass over the taste buds to allow the specific taste to be per-

ceived. The background *taste* of saliva is ignored as a product of habituation, however this background will change with age as a result of the alterations in ionic composition of the fluid and the mucin balance. This change may go some way to explaining the variations in taste perception with increasing age.

The variations in taste perception are variable in their manifestation between individuals and comprise both reductions in the ability to detect a taste-ant compared with water (taste discrimination) and in recognition of different tastes. In addition, older people are less able to discriminate between taste qualities in a food compared with the young. There are five principal tastes: bitter, salty, sour, sweet and unami (unami is the fifth taste modality often described as the taste of savoury). Four of these are affected by ageing in healthy, unmedicated adults: bitter, salt, sour and to a lesser extent sweet. There is some controversy in the literature relating to the methods used to measure taste thresholds and the impact of the method on the result. There is some evidence that the age-associated changes seen with tasteants dissolved in water are modified when the same tastes are present in food products, and also when the taste test is undertaken with or without a nose clip (Mojet *et al.* 2003, 2004; Ng *et al.* 2004).

These effects are amplified in people who take multiple medications and in those who are chronically ill (with a considerable overlap between the two groups). This amplification effect may well be the consequence of salivary changes seen in such individuals as a consequence of their medication use. The effect of polypharmacy extends to all the principal tastes, with increase in detection thresholds of 11.6-fold for sodium salts, 7-fold for bitter, 5-fold for unami, 4.3-fold for acids and 2.7-fold for sweeteners.

Taste will also be changed in people who wear complete or partial dentures that cover the palatal vault and in people who are suffering from xerostomia.

There is limited evidence of alterations in appetite and nutrient intake in individuals with reduced taste perception or loss of taste (dysgeusia) (Ritchie 2002). Mattes-Kulig and Henkin (1985) showed lower intakes of vitamins A and C and calcium in people with dysgeusia compared with controls.

A number of studies have looked at the effects of flavour enhancement on food consumption in residential homes and hospitals. Beneficial effects have been noted, either in the form of arresting decline in food consumption (the experimental group maintained their dietary intake compared with decline in the controls) or overt increases in energy intake and even increases in body weight (Schiffman and Warwick 1993; Schiffman and Graham 2000).

3.4.2 Alterations in olfactory perception with age

Reductions in olfaction with age are generally more profound and more consistent than changes in taste.

Olfactory change is relatively common, with nearly two-thirds of all adults over the age of 80 showing some level of disturbed sense of smell, with increased rates among men, current smokers and those with stroke or epilepsy. Self-reports of changes in olfaction are unreliable and become increasingly unreliable with increasing age. Olfactory thresholds are elevated for all odours by between two- and 15-fold when younger populations are compared with the old. Central nervous system pathology will also impact on olfactory perception including facial trauma and both Alzheimer's and Parkinson's disease. Indeed, reduced olfactory ability has been suggested as a marker for cognitive decline (Hawkes 2006).

Reductions in olfactory ability can result in altered food choice and reduced energy intake; it has also been suggested that individuals may also be at increased risk of food poisoning as they would not be able to detect rotten foods by their smell.

3.5 Texture

Food's texture plays an important part in an individual's ability to process the food in their mouth. There are changes with increasing age, associated with changes in oral status and with diminution in muscle bulk reducing chewing strength (Kohyama *et al.* 2003). Older subjects attempt to compensate for these alterations in masticatory function by increasing the number of chewing strokes they use to process a bolus of food. However, these attempts at compensation appear incomplete and there is evidence that older subjects swallow a bolus with lower levels of comminution of the food than younger cohorts (Mioche *et al.* 2004; Yven *et al.* 2006). Another coping strategy is for individuals with limited masticatory function to avoid foods whose texture makes them difficult to chew and swallow. Foods that are avoided are those that require high forces or prolonged chewing to reduce them to a state suitable for swallowing, as well as those that adhere to dentures and/or teeth (Sheiham *et al.* 2001b; Kalviainen *et al.* 2002). Roininen and co-workers (2004) conclude that both older and young respondents found fruit and vegetables easy to eat if they were ready-to-eat, but those that were hard, fibrous, adhere to the teeth and require preparation were perceived as troublesome for all. Finally, there is some evidence that, with reducing numbers of teeth, individuals alter the way that they prepare foods, presumably to cope with difficulty in chewing (Hung *et al.* 2003). Such alterations in food preparation (*e.g.* changing from eating raw carrot to consuming processed cooked carrot) may influence the stability and bioavailability of nutrients from such foods.

One final variable that also influences perceived texture in the oral environment is salivary function. Individuals with poor salivary flow have more difficulty chewing and swallowing foods in general, as the lubricating and binding actions of the saliva are reduced (Ono *et al.* 2003). This will have its greatest effect with foods that are perceived more difficult to chew.

3.6 Key points

- The oral health status of older people is changing dramatically and rapidly with fewer older people being edentulous and a much larger proportion having some natural teeth.
- With natural teeth come the diseases associated with the dentate, notably tooth decay and periodontal (gum) disease.
- With increasing age the roots of teeth become exposed into the mouth. The root is made from dentine which is softer and more susceptible to decay than the enamel of the crown of the tooth.
- Fluoride has a key role in helping to prevent disease, particularly in topical applications in older people. Community fluoridation schemes have a significant benefit for older dentate people because of the topical effect of an all-pervasive fluoride.
- Personal oral hygiene is a challenge for many older people as their dexterity and sight fail and the architecture of the mouth becomes more complex.
- There are minor changes in salivary flow with age, particularly in post-menopausal women. These are probably of limited clinical significance. However, reductions in salivary flow associated with disease of the glands or polypharmacy are a significant source of xerostomia in older people, leading to tooth decay, tooth wear and difficulty in chewing and swallowing foods.
- Frequency of intake of simple carbohydrates is linked to tooth decay; this includes even small quantities of sugar used to sweeten drinks. This can be a problem when people are taking drugs with prolonged oral clearance, high-energy syrup food supplements and other forms of between-meal snacks.
- Chewing gum has a useful role in stimulating salivary flow and moderating the acidogenic response of dental plaque to sugars.
- Some micronutrients are important for oral mucosal health, notably the B group vitamins and iron.
- Iron deficiency, alcohol and tobacco in various forms are all associated with oral cancer. Chewing tobaccos and quid particularly increases risk.
- The number and distribution of teeth influence food choice, with people who have few teeth tending to eat an 'unhealthy' diet low in fruit and vegetables and potentially higher in fat.
- Dental intervention alone has little impact on changing diet. However when teamed with tailored dietary advice a significant effect can be seen.
- Both the ability to taste and to smell deteriorate with age; this may also influence dietary selection. There is limited evidence of the benefits of taste enhancers (monosodium glutamate) in improving dietary intake in older people.
- Reductions in chewing efficiency, possibly linked with alterations in the availability of salivary mucin, result in older people with limited dentitions chewing food less efficiently, giving coarser particles in the food bolus prior to swallowing. Texture preferences change among older people, towards smooth, moist and slippery textures, rather than hard, crunchy or fibrous foods.

3.7 Recommendations for future research

- Further research is needed to determine the optimum combination of preventive strategies for dental caries, particularly in people with dry mouth; and the most effective methods for personal oral hygiene for older people with altered dental architecture.

- It remains to be clarified whether the alterations in nutrient uptake from foods in dentate compared with edentulous subjects are associated with their altered ability to chew foods.

- Studies should investigate the ability of dietary intervention/supplementation to influence the severity or progression of periodontal disease.

- Studies are also required to determine whether tailored dietary interventions delivered in a dental primary care setting can achieve meaningful and sustained changes in dietary patterns for patients whose masticatory function is compromised through lack of teeth.

- Other research questions that need to be addressed include whether edentulous people suffer greater levels of chronic disease and die earlier because of their altered dietary pattern; if taste enhancement can improve the perceived quality of foods for older people and, if it does, whether enhancers can be used in association with dietary intervention to bring about improvements in dietary quality and improvements in quality of life.

- It remains to be clarified whether reported changes in preferences for food texture are associated more with altered oral function than ageing.

3.8 Key references

Bradbury J, Thomason JM, *et al.* (2006) Nutrition counseling increases fruit and vegetable intake in the edentulous. *Journal of Dental Research*, **85**, 463–8.

Ghezzi EM and Ship JA (2003) Aging and secretory reserve capacity of major salivary glands. *Journal of Dental Research*, **82**, 844–8.

Locker D (2003) Dental status, xerostomia and the oral health-related quality of life of an elderly institutionalized population. *Special Care in Dentistry*, **23**, 86–93.

Ritchie CS (2002) Oral health, taste, and olfaction. *Clinics in Geriatric Medicine*, **18**, 709–17.

Walls AW and Steele JG (2004) The relationship between oral health and nutrition in older people. *Mechanisms of Ageing and Development*, **125**, 853–7.

4
Healthy Ageing: Bone Health

4.1 Introductory remarks

4.1.1 Defining bone health

Bones break because the loads placed on them exceed the ability of the bone to absorb the energy involved. This may be the result of a number of factors, including a reduction in bone mass, a change in the distribution of bone, loss of cancellous or cortical micro-architecture, an accumulation of damaged bone or a change in the material properties of the remaining bone (Parfitt 1990). Throughout life, the skeleton requires optimum development and maintenance of its integrity since the resultant effect of poor bone health is osteoporotic fracture. Osteoporosis is currently defined as a metabolic bone disease which has two predominant characteristics: low bone mass and micro-architectural deterioration of bone tissue. Both factors lead to enhanced bone fragility and a consequent increase in fracture risk (Consensus Development Conference 1991). Bone 'weakness' refers to both poor structural quality and decreased bone mass. An illustration of 'normal' and 'osteoporotic' bone can be seen in Figure 4.1.

4.1.2 Implications of osteoporosis from a public health perspective

Current figures estimate that one in three women and one in 12 men over the age of 55 will suffer from osteoporosis in their lifetime. Approximately 200,000 osteoporotic fractures occurred in the UK alone in 2000 (National Osteoporosis Society), with costs to the NHS in excess of £1.7 billion per annum

(Torgerson *et al.* 2001). This cost is a significant contributor to the financial implications of osteoporosis in Europe (€13.9 billion) and is substantially lower than that for the US ($17.9 billion) (O'Neill 2007). Hip fractures are believed to account for over a third of the total figure and are a reflection of the inpatient (hospital) and outpatient (nursing home) care required for patients with osteoporosis. In the context of other conditions, osteoporosis is grossly under-funded when compared to other diseases such as cardiovascular disease and cancer (Royal College of Physicians 2000). Osteoporotic fractures are continually associated with both increased mortality and morbidity, giving rise to a huge burden to the health care system, notwithstanding the tremendous pain and discomfort to the people with osteoporosis. The lifetime risk of a fragility fracture in the UK is considered to be 53.2% in women and 20.7% in men at the age of 50 years (Dennison and Cooper 2007).

Given the projected rise of osteoporotic fracture worldwide to 6.26 million in the year 2050 (compared with 1.66 million in 1990) (World Health Organization 1994), there can be no doubt that the future economic impact of osteoporosis will be phenomenal.

4.1.3 Change in bone mass with ageing

As we age, the risk of hip fracture increases approximately ten-fold every 20 years. While areal bone mineral density (aBMD; measured as mineral content/area) declines with age, age still has an independent and strong effect on fracture risk after adjusting for aBMD (World Health Organization

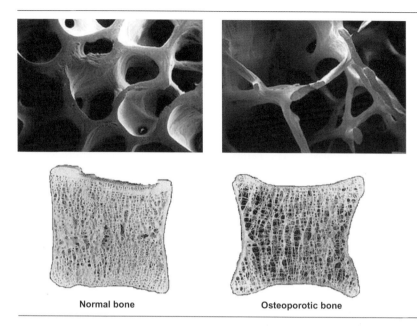

Figure 4.1: Normal and osteoporotic bone under the microscope.

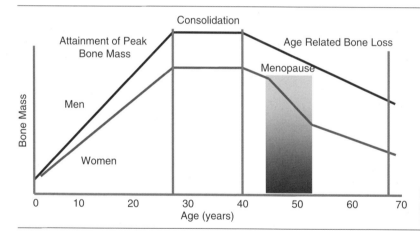

Figure 4.2: Changes in skeletal mass throughout the lifecycle.

1994). Thus, even though an 80-year-old may have the same aBMD as someone 20 years younger, they have an increased risk of fracture, which is probably related to an increased risk of falling as well as changes in bone architecture. With age, the width of long bones (including the femoral neck) is constantly increasing, presumably because the outer surface of the bone is subjected to the highest strains, which in turn promotes bone formation. In biomechanical terms increasing the width of a bone means that the resistance to bending (measured by engineers as

section modulus, Z) can be maintained with less bone. Recent studies have indicated that the decline in aBMD with age is the result of the distribution of bone over a greater area as well as a loss of bone (Lenchik *et al.* 2004).

An example of the changes that occur in bone mass (aBMD) in men and women with ageing can be seen in Figure 4.2. Considerable alterations occur within the skeleton throughout an individual's life and it is now well established that there are two principal mechanisms determining adult bone health: the maximum attainment of peak bone mass (PBM), which is achieved during growth and early adulthood; and the rate of bone loss with advancing age, with the menopausal years being a time of considerable concern for women.

Throughout early childhood, bone mass increases linearly with skeletal growth. This is clearly a critical time point for bone health. There is a rapid increase in bone density during the pubertal years (by as much as 40–70%), although it is known to vary according to skeletal site (Bonjour *et al.* 1991). The pubertal stage is an all-important time for skeletal development and careful consideration should be given to the design of studies examining the influences of the modifiable factors (such as nutrition/exercise interventions) on bone health during this period (Bass *et al.* 2007). The optimum time (*i.e.* pre-, peri- or post-pubertally) for intervention with such exogenous factors remains unquantified.

Bone density continues to increase for several years after the cessation of growth until maximum bone mass (or PBM) is achieved (Osteoporosis Prevention). The exact age at which PBM is attained remains controversial, but is generally believed to be around the late second to early third decade (*i.e.* late teens/early twenties), although it is known to vary between the sexes and according to skeletal site.

Following attainment of PBM and with the onset of the menopause, rapid bone loss occurs, which is believed to average approximately 2–3% over the next 5–10 years, being greatest in the early postmenopausal years. This is a further 'critical time' for bone health, as indicated in Figure 4.3 (Department of Health 1998a). Bone mass continues to decline with ageing, but at a slower rate than during the

early menopausal time. In some older individuals, there is evidence that under-nutrition is a problem and that these individuals may enter the 'danger zone' with respect to increasing their risk of fracture (Department of Health 1992).

4.1.4 Determinants of bone health: modifiable vs. non-modifiable factors

The pathogenesis of osteoporosis is multifactorial. Both the development of PBM in the younger population and the rate of bone loss in postmenopausal women and older people are determined by a combination of genetic, endocrine (see Chapter 13, Sections 13.2.5 and 13.3.5), mechanical and nutritional factors, with evidence of extensive interactions within and between these groups (Figure 4.3) (Bonjour *et al.* 2003).

Endogenous factors have a very important influence on the skeleton. Research focusing on monozygotic and dizygotic twins, as well as comparisons between mother and daughter pairs, indicate a genetic influence on bone health of around 75% (Eisman 1999). The skeletal determinants of osteoporotic fracture risk, such as aBMD, bone geometry and bone turnover, are all subject to strong genetic influences. It has been estimated from twin studies that 60–85% of the variance in aBMD is genetically determined (Krall and Dawson-Hughes 1993), and heritability estimates for other risk factors such as quantitative ultrasound, femoral neck geometry and bone turnover markers range between 50% and 80% (Arden *et al.* 1996; Garnero *et al.* 1996). Although a family history of fracture is a risk factor (Keen *et al.* 1999), the heritability of fracture itself is relatively low (25–35%) (Deng *et al.* 2000), reflecting both the importance of fall-related factors and the possible effects in the pathogenesis of fracture.

Major advances in our knowledge of the genetic determinants of osteoporosis include the discovery of genes responsible for monogenic bone diseases associated with abnormal bone mass (Little *et al.* 2002); the identification of quantitative trait loci for bone mass in the general population and in mice; and the characterisation of several candidate genes for osteoporosis. To date, over 40 candidate genes have been identified as having an important effect on bone mass (Liu *et al.* 2003; Ralston 2003). These range from genes encoding calciotropic hormones (*e.g.* parathyroid hormone, PTH and calcitonin) (see

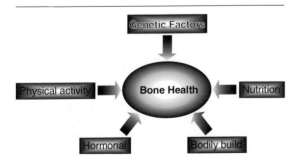

Figure 4.3: Endogenous vs. exogenous factors affecting bone health.

Table 4.1: Nutritional strategies for populations and individuals

Strategic level of prevention	Nutritional recommendations
Universal primary prevention Males and females of all ages	A balanced diet satisfying all nutritional needs for the major food groups, minerals and micronutrients should be provided throughout the life-course
High-risk groups Examples: those with a family history of osteoporosis, some ethnic populations, the oestrogen-deficient, the physically inactive, the housebound, the lactose intolerant, those with low energy intakes or eating disorders, alimentary malabsorption problems, renal failure and patients requiring corticosteroids or anticonvulsants	People identified as having above-average risks of developing thin bones for reasons of genetic inheritance, ethnicity, disease or behaviour should be encouraged to pay special attention to nutrition; they may require specific supplements or foods fortified with particular nutrients
Individuals with osteoporosis Particularly those with any history of minimal trauma fractures, poor balance, musculoskeletal problems or a history of frequent falling	Dietary interventions should be instituted to correct under-nutrition, particular deficiencies and to counter excessive bone loss. Over-consumption of urinary calcium-wasting agents (*e.g.* sodium chloride, caffeine) should be avoided. For those on bone-sparing anabolic therapies extra nutrients may be required to meet the demands of new bone (calcium, vitamin D, protein)

Source: Reproduced from Goulding (2003) by permission of the Royal Society of Chemistry.

Chapter 13, Section 13.2.5), hormone receptors (*e.g.* those for vitamin D and oestrogen), bone matrix proteins (*e.g.* COL1A1 and osteocalcin), local regulatory factors (*e.g.* TGFβ1, IGF-1 and osteoprotegerin) to those that may alter bone cell differentiation (*e.g.* PPAR-γ and LRP5). Although there are concerns regarding the statistical power of a number of published studies, with the resultant reports of both positive and negative findings for a particular gene, it is clear that a few of these genes have consistent effects on bone mass and possibly bone fragility. In the case of the haplotypes for COL1A1 and oestrogen receptor-α, there appears to be dissociation between gene effects on fracture risk and on BMD. What are generally lacking, however, are plausible biological mechanisms whereby some genes might contribute to femoral neck fragility (Ralston 2007).

4.2 Nutritional influences on bone health

4.2.1 General

Sensible and simple nutritional advice, based on sound scientific evidence, is of paramount impor-

tance to encourage the optimisation of bone health throughout the lifecycle (Goulding and Grant 2007). Even a small or modest effect on bone health is likely to have a significant impact on fracture prevention. For example, an increase in bone mineral density by one standard deviation unit is likely to result in a 50% reduction in fracture rates (Melton 1995). As noted by Goulding (2003), the application of dietary advice needs to be given at three levels: 1) universal primary prevention; 2) selective prevention in high-risk groups; and 3) targeted prevention in individuals (Table 4.1; Figure 4.4).

4.2.2 Calcium

4.2.2.1 Peak bone mass attainment

Calcium absorption and bone calcium deposition rates peak in girls shortly before menarche. Thus, low calcium intake during growth and late menarcheal age may affect PBM, and consequently fracture risk later in life (Abrams 2003). There is evidence in the literature to show that adolescent girls are less likely than boys to meet the current recommended dietary levels for calcium and that

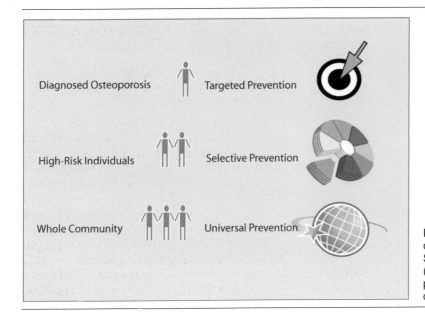

Figure 4.4: Application of dietary advice to the population. Source: Adapted from Goulding (2003). Reproduced by permission of the Royal Society of Chemistry.

calcium intake in girls may begin to decline around the time of puberty (Matkovic *et al.* 1994).

To date, clinical trials investigating the effect of increased calcium intake (either through foods or supplements) on PBM development have been of relatively short duration, and it has been difficult to determine whether the positive effects of calcium supplementation on bone are maintained. This is an area that requires urgent attention.

Matkovic and colleagues (2005) have examined the effect of calcium intake over an extended period. They reported the results of a four-year randomised clinical trial that involved 354 girls at stage 2 of puberty. The study was optionally extended for a further three years. Calcium-supplemented participants received an additional 670 mg/day of calcium over and above a mean intake of 830 mg/day over the seven-year period. Calcium supplementation significantly influenced bone accretion in girls during the pubertal growth spurt. The effect diminished in young adulthood but, in tall girls, the significant effects remained at the metacarpals and at the forearm. Thus, calcium requirements for maximum skeletal development may be associated with bone size.

An eight-year follow-up of calcium supplementation in pre-pubertal girls showed that pre-pubertal calcium intake may have a key effect on menarche timing (Chevalley *et al.* 2005). This double-blind, randomised trial followed girls from a mean age of 7.9 years to a mean age of 16.4 years. The initially enrolled 149 participants were allocated to receive either calcium-enriched foods or a placebo for 48 weeks; approximately 7.5 years later, 125 of these participants were re-examined. Findings at baseline and at 7.5 years after the end of the intervention were compared. There was no significant difference between placebo and calcium groups in terms of standing height or bodyweight. However, there was a significant difference between groups with regard to menarcheal age: girls in the calcium-supplemented group were found to have started menarche approximately five months earlier. In addition, there was a tendency for the BMD gain at all of the sites measured to be greater for the calcium group compared with the placebo group. The aBMD gain between 7.9 and 16.4 years of age was inversely related to menarcheal age at both the axial and appendicular skeletal sites.

Sub-group analysis on the basis of menarcheal age revealed that the mean aBMD gain from baseline remained significantly greater in girls with early menarche (<13 years) who were supplemented with calcium compared with placebo, at all sites measured, except at the lumbar spine, whereas for girls with late menarche (>13 years) no lasting effect of calcium supplementation on BMD was observed (Chevalley *et al.* 2005). The authors hypothesise that calcium supplementation in pre-pubertal girls may accelerate the onset of pubertal maturation and that factors known to determine the timing of pubertal maturation may also affect the duration of response (*i.e.* bone mineral mass accrual) to calcium supplementation. Again, this is an area for further research.

4.2.2.2 Effect of oligosaccharides on calcium absorption

For maximum attainment of PBM, absorbing an adequate amount of calcium is particularly important. There are data to show that intestinal calcium absorption is a critical factor determining the retention of calcium. There is now an increasing body of evidence in the animal model, and more recently in humans, that a daily consumption of short- and long-chain inulin-type fructans can significantly increase calcium absorption in adolescents (van den Heuvel *et al.* 1999; Abrams 2005) and postmenopausal women (van den Heuvel *et al.* 2000), as well as enhance the mineralisation of bone during the stages of pubertal growth (Abrams, 2005).

4.2.2.3 Postmenopausal bone loss

There are good data to suggest that calcium supplements are effective in reducing bone loss in late menopausal women (>5 years post-menopause), particularly in those with low habitual calcium intake (<400 mg/d). The study published by Professor Bess Dawson-Hughes and colleagues (1990) marked the turning point for studies differentiating between early and late postmenopause. In addition, a meta-analysis of 15 trials indicated that calcium supplementation at levels between 500 and 2000 mg/day reduced postmenopausal bone loss (Shea *et al.* 2004). It is important to note that in the US, 1200 mg/day is considered an optimal calcium intake for women 51 years and older, with recommendations being lower in the UK and other European countries (between 700 and 1000 mg/day). The findings of calcium supplementation studies in the early stages of the menopause are conflicting. This is clearly an important area for research given the findings of the Women's Health Initiative study, which has indicated that long-term menopausal hormone therapy should no longer be recommended because of the likely increased risk of cardiovascular disease and breast cancer (Rossouw *et al.* 2002).

4.2.2.4 Calcium and vitamin D in fracture prevention

In younger postmenopausal women who are not vitamin D-deficient, vitamin D supplementation has little effect on BMD (Bischoff-Ferrari *et al.* 2006).

Vitamin D supplementation alone seems to be marginally, if at all, effective in preventing fractures in the elderly if the dosage is not sufficient. In a Norwegian supplementation trial using cod-liver oil containing 10 μg/d of vitamin D (400 IU/d), fractures in 1144 nursing home residents were not prevented (Meyer *et al.* 2002). This dosage would be considered sub-optimal on the basis of the 2005 meta-analysis by Bischoff-Ferrari and colleagues (2005), which shows that the dosage of oral vitamin D supplementation is critical. Their results indicate that a daily dose of 17.5–20 μg/d (700–800 IU) reduces the risk of hip and any non-vertebral fractures in ambulatory or institutionalised older persons, but 10 μg/d (400 IU/day) is not sufficient for fracture prevention.

Supplementation with 2500 μg (100,000 IU) of oral vitamin D_3 given every fourth month for five years has been shown to significantly (−22%) reduce the number of fractures of the hip, wrist, forearm and spine compared with placebo in British men and women aged 65–85 years (Trivedi *et al.* 2003). However, in another study in the UK, three injections of 7500 μg (300,000 IU) of vitamin D_3 per year yielded no reduction in fracture risk in 9000 healthy ambulatory older men and women and, if anything, showed that the vitamin D_3 *increased* the risk of fracture ($P < 0.06$) (Smith *et al.* 2007).

However, vitamin D and calcium supplementation studies have been shown to reduce fracture rates in institutionalised older people (Chapuy *et al.* 1992; Bischoff-Ferrari *et al.* 2005). Results of the study by Professor Meunier's group are shown in Figure 4.5. There are also data to suggest an effect in free-living older populations. A group of older American men and women (mean age 71 years) given daily treatment with 500 mg of calcium and 20 μg (800 IU) of vitamin D_3 had a significantly reduced total number of non-vertebral fractures (Dawson-Hughes *et al.* 1997). However, it is

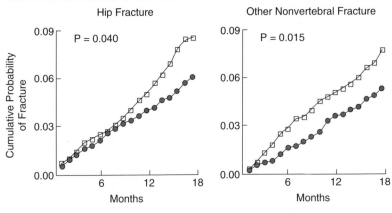

Figure 4.5: Effectiveness of calcium and vitamin D on fracture prevention in elderly women living in nursing homes. Source: Chapuy *et al.* (1992) © Massachusetts Medical Society 2006. All rights reserved.

Cumulative probability of hip fracture and other nonvertebral fracture in the placebo group (□—□) and the group treated with vitamin D₃ and calcium (●—●), estimated by the life-table method and based on the length of time to the first fracture

important to bear in mind that the study was not specifically powered to look at fracture reduction.

In a factorial, cluster-randomised, pragmatic intervention study of 9605 community-dwelling residents living in Denmark, a daily supplement of calcium carbonate (1000 mg) and vitamin D (10 µg or 400 IU) over a period of three years resulted in a 16% reduction in fracture incidence rate (relative risk, RR: 0.84 (95% CI: 0.72–0.98)) in treated subjects compared with those offered no supplement but who participated in an environmental and health programme (Larsen *et al.* 2004).

However, in a pragmatic, open, randomised trial conducted in the UK with 3314 women aged 70 years and older who had risk factors for hip fracture (any previous fracture, low bodyweight, smoker, family history of hip fracture or poor or fair self-reported health), supplementation with calcium (1000 mg/day) and vitamin D₃ (20 µg/d or 800 IU) apparently failed to reduce the risk of fracture in women with at least one risk factor for hip fracture, although the confidence intervals were wide (Port-house *et al.* 2005). The odds ratio (OR) for hip fracture was 0.75 (95% CI: 0.31–1.78) after a median follow-up of 25 months. There was no evidence of an effect on falls at either six months (OR: 0.99 (95% CI: 0.81–1.20)) or one year (odds ratio 0.98 (95% CI: 0.79–1.20)). The authors note that the adherence rate was just over 60% at 12 months (an adherence

level that is to be expected in a general practice setting).

The findings of another trial (Grant *et al.* 2005) conducted in the UK do not support routine oral supplementation with calcium and vitamin D₃, either alone or in combination, for the prevention of fractures in older men and women with previous fracture. In this factorial-design trial of 5292 men and women aged 70 years or older, who were mobile before developing a low-trauma fracture, calcium (1000 mg) or vitamin D (20 µg or 800 IU), either alone or in combination, did not significantly reduce the incidence of new, low-trauma fractures after 24 months. However, a number of concerns have been raised about these results, particularly the low compliance with treatment and the small number of subjects measured for vitamin D status (Sambrook 2005).

The 2005 Cochrane Review (which includes some of the most recent vitamin D trials showing a negative effect) reported a reduced risk for hip fracture (RR: 0.81 (95% CI: 0.68–0.96) for seven trials) and non-vertebral fractures (RR: 0.87 (95% CI: 0.78–0.97) for seven trials). However, the effect may be restricted to those living in institutional care (Avenell *et al.* 2005). There was no significant effect on vertebral fractures.

In conclusion, combined calcium and vitamin D supplementation can impact beneficially on frac-

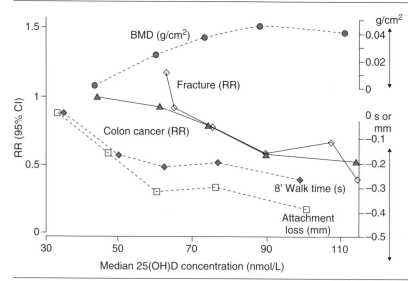

Figure 4.6: Thresholds for 25 OHD status and health outcomes.
BMD: bone mineral density; CI: confidence interval; RR: relative risk.
Source: *American Journal of Clinical Nutrition* (2004, 291: 1999–2006); American Society for Nutrition; Bischoff-Ferrari *et al.* (2006).

tures in older subjects, although the evidence is not consistent. Adequate dose of vitamin D and pre-existing status are likely to be important.

4.2.3 Vitamin D status and health

The vitamin D supplementation studies referred to above have highlighted the need to reconsider the definition of adequate vitamin D status. Currently in the UK, the definition is linked with the rickets/osteomalacia prevention threshold of 25 nmol/L as 25 hydroxyvitamin D (25 OHD), but recent work suggests that a higher threshold (about 75 nmol/L or 30 ng/ml of 25 OHD) may be required for optimum health (Bischoff-Ferrari *et al.* 2006; Holick 2007; Vieth *et al.* 2007) (Figure 4.6).

There is a considerable gap in our knowledge of exactly what dietary intakes and associated plasma levels of vitamin D define sufficiency, insufficiency and deficiency. These gaps are especially evident in ethnic groups, as highlighted in the UK Scientific Advisory Committee on Nutrition (SACN) Vitamin D report (2007c). Findings of the National Diet and Nutrition Surveys (NDNS) (4–18 years; 19–64 years; 65 years and over) indicate that vitamin D deficiency (defined as a plasma 25 OHD level less than 25 nmol/L or 10 ng/ml) is a problem (*e.g.* 24% of men and 28% of women in the 19–24 years age groups have levels below 25 nmol/L) (Ruston *et al.* 2004). Data

from the 1958 British birth cohort (n = 7437) also shows extensive hypo-vitaminosis D in subjects at 45 years of age (25 OHD levels <25, <40 and <75 nmol/L were found in 15.5%, 46.6% and 87.1% of the population respectively) (Hypponen and Power 2007).

Currently in the UK there is no dietary reference value (DRV) for vitamin D for 4–64 years unless sunlight exposure is considerably restricted (Department of Health, 1991). However, in the US adequate intake (AI) recommendation for 0–50 years is set at 200 IU/d (5 μg/d); and 600 IU/d (15 g/d) for 70 years and over (Food and Nutrition Board. Institute of Medicine 1997).

4.2.3.1 Defining vitamin D status

Sources of vitamin D: Vitamin D is the generic term for two molecules, egocalciferol (vitamin D_2) and cholecalciferol (vitamin D_3). The former is derived by UV irradiation of the ergosterol which is widely distributed in plants and other fungi, whereas the latter is formed from the action of UV irradiation on the skin. The action of sunlight on the skin converts 7-dehydrocholesterol to previtamin D, which is then metabolised to vitamin D (3 or cholecalciferol) by a temperature-dependent isomerisation. Vitamin D is then transported via the general circulation to the liver, where the enzyme 25-hydroxylase converts it to 25 OHD. Further conversion to 1,25 hydroxyvitamin D (1,25 (OH)$_2$ D$_3$) occurs in the kidney. 25 OHD is the main circulating vitamin D metabolite and is the best indicator of clinical status, whereas 1,25 hydroxyvitamin D is the active form of the vitamin which is involved in calcium homeostasis (Holick 2004).

Dietary effects on vitamin D status: There are few dietary sources of vitamin D, the major providers being fat spreads (which are fortified with vitamin D), fish, eggs, pastry products, fortified breakfast cereals and meat (Food Standards Agency 2002). Recent changes in EU regulations have resulted in a number of cereal manufacturers removing the vitamin D fortification.

Climate effects on vitamin D status: Much of the UV in sunlight is absorbed by clouds, ozone and other forms of atmospheric pollution. Thus, due to the reduced zenith angle of the sun and increased path length of sunlight through the atmosphere, the effective level of UV energy decreases north–south distance from the seasonally varying latitude at which the sun is directly overhead. In the UK, there is no UV radiation of the appropriate wavelength (280 mm–310 mm) from the end of October to the end of March and for the remaining months of the year the main percentage of the effective UV radiation occurs between 11.00 am and 3.00 pm.

4.2.3.2 Importance of vitamin D to bone

Vitamin D is critical to bone. It is known to stimulate matrix formation and bone maturation, enhance osteoclastic activity and may influence differentiation of bone cell precursors. Together with PTH, it regulates calcium and phosphorus metabolism and promotes calcium absorption from the gut and kidney tubules. It has been shown that fractional calcium absorption increases with serum 25 OHD concentrations within the reference range, up to a level of 80 nmol/L, reaching a plateau above that level (Heaney *et al.* 2003). There are also data to suggest even lower absorption among individuals with serum concentrations of vitamin D below the reference range (Barger-Lux and Heaney 2002). Vitamin D is key to PBM attainment, postmenopausal bone loss and skeletal integrity in our ageing population (Dawson-Hughes *et al.* 2005).

4.2.3.3 Vitamin D and risk of falling

Low vitamin D status has been implicated in an increased risk of falling, and a meta-analysis has shown that vitamin D supplementation reduces the risk of falls among institutionalised and free-living older people (OR: 0.78 (95% CI: 0.64–0.92) for five studies) (Bischoff-Ferrari *et al.* 2004). The results of a randomised trial also suggest that vitamin D supplementation for two years in institutionalised older people can reduce falls, even if they are not initially vitamin D-deficient (Bischoff-Ferrari *et al.* 2005). Mechanisms of action need further elucidation, but a beneficial effect on muscle weakness, which can affect balance and mobility, has been implicated (see Chapter 6, Sections 6.3 and 6.11). Vitamin D (and calcium) supplementation may be helpful in reducing falls by improving body sway and by normalising blood pressure (Pfeifer *et al.* 2001).

4.2.4 Protein intake and bone health

4.2.4.1 General

There has been controversy concerning the relationship between dietary protein (especially protein derived from animal sources) and bone metabolism. Excess dietary protein can result in urinary calcium loss, negative calcium balance and increased bone loss. Cross-sectional and longitudinal epidemiological studies examining the effect of protein intake on BMD, bone loss and risk of fracture have produced mixed results, with some studies showing that high protein intake may be detrimental to bone health and others finding a beneficial effect (including improvement in recovery from hip fracture), whereas others have shown no effect (Massey and Whiting 2003). It is very important to note, however, that protein-energy under-nutrition is a risk factor for bone loss, osteoporosis and fracture, and older people in particular are at risk of protein undernutrition (Rizzoli *et al.* 2003).

4.2.4.2 Animal vs. vegetable protein intake: impact on bone

Ecological studies have shown that worldwide per capita consumption of animal protein has been associated with a higher risk of hip fracture in women aged >50 years (Abelow *et al.* 1992). More recently, the correlation has been shown to be stronger with the ratio of animal protein to vegetable protein in a study that adjusted for important cultural differences (Sellmeyer *et al.* 2001). It is important to note, however, that in these ecological studies, the unit of measurement is country, not individual, and as such these types of studies have a number of limitations that must be considered in the interpretation of such data.

The effect of a high dietary ratio of animal protein to vegetable protein on bone loss and risk of fracture has been investigated in a prospective cohort of 1035 women who participated in the Study of Osteoporotic Fractures. Women with a higher ratio of animal to vegetable protein intake had a higher rate of bone loss at the femoral neck than did those with a low ratio, as well as a greater risk of hip fracture (RR: 3.7). The authors conclude that a reduction in animal protein and an increase in vegetable protein may decrease bone loss and risk of hip fracture, although this has been a topic of some debate.

Other published studies which present data specifically examining animal vs. vegetable protein effects on bone include the IOWA Women's Health Study and the Framingham Study. Munger *et al.* (1999) report that higher intakes of animal sources of protein were associated with a 70% reduction in hip fracture, which is in stark contrast to the findings of the Study of Osteoporotic Fractures (Sellmeyer *et al.* 2001) and highlights the degree of inconsistency with results. Hannan *et al.* (2000b) found that the lowest quartile of animal protein consumption was significantly related to hip and spine bone loss in men and women aged 67–93 years. Both population groups had adequate calcium intakes.

4.2.5 Vitamin K

4.2.5.1 General

Vitamin K refers to a family of compounds with a common chemical structure, 2-methyl-1,4 naphthoquinone. Phylloquinone (known as vitamin K_1) is present in foods of plant origin. Bacterial forms of vitamin K, referred to as the menaquinones or vitamin K_2, differ in structure from vitamin K_1. Different forms of vitamin K have a tissue-specific distribution. Vitamin K mediates the γ-carboxylation of glutamyl residues on a number of key bone proteins, especially osteocalcin, to produce γ-carboxy-

glutamyl (Gla) residues (Shearer *et al.* 1996). Vitamin K has an important function for the skeleton; it acts as a co-factor in the post-translational carboxylation of several bone proteins, with osteocalcin being the most abundant. Deficiency of vitamin K results in the synthesis of under-carboxylated osteocalcin (ucOC). There are data to show that low serum concentrations of either vitamin K_1 or ucOC are associated with low bone mineral density and increased risk for osteoporotic fractures (Booth *et al.* 2003).

4.2.5.2 Vitamin K supplementation and bone quality in younger and older women

In an important study by Braam *et al.* (2003), the effect of vitamin K_1 on bone mineral density was examined in 181 healthy postmenopausal women aged 50–60 years, with 155 completing the 36-month treatment period. The study was designed using a double-blind, placebo-controlled intervention protocol to examine the potential complementary effect on postmenopausal bone loss of vitamin K_1 (at a dosage of 1 mg/d) and vitamin D (at a dosage of 8 μg/d) and mineral supplement. The minerals included magnesium (150 mg/d), calcium (500 mg/d) and zinc (10 mg/d). The main outcome measures were change in BMD at the femoral neck and lumbar spine sites.

Results indicated a positive effect of the vitamin K_1 supplement on bone loss at the femoral neck (Table 4.2). This is the first supplementation study examining the effect of vitamin K_1 supplementation on indices of bone health in postmenopausal women. The results are important from a clinical point of view for a number of reasons. The vitamin K_1 supplement showed almost complete protection of the skeleton during the first year of the intervention study and subsequently a partial but nonetheless persistent protective effect on bone mass, leading to a 35% reduction in bone loss when compared with placebo after 36 months. The sharp decrease in circulating ucOC after the vitamin K_1 supplementation indicates that the subjects were in a sub-optimal state with regard to their vitamin K status. Hence, it might be a useful pointer to examine for vitamin K nutrition in the ageing population, but especially among those who are at an increased risk of osteoporosis. The results are confined to the femoral neck (a key osteoporotic site); the lack of an effect at the

Table 4.2: Mean percentage change from baseline in femoral neck bone mineral density (BMD) between the placebo group (n = 60), minerals and vitamin D group (MD) (n = 46) and minerals, vitamin D and vitamin K group (MDK) (n = 56)

	Length of follow-up								
	12 months			24 months			36 months		
	Placebo	MD	MDK	Placebo	MD	MDK	Placebo	MD	MDK
Change (%) in femoral neck BMD from baseline	−0.2	−1.0	−0.2	−2.1	−3.6	−1.8	−4.9	−5.5	−3.5*

*MDK group was significantly different to placebo and MD groups at 36 months ($P < 0.05$).
Source: Adapted from Braam *et al.* (2003). Reproduced with kind permission from Springer Science and Business Media.

lumbar spine is interesting and perhaps reflective of problems with vertebrae measurements in the elderly, such as osteoarthritis (with occurrence of osteophytes) or extensive aortic calcification.

More recently, the effect of 200 µg of vitamin K_1 supplementation on postmenopausal women's bone health, in combination with calcium (1000 mg) and vitamin D (10 µg), was investigated over a two-year period in a randomised, placebo-controlled study design (Bolton-Smith *et al.* 2007). Bone mineral density was assessed at the hip and wrist. Subjects who took the combined phylloquinone (vitamin K_1) and vitamin D plus calcium supplement showed a significant increase in ultra-distal bone mineral density and bone mineral content. This is the first randomised trial using a dosage of vitamin K_1 that is possibly attainable from the diet (200 µg is obtainable from a 50 g portion of leafy green vegetables). There is also good evidence to show that vitamin K_2 supplementation is effective in improving markers of bone health, although it is important to note that the doses of vitamin K_2 used could not be achieved via the diet (Knapen *et al.* 2007). A recent meta-analysis examining the effect of vitamin K_2 supplementation on vertebral and hip fracture shows a convincing effect of pharmacological doses of vitamin K_2 on fracture rates (Cockayne *et al.* 2006; Shearer *et al.* 2007). As shown in Figures 4.7 and 4.8, Vitamin K_2 significantly reduced fracture rates.

Further research is required in older population groups, but these data suggest that vitamin K nutrition is absolutely critical for skeletal integrity. Interestingly, key dietary sources of vitamin K are vegetables, so this is another good reason to encourage a high vegetable intake for maximising skeletal strength.

4.2.6 The effect of fruit and vegetables on bone health

4.2.6.1 Observational studies

A variety of population-based studies published in the latter part of the twentieth century and more recently between 2001 and 2006 have demonstrated a beneficial effect of fruit and vegetable/potassium intake on indices of bone health in young boys and girls (Tylavsky *et al.* 2004; Prynne *et al.* 2006), premenopausal women (New *et al.* 1997), perimenopausal women (Macdonald *et al.* 2004), postmenopausal women and older men and women (Tucker *et al.* 1999).

4.2.6.2 Dietary intervention studies

Further support for a positive link between fruit and vegetable intake and bone health can be found in the results of the Dietary Approaches to Stop Hypertension (DASH) and DASH-sodium intervention trials (Appel *et al.* 1997; Sacks *et al.* 2001). In DASH, diets rich in fruit and vegetables were associated with a significant fall in blood pressure compared with baseline measurements (see Chapter 10, Section 10.7.6.1, Chapter 8, Section 8.2.2 and Chapter 14, Section 14.3.6). However, of particular interest to the bone field were findings that increasing fruit and vegetable intake from 3.6 to 9.5 daily servings decreased the urinary calcium excretion from 157 mg/d to 110 mg/d. Bone turnover markers were

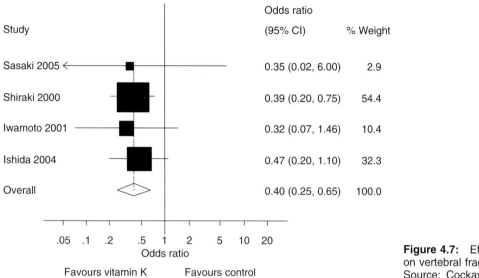

Study		Odds ratio (95% CI)	% Weight
Sasaki 2005		0.35 (0.02, 6.00)	2.9
Shiraki 2000		0.39 (0.20, 0.75)	54.4
Iwamoto 2001		0.32 (0.07, 1.46)	10.4
Ishida 2004		0.47 (0.20, 1.10)	32.3
Overall		0.40 (0.25, 0.65)	100.0

.05 .1 .2 .5 1 2 5 10 20
Odds ratio

Favours vitamin K   Favours control

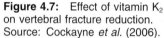

Figure 4.7: Effect of vitamin K_2 on vertebral fracture reduction. Source: Cockayne *et al.* (2006).

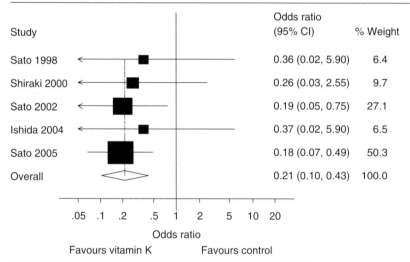

Study		Odds ratio (95% CI)	% Weight
Sato 1998		0.36 (0.02, 5.90)	6.4
Shiraki 2000		0.26 (0.03, 2.55)	9.7
Sato 2002		0.19 (0.05, 0.75)	27.1
Ishida 2004		0.37 (0.02, 5.90)	6.5
Sato 2005		0.18 (0.07, 0.49)	50.3
Overall		0.21 (0.10, 0.43)	100.0

.05 .1 .2 .5 1 2 5 10 20
Odds ratio

Favours vitamin K   Favours control

Figure 4.8: Effect of vitamin K_2 on hip fracture reduction. Source: Cockayne *et al.* (2006).

not measured. However, more recently, P.H. Lin and colleagues (2003) reported the findings of the DASH-sodium trial. The impacts of two dietary patterns on indices of bone metabolism were examined. The DASH diet emphasises fruits, vegetables and low-fat dairy products and is reduced in red meats. In this DASH-sodium trial, three levels of sodium intake were investigated: 50, 100 and 150 mmol/L (Sacks *et al.* 2001). Subjects consumed the control diet at the 150 mmol sodium intake/d level for two weeks and were then randomly assigned to eat either the DASH diet or the control diet at each of three sodium levels (in random order) for a further four weeks. The DASH diet compared with the control diet was found to significantly reduce bone formation (by measurement of the marker osteocalcin) by 8–10% and bone resorption (by measurement of the marker CTx) by 16–18%. Interestingly, sodium intake did not significantly affect the markers of bone metabolism. This is an important intervention study which shows a benefit of the high intake of fruit and vegetables on markers of bone metabolism.

Buclin and colleagues (2001) have examined the effect of dietary modification on calcium and bone metabolism. The 'acid-forming' diet (rich in protein sources, bread and butter) increased urinary calcium excretion by 74% and bone resorption, as measured by C-terminal peptide excretion, by 19% in comparison to the alkali-forming diet (rich in fruit and vegetables), both at baseline and after an oral calcium load.

Research is now required to determine the long-term clinical impact of the DASH diet on bone health and fracture risk, as well as clarification of the exact mechanisms involved with respect to this diet on skeletal protection.

4.2.6.3 *Clinical studies*

The clinical application of the effect of normal endogenous acid production on bone is of considerable interest. Sebastian and colleagues (1994) demonstrated that potassium bicarbonate administration resulted in a decrease in urinary calcium and phosphorus, with overall calcium balance becoming less negative (or more positive) (Table 4.3). Changes were also seen in markers of bone metabolism, with a reduction in urinary excretion of hydroxyproline

(bone resorption) and an increased excretion of serum osteocalcin (bone formation).

More recently, the Aberdeen Prospective Osteoporosis Screening Study (APOSS) has undertaken a two-year investigation into the effect of potassium citrate supplementation on markers of bone turnover (Macdonald *et al.* 2006). Results did not show a beneficial effect of either the high-dose potassium citrate (55.6 mEq potassium citrate) or the low-dose potassium citrate (18.5 mEq potassium citrate) supplementation and would therefore suggest that any long-term benefits of fruit and vegetables on the skeleton are unlikely to be due to the alkaline salts they provide in the healthy postmenopausal population. However, it is important to note that although the results of the APOSS long-term potassium citrate supplementation study do not support the postulated acid-base/bone hypothesis in the healthy population, short-term studies (3–6 months) do indicate an effect (Sebastian *et al.* 1994; Sellmeyer *et al.* 2002). New data (Jehle *et al.* 2006) shows that potassium citrate may be beneficial to bone health in postmenopausal women with established osteopenia. Longer-term studies of the effect of DASH-style diets or specific types of fruit and vegetables on bone health markers (including fracture risk) are now urgently needed (Lanham-New 2007; Rafferty and Heaney 2008). Clearly, fruit and vegetables contain a number of nutrients (including vitamin C, vitamin K, magnesium, carotenoids, fibre, *etc.*) all of which may have independent effects on the skeleton (Lanham-New 2006).

Table 4.3: Clinical application – potassium bicarbonate supplementation study

	Before potassium bicarbonate supplementation (mean ± SD)	During potassium bicarbonate supplementation (mean ± SD)	Change (mean ± SD)
Calcium balance (mg/day/60 kg)	−180 ± 124	−124 ± 76	+56 ± 76
Phosphorus balance (mg/day/60 kg)	−208 ± 127	−161 ± 92	+47 ± 64
Serum osteocalcin (ng/ml)	5.5 ± 2.8	6.1 ± 2.8	+0.6 ± 0.48
Urinary hydroxyproline (mg/day)	28.9 ± 12.3	26.7 ± 10.8	−2.2 ± *
Net renal acid excretion (mmol/day)	70.9 ± 10.1	12.8 ± 21.8	−58.1 ± *

*SD not reported in publication.
Source: Adapted from Sebastian *et al.* (1994).

4.2.7 Vegetarianism and bone health

4.2.7.1 *Earlier studies in vegetarian populations*

A number of population-based cross-sectional studies were undertaken investigating the effect of lacto-ovo-vegetarian diets on bone mineral mass. Earlier studies found BMD to be higher in the vegetarian group compared to the non-vegetarians. However, it is important to note that in Ellis *et al.* (1972), there was a fundamental error in the interpretation of the photographic density measurements and their conclusions should have been the opposite of what they reported. Furthermore, the subjects studied in several of the published studies were Seventh Day Adventists (SDA), who had a significantly different lifestyle from that of the omnivorous group. For example, the SDA group refrained from smoking and caffeine intake, and physical activity levels were higher. This difference is likely to have been an important confounding influence, which may have, in part at least, biased some of the study findings (New 2004).

4.2.7.2 *Later (post-1984) studies in vegetarian populations*

Cross-sectional and longitudinal population-based studies published in the last two decades suggest no differences in BMD between vegetarians and omnivores. Lloyd *et al.* (1991) found no differences in lumbar spine BMD between omnivorous and vegetarian premenopausal women. In another study (Tesar *et al.* 1992) differences in nutrient intake and trabecular/cortical bone density were examined in postmenopausal Caucasian vegetarian and omnivorous women. The vegetarian group were found to consume greater quantities of carbohydrate (in absolute terms and as a proportion of energy intake), fibre, magnesium, ascorbic acid and copper, and lower amounts of protein (in absolute terms and as a proportion of energy intake), niacin, alcohol, vitamin B_{12} and cholesterol; but neither cortical nor trabecular bone mass was affected by a lacto-ovo-vegetarian diet. In a five-year prospective study of changes in radial bone density of white American women (mean age 81 years) living in residential communities, no differences were seen in bone loss rates between the lacto-ovo-vegetarians and the omnivorous group (Reed *et al.* 1994). On the other hand, in

the most recently published studies, bone mass was found to be significantly lower in the groups consuming vegetable-based diets (New 2004).

4.2.7.3 *Studies in Inuit populations*

Few data are available on bone health in populations consuming a diet highly dependent on animal foods, particularly meat and fish. Mazess and Mather (1974) examined forearm bone mineral content (BMC) in a sample of 217 children, 89 adults and 107 older Inuit natives of the north coast of Alaska. Inuit children were found to have a 5–10% lower BMC than US white children, a finding that was consistent with smaller body and bone size. In the young adult population (age 20–39 years), BMD was similar to the white population. However, after the age of 40 years, the Inuit of both sexes were found to have a 10–15% deficit of bone mineral relative to white standards. The authors note that ageing bone loss, which occurs in many populations, was found to have an earlier onset and greater intensity among the Inuit population. Similar results (showing an even greater bone loss) have also been found in Canadian Inuit (Mazess and Mather 1975a). These findings are of interest with regard to the discussion on regulation of systemic acid-base balance (see Section 4.2.5).

However, it is important to note that the studies of the Inuit populations have a number of limitations and thus interpretation of these data should be treated with some caution; there is no internal comparison group and statistical control for major confounders is insufficient (Mann 1975; Mazess and Mather 1975b). For example, the Inuit population consume a diet that is extremely low in calcium (approximately 200 mg/d), which is likely to impact on the effect of dietary protein on indices of bone health.

4.2.8 Isoflavones and bone health

Soya isoflavones have a chemical structure similar to that of oestradiol and have been shown to possess weak oestrogenic activity (see Chapter 13, Section 13.4.4) (Sacks 2006). Hence, theoretically they may have a beneficial effect on bone loss reduction in postmenopausal women. In animal studies, comparable effects on bone have been shown with 17β-oestradiol and the soy protein isolates genistein and daidzein (Cai *et al.* 2003). A recent study using the ovariectomised rat model suggests that isoflavones may influence tibial microstructural properties rather than bone mass (Devareddy *et al.* 2006).

Data from epidemiological studies looking at the association between soya product consumption and fracture rates look promising. A large prospective cohort study that examined the relationship between soya consumption and fracture incidence in 24,403 Chinese postmenopausal women, who had no history of fracture or cancer, found that soya consumption reduced the risk of fracture in postmenopausal women (Zhang *et al.* 2005). The effect was particularly marked in those in the early stages of menopause. However, clinical trials using a range of intakes of soy isoflavones from 54 mg to 300 mg (although the majority of studies have used 80–110 mg) and either direct measurement of bone density/content or biochemical indices of bone turnover have yielded conflicting results. For example, soy isoflavones reduced bone loss over a period of 6–24 months in two studies (Morabito *et al.* 2002; Nikander *et al.* 2004), but this was not a consistent finding, with three other trials showing no effect over the same duration (Khalil *et al.* 2002; Dalais *et al.* 2003; Kreijkamp-Kaspers *et al.* 2004). Hence, there is an urgent need for further clinical trials which have a substantial sample size and are of 24–36 months in duration.

4.2.9 Vitamin A and bone

Vitamin A refers to a family of essential, fat-soluble compounds called retinoids. Retinol is the principal dietary form of vitamin A. The main natural sources of vitamin A are animal foods, such as liver, meat, milk products, eggs and fatty fish. In addition, some foods are fortified with vitamin A. Cod liver oil (which is commonly used in a number of population groups, particularly postmenopausal women/older people) also contains high levels of vitamin A. It is important to note that pure cod liver oil can provide as much as 1200 µg of retinol equivalents in a 10 ml dose. Vitamin A can also be made in the body from carotenoids such as β-carotene. There are about 600 or so carotenoids, with approximately 10% of these having provitamin A activity (Melhus 2003).

Vitamin A is necessary for normal bone growth. However, intakes of vitamin A >1500 µg of retinol equivalents have been associated with lower BMD

and higher fracture risk in populations in the US and Sweden (Feskanich *et al.* 2002; Michaelsson *et al.* 2003). In both countries, dairy products and cereals are generally fortified with vitamin A and so habitual intake is likely to be higher than that found in the UK. No such detrimental effects of vitamin A have been found in the UK population (Barker *et al.* 2005). However, advice for the UK population has been published by the Scientific Advisory Committee on Nutrition (SACN) (2005a).

4.2.10 Folate and osteoporosis

There is increasing evidence at the experimental, clinical and epidemiological levels that elevated homocysteine is associated with increased fracture risk (see Chapter 8, Section 8.2.3; Chapter 10, Section 10.4.2.2). Two studies have shown that elevated homocysteine levels are associated with increasing risk of fracture in Dutch and American populations. In the Dutch study, a homocysteine level in the highest age-specific quartile was associated with a 1.9-fold increase in the risk of fracture. The associations between homocysteine and risk of fracture seemed to be independent of BMD and other potential risk factors for fracture (van Meurs *et al.* 2004). In the American study, men and women in the highest quartile of plasma homocysteine level had a greater risk of hip fracture than those in the lowest plasma homocysteine quartile, with the risk being four times higher for men and 1.9 times higher for women (McLean *et al.* 2004).

There seems to be little evidence for a direct effect of homocysteine on bone, but there are some suggestions that high levels of homocysteine in the serum may weaken bone by interfering with collagen cross-linking, thus increasing the risk of osteoporotic fracture (Raisz 2004b). The homocysteine/fracture risk link suggests the potential for a positive effect of vitamin B complex on the skeleton. Elevated homocysteine levels can be reduced simply and inexpensively through folic acid supplementation. Care should be taken with high doses of folic acid supplements in older people as it can alleviate or mask anaemia associated with vitamin B_{12} deficiency (see Chapter 8, Section 8.3.2). In the absence of specific folic acid/fracture reduction trials, we cannot say whether certain B vitamins may provide an effective strategy for osteoporosis prevention, but it is certainly an area for research.

4.2.11 Sodium

There are not enough data currently to support the claim that salt intake is a significant risk factor for osteoporosis. However, high salt intakes have been associated with increases in urinary calcium loss. For example, it has been estimated that a 100 mmol increment in daily sodium intake is associated with an average loss of urinary calcium of approximately 1 mmol in free-living normo-calciuric healthy populations (Nordin *et al.* 1993). This loss has not been specifically correlated to bone loss; some studies have shown an effect (*i.e.* higher sodium intake, higher bone turnover), but others have found no difference (Cashman and Flynn 2003). In one study, urinary excretion of deoxypyridinoline (a marker of bone resorption) was found to be higher in post-menopausal women on a high sodium diet (300 mmol/d; 6900 mg/d) compared with a low sodium diet (50 mmol/d, 1150 mg/d), but this was not found in premenopausal women (Evans *et al.* 1997). Another study has shown a significant increase in urinary calcium excretion and bone resorption in postmeno-pausal women randomised to a four-week, high salt (225 mmol/d sodium, 5175 mg/d) diet. Notably, the addition of oral potassium citrate to the high salt diet prevented the increased urinary calcium excretion and bone resorption (Sellmeyer *et al.* 2002). The DASH-sodium trial showed no effect of different levels of salt intake on bone turnover markers (P.H. Lin *et al.* 2003).

4.2.12 Alcohol and caffeine

4.2.12.1 Alcohol and osteoporosis risk

There is evidence in the literature that chronic alcohol abuse is a key risk factor for osteoporosis and osteo-porotic fracture (Crilly *et al.* 1988). Alcohol in large amounts is directly toxic to osteoblasts (hence bone formation is reduced) and may also have a direct effect on bone density by impairing liver function and altering vitamin D and calcium metabolism (Pepersack *et al.* 1992). Falls related to alcohol excess are also a key risk factor for osteoporosis.

However, moderate alcohol consumption has been shown in some studies to have a positive effect on bone mass. Social drinking was found to be asso-ciated with higher bone mass in men and women in prospective cohort study (Holbrook and Barrett-Connor 1993). In a study by Rapuri *et al.* (2000), moderate alcohol consumption was associated with higher bone density in a population of 489 women aged 65–77 years. However, this finding is not con-sistent in all studies and clarification of the mecha-nisms involved is needed.

4.2.12.2 Caffeine consumption and bone health

Caffeine does not directly affect bone, but does alter metabolism by antagonising the adenosine receptors (Bergman *et al.* 1990). Hence, it has an impact on calcium metabolism by its hypercalciuric effect on the kidney, and a possible link to decreasing intesti-nal calcium absorption. Long-term effects on bone are conflicting and require further elucidation. Con-sumption of recommended amounts of dietary calcium may offset the small calcium losses which may be caused by caffeine (Dickerson *et al.* 2003).

4.2.13 Polyunsaturated fatty acids and bone health

Polyunsaturated fatty acids have been suggested to influence bone growth and modelling in humans, but data remain sparse, particularly in older groups. There is some evidence that appropriate amounts of omega-3 (*n*-3) polyunsaturates have a beneficial effect on bone health. For example, a recent cohort study of 78 healthy young men showed positive associations between *n*-3 fatty acids, especially docosahexaenoic acid (DHA), and bone mineral accrual between 16 and 22 years of age and with total and spine BMD at 22 years (Hogstrom *et al.* 2007). Weiss *et al.* (2005) investigated the associa-tion between the ratio of *n*-6 (omega-6) to *n*-3 fatty acids and bone mineral density in a group of 1532 community-dwelling men and women aged 45–90 years. A higher ratio of *n*-6 to *n*-3 fatty acids was associated with lower BMD at the hip in both sexes, suggesting that the relative amounts of dietary poly-unsaturated fatty acids may play some role in pre-serving skeletal integrity in older age.

4.2.14 Other key factors affecting bone health

4.2.14.1 Physical activity

Principal concepts: More than a century ago, a German, Julius Woolf, stated the theory which is now called Woolf's Law: 'bone accommodates the forces applied to it by altering its amount and distribution of mass'. More recently, this concept has been refined to a general theory of bone mass regulation, known as the mechanostat model (Frost 1987, 1992). It is well known that in the absence of weight-bearing exercise bone loss will occur at both axial and appendicular skeletal sites. In a recent study examining bone loss in 15 Russian cosmonauts, in the weight-bearing tibial site, cancellous BMD loss was present after the first month in space and deteriorated with mission duration (Vico *et al.* 2000). In those cosmonauts who spent six months in space losses ranged up to 23%; this is clearly a serious problem which may ultimately substantially affect plans for long-distance space travel (Holick 2000).

Whilst the exact mechanism whereby mechanical loading affects bone remains to be clarified, the literature supports a positive relationship between physical activity, physical fitness, muscle strength and bone mass at the lumbar spine and femoral neck sites (Pocock *et al.* 1989).

Role of exercise in PBM development, postmenopausal bone loss reduction and fracture prevention: There is evidence which supports a positive relationship between weight-bearing exercise and bone mass in children (Slemenda *et al.* 1991), young women (Recker *et al.* 1992), premenopausal women (Jonsson *et al.* 1992) and postmenopausal women (Kohrt *et al.* 1995). There is also a relationship between past physical activity levels and bone density in young women (Tylavsky *et al.* 1992), premenopausal women (Halioua and Anderson 1989) and postmenopausal women (Kriska *et al.* 1988).

Very little information is available on the relationship between exercise and fracture. Lau *et al.* (1988) reported a significantly decreased relative risk of hip fracture in those who undertook regular walking activities (Lau *et al.* 1988), and in a parallel study Cooper *et al.* (1988) noted that increased daily activity was a protective factor against hip fracture in both males and females (Cooper *et al.* 1988).

There are, however, data to support a specific role for high-impact exercise in increasing bone density in premenopausal women (Snow-Harter *et al.* 1992; Bassey and Ramsdale 1994; Lohman *et al.* 1995), postmenopausal women (Kohrt *et al.* 2004) and in both middle-aged and older men (Menkes *et al.* 1993). Interestingly, in one study, pre- and post-

menopausal women were found to respond differently to the same high-impact activity (Bassey *et al.* 1998).

Whilst exercise is clearly of benefit to the skeleton, what remains undefined is exactly the type, intensity and duration of weight-bearing physical activity required for optimum bone health. Furthermore, exercise may be of benefit in the prevention of osteoporosis, not necessarily via the mechanism of increasing bone mass but by increasing muscle strength, coordination, flexibility and balance, and thus reducing the tendency to fall (see Chapter 6, Section 6.10).

4.2.14.2 Bodyweight

There are good data to show that bodyweight has a direct effect on bone mass (Shapses and Cifuentes 2003). A lower bodyweight tends to be associated with lower bone mass and a consequent increase in fracture risk (Edelstein and Barrett-Connor 1993). Conversely, a higher bodyweight is associated with a lower risk of osteoporosis, although from a public health perspective, obesity should not be seen as a protective factor against poor bone health (Hannan *et al.* 2000a). However, it is important to recognise that weight reduction, which is consistently and continuously encouraged in populations with obesity problems, is likely to result in some bone loss (Ricci *et al.* 2001).

4.2.14.3 Smoking

There are a number of epidemiological studies which show that bone mass is lower in both men and women who are smokers compared with their non-smoking counterparts (Jones *et al.* 1995). It is important to note, however, the likely interaction with low bodyweight, particularly in women, which is likely to exaggerate the detrimental effects (Johnell 2003). Certainly, smoking appears to result in a low bone mineral density and has been found to be a significant risk factor for osteoporosis in some (Paganini-Hill *et al.* 1991) but not all population groups (Hoidrup *et al.* 1999).

4.3 Discussion

The effects of nutrition on the skeleton are powerful and wide-ranging. There is evidence to suggest that such effects begin *in utero* and remain throughout the entire lifespan. It is widely recognised that there are genetic, environmental, lifestyle and dietary determinants of risk of osteoporotic fracture, as well as interactions between them. Given the fact that, by 2030, 25% of the adult population will be elderly, it is absolutely critical that special attention is given to nutritional strategies for the optimisation of bone health throughout the lifecycle. The key to primary prevention is to understand both the pathological and physiological basis of bone fragility. The key to secondary prevention is to understand how these components can be integrated into an effective assessment of the major risks when a fracture has already occurred. It is not unreasonable to suppose that in countries such as the UK and North America our limited and stereotypical patterns of locomotion from middle age onwards may offer considerably less protection than, for example, the more physically demanding activity of subsistence farming.

This provides us with clear target audiences on whom we can focus our nutrition and bone health messages. On the dietary front, calcium and vitamin D are clearly key nutrients for optimal bone health. At all costs, we must protect against sub-optimal intakes and look to dietary fortification strategies, if necessary, for particularly vulnerable groups such as older people, postmenopausal women, adolescent females and amenorrhoeic women. Recent data suggest that calcium works synergistically with physical activity to enhance PBM development and both should be on the agenda as recommended strategies for maximising PBM attainment during growth. At the other end of the age spectrum, calcium and vitamin D have been shown to be effective strategies for fracture prevention in the elderly, particularly for those populations where vitamin D insufficiency is rife.

Data continue to accumulate showing a positive impact of dietary potassium/fruit and vegetables on skeletal integrity. Although further long-term intervention trials are urgently required, it is sensible to promote a high potassium intake because potassium has been shown to conserve calcium (see Section 4.2.6.3). A high intake of fruit and vegetables is likely to have numerous other health-related benefits (see Chapter 14). In recent years, evidence has emerged for a role for vitamin K in bone health. Although isoflavones have also been the target of research, data have been less consistent.

Further data are urgently required to enable a fuller understanding of the complex interaction between dietary factors and bone health. Whilst there are plausible mechanisms for the effect of other micronutrients on bone health, such as magnesium, trace elements and vitamin C, more research is required on the specific effects of these nutrients on markers of bone health before any conclusions can be drawn. The same applies to dietary alkali.

Furthermore, there is evidence that modest protein under-nutrition is common in older people and an important additional risk factor for an increased propensity to fall and hence suffer an osteoporotic fracture via an effect on skeletal muscle. Simple protein supplementation in at-risk groups via dietary means might reduce this risk. As well as these potential interventions, it is timely to undertake a comprehensive epidemiological study of the relationship between nutrition and fractures in an older population to ascertain the role of other key nutrient factors (including vitamin K, potassium (acid-base link), vitamin A, magnesium, copper and zinc) in fracture causation/prevention.

In this era of functional genomics, data are now urgently required to characterise the key nutrient–gene interactions that are likely to affect bone health in both younger and older population groups. Targeting dietary advice at those who are genetically susceptible to osteoporosis is likely to become a useful approach for the practising clinician.

4.4 Key points

- It is critical that the body is supplied with the nutrients required for the growth, mineralisation and repair of bone. Hence consumption of a balanced diet is crucial throughout the lifecycle.

- Adequate intakes of calcium and vitamin D are key for optimisation of PBM attainment, reduction of postmenopausal bone loss and prevention of osteoporotic fractures.

Continued

- There is evidence of widespread vitamin D insufficiency, particularly in the vulnerable elderly. This urgently requires a public health strategy.
- Conflicting data exist for the effects of protein on the skeleton, with both high protein consumption (especially without a good calcium/alkali intake) and low protein intake (*e.g.* with respect to older people and vegan diets) being detrimental to bone. More longer-term studies are urgently required, as well as a meta-analysis of the evidence.
- There is evidence in the literature that low vitamin K intake and/or status are associated with low bone mass and increased fracture risk. Intervention studies, with fracture reduction as the clinical end-point, are now needed.
- There is support in the literature from a combination of observational, experimental, clinical and intervention studies of a positive link between fruit and vegetable consumption and bone health, but more longer-term intervention studies are required before firm conclusions can be drawn.

- Particular attention should be given to the benefits of impact-loading exercise (*e.g.* brisk walking, jogging, running, step aerobics, light gymnastics) for helping maintain a healthy skeleton. There is a positive relationship between weight-bearing exercise and bone mass in children and adults, and being active may also protect against osteoporosis via effects on muscle strength, coordination, flexibility and balance.
- High sodium chloride (salt) intake is associated with an increase in urinary calcium excretion, but there is limited data for a long-term adverse effect on bone. Further research in this area is urgently required.
- A high intake of vitamin A (from animal sources) may be associated with low bone mineral density and increased risk of osteoporotic fracture in certain populations. High consumption ($>1500\,\mu g$ retinol equivalents) should be avoided.
- At a cellular level vitamin C, B vitamins, copper, zinc and magnesium all have a role to play in skeletal development, but specific mechanisms need to be identified.

4.5 Recommendations for future research

- Standardised methodologies for measuring vitamin D status are needed, combined with assessment of the relationship between biochemical status and health outcomes.
- Longer-term studies of the effect of different dietary patterns (such as the Dietary Approaches to Stop Hypertension or DASH diet) or specific types of fruit and vegetables on bone health markers (including fracture risk) are urgently needed. It remains to be established which nutrients or combination of nutrients may be responsible for any beneficial effect (*e.g.* vitamin C, vitamin K, magnesium, carotenoids, fibre, phytonutrients, *etc.*).
- Long-term studies of the effects of protein and sodium intake on bone health are required.
- Intervention studies are needed to elucidate the effects of vitamin K intake/status on fracture

reduction. The role of other micronutrients also remains to be clarified.
- Whether polyunsaturated fatty acids, particularly *n*-3 fatty acids, alter biochemical and molecular processes involved in bone modelling and bone cell differentiation warrants further research.
- In this era of functional genomics, data are now urgently required to characterise the key nutrient–gene interactions that are likely to affect bone health in both the younger and older population groups.
- The effects of different types of physical activity on fracture risk in older people should be investigated and work carried out to clarify the exact mechanism whereby mechanical loading affects bone.

4.6 Key references

Favus M (ed.) (2006) *Primer on the Metabolic Bone Diseases and Disorders of Mineral Metabolism.* New York, The American Society for Bone and Mineral Research.

Holick M and Dawson-Hughes B (eds) (2004) *Nutrition and Bone Health.* New Jersey, Humana Press.

Lanham-New S, O'Neill T, Morris R and Sutcliffe A. (eds) (2007) *Managing Osteoporosis.* Oxford, Clinical Publishing.

New S and Bonjour J-P (eds) (2003) *Nutritional Aspects of Bone Health.* Cambridge, Royal Society of Chemistry.

Rosen C, Glowacki J and Bilezikian J (eds) (1999) *The Aging Skeleton.* London, Academic Press.

5
Healthy Ageing: The Joints

5.1 Introduction

5.1.1 Background

Our current culture views musculoskeletal problems as a natural part of ageing. This is apparent from the widespread use of images like the road sign that warns us that older people are in the vicinity, which shows an older couple bent over and using walking aids (Figure 5.1).

Musculoskeletal pain and impairment are very common in older people: a survey of the prevalence of pain in the UK (Elliott *et al.* 1999) found that 50.4% of all adults self-reported chronic pain, and that the prevalence rose with increasing age, resulting in 62% of those over 75 years reporting chronic pain, most of which was musculoskeletal in origin. Similarly, a health survey from the UK Office for National Statistics (ONS) (2002) indicated that pain and disability attributable to musculoskeletal problems were highly prevalent in the population, particularly among older people. The problem of chronic musculoskeletal pain associated with increasing age is also found in other countries. A large survey of adults in the Netherlands found that some 50% reported chronic pain, with a relationship to age, and with the commonest sites affected being the back, shoulder, neck and knee (Picavet and Schouten 2003). Similar findings have been reported from the US (Barkin *et al.* 2005).

This high prevalence of musculoskeletal pain and disability could result from numerous age-related changes in body structure and function, or from several different diseases. Age-related changes in muscles, bones and the nervous system probably contribute extensively (Dieppe and Tobias 1998). However, it is customary to attribute the majority of the problems to joint disease (*i.e.* 'arthritis'). Over 200 forms of arthritis have been described, but relatively few of these occur commonly. They can be classified into two main categories: the inflammatory arthropathies, such as rheumatoid arthritis (RA), and age-related conditions, such as osteoarthritis (OA) (Table 5.1). Interestingly, the differences in the incidence rates among men and women of these major forms of arthritis appear to decline with age.

Inflammatory forms of arthritis, such as RA, ankylosing spondylitis, psoriatic arthritis and gout, affect about 1% of the UK population. They are chronic diseases that are generally not fatal and, therefore, tend to become more prevalent in older people even when the main incidence occurs at a younger age. OA is a much more common condition that is strongly age-related, causing pain and disability in over 10% of those over the age of 65 (Felson *et al.* 2000). Although there are other, less common age-related rheumatic disorders (*e.g.* polymyalgia rheumatica), no other joint disease is as important as OA in terms of public health or as closely linked with nutrition. For these reasons the majority of this chapter will be concerned with OA, although some relevant aspects of the inflammatory arthropathies, particularly rheumatoid arthritis and gout, will be considered first.

5.1.2 Principles relating to associations between diet and arthritis

The majority of people with arthritis wonder if their diet might cause, cure or alleviate their disease or

Table 5.1: A classification of the most common forms of arthritis and their incidence in different age and sex groups

| Age group | Gender | | |
	Males > Females	Males approx = Females	Females > Males
Young adults	Ankylosing spondylitis Reactive arthritis		Rheumatoid arthritis Systemic lupus erythematosis
Middle age	Gout	Psoriatic arthritis	Rheumatoid arthritis Osteoarthritis
Older people		Osteoarthritis Pyrophosphate arthropathy Polymyalgia rheumatica Rheumatoid arthritis	

Figure 5.1: Road sign for older people from the Highway Code.
The road sign that indicates that accommodation for older people is nearby. Note the depiction of the older people as frail and suffering from musculoskeletal disease, apparent from one being bent over and the other having to use a walking aid. This illustrates our cultural belief that advancing age is associated with inevitable arthritis, pain and musculoskeletal disability.

illness. For example, it has been reported that between 33% and 75% of patients with RA believe that food plays an important part in their disease and some 20–50% try dietary manipulation to alleviate symptoms (Martin 1998; Salminen *et al.* 2002). A visit to any bookshop will reveal shelves of books on diet and arthritis, all of them strongly recommending something completely different, with little or nothing to support these claims other than anecdotal evidence. Similarly, a visit to a high street pharmacy will reveal shelves full of a variety of different dietary products recommended for the treatment of 'arthritis'. These phenomena are an index of the public belief in and demand for dietary treatments for arthritis (and also, perhaps, of their gullibility). Science and modern medicine has not yet caught up with these public needs and beliefs. We still know relatively little about the value (or not) of different dietary manipulations in either the cause or treatment of arthritis, their possible mechanisms of action remain unclear, and even when we do have evidence of potential value, we are not implementing public health policies to improve the diets of people with arthritis (Stamp *et al.* 2005).

There are many recommended diets for arthritis and many different aims (Table 5.2). Unfortunately, these different types of diet and aim get confused, not only in the minds of the patients, but all too often in those of the health care professionals and even in the minds of those investigating the subject.

5.2 The inflammatory arthropathies

Inflammatory forms of arthritis are characterised by chronic inflammation of the synovial lining of the joint (synovitis), and/or inflammation at the points at which ligaments and tendons insert into the bone (enthesitis). Enthesitis is particularly characteristic of the so-called sero-negative spondarthropathies,

Table 5.2:   Some principles of the use of diets
in arthritis

Three types of diet:
1. A diet may *eliminate* a foodstuff that is thought to
   contribute negatively.
2. A *supplement* might be added to the diet if it is
   thought to be beneficial.
3. A food supplement might be used to create *tolerance*
   to an antigen if this is thought to be driving an
   immune process responsible for arthritis.

Three possible reasons for dietary manipulation:
1. Diets might be recommended to *prevent* arthritis.
2. A dietary manipulation might be used to *control the
   disease process.*
3. Diets can be used to *relieve the symptoms* of arthritis.

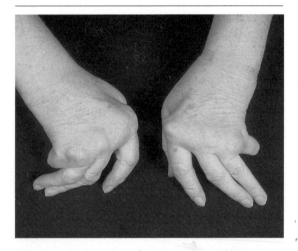

Figure 5.2:   The hands of someone with advanced
rheumatoid arthritis showing severe joint damage
caused by erosion and destruction of the bone and
soft tissues caused by the inflamed synovium of the
joints.
Source: Courtesy of Professor Michael Doherty,
Nottingham University.

such as ankylosing spondylitis, psoriatic arthritis
and reactive arthritis, whereas in RA, synovitis is the
dominant pathology. In each case, the inflammation
can lead to damage to the adjacent bone, cartilage
and soft tissues. A pathognomonic feature of RA is
erosion of the bone at the margins of the joint due
to invasion of the inflammatory synovium; this can
lead to severe joint damage, deformity and loss of
function, as well as pain (Figure 5.2).

Other, uncommon forms of inflammatory joint
disease include septic arthritis and the arthritis that
accompanies several systemic multi-system, autoimmune disorders such as systemic lupus erythemato-
sis. Finally, there are the crystal-related arthropathies,
including gout, where inflammation is caused by
micro-crystals of monosodium urate monohydrate,
and pyrophosphate arthropathy, in which the
villains are crystals of calcium pyrophosphate
dihydrate.

The inflammatory arthropathies are complex diseases, caused by a mixture of multiple genetic sus-
ceptibilities and environmental factors (Silman and
Pearson 2002; Padyukov *et al.* 2004). Genetic susceptibility is important, but it is far from the whole
story; having a parent with a susceptibility gene or
with arthritis may double the risk, but the resulting
risk will only be around 1:50, as opposed to, say,
1:100. Therefore, environmental factors must also
be crucial, and these diseases are probably caused
by a complex interaction between genetic susceptibility and life-course exposures, such as smoking
and possibly diet.

The 'downstream' inflammatory synovitis that
characterises RA and most of the other conditions
in the group (apart from septic arthritis and crystal-
induced arthropathies) is clearly immune-driven and
a variety of abnormalities of immune function occur,
including the overproduction of certain antibodies.
High serum levels of some of these antibodies, such
as rheumatoid factor (an antibody directed against
the body's IgM antibodies) and anti-citrullin antibodies, can be helpful in both the diagnosis and
prognosis of RA. Many of the most useful therapies
for RA, such as anti-tumour necrosis factor (anti-
TNF) drugs, are immunomodulators, and, as discussed in Chapter 11, Section 11.7, a variety of
nutritional factors can also be immunomodulatory.
Immune-related diseases are characterised by variable activity, resulting in periods of relative remis-
sion interspersed with what are commonly known as
flare-ups of arthritis. We have little understanding
of what causes these episodes of increased disease
activity. Not surprisingly, many people who have
RA or another inflammatory arthropathy believe
that certain specific dietary factors are likely to be
responsible for flare-ups of their inflammatory
disease. (See Chapter 11 for other examples of
inflammatory diseases in which flare-ups happen
periodically.)

5.2.1 Diet and rheumatoid arthritis

This topic has been well reviewed (Choi 2005; Stamp *et al.* 2005). A vast array of elimination diets, supplements and oral tolerance regimens have all been used in an attempt to prevent or treat RA. Coffee and tea drinking have been considered as possible risk factors for the disease, as have diets rich in red meat, those lacking fish and fish oil, or lacking in minerals such as selenium or vitamins including vitamins C, D and E. Attempts have been made to make patients tolerant to collagen (based on the hypothesis that collagen may provide the antigenic drive for chronic inflammation in the joints) in order to control their arthritis, and a large number of elimination diets (removal of a specific type of food thought to affect the inflammatory response) and supplements have been tested for their ability to relieve symptoms (Choi 2005; Stamp *et al.* 2005). Different dietary supplements go through periods of popularity for the treatment of RA and other diseases. For example, a few years ago the green-lipped mussel was in high demand, whereas recently there has been a surge of interest in the possible value and immunomodulatory effects of turmeric (Funk *et al.* 2006). It is difficult to conduct well-designed studies in this area for several reasons. These include the fact that everyone with a diagnosis of RA will be on a variety of drugs that may affect dietary manipulation, and the inherent problems of funding and carrying out large-scale definitive randomised controlled trials of diet for arthritis, when research and research funding is so dominated by the pharmaceutical industry.

There is weak evidence to link high meat/protein diets, as well as those low in fish and fish oil, with an increased risk of acquiring RA, but the data appear to be conflicting, as well as lacking in power (Choi 2005; Stamp *et al.* 2005). The so-called Mediterranean diet, which is relatively low in meat and high in fish oil and other 'good' dietary fatty acids, may have a weak beneficial effect in both the prevention of RA and the treatment of established disease (Hagfors *et al.* 2003). Most of the published trials investigating the effect of elimination diets have shown little effect, although they may mask a large benefit to a very small number of patients. Problems inherent in the investigation of elimination diets include the fact that different patients blame different foods, without any clear pattern emerging, and

the finding that relative starvation relieves RA by immunosuppression. The studies of diets to achieve tolerance to collagen also provide conflicting data, but appear to show little or no effect overall. Similarly, trials with supplements or vitamins and minerals have generally been disappointing. The most data, and the most promising findings, relate to the use of dietary fatty acid supplements used to manipulate the inflammatory response in established arthritis. Therefore, this area is considered in more detail.

5.2.2 Dietary fatty acids and inflammatory arthritis

The amount of the different types of fatty acids in the diet can affect a large number of mediators of inflammation (see Chapter 11, Section 11.7), most notably the eicosanoids (prostaglandins and leukotrienes), through their incorporation into cell membranes. Stamp and colleagues (2005) reviewed 14 published randomised controlled trials of the effects of dietary supplementation with *n*-3 (omega-3) fatty acids on the symptoms and course of rheumatoid arthritis. They concluded that there was evidence of a weak beneficial effect, provided that the dose of the dietary supplement was high enough. They recommended doses of fish oil containing 2.7–4 g of eicosapentaenoic acid (EPA) and docosahexaenoic acid (DHA) per day, coupled with advice to avoid *n*-6 (omega-6)-rich foods (*e.g.* vegetable oils such as sunflower, safflower and corn oils, and products made from these, see Chapter 10, Table 10.3). For comparison, current dietary recommendations for combined EPA and DHA are 0.45 g/day (Scientific Advisory Committee on Nutrition 2004). This level of supplementation may be both difficult to achieve and expensive to implement, and may cause problems with taste as well as gastrointestinal upsets. However, the benefits may be worthwhile, particularly as people with RA have an increased risk of cardiovascular disease, which might also be reduced by a diet rich in long chain *n*-3 fatty acids (Myllykangas-Luosujarvi *et al.* 2000; Snow-Marcus and Mikuls 2005) (see Chapter 10, Section 10.7.3.6). In most of the formal trials, long chain *n*-3 fatty acids have been provided as supplements to the usual diet in the form of capsules. However, fish oils, olive oil and the Mediterranean diet have also been tested in RA, with modest beneficial effects in some cases

(Belch 1990; Berbert *et al.* 2005). There are many practical issues concerning the best way to administer *n*-3 fatty acid supplements that need to be addressed, in addition to the need for more research on their benefits and mode of action.

5.2.3 Nutritional problems resulting from severe inflammatory arthritis

Any severe inflammatory condition can result in cachexia (general physical wasting and malnutrition), and severe weight loss can be a result of active RA. Disability caused by joint damage can complicate the issue. For example, if an older person with disabling arthritis is unable to leave their house and their diet is poor, they may not get enough exposure to sunlight to maintain adequate vitamin D status (see Chapter 1, Section 1.6.2; Chapter 4, Section 4.2.3 and Chapter 14, Section 14.3.2). As osteoporosis occurs as a result of immobility anyway, added problems from low vitamin D levels can contribute to secondary fractures. In the most severely disabled, there may even be problems with feeding, due, for example, to the individual's inability to cut up food or get a fork or spoon to their mouth. However, this is uncommon.

5.2.4 Gout and nutrition

Gout is characterised by severe, acute, self-limiting attacks of inflammation in joints. Most attacks are confined to one site, and the joint at the base of the big toe is the one most often affected (Agudelo and Wise 2001). The cause of the inflammation is the release of crystals of monosodium urate monohydrate from preformed deposits in and around the joints. Uric acid, a natural product of metabolism, is the substrate for the formation of the crystals, and serum levels above the natural saturation level (around 0.42 mmol/L) are common, particularly in men. High levels of serum uric acid (hyperuricaemia) usually result from relatively poor renal excretion, but other causes include overproduction within the body, and diets that stimulate more production of uric acid or those that are excessively rich in its precursors of urate, such as purines.

It is widely known that there are associations between diet and gout, and the supposed links with excessive drinking and the consumption of port are common knowledge. Alcohol consumption does contribute to gout, although these days the main culprit is beer rather than port. The association with port and madeira stems from Georgian days in England, when it was probably largely due to the tendency to sweeten these wines with lead shot; chronic low grade lead poisoning being a risk factor for gout. However, the consumption of any form of alcohol can increase the production of uric acid in the body, as well as contributing to obesity, another independent risk factor for gout (Fam 2005). Diets rich in purines can also raise serum uric acid levels, and dietary restriction of foods rich in them, such as anchovies, are often advised for people who have gout (Zhang *et al.* 2006).

5.3 Osteoarthritis

5.3.1 What is osteoarthritis (OA)?

OA can be defined as a pathological state of a synovial joint characterised by focal areas of destruction of articular cartilage associated with the formation of new bone at the joint margins (osteophytosis), remodelling of subchondral bone, capsular fibrosis and variable degrees of mild inflammation of the synovial lining (synovitis). When severe, this pathology appears on radiographs as narrowing of the joint space (due to cartilage loss), osteophyte formation and subchondral bone sclerosis (hardening) or cyst formation (Brandt *et al.* 2003; Dieppe and Lohmander 2005).

The radiograph is the technique most often used to define OA for epidemiological or clinical research purposes, in part because of the absence of clear clinical criteria for definition (Watt and Doherty 2003; Dieppe and Lohmander 2005). OA can occur in any synovial joint in the body, although the only frequently affected sites are the spinal apophyseal joints, the interphalangeal joints of the hands, the knees and hips. Hip and knee OA are frequent causes of severe pain and disability and account for some 85% of the huge burden of need for total joint replacement (Petersson 1996; Jones, Beaupre *et al.* 2005). The joint distribution of OA has been explained in evolutionary terms; the most frequently affected joint sites being those that are not well designed for the change from primate usage to the upright posture and prehensile grip (Lim *et al.* 1995).

Although there are no clinical criteria for the diagnosis of OA, there are agreed characteristic clinical features (Altman 1991). These include use-related joint pain, short-lasting stiffness or 'gelling' of joints after inactivity, a reduced range of movement with pain at the end range, firm swellings at the joint margins and audible or palpable crepitus (a crackling or grating feeling or sound in the joints) on movement.

The pathogenesis of the condition remains ill understood and is beyond the scope of this chapter; interested readers are referred to recent comprehensive texts (Hascall and Kuettner 2002; Brandt *et al.* 2003). In brief, OA appears to be a condition caused by abnormal biomechanics and mediated by changes in the normal turnover of connective tissue components (Figure 5.3). The current thinking is that subtle abnormalities of joint loading trigger a process of dysregulation of the balance of synthesis and degradation of matrix components of the articular cartilage and subchondral bone, such as proteoglycans and collagens, leading to loss of volume of cartilage and bone remodelling. Thus OA can be regarded as the response of the joint to abnormal loading, and an attempted, albeit aberrant, repair response of the joint. This response causes pain and can sensitise the joint to pain on normal joint use. The disease process is quite often 'successful', in the sense that it can contain the mechanical abnormality, resulting in a stable, but abnormal joint. However, as pain sensitisation may have occurred during the phase in which joint anatomy is changing, pain can continue even if the disease process is no longer active. In some cases, joint damage may continue unchecked leading to severe joint destruction.

5.3.2 Incidence and prevalence of OA

OA is common in all parts of the world and is known to have been common throughout history (Rogers and Dieppe 2003). Its strong age relationship means that most older people in the developed world will have acquired OA in some of their joints before death. There are, however, differences in the incidence and prevalence of the disease in different age, sex and ethnic groups. The ethnic differences have not been fully described, although knee OA appears to be particularly common in black Americans, and hip OA relatively uncommon in Chinese people, perhaps due to subtle differences in pelvic anatomy (Nevitt *et al.* 2000). Reliable incidence figures are also hard to come by, but the prevalence of OA in different joints is well described by age and sex in Caucasians (van Saase *et al.* 1989).

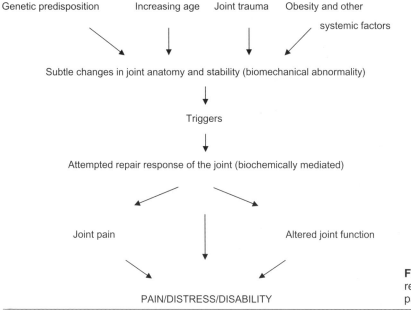

Figure 5.3: Schematic representation of the pathogenesis of osteoarthritis.

5.3.3 Risk factors for OA

The main risk factors for OA include increasing age, sex, genetic predisposition, joint trauma, certain forms of repetitive activity and obesity (Felson *et al.* 2000) (Figure 5.3). However, the balance of risk factors varies according to joint site. For example, symptomatic OA of the hand and knee is much more frequent in women than in men, but for hip OA the sex ratio is roughly equal. A generalised form of the disease has been described, and this is thought to have a particularly strong genetic predisposition (Kellgren and Moore 1952).

5.3.3.1 Age as a risk factor for OA

OA is unheard of in childhood, infrequent in early adulthood and practically universal in older people. Age itself produces changes in joints, including thinning of articular cartilage and reduced joint movement. The literature contains extensive discussion of the link between 'pure' age-related change and the 'disease' osteoarthritis (Loeser and Shakoor 2003). However, it is now clear that the biochemical changes that characterise the older joint are fundamentally different from those of OA, and it has been calculated that people might have to live to the age of 200 or more before age-related changes alone would lead to the sort of damage seen in a joint with established OA.

5.3.3.2 Obesity and the risk of OA

Obesity is a strong risk factor for OA, particularly of the knee. Females with severe obesity have an approximately nine times increased risk of getting knee OA (Cooper *et al.* 1994). The most obvious explanation for this would be that obesity results in excess mechanical loading of the joint, and this is likely to be part of the explanation (McAlindon and Biggee 2005). But this is probably only part of the story. Obesity has relatively little effect on the risk of hip OA, but is a major risk factor for hand and wrist OA (Carmen *et al.* 1994). The association between obesity and OA may be mediated in part through systemic factors such as altered oestrogen, lipid or leptin metabolism and the effects of this on connective tissue turnover.

5.3.3.3 Other nutritional factors as risk factors for OA

There is much current interest in the fetal origins of disease. It has recently been suggested that OA, although a disease of older people, may have its origins in maternal and fetal nutrition, through 'programming' of connective tissue turnover and the response of the tissues to mechanical insults (Sayer *et al.* 2003).

The associated concept that chronic diseases of later life, like osteoarthritis, might result in part from lifelong exposures to environmental factors, including diet, with that exposure beginning to confer risk from time spent *in utero* is intriguing, but very difficult to research. Clearly, lifelong nutrition could be important: for example, peak bone mass in early adulthood, which is partly dependent on diet (see Chapter 4, Section 4.2), is a strong predictor of subsequent age-related osteoporosis. Similarly, it is possible that the final shape of the joints, the characteristics of subchondral bone and the thickness of articular cartilage achieved at the point of skeletal maturity, could all be dictated by diet and be of importance to the pathogenesis of OA. All these features could depend on both nutrition and exercise, although there is as yet no good evidence to support such hypotheses. Finally, there is indirect experimental and epidemiological evidence to suggest that deficiencies of vitamins C, D or E and minerals such as selenium could be a risk factor for the development of OA (McAlindon and Biggee 2005).

5.3.4 Incident OA and progressive OA

Although most people will develop OA in at least some joints if they live to the age of 65 or over, far fewer will get severe joint damage or be in need of a joint replacement. For example, while some 20% of those over 65 have radiographic knee OA it has been estimated that only some 2% will ever need a total knee replacement. In other words, most people get the condition, but in the majority it does not progress to cause severe problems.

There are some data to suggest that the risk factors for incident and progressive disease are different. For example, Cooper and colleagues (2000), examining data from a community cohort in the south-west of England, found that while the classic risk factors for OA (age, obesity, Heberden's nodes as a proxy for genetic predisposition and selected activities) all influenced incident disease at the knee joint, only obesity was a risk factor for radiographic progression. Similarly, Zhang and colleagues (2000) found that incident and progressive radiographic changes had different risk factors, suggesting that osteoporosis might be a negative risk factor for incident OA but a positive risk factor for progressive changes. Very little is known about the possible influence of nutritional factors, other than obesity, on OA progression, but it is possible that the link to vitamin D, which might be mediated by bone metabolic changes, may influence progression rather than incidence.

5.3.5 Clinical features of OA

The main clinical problems associated with OA are pain and physical disability. The severity of joint damage has some influence on the degree of pain and disability, but many other factors are also important. If the association between joint damage and symptoms was good, research energy could be directed at the prevention or treatment of joint damage, and if there was no association, there would be no need to worry about joint damage at all. The 'problem' with OA is that the association is partial. This means that, for the purposes of this discussion, we need to consider whether pain and disability might have nutritional determinants that are separate from those related to OA, when defined as a pathological entity.

5.3.6 Joint pain in older people

The high prevalence of joint pain in older people has already been mentioned (Elliott *et al.* 1999). Most of this pain is localised (the neck, back, shoulder and knee being the commonest sites), and OA is the usual label given to an older person complaining of localised joint pain. But in many people it is more generalised, in which case 'fibromyalgia' or a systemic condition like hypothyroidism might be diagnosed.

The main pathological changes of OA centre on the articular cartilage. This is a tissue without nerve endings, blood or lymphatic vessels, which cannot generate pain directly. The nocioceptive drive to pain (direct stimulation of receptors in and around joints) must come from other tissues, such as subchondrial bone, synovium, capsule or periarticular tissues (Felson 2005). This may explain why OA is not necessarily painful. Many investigators have explored the relationship between radiographic evidence of OA in a particular joint site and the presence or absence of pain. The seminal observation was made by Lawrence and colleagues (1966), based on a community cohort in the Manchester area. They found that while radiographic changes clearly made pain more likely, there were large numbers of people in the community with severe radiographic changes but no pain. This observation has been corroborated and extended by others, including Creamer and colleagues (1999), who suggest that any degree of joint damage predisposes to pain, but is not a sufficient cause for it; however, that the degree of joint damage has little or no effect on the likelihood or severity of pain. Other factors associated with localised joint pain include depression, anxiety and social isolation.

Recent work by at least four groups (Farrell *et al.* 2000; Bajaj *et al.* 2001; Kidd *et al.* 2004; Oderberg 2004) suggests that one of the main mechanisms of joint pain in older people might be pain sensitisation (where the pain message gets amplified and distorted, resulting in a painful condition that is severe and out of proportion to the disease or original injury). These findings suggest that OA pain might be caused through the pathology predisposing some people to local pain sensitisation, leading to a situation in which normal joint use becomes painful in those individuals (Kidd *et al.* 2004; Oderberg 2004; Dieppe and Lohmander 2005). If this were the case, then those in pain would perhaps remain in pain even if the OA process was quiet and non-progressive, whereas in other cases progressive joint damage remains asymptomatic because in that individual the changes have not led to pain sensitisation.

Age is clearly a risk factor for painful OA. Currently, there are no data that distinguish between dietary (or other) risk factors for joint pain and from those that predispose to joint damage. However, it is conceivable that nutrition might affect pain independently of joint damage. Perhaps age or nutritionally-related changes to the peripheral and central nervous system are as important as factors directly affecting the joint when it comes to pain, as opposed to joint damage.

5.3.7 Musculoskeletal disability in older people

The common impairments associated with OA of the hip or knee are difficulties with locomotion, particularly problems with walking and step/stair climbing, and in getting in and out of a low chair and on and off the toilet. Upper limb joint OA can lead to problems with reach, grip and manual dexterity.

Pain is one of the main determinants of physical disability in people with OA, but many other factors are also involved. The extent of 'disability' is in part a consequence of impairment, but it is also influenced by other factors such as the degree of motivation and degree of need (*e.g.* presence of carers), so psychological factors are *de facto* associated with disability (Nusselder *et al.* 2005). In addition, muscle strength is very important. Recent data suggest that muscle weakness may predispose to the development of OA (Slemenda *et al.* 1997). It is also an important consequence of the condition; joint pain and immobility lead to localised muscle-wasting and consequent weakness. For these reasons, age-related sarcopaenia is of major relevance to OA and to the joint problems and disability experienced by older people.

Therefore, just as the effect of nutritional factors on the immune response (see Chapter 11, Section 11.8 and Chapter 14, Section 14.3.9) may affect inflammatory arthropathies, the effects of nutritional factors on muscle (see Chapter 6 and Chapter 14, Section 14.3.4) may be important determinants of both the cause and effects of osteoarthritis.

5.3.8 The prevention and treatment of OA

OA is a major public health problem. Its prevalence is increasing fast in the developed and developing world, due in part to longer lifespans, as well as to the increase in obesity. A recent World Health Organization/World Bank report suggested that it would soon become the world's fourth most important cause of disability (Murray and Lopez 1996). Prevention and treatment are therefore of great importance.

5.3.8.1 Prevention

Epidemiologists look for the effect size of modifiable risk factors. The most obvious one for OA is obesity, and it has been estimated that 20–30% of knee OA would be prevented if severe obesity were avoided (Felson and Zhang 1998). Joint injury is another potentially preventable risk factor; as with obesity, the prevalence of significant injuries, such as knee cruciate ligament rupture, appears to be increasing rather than decreasing (as we take more skiing holidays, for example). It has also been suggested that more regular exercise to keep muscles strong and increase joint usage might help prevent OA, as muscle weakness (see Chapter 6) may be a cause as well as an effect of OA (Slemenda *et al.* 1997), and in the light of the hypothesis that under-use rather than over-use of joints might predispose to OA (Alexander 2004). However, there is no direct evidence to support this hypothesis, and such data would be very difficult to obtain. The other major risk factors for OA – age and genetic predisposition – are, of course, unlikely to be modifiable.

Dieppe and Brandt (2003) suggest that the prospects for prevention of OA were poor in our culture, because it would require major changes in behaviour of the type that we seem unprepared to consider (less obesity, less risk of joint injury and more general physical activity) and do not know how to implement.

5.3.8.2 Principles of OA management

The principles of OA management have been reviewed in several publications (Brandt *et al.* 2003; Dieppe and Brandt 2003; Barnes and Edwards 2005; Dieppe and Lohmander 2005; Sarzi-Puttini *et al.* 2005), and a guideline from the National Institute for Health and Clinical Excellence (2008) in the UK. Most authorities believe that a pyramidal approach, of the sort illustrated in Figure 5.4, is appropriate.

However, the evidence base is weak for most interventions; and the effect sizes of individual types of treatment small (Dieppe and Lohmander 2005; Juni *et al.* 2006). As shown by Chard and colleagues (2000), only drugs have had detailed investigation, and it is clear that the pharmaceutical industry has an inappropriately large influence on research into the management of OA (Tallon *et al.* 2000), resulting in other interventions, such as physiotherapy, being under-used (Jordan *et al.* 2004). Furthermore, there are very few data on the effect of packages of care (combinations of different pharmaceutical and non-drug interventions), of the sort most com-

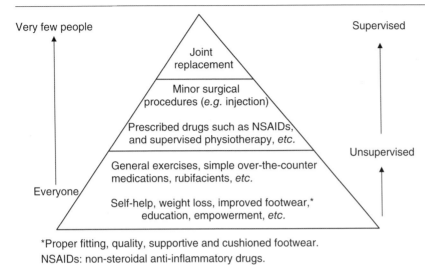

Very few people

Supervised

Unsupervised

Everyone

Joint replacement

Minor surgical procedures (*e.g.* injection)

Prescribed drugs such as NSAIDs, and supervised physiotherapy, *etc.*

General exercises, simple over-the-counter medications, rubifacients, *etc.*

Self-help, weight loss, improved footwear,* education, empowerment, *etc.*

*Proper fitting, quality, supportive and cushioned footwear.
NSAIDs: non-steroidal anti-inflammatory drugs.

Figure 5.4: The pyramidal approach to OA management. Everyone with symptomatic OA should be empowered to help themselves through education, appropriate dietary change (such as weight loss in the obese), footwear alterations and other walking aids, as necessary. Some will need supervised care from doctors or therapists, involving drugs or physical therapy, for example a few may need surgical interventions, such as joint replacement. Source: Dieppe and Lohmander (2005). Reproduced with permission from Elsevier.

monly used in routine practice (Dieppe and Brandt 2003).

Patients with pain, disability and distress attributable to OA need to be empowered to take some control over their own disease, rather than being over-prescribed with drugs. There is, therefore, a great need for sensible, evidence-based dietary advice, along with the use of exercise and safe complementary and alternative medicines, instead of drugs and surgery.

5.3.8.3 Nutrition and the treatment of OA

This subject has been reviewed by McAlindon and Biggee (2005). Jordan and colleagues (2004) have also surveyed patients in the UK to ascertain how much use they are making of the most common forms of dietary intervention used in OA, and to compare such utilisation with that of common drugs. They undertook a postal survey of 828 people with a diagnosis of knee OA ascertained from two general practice lists in southern England. Data on the use of the most commonly prescribed drugs and most often used nutritional supplements are shown in Table 5.3. It is clear that the use of glucosamine and cod-liver oil is extensive but, as outlined below, the evidence base to support their use is poor. Morelli and colleagues (2003) report that Americans spend more on natural remedies for OA (mostly dietary, including glucosamine, chondroitin and

Table 5.3: Estimate of the numbers of people with knee OA using different types of therapy

Number (%) of patients with symptomatic knee osteoarthritis using common drugs and dietary supplements in a UK survey:

Non-steroidal anti-inflammatory drugs	45.5%
Paracetamol	42.5%
Cod-liver oil	38.2%
Glucosamine	15.9%
Chondroitin	5.4%

Source: Jordan *et al.* (2004). Reproduced by permission of Oxford University Press.

s-adenosylmethionine) than for any other medical condition.

The two most commonly used dietary interventions in OA are 'diets', in other words attempts to lose weight, and the use of dietary supplements in an attempt to treat symptoms or the disease process. Most of the supplements used in OA are naturally occurring and are sometimes referred to as 'nutraceuticals'. They include glucosamine, chondroitin, vitamin supplements, avocado-soybean, cod-liver oil, s-adenosylmethionine and ginger extracts. Recent data on the efficacy of each of these interventions is summarised below.

Weight reduction: The strong association between obesity and knee OA has already been mentioned,

Table 5.4: The results of the 'ADAPT' (the Arthritis, Diet and Activity Promotion Trial), a randomised controlled trial of overweight patients with symptomatic knee OA

	Change from baseline at 18 months	
	Weight loss	Pain reduction*
Healthy lifestyle group (n = 78)	1.2%	1.23%
Diet only group (*n* = 82)	4.9%†	1.07%
Exercise only group (*n* = 80)	3.7%	0.40%
Diet and exercise group (n = 76)	**5.7%†**	**2.20%†**

The table shows the percentage reduction in weight and in self-reported pain over the 18 months, in each of the four groups within the trial. Although the changes are not large, taken in conjunction with the other data mentioned in the text, they suggest a dose–response effect of weight reduction on the symptoms of OA. *Self-reported using the Western Ontario and McMaster Universities Osteoarthritis Index with a scale of 0 (none)–4 (extreme). †$p < 0.05$ vs. healthy lifestyle. Source: Messier *et al.* (2004).

as has the fact that this is likely to be due, at least in part, to direct mechanical effects on the joint. Therefore, it is reasonable to assume that weight loss in obese people might help prevent OA. Whether or not weight loss might also reduce symptoms in those with established OA is less clear. However, recent trials suggest that it does.

Two recently published trials have concluded that weight loss reduces pain and disability in patients with knee OA. Messier and colleagues (2004) reported data from a trial comparing routine treatment with exercise alone or diet and exercise (Table 5.4). Those in the diet and exercise group had better outcomes than the other two groups. Christensen and colleagues (2005) compared the effects of two diets and found that those randomised to a low-energy diet resulting in rapid weight loss improved more than the comparative group.

Data from a further trial of weight loss has also been reported with positive outcomes (Miller *et al.* 2006), and in a recent, small study of the effect of bariatric surgery to achieve major weight reductions in the very obese, large improvements in joint pain were also seen (Hooper *et al.* 2007). As McAlindon

and Biggee (2005) point out, there are potential criticisms of the design and analysis of these studies, but the consistency of the outcomes is impressive.

Glucosamine and chondroitin: Data from Jordan and colleagues (2004) suggest that some 20% of people with OA in the UK are using glucosamine or chondroitin, although it is likely that this is now an under-estimate. Over recent years these products have had extensive media coverage and massive advertising campaigns to promote their use in the prevention and treatment of arthritis, in spite of a weak and largely negative evidence base.

There have been several trials of these agents, many of which have suggested that they reduce pain in people with established OA (mostly of the knee joint), and some of which even suggest that they might have a beneficial effect on radiographic changes (Reginster *et al.* 2001). However, these studies are fraught with difficulties. First, there are lots of different preparations and they may have different efficacy; second, there is strong evidence of publication bias and industrial bias: for example, all trials sponsored by the manufacturers of these agents are positive, whilst all independent trials are negative (Chard and Dieppe 2001). Further confusion is thrown into the field by the finding that when supplements of glucosamine are taken orally, the amount entering the blood or the joints is very small, casting doubt on the whole rationale for their use. Reichenbach and colleagues (2007) have recently carried out a meta-analysis of all large (>100 patients) trials of chondroitin, and found very little evidence for efficacy, and a recently published trial from the US failed to find any effects of glucosamine, chondroitin or a combination of the two (Clegg *et al.* 2006). Although controversy remains on the value of these agents, in our view, while relatively safe, they have little or no greater value than that of a placebo (Juni *et al.* 2006).

Cod-liver oil: Cod-liver oil supplements are among the most widely used dietary interventions by patients with OA (Jordan *et al.* 2004). But there is almost no rationale and very little evidence to support their use. There is a good rationale for the use of *n*-3 fatty acids in inflammatory arthritis, but OA is not primarily an inflammatory condition.

Only one trial testing the clinical efficacy of cod-liver oil in OA has been found (Stammers *et al.* 1992), and this randomised controlled trial of 86 patients found no effect whatsoever.

Avocado-soybean: Avocado-soybean unsaponifiables are oil extracts that have been shown to have a variety of effects on connective tissue metabolism and inflammation (Henrotin *et al.* 2003). They have been available on prescription in France for some years and have been used to treat a variety of diseases. There have been several trials of avocado-soybean extracts in OA. One systematic review (Ernst 2003) identified four high-quality trials, three of which suggested some modest symptomatic benefit from use of this dietary supplement in patients with hip or knee OA. However, the one longer-term trial showed no effect.

Vitamins: There has been interest in the possible value of vitamin C in OA for many years, the rationale being that antioxidants might help prevent age-related degeneration of joints. An observational study suggested that vitamin C deficiency might be a factor affecting the incidence or progression of OA, but there seem to have been no formal randomised clinical trials (McAlindon *et al.* 1996). Furthermore, a study in an animal model of OA suggested that vitamin C supplementation might paradoxically make the disease worse (Kraus *et al.* 2004).

Vitamin D has also been the subject of study in OA and its treatment, in view of the importance of bone in both the progression of structural changes and in the generation of pain (Dieppe 1999). Randomised controlled trials of the possible benefit (on both structure and symptoms) of vitamin D supplements in OA are currently underway in Europe and North America, but it will be some years before the data from these are available.

Ginger extracts: Two clinical trials of the effects of supplementing the diet with ginger extracts have been reported in patients with OA (Altman and Marcussen 2001; Wigler *et al.* 2003). Both indicated that there might be a small beneficial effect, but these trials were small.

S-adenosylmethionine: S-adenosylmethionine is the universal methyl donor for most methylation

reactions which has a variety of biological effects, including stabilisation of cell membranes. It is a food component which has been used in a number of situations, including in the treatment of OA. A systematic review by Soeken and colleagues (2002) suggests that it does result in a very small symptomatic benefit, but only two trials met the inclusion criteria for the meta-analysis that came to this conclusion.

Others: Perhaps as a result of the public belief in, and need for, dietary answers to arthritis, new dietary products are continually being tested and marketed. One example of a 'new entry' to the field is 'LitoZin', a supplement derived from the seeds and husks of rosehips (Warholm *et al.* 2003). The problem with this, and other products, is the paucity of either a good rationale for use or of large high-quality clinical trials to demonstrate its efficacy.

5.4 Conclusion

Nutrition is important in the development and maintenance of healthy bones, muscles and joints. It is likely that lifelong dietary exposures affect the chances of older people acquiring major problems with arthritis, but research to address this hypothesis and identify which dietary factors matter most is largely absent. Once arthritis has been diagnosed, be it an inflammatory form or osteoarthritis, diet can also affect symptoms and disease progression. This is an area of great public interest, surrounded by many myths, but relatively lacking in definitive evidence. However, there is good evidence to support at least two conclusions:

- Loss of weight by those who are obese will reduce the risk of acquiring osteoarthritis, and improve symptoms in those with the disease.
- Dietary supplementation with relatively large doses of long chain *n*-3 fatty acids is of value in reducing symptoms and inflammation in those with inflammatory arthropathies such as rheumatoid arthritis.

Many of the other commonly marketed dietary remedies, such as supplements of cod-liver oil, vitamins and glucosamine, are of doubtful value.

5.5 Key points

- Musculoskeletal pain and impairment are very common in older people; prevalence increases with age. This could be due to numerous age-related changes or result from the concomitant presence of several different diseases but is customarily attributed to joint disease (arthritis).
- Two main categories of arthritis exist: inflammatory arthropathies, such as rheumatoid arthritis (RA) and gout, and age-related conditions such as osteoarthritis (OA). Inflammatory forms are characterised by chronic inflammation of the synovial lining of the joint; their aetiology is complex, involving both genetic susceptibility and environmental factors.
- Many different dietary manipulations have been tried to either prevent, or treat, RA. While there is weak evidence to link high meat/protein diets, as well as those low in fish and fish oils, with an increased risk of acquiring RA, the data are conflicting and lacking in power. The bulk of the data and the most promising findings relate to the use of dietary fatty acid supplements to manipulate the inflammatory response in established arthritis. A recent review of 14 published randomised controlled trials concluded that there was evidence of a weak beneficial effect of fish oils (at levels of 2.7–4 g EPA and DHA/day).
- Gout is an inflammatory arthritis caused by crystals of uric acid. Obesity and alcohol intake, as well as diets rich in purines, are risk factors for this disease, and dietary manipulations to reduce them are a part of the disease management.
- In OA there are local areas of destruction and damage to the joint and related tissues, such as cartilage, which commonly affects the spine, hands, knees and hips. It is thought to be triggered by subtle abnormalities in joint loading.
- Risk factors for OA include increasing age and obesity, and genetics play a part. Weight reduction may be effective in reducing pain and disability in patients with knee OA, but the link with obesity is not simply mechanical loading; systemic factors such as oestrogen, lipid or leptin metabolism are also thought to be important.
- A wide range of dietary supplements are also commonly used by those with OA despite a paucity of good evidence demonstrating a beneficial effect.

5.6 Recommendations for future research

- Given the importance of arthritis in older people and the paucity of good evidence on how dietary factors influence risk, progression and symptom relief, there is an immediate need for much better studies to address this.
- Given the public's appetite for, and belief in, dietary modulation it is important that the scientific/medical community pushes for funding of better studies, if only to counter the claims of the commercial suppliers who may (wittingly or inadvertently) be selling ineffective products.
- Diet–gene interactions may be very important as small studies are almost certain to yield conflicting results because each 'sample' will contain different proportions of responders and non-responders. This needs to be addressed in research.

5.7 Key references

Goldberg RJ and Katz J (2007) A meta-analysis of the analgesic effects of omega-3 polyunsaturated fatty acid supplements for inflammatory joint pain. *Pain*, **129**, 210–23.

McAlindon TE (2006) Nutraceuticals: do they work and when should we use them? *Best Practice Res Clin in Rheumatology*, **20**, 99–115.

McAlindon TE, Biggee BA (2005) Nutritional factors and osteoarthritis: recent developments. *Current Opinion in Rheumatology*, **17**, 647–52.

Serra-Majam L, Roman B, Estruch R (2006) Scientific evidence of interventions using the Mediterranean diet: a systematic review. *Nutrition Review*, **64**, S27–47.

Stamp LK, James MJ, Cleland LG (2005) Diet and rheumatoid arthritis: a review of the literature. *Seminars in Arthritis & Rheumatism*, **35**, 77–94.

6
Healthy Ageing: Skeletal Muscle

6.1 Introduction

This chapter provides information, within a nutritional context, on the changes that occur with increasing maturity and ageing in the amount and composition of skeletal muscle, in its functions (both mechanical and metabolic), the mechanisms underlying some of these changes and the dietary implications and recommendations for the maintenance of mass and function (and thus independence and quality of life) during ageing. We discuss what we believe to be the most robust research findings, but have not been exhaustive in attempting to adjudicate between differing views, except where the topic is of particular importance.

6.2 Functions of skeletal muscle

The principal functions of skeletal muscle are to enable the body to move and to maintain posture, functions which depend on an adequate mass and appropriate composition of muscle and a properly functioning motor-control system. Muscle has an astonishingly diverse range of metabolic power output, being able to increase its metabolic rate from an almost quiescent state at rest by ~25-fold in terms of oxygen consumption and to increase its adenosine triphosphate (ATP) turnover, buffered by creatine phosphate, by many times more than this.

Muscle has other metabolic functions as a store of fuel (*e.g.* glycogen, used locally as an energy source or, after glycolysis and conversion to lactate, exported for use by the heart or brain for gluconeogenesis). Skeletal muscle is probably the most important tissue for glucose disposal in the body. This has important implications as the processes of glucose transport, glycogen synthesis and glucose oxidation all appear to be vulnerable to deterioration with ageing, resulting in hyperglycaemia and insulin resistance or insensitivity. Skeletal muscle fibres also contain triglyceride (so-called intramyocellular lipid [IMCL], to distinguish it from lipid in interstitial spaces), which appears to be a major source of fuel for muscle (Schrauwen-Hinderling *et al.* 2003). Together with the heart, skeletal muscle accounts for most of the fatty acid oxidation in the body and diminished or inefficient fatty acid oxidation is associated with glucose intolerance and insulin resistance. Muscle also contains the greatest mass of protein-bound amino acid in the body (more than 80%) and the processes of protein synthesis and breakdown which service this account for between a quarter and a half of all protein turnover in the body, depending on the state of feeding.

The protein mass of muscle (which some workers resist calling a 'store' because the constituent proteins all have other functions) acts as a reserve of amino acids which can be used elsewhere in the body for wound healing or, in the cases of the amino acid glutamine (which is mainly synthesised in muscle from glutamate and branched chain amino acids released from protein or delivered after meals), as a fuel for rapidly turning over cells, including those of the immune system. Glutamine also provides a substrate for nucleic acid base synthesis and is a source of ammonia for acid-base regulation. Also, branched chain amino acids function as fuels for the heart and muscle, though contributing no more than ~15% to the total fuel requirements during exercise. In addition, muscle is a factory, detoxifying the branched chain amino acids and in the process producing keto acids which are themselves used as fuel and synthesising glutamine and alanine, both of which are gluconeogenic precursors.

Thus, maintenance of an adequate skeletal mass is vitally important for the control of blood sugar as well as for fat and protein homeostasis. It is becoming apparent that skeletal muscle may also have a humoral role, in as much as it expresses the cytokine interleukin-6 (IL-6) which has autocrine and paracrine functions in muscle itself and may also have endocrine functions in influencing the metabolism of adipose tissue (see Chapter 13, Section 13.1).

6.3 Sarcopenia

The term sarcopenia was coined to describe age-related loss of skeletal muscle, but has since been adopted to describe muscle wasting occurring in a variety of chronic clinical conditions (Rosenberg 1997). Sarcopenia seems to be an inevitable consequence of ageing and affects both sexes and all races, although not necessarily to the same extent. Like most multifactorial physiological and pathophysiological processes, it is likely that about 50% of its origin is genetic and about 50% due to environmental factors. Although substantial progress has been made in identifying genetic factors important for longevity in fruit flies, round worms and rodents (Browner *et al.* 2004), the relevance of these to human ageing remains unclear; in particular the nature of the interaction between genetic and environmental factors is a crucial issue which remains to be teased out (see Chapter 2).

Whatever the causes, the effects of loss of muscle mass and alteration of its fibre type composition can have a dramatic effect on muscle function. Loss of strength and increased fatigue lead to an inability of older individuals to carry out simple tasks as effectively as younger persons do, a decline in body stability, particularly at the ankles, knees and hips, and thereby an increased risk of falls and fractures. These lead not only to a loss of quality of life and a threat to independence, but are also associated with substantial increases in morbidity and mortality (Janssen *et al.* 2004). The subsequent costs of sarcopenia have been calculated to be of the order of $18.5 billion in the US (Janssen *et al.* 2004), *i.e.* excess costs of ~$900 per individual (at 2003 prices). The costs are likely to be of the same order of magnitude in the UK, with hip fracture alone costing approximately £280 million per annum in the UK (Hollingworth *et al.* 1995).

6.3.1 Definition of sarcopenia and its prevalence

Ideally, diagnostic criteria should be based on knowledge of the distribution across all relevant ethnic populations of actual muscle mass, measured using techniques which are accurate, precise and reproducible – and if possible inexpensive and easily clinically applicable. A major problem is that no method measures the mass of active skeletal muscle cells *per se*; all use a model based on how much there is of, say, some structural component of muscle or product of muscle metabolism, such as phosphocreatine (see Table 6.1). The degree to which the model accurately reflects living muscle is variable with the best method, magnetic resonance imaging (MRI), having been validated against anatomical analysis of cadavers and shown to be associated with errors of as little as 2% (Engstrom *et al.* 1991; Mitsiopoulos *et al.* 1998). Computerised tomography, the next best method, seems to underestimate skeletal muscle mass, possibly by as much as 8% (Heymsfield *et al.* 2005).

Unfortunately, the usefulness of the validation is only as good as the 'gold standard' used. In the case of ageing muscle, the problems of a shift with age in the amount of the measured muscle surrogate (whether this is the longitudinal relaxation time of water protons or tissue electrical impedance), due to alterations in distribution of water between compartments, loss of cytoplasm and increase of extracellular matrix, inevitably affect the calculated muscle mass. The errors are likely to increase with age and to a greater extent in methods validated indirectly (*e.g.* impedance).

A further difficulty is that mass of muscle determined by whatever means does not necessarily predict *functional* muscle mass. Alterations in muscle fibre components (*e.g.* actin and myosin amounts and isoforms) and myofibre function or metabolic characteristics (*e.g.* creatine phosphate content or mitochondrial oxidative capacity) may not map onto pure mass measures.

MRI appears to be the technique most likely to produce accurate, sensitive and reproducible values, and it is safer than quantitative computer tomography (qCT) because of the lack of any radiation risk.

Table 6.1: Comparison of body composition measurement tools

	Benefits	Limitations
Magnetic resonance imaging (MRI)	• Gold standard (cadaveric anatomical validation) for accuracy and precision • No radiation exposure • Direct measurement of skeletal muscle mass is possible • Low field MRI (for limbs only) is near-perfect, much less expensive and easy to operate	• Expensive (~£300 per scan) due to high initial capital costs (~£200,000), maintenance and service costs (cryogenic gases in particular) • Highly trained technical staff required – no standard software for body composition analysis • Subject acceptability – noise and claustrophobia
Computer tomography (CT)	• Good precision and accuracy • Direct measurement of anatomical skeletal muscle mass is problematic • Routinely used in clinical practice	• Substantial radiation exposure • Expensive, but running costs less than MRI • Highly trained technical staff required – no standard software for body composition analysis
^{40}K – whole body potassium counting	• Good precision and accuracy for LBM and skeletal mass, validated against MRI and cadaveric analysis • Direct measurement of LBM • No radiation exposure (^{40}K occurs naturally within the body) • Subject-friendly – fasting is not required and there is no noise or movement by the scanner	• Dedicated facilities required (~30 centres worldwide) • Skeletal muscle mass is estimated using the ratio of total body potassium content to that in skeletal muscle – a relatively stable index in healthy adults, but not fully validated in wasting disorders
DXA	• Reasonable precision and accuracy (within 1.5 and 4% respectively for LBM) • Particularly useful for longitudinal change • Less expensive than MRI and CT (~£50 per scan) • Standard software for body composition analysis available • Minimal radiation exposure • Minimal operator training required	• High initial capital costs (£60,000) • LBM is determined indirectly based on adipose and bone mass and thus is affected by hydration status and intramyocellular fat • Skeletal muscle mass is not determined • No tomographic (*i.e.* cross-sectional) information
Bioelectrical impedance analysis (BIA)	• No radiation exposure • Portable • Inexpensive equipment • Minimal operator training required	• Poorer precision and accuracy • Very model-dependent – hydration status and pre-test exercise affects measurements • LBM over-estimation in obesity • Few validations in ageing population
Urinary excretion of 3-methylhistidine or creatinine	• Inexpensive • Home urine collections enable recruitment of house-bound subjects • In healthy subjects, predominantly measures muscle mass (contribution from gut, *etc.*, is small)	• Relies on subject compliance to meat-free diet and complete urinary collection for ≥72 hours • Insensitive measure (CV ~5% despite strict supervised subject compliance) • Inaccuracies amplified when body mass is low
Total body water by isotope dilution – deuterium oxide (D_2O) or $H_2{}^{18}O$	• Accuracy and precision of total body water estimates are reasonable (<1% and <4% respectively) • No radiation	• Expensive (isotope and analysis costs) • LBM is an estimate based on a constant distribution of water in LBM • $H_2{}^{18}O$ overestimates total body water by ~1%, as it can bind to non-exchangeable sites such as acidic amino acids, and D_2O by 5% as take up into lipid • Typical protocols take up to 6 h for complete equilibrium

CV: coefficient of variation; DXA: dual energy X-ray absorptiometry; LBM: lean body mass.

A disadvantage is that it is expensive (~£300 per investigation in most NHS establishments), although the development of fixed magnet low field (0.2 Tesla) scanners means that MRI is likely to be more widely used in future (Morse *et al.* 2005).

Dual energy X-ray absorptiometry (DXA) is a much more cost-effective approach (~£50 per investigation), but it is less useful in imaging muscle tissue than MRI partly because muscle is relatively X-ray transparent and complicated calculations need to be used to subtract for bone and fat masses; also intramyofibrillar fat, for example, is registered as muscle, hence the method's lower accuracy and precision. DXA has a further disadvantage in that it cannot be used tomographically *i.e.* no cross-sectional images can be produced, only integrated plan views of density of a volume. Furthermore, the errors for muscle or appendicular lean tissue are greater than for MRI.

The proponents of multiple frequency bioelectrical impedance analysis (BIA) have made substantial strides in answering criticism of its model dependence (Rubiano *et al.* 2000), but substantially greater imprecision and inaccuracy persist with this method in comparison with its rivals. Nevertheless, BIA has major advantages in being inexpensive, portable and easily applicable in epidemiological studies by relatively untrained staff.

Measurement of muscle mass on the basis of creatinine and 3-methylhistidine excretion (on the assumption that they are derived from muscle) demands a high degree of subject compliance to ensure adherence to a meat-free diet and complete 24 h urine collection. The validity of 3-methylhistidine as a marker is a problem when total body mass is low because of the persistent contribution of 3-methylhistidine produced from the skin and smooth muscle in the gut (Afting *et al.* 1981; Rennie and Millward 1983). Furthermore, creatinine, when used as a measure of muscle mass in the elderly, gives higher values than DXA or deuterated water dilution (Proctor *et al.* 1999).

Even in the US and Scandinavia, only relatively small numbers of the population (especially of sex- and ethnic-specific sub-groups) have been examined by any method and even fewer have been measured using near-'gold standard' methods such as MRI or qCT. It has been calculated that in order to construct percentile charts of muscle mass at five-year intervals that would be accurate and clinically useful, some 300–400 people of any particular group at each five-year point would be needed (Guo *et al.* 2000). The biggest sample size examined so far with a reliable method is of the order of 1800 individuals with a mean age of 74 years (Goodpaster *et al.* 2006). No diagnostic definitions presently include any consideration of the alterations in muscle fibre type composition, which is rarely assessed as a factor changing independently. There is thus a major gap, which for most developed and developing countries needs to be filled soon or we will not be able to judge what is 'normal' and what is aberrant as the current population changes its lifestyle and ages at a different rate from previous generations.

All of the current definitions of sarcopenia require a comparison of lean body mass or skeletal muscle mass of the subject under consideration with those of height- and weight-matched young adults. Some workers take two standard deviations below the mean as defining significant sarcopenia (Gallagher *et al.* 1997; Baumgartner *et al.* 1998). This results in estimates of prevalence of 13–24% for men and women aged 65–70 years and >50% in those aged 80 years and over.

Janssen *et al.* (2004) used assigned thresholds for both sexes in relation to the skeletal mass index ratio (*i.e.* lean body mass per height squared), a modification of body mass index. This is said to denote sarcopenia at values of 5.75 kg/m^2 for women and 8.5 kg/m^2 for men according to Janssen and co-workers, who identified these cut-offs for risk of disability using epidemiological data. The muscle mass of the limbs (the so-called appendicular lean tissue mass) (J.Z. Kim *et al.* 2002) has been used in relation to height squared (or more rationally to height alone, since this effectively removes height as a variable in the final quotient) to produce an index which is clinically useful.

6.3.2 Onset of sarcopenia

There is broad agreement from cross-sectional studies that diminution of muscle mass and function starts in the third decade of life, with the process accelerating markedly by the fifth decade (Larsson *et al.* 1979; Melton *et al.* 2000; Marcell 2003; Janssen *et al.* 2004) (Figure 6.1). However, the rate of decline is not clearly defined; researchers interpreting cross-sectional studies have obtained rates varying by an order of magnitude. Nevertheless, there is some

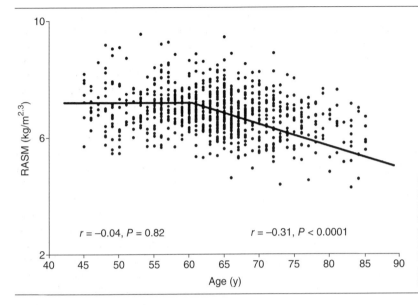

Figure 6.1: Relative appendicular skeletal muscle (RASM) mass index according to age in 845 men aged 45–85 years who belonged to the MINOS cohort.
Source: Szulc *et al.* (2004), by permission of the American Society for Nutrition.

consensus that the period of the fastest decline is from 60 years onwards at ~0.5–2% per year, depending on the muscle, its anatomical location and its fibre type composition (Frontera *et al.* 2000; Sehl and Yates 2001; Hughes *et al.* 2002; Visser *et al.* 2003). Loss of strength and power is reportedly up to three times that of mass (Goodpaster *et al.* 2006), with reports of 1–2% per annum in isometric strength but almost double this in leg extensor power (Jubrias *et al.* 1997). This may be due to selective loss of muscle components (*e.g.* speed of contraction), which is affected by the amount of actin and components of the sarcoplasmic reticulum, such as calcium pumps.

There are few longitudinal studies of either muscle mass or function, and many of those that do exist (Forbes 1999; Frontera *et al.* 2000; Gallagher *et al.* 2000; Hughes *et al.* 2002; Visser *et al.* 2003) suffer from small sample sizes and demonstrate great variability in the rates of loss of function and mass, possibly due in part to innate biological variability but also to differing degrees of habitual physical activity, nutritional state and independence in activities of daily living.

The Health ABC study cohort (Goodpaster *et al.* 2006) assessed body composition and strength changes in 1880 older men and women over a three-year period. Strength changes, in terms of isokinetic knee extension, were three times greater than losses of lean mass, which averaged 1% per annum. Racial differences in the rate of strength decline were also observed in this cohort in which over a third of participants were black: African Americans lost 28% more strength than their Caucasian counterparts, regardless of gender. Changes in body composition accounted for approximately 5% of these functional changes; a loss of 3% or more of baseline body-weight resulted in a greater decline in muscle function and mass, whereas weight gain yielded a slight improvement in lean mass but not strength.

A further longitudinal study of isokinetic strength of knee and elbow extensors and flexors, muscle mass, physical activity and health, originally examined in 120 subjects aged 46–78 years and re-examined after ~10 years in 68 women and 52 men, demonstrated more modest rates of decline in isokinetic strength, which averaged 1.4% per annum for knee extensors and 1.6% per decade for knee flexors in men and women (Hughes *et al.* 2001). Women demonstrated slower rates of decline in strength of elbow extensors and flexors (2% per decade) than men (12% per decade), and in older subjects the rate of decline was accelerated. In men, longitudinal rates of decline of leg muscle strength were approximately 60% greater than estimates predicted from a cross-sectional analysis in the same population.

The largest study of strength decline measured hand grip and involved over 8000 Japanese-

American men, of whom 3680 were followed up over an average of 27 years (Rantanen *et al.* 1998). Average annual grip strength decline was 1% per annum; although the rate of decline is dependent on age, greater age results in a more rapid decline in strength. Of note, strength was completely preserved throughout the follow-up period in 40 participants (1.1%). Nevertheless, another report concerning a much smaller group (Greig *et al.* 1993) (14 healthy physically active survivors of a group of people aged 79–89 years, first investigated eight years previously) suggested that muscle strength was well preserved: the median change in the strength of the stronger quadriceps was −0.3% per annum.

A further longitudinal study spanning 12 years (Frontera *et al.* 2000) revealed a reduction in the cross-sectional area (determined by CT) of the whole thigh (12.5%) and all thigh muscles (14.7%) – both extensors (16.1%) and flexors (14.9%); initial strength was an independent predictor of final strength. MR cross-sectional area data collected from 19 older men and 12 young controls (mean ages 73.8 years and 25.3 years respectively) suggests the decline is greater with a decrease in thigh volume of 25% and muscle cross-sectional area of 17% (Morse *et al.* 2005).

Risk factors for sarcopenia are listed in Table 6.2.

6.3.3 Sex differences

The prevalence of sarcopenia is greater in women than men but, puzzlingly, the rate of appendicular

Table 6.2: Risk factors for sarcopenia

Established risk factors
Advancing age
Low bodyweight
Physical inactivity
Female sex
Low birthweight
Impaired lower limb function
Co-morbidities: diabetes mellitus, rheumatoid arthritis, congestive cardiac failure, chronic obstructive pulmonary disease, malignancy, cirrhosis, renal disease

Possible risk factors
Smoking
Excessive alcohol intake
Stress – increased endogenous corticosteroid secretion
Chronic low-grade inflammation

(*i.e.* limb) muscle mass loss with age is said to be twice as great in men as in women, for reasons which are not entirely clear (Gallagher *et al.* 1997; Zamboni *et al.* 2003). Nevertheless, some workers (Bassey and Harries 1993; Lindle *et al.* 1997) report that appendicular muscle declines in *strength* (which should be almost directly related to muscle mass) at about 15% per decade in both sexes, which appears inconsistent with the greater rate of decline of muscle mass in men. However, Goodpaster *et al.* (2006) report a twofold greater decline in absolute strength in men compared with women, which is more in keeping with the changes seen in muscle mass, although individuals with preservation of body composition over the three-year study period also demonstrated strength decline, reiterating the importance of muscle quality. Despite these findings, there is a twofold greater prevalence of physical disability in women than in men, possibly reflecting the smaller peak muscle mass at the onset of sarcopenia in women (Janssen *et al.* 2004).

Hormonal differences between the sexes before the menopause clearly contribute to the ability to maintain muscle mass (see Chapter 13, Sections 13.2.6 and 13.3.6). Although the concept of the andropause has been severely criticised, there is no doubt that production of testosterone diminishes with age in men (Harman *et al.* 2001) and hypogonadism and low testosterone production are associated with a greater risk of sarcopenia in older men (Szulc *et al.* 2004). Nevertheless, testosterone replacement therapy appears to have only a small effect in significantly hypogonadal men (Wittert *et al.* 2003). In women, the decline of muscle mass is greatest after the menopause, possibly because oestradiol conversion to testosterone is diminished, accounting for the relative preservation of muscle mass with the use of hormone replacement therapy (Cauley *et al.* 1987; Greeves *et al.* 1997).

6.3.4 Impact of birthweight

There is emerging evidence that intrauterine influences affect muscle mass in later life. A positive correlation between birthweight and fat-free mass has been found in men and women living in geographically distinct areas within the UK (Gale *et al.* 2001; Sayer, Syddall, Dennison *et al.* 2004). Adult grip strength also shows a strong positive correlation with birthweight (Kuh *et al.* 2002; Sayer,

Syddall, Gilbody *et al.* 2004). Aside from genetic constraints, maternal age (less than 17 and above 35 years), poor nutrition (especially a low protein diet), smoking, alcohol consumption and parity all reduce birthweight in otherwise healthy pregnancies, and hence may play a role in modelling gestational muscle development, and thus setting future risk of sarcopenia.

6.3.5 Effects of co-morbidity and smoking

Muscle wasting due to ageing differs from that of illness in its rate of progression and possibly patho-physiology. Despite these disparities, periods of disease have a profound effect on total muscle bulk, which cannot be effectively restored on recupera-tion. Any condition associated with relative anorexia, low physical activity or inflammation increases the risk of muscle wasting and therefore chronic dis-eases: rheumatoid arthritis, congestive cardiac failure and chronic obstructive pulmonary disease are significant risk factors for sarcopenia (Poehlman *et al.* 1995; Kyle *et al.* 2002). The profound effects of chemotherapy and malignancy on muscle mass were confirmed from CT data of lung cancer patients

at post-mortem, which suggests a 75% prevalence of sarcopenia across all ages (Baracos 2005).

Smoking cessation has not been studied directly with regard to sarcopenia management, but a posi-tive association between smoking and low muscle mass has been described (Szulc *et al.* 2004). Further-more, smoking decreases oxidative capacity and increases type IIx fibre proportion in muscle (Orlander *et al.* 1979).

6.4 Muscle fibre type composition and ageing

The various muscle fibre types are listed in Table 6.3. Muscle fibre type composition depends in part on the anatomical location of the muscle. For example, muscles deeper within limbs and anti-gravity muscles (*e.g.* knee and hip extensors) contain more type I fibres, whereas muscles involved in kinetic move-ments and superficial muscles, such as the triceps or plantaris, usually contain more type II fibres. In addition, there is a substantial range of variability between individuals in fibre type distribution, in the range of 15–85% of a particular fibre type, which

Table 6.3: Overview of muscle fibre types

Myosin heavy chain	Contractile speed	Fibre cross-sectional area	Colour	Changes with ageing	Characteristics
Type I	Slow twitch	Small	Red	Proportional increase	Found in high proportions in anti-gravity muscles as they are resistant to fatigue and contraction velocities are slow. ATP generation capacity is great.
Type IIA	Fast twitch	Medium	Red	Proportional increase	Resistant to fatigue, although less so than type I fibres. Muscle contraction velocities are fast and fibres have moderate ATP generation properties, enabling prolonged anaerobic activity.
Type IIx	Fast twitch	Large	White	Proportional loss, mostly in proximal muscle groups	Good for short-lived anaerobic activity, found in high proportions in the upper limbs. Contraction velocities are fast, but fibres readily fatigue and have poor ATP generation capacities.

ATP: adenosine triphosphate.
Source: Adapted from Spangenburg and Booth (2003).

is mainly genetically determined (Simoneau and Bouchard 1995). Superimposed on this pattern are the effects of sustained dynamic physical activity so that low-intensity, repeated long-term exercise leads to phenotypic changes such that more type I myosin heavy chain proteins are expressed and repeated, high-intensity, fast movements lead to a greater expression of type II myosin.

It was generally accepted, as a result of work carried out over 25 years ago, that ageing was associated with a loss of type II muscle fibres, with the consequent functional sequelae overall of a diminution of muscle strength and speed of contraction resulting in a loss of power (Larsson *et al.* 1979) (Figure 6.2). This is now seen as oversimplified and there appear to be differences in fibre changes with anatomical site, the more distal muscles probably showing greater type II fibre atrophy than more proximal muscles in limbs. It is likely that there are also differences between men and women, for instance, marked atrophy of type II fibres is seen in the deltoid muscle of ageing women, but without significant change in muscle fibre type distribution compared with that in men, in whom the relative proportion of type IIb fibres reduces with ageing but without apparent atrophy (Fayet *et al.* 2001).

Whether the loss is neurogenic or myogenic remains controversial. With ageing, the apparently random, checkerboard distribution of muscle fibres of histochemically distinct types changes to one in which there is substantial fibre type grouping, with clusters of each fibre type appearing together

(Nygaard and Sanchez 1982; Lexell *et al.* 1986). The prevailing view of the underlying mechanism is of a process of denervation and re-innervation, in which motor units first become denervated through nerve damage (through whatever cause) followed by sprouting of neighbouring axons to develop collateral nerves which partially re-innervate contiguous fibres. Because a major influence on muscle fibre phenotype is the nature of the motor nerve activity it receives, re-innervation tends to reinforce the presence of muscle fibres of a particular type, supplied by previously damaged nerve(s). Thus, whether there is actually a reduction in fibres of a particular genotype or some phenotypic change remains controversial but certainly co-expression of myosin heavy chain types I and IIA appears to increase with fibre grouping in older people (Andersen *et al.* 1999).

The correct interpretation of data obtained using histochemistry is complicated by the alteration of the typography of muscle fibres, with type II fibres being more susceptible to compression or flattening than type I fibres, which tend to retain their hexagonal shape (Andersen 2003). Thus, any loss of fibre area will lead to a more apparent diminution of type II fibre areas. Reduction of fibre size also affects interpretation of capillary density changes with age. Some authors report a reduction in the ratio of capillary density to muscle fibre (Coggan *et al.* 1992; Frontera *et al.* 2000) (*i.e.* a change in the opposite direction to that which might be expected as type II fibres are lost), when in fact capillary density per

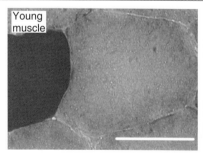 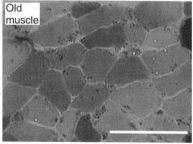

Figure 6.2: Muscle fibre changes with ageing. Young and old human skeletal muscle fibres with ATPase staining. Note retention of hexagonal shape with type I fibres (stained dark) and flattening of type II fibres (stained light). Bar represents 50 μm.
Source: Andersen (2003), by permission of Blackwell Publishing.

cross-section of muscle (not per muscle fibre) may actually be slightly increased (Andersen 2003).

Force generation is determined by the total number of active cross-bridges and the maximum force generated by muscle is independent of its muscle fibre composition (unlike the maximal power, which is greater for muscles containing faster muscle fibres). Also, force is substantially dependent on the orientation of muscle fibres, whether parallel to the main axis of the muscle, pennate (where the muscle fibres run diagonally over the length of the muscle) or bipennate (where the fibres have a herring bone pattern). The physiological cross-sectional area of the muscle is the muscle area multiplied by the cosine of the angle of pennation. As muscle fibre area diminishes, so the angle of pennation is reduced. This is demonstrated in older men where the angle of pennation is 13% and physiological cross-sectional area is 15% less than in younger counterparts (Kubo *et al.* 2003; Narici *et al.* 2003; Morse *et al.* 2005). Paradoxically this should *increase* the specific force per cross-sectional area of muscles, which may compensate to some extent for fibre area loss.

In some cases, neuropathic changes (almost certainly following inflammatory damage) may lead to marked damage of nerve and muscle fibres, with consequent rapid loss of muscle fibres, which in addition to the shrinkage of the fibre cross-sectional area may result in a further diminution in muscle size. Such changes occur rapidly (3–4% loss of cross-sectional area per day for type 1 and 2 fibres respectively) in patients who are critically ill, especially those with sepsis (Helliwell *et al.* 1998).

Other changes, beyond the scope of this chapter (*e.g.* alterations in patterns of motor unit recruitment, excitation-contraction coupling, alterations in the relative proportions of actin and myosin), may also contribute to the changes in muscle function with age.

It is not known to what extent the alteration in human muscle fibre composition during ageing is of functional importance for muscle metabolism. It has been long recognised that type I fibres are more oxidative and more dependent on blood-borne fuels than type II fibres (Essen *et al.* 1975), although the difference for some components such as glycogen is much less than it is in animal muscle (Gollnick *et al.* 1972). It has recently been shown that the rates of protein turnover in human muscles of different types are inconsequential biologically (at least in young adults), suggesting that fibre type has very little influence on muscle protein metabolism (Mittendorfer *et al.* 2005). Thus, loss of a particular fibre type is unlikely to impinge on protein metabolism in muscle or the whole body.

6.4.1 Muscle collagen

In rodents the extracellular matrix in muscle increases in amount with ageing, relative to the total muscle fibre mass (Kjaer 2004); thus, changes in the whole tissue may be exaggerated on a specific weight basis as the muscle tissue itself shrinks. Paradoxically, the collagen in older human beings, being less cross-linked than in younger subjects, may turn over more rapidly than in the young (Babraj *et al.* 2005). The prevalence of 'immature', possibly physically incompetent collagen fibres in the perimysium of muscle may predispose elderly muscle to increased damage on unaccustomed physical activity. Oddly, given the marked sensitivity of myocellular protein turnover to postprandial supply of amino acids and insulin, muscle collagen turnover seems to be insensitive to feeding (Babraj *et al.* 2005). It may be that the extracellular matrix size is under the control of the size and activity of muscle in a secondary fashion, mediated through muscle tension acting on fibroblasts. This would certainly tie muscle structure with function.

6.5 Proximal causes of age-related changes in skeletal muscle

6.5.1 Free radical theory of ageing

This theory, which first evolved in the 1950s, states that reactive oxygen species (ROS) generated as part of normal oxygen consumption by mitochondria cause damage to intracellular proteins, lipid and DNA, resulting over time in cellular dysfunction (Harman 1956) (see Chapter 2, Section 2.3). The effects of ROS are moderated by the scavenger enzyme superoxide dismutase (SOD); SOD overexpression by transgenic mutation in fruit flies and worms results in delayed ageing (Parkes *et al.* 1998; Tower 2000). In vertebrates life expectancy has been inversely correlated with free radical production from isolated mitochondria (Melov *et al.* 2000).

6.5.2 Mitochondrial damage theory

Most cells of skeletal muscle, heart and the central nervous system are post-mitotic, with the exception of a small number of stem cells in these tissues. Although these amitotic cells do not divide, they are capable of nuclear transcription and mRNA synthesis. Nevertheless, their genomic content is not necessarily stable because mitochondria, the numbers and composition of which are able to alter throughout life (most obviously in muscle), contain a small amount of circular DNA, inherited maternally, which codes for a number of mitochondrial proteins of great importance, such as cytochrome C oxidase and other electron transport chain proteins and associated proteins such as the F_1-sub-unit of the ATPase of the proton pump. Not all of the enzymes involved in mitochondrial metabolism are coded however, for in the mitochondrial genome and among the most important nuclear transcripts (which need to be transported into the mitochondria to allow successful metabolism) is a form of DNA polymerase which is almost entirely responsible for mitochondrial DNA (mtDNA) metabolism, including DNA synthesis and crucially, DNA repair.

There is now substantial evidence suggesting that in many animal tissues, from nematodes to human beings, ageing is associated with an accumulation of mitochondrial genomic defects, including point mutations and deletions (Linnane *et al.* 1989; Kovalenko *et al.* 1997; Ozawa 1998) (see Chapter 2, Section 2.3.3). The deletions inevitably result in the linearisation of the mitochondrial genome, although the total amount of mitochondrial DNA (mtDNA) lost is usually small. Nevertheless, electron transport chain damage results in leakage of ROS and further damage to mitochondrial proteins and DNA, completing a vicious circle; indeed accumulation of damaged proteins and linearised DNA is seen in ageing mitochondria.

The difficulty of assigning cause and effect in relation to mtDNA mutations has been recently clarified by an elegant study in which a modified subunit of DNA polymerase was 'knocked in' to mice, in order to test the hypothesis that loss of the DNA repair function in mitochondria would result in an increased rate of point mutation and deletion (Trifunovic *et al.* 2004). This did indeed occur early in the life of the mice (at ~25 weeks). Puzzlingly, however, although the total amount of mtDNA disruption was large, it did not increase over the shortened life of the affected animals. Nevertheless, they died at about 50% of the expected wild type lifespan (48 weeks instead of 90–100 weeks) and from 25 weeks onwards had substantial visible natural and functional defects such as alopecia, kyphosis, osteoporosis, reduced mobility and both sarcopenia and lipodystrophy. These gross changes are thought to be the results of mitochondrial dysfunction, especially in highly energetic tissues such as skin dermis, nerve, cardiac and skeletal muscle tissue.

Age-related functional deficits have been observed in some, but not all, studies of ageing mitochondria, lending support to the mitochondrial damage theory. Muscle mitochondrial oxidative enzymes are diminished, resulting in a reduction in fatty acid oxidation (Rasmussen *et al.* 2003) and ATP production (Trounce *et al.* 1989; Petersen *et al.* 2003). Mitochondrial protein synthesis is reportedly diminished in the middle-aged and elderly, resulting in diminished oxidative capacity (Rooyackers *et al.* 1996). This decrease in mitochondrial function with ageing appears to be relatively specific in that the decrement is greater than would be expected simply on the basis of loss of muscle mass.

A major effect of mitochondrial dysfunction is said to be an appropriately high generation of ROS and proton leakage, resulting in a diminution of ATP production in relation to electron input from mitochondrial metabolism. Leaked ROS and protons cause damage to a wide range of macromolecules, including enzymes, nucleic acids and membrane lipids within and beyond mitochondria, and thus are consistent with the inflammation theory of ageing as being proximal events triggering the production of pro-inflammatory cytokines. There is good evidence that ageing skeletal muscle is associated with decreased efficiency and capacity for ATP synthesis, the most robust coming from ^{13}C and proton NMR spectroscopic studies of young and older muscle (Petersen *et al.* 2003). But some workers have suggested that the deficits in mtDNA that can actually be seen in human beings are relatively small and most of the anabolic alterations are due to a lack of physical conditioning. In this context it is interesting that physical training, while having no apparent effect on amounts of DNA deletions in mitochondria, is associated with a decrease in the production of oxidised products of deoxyguanine, which can be measured in urine, indicating that

DNA damage as a whole (without specifically identifying damaged mtDNA) is less common in physically fit individuals (see Section 6.10 for more on the effects of physical activity).

6.5.3 Inflammation theory of ageing

Since it was first mooted, the inflammation theory of ageing has gained broad credence, with a substantial amount of experimental evidence in its favour gathered from studies in animal models, isolated cells and tissues, and physiological and clinical investigations in human beings. The idea is relatively simple: toxic materials of whatever source – and there is a substantial list of potential candidates (*i.e.* not just free radicals) – are thought to initiate pre-inflammatory changes in target tissues and in immune cells, as well as other contiguous target tissues such as vascular epithelium.

The major pro-inflammatory cytokines involved appear to be tumour necrosis factor-α (TNF-α) and interleukin-6 (IL-6) (Visser *et al.* 2002), although other pro-inflammatory cytokines, such as interleukin-1β, are also likely to be involved (see Chapter 11, Section 11.2.7).

TNFα and IL-6 have been implicated in a substantial number of cellular processes, either directly or indirectly, leading to alteration of nuclear transcription, both up- and down-regulation of signalling proteins, alteration of 26 S proteosome activity (some of which may be adaptive and some destructive) and other important cellular processes. In addition, manoeuvres that block pro-inflammatory cytokine action or production, or decrease their availability in some other way, such as control of hyperglycaemia and hyperlipoproteinaemia, are associated with improvements in muscle histological appearance and function, both mechanically and metabolically.

A number of workers have identified increases in pro-inflammatory cytokines (particularly TNFα and IL-6) in conditions associated with muscle wasting. Even in healthy older men the expression of NFκB (necrosis factor κB) protein and TNFα and IL-6 mRNA are elevated compared to values in the muscle of younger men (Cuthbertson *et al.* 2005). The ultimate cause of the inflammatory response is not understood, but hyperglycaemia, hyperlipidaemia, alteration of endothelial membrane function and production of pro-inflammatory agents appear

to be functionally linked. It may be that some of the changes derive from alterations in the production of ROS due to the dysfunction of muscle mitochondria. The difficulty is in deciding whether or not the changes seen in pro-inflammatory cytokine expression represent cause or effect. Certainly it is possible to associate increases in pro-inflammatory cytokines with metabolic disruptions such as hyperglycaemia, hyperlipidaemia, increased IMCL and associated disruption of cell structure and function. However, whether these associations are causative or correlative remains controversial.

6.6 Ageing and glucose metabolism

A reduction in the total amount of skeletal muscle will decrease the ability of the body to handle an exogenous glucose load adequately, potentially diverting more of the glucose, which would otherwise be oxidised, to fat and liver stores. In ageing, the effect on glucose metabolism of loss of muscle mass is exacerbated because muscle becomes insulin-resistant, with the development of insulin resistance of gluconeogenesis, hepatic glycogen synthesis and also lipolysis in adipose tissue. There is now a general acceptance that, even in individuals with few objective signs of glucose intolerance (*i.e.* fasting hyperglycaemia and elevated insulin/glucose ratios), there may nevertheless be incipient insulin resistance. Glucose disposal in skeletal muscle in older individuals is characterised by decreases in: amounts and requirements of the glucose transporter (GLUT 4), insulin receptors, glycogen synthase activity and glucose oxidation. It is well known that even a small amount of exercise (traditionally endurance exercise, but more recently resistance exercise) increases the storage capacity of skeletal muscle and the activities of GLUT 4 and glycogen synthase, which have been associated with increased glucose tolerance and decreased insulin resistance. The alterations in insulin resistance appear to be rapid, with a single strenuous bout of exercise being sufficient to increase insulin sensitivity in leg muscle and the effect disappearing within 48–72 hours (Wojtaszewski *et al.* 2002).

The causes of increased insulin resistance in the elderly remain a mystery. There is little doubt that there is a genetic propensity for inheritance of a range of metabolic abnormalities (the metabolic syndrome), among which glucose intolerance and type 2 diabetes are important characteristics. However, what causes insulin resistance in muscle itself remains a mystery. The accumulation of IMCL has been a favoured candidate for some years, and now that it is possible by the use of MRI to obtain much more sensitive and precise measurements of IMCL, it has been possible to show definitively that a high-fat diet can cause increases in IMCL associated with decreases in insulin action in muscle of sedentary individuals (Bachmann *et al.* 2001). Furthermore, good correlation has been observed between the IMCL concentration in human soleus, increasing age and glucose intolerance (Cree *et al.* 2004).

The fly in the ointment for this proposed aetiology of insulin resistance in skeletal muscle is the observation that endurance-trained athletes, who have been known for many years to increase their intramuscular stores of glycogen, also show increased stores of IMCL juxtaposed to the mitochondria (Goodpaster *et al.* 2001). In these individuals glucose tolerance is extremely good, with no sign of insulin resistance at rest or during exercise. This finding makes it impossible to link the presence of IMCL *per se* to insulin resistance and it may be that decreased capacity to liberate and oxidise free fatty acids from IMCL in the muscle of sedentary older subjects is more important than lipid accumulation *per se*. To what extent the type of lipid accumulated is important is not well understood, but there are indications that polyunsaturated fatty acids of the omega 3 (*n*-3) variety (but not *n*-6) may be relatively protective against insulin resistance (Haugaard *et al.* 2006) (see Chapter 13, Section 13.4.5 for further discussion).

It has been suggested that the proximal events in the development of insulin resistance actually occur in the liver, due to oxidative stress at the endoplasmic reticulum (Ozcan *et al.* 2004). The changes instituted here are said to be associated with alterations of insulin signalling, including changes to insulin receptor action. How these changes would cause alterations in skeletal muscle is unknown but it may be that adipokines released by the liver (and possibly more likely by adipose tissue) trigger the characteristic changes in muscle.

6.7 Protein turnover

6.7.1 Muscle protein synthesis

Most workers agree that age-related changes in whole body protein turnover are small and when data that show a low rate of whole body protein synthesis are normalised for fat-free mass, the age effect largely disappears, although some workers claim that there is an age-related decline of as much as 20% in whole body protein turnover in older subjects (Dorrens and Rennie 2003). Increases and decreases in muscle protein mass are mainly due to alterations in protein synthesis as a facilitative process, with only adaptive changes in muscle protein breakdown, except in circumstances where there is rapid loss of tissue (*e.g.* sepsis and burn injury), when breakdown appears to dramatically exceed synthesis, which may itself be elevated (Smith and Rennie 1996).

The idea that there is a reduction in basal muscle protein synthesis in older people has been proposed (Welle *et al.* 1995; Balagopal, Rooyackers *et al.* 1997; Hasten *et al.* 2000). However, others disagree, having found that basal muscle protein synthesis does not change significantly with age (Volpi *et al.* 2000). The Mayo Clinic group (Short *et al.* 2004) suggests that the age-related difference in mixed muscle protein synthesis is actually rather small and, although they claim statistical significance, it appears to be biologically rather small. There are occasional oddities and discrepancies in the published literature. Hasten *et al.* (2000) found a marked decrease in the synthetic rate of myosin heavy chain (MHC) by about 40% with ageing, but without any differences in mixed muscle protein or actin synthetic rates and Balagopal, Ljungqvist and Nair (1997) reported lower rates of synthesis of myosin heavy chain and mixed muscle protein, but sarcoplasmic synthetic rates were similar in the young and the elderly. There are many reasons why these discrepancies might exist – the relative frailty of the subjects, their state of physical fitness, the plane of preceding diet and the amount of dietary protein ingested in the previous 24 hours. The arguments put forward by Volpi and colleagues (2001) seem to be consistent with our measurements of muscle protein synthesis, in that there are no statistically significant differences between young subjects and older subjects in the basal state.

However, it may be that there are differences in the responsiveness to feeding. We know that muscle protein synthesis rates in human skeletal muscle increase as a result of feeding a mixed meal; hyperaminoacidaemia *per se* stimulates fractional protein synthesis and net muscle accretion (Bennet *et al.* 1990). Increasing amino acid availability certainly stimulates the net incorporation of amino acids into muscle protein in older individuals, although there is the rather paradoxical finding that muscle anabolism is blunted in older people during the intake of an amino acid/glucose mixture (Volpi *et al.* 2000).

Our group (Cuthbertson *et al.* 2005) has tackled this problem by investigating the dose responsiveness of skeletal muscle to oral essential amino acids (since muscle protein synthesis can be stimulated for a short period without the presence of the non-essential amino acids) and conducted the studies during an insulin clamp in order to exclude any effects of insulin on muscle protein synthesis. We found not only decreased responsiveness in total, but a decreased sensitivity in the relationship between muscle protein synthesis and oral amino acids (Figure 6.3). When the results were transformed to take into account the plasma amino acid concentrations, the differences were exacerbated. In other words, there appeared to be an anabolic resistance to amino acids in skeletal muscle in otherwise apparently healthy older men. These results were accompanied by decreases in both the amounts and the ability of exogenous amino acids to stimulate phosphorylation of the anabolic signalling pathways involving a cellular protein, mammalian target of rapamycin (mTOR), and the 70 kDa subunit of ribosomal s6 kinase (p70 s6 kinase) (see Kimball and Jefferson [2006] for more information on muscle signalling pathways). mTOR appears to be the key cellular protein involved in the recognition of amino acid availability. Through phosphorylation, mTOR activates downstream kinases involved in transcription initiation, including p70 s6 kinase, thereby enabling protein synthesis. These results suggest that, in older subjects, the ability to acquire muscle protein is likely to be less at a given availability of amino acids than in the young. These data are at variance with previously published studies in which no account was taken of possible differences in insulin availability between the young and the elderly.

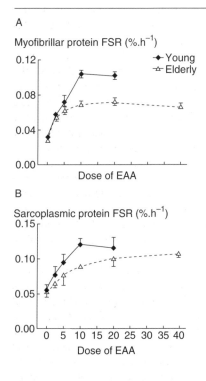

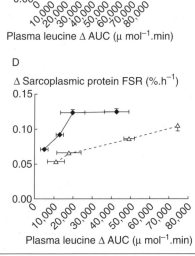

Figure 6.3: Muscle protein synthesis in young and elderly subjects.
Dose–response relationships between rates of protein synthesis in myofibrillar and sarcoplasmic protein and oral dose of essential amino acids (EAA; *A* and *B*) and plasma leucine availability expressed as area under the curve (AUC) (*C* and *D*) during insulin clamped studies in young and older men.
FSR: fractional synthesis ratio.
Source: Cuthbertson *et al.* (2005). Reproduced by permission of Elsevier.

The importance of insulin availability is debateable. It appears to have a permissive role in nutrient stimulation of protein synthesis in that a background low level is required, but hyperinsulinaemia causes no added increase in protein synthesis (Louard *et al.* 1992).

Despite early reports, growth hormone seems to have little anabolic effect on healthy adult human skeletal muscle (Rennie 2003). Indeed, growth hormone supplementation in older men and women had no effect whatsoever on muscle strength or fibre size, although myosin heavy chain characteristics switched from slow to fast (Lange *et al.* 2002).

Insulin-like growth factor (IGF-1) appears to be a key hormone in muscle signalling, acting in both a paracrine and endocrine manner. IGF-1 is expressed predominantly by liver tissue. The role of liver derived IGF-1 in muscle repair is unclear and production also occurs in skeletal muscle and other tissues, where (according to studies in animal muscle) it appears to have a very important role in proliferation of muscle cells via satellite cell activation, fibre type differentiation and muscle hypertrophy. However, the roles of IGF-1 in human muscle are much less clear and its possible modulatory effects in ageing muscle are undefined (Adamo and Farrar 2006).

IGF-1 receptor binding is impaired by both TNFα (often increased in ageing) and corticosteroids, further limiting possible activity. Testosterone can stimulate muscle growth in older men by mechanisms that include activation of IGF-1 mRNA transcription (Urban *et al.* 1995). Vitamin D can directly activate the IGF-1 receptor, presumably also stimulating muscle growth, suggesting a further cause of sarcopenia in vitamin D-deficient elderly (see Chapter 1, Section 1.6.2; Chapter 4, Section 4.2.3 and Chapter 14, Section 14.3.2 for more about vitamin D).

IGF-1 is also increased following administration of the steroid hormone dehydroepiandrosterone (DHEA), possibly accounting for its effects on muscle mass during resistance exercise. Plasma concentrations of DHEA and its sulphated forms (DHEAS) are markedly reduced with ageing, but replacement therapy in sedentary volunteers confers no benefit over placebo (Percheron *et al.* 2003; Villareal and Holloszy 2006). However, when combined with resistance exercise, DHEA therapy produced significant improvements in muscle strength and mass compared with placebo.

6.7.2 Muscle protein breakdown

The net accretion of protein depends on the balance between muscle protein breakdown and muscle protein synthesis. It has been shown that whole body protein breakdown (measured as rate of appearance of unlabelled amino acids) is less sensitive to the normal inhibitory effects of insulin in the elderly than in the young (Boirie *et al.* 2001; Guillet *et al.* 2004). It is not known to what extent the blunting of the insulin-mediated inhibition of whole body protein breakdown is due to changes in skeletal muscle mass, although this seems highly likely since skeletal muscle protein breakdown contributes about 50% of the whole body breakdown. The degree to which feeding alone stimulates muscle protein breakdown (*i.e.* without the confounding effect of circulating insulin available at postprandial concentrations) and the impact of age on this process are both unknown.

6.8 Implications for protein requirements

Our results suggest that, contrary to predictions that people require more protein as they get older, they would in fact be unable to utilise any increase and therefore the requirements would probably fall. This is in line with information obtained concerning postprandial protein utilisation (PPU), a concept developed by Millward (2000) specifically to describe the amount of food protein taken into tissues after meals. Investigation of young and old subjects showed no significant age effect, but the metabolic demand in older subjects was markedly reduced per kg bodyweight or per kg fat-free mass compared to the younger control subjects. With no change in the efficiency of protein utilisation but a decreased metabolic demand, the apparent protein requirements calculated from these values were substantially lower in the older subjects (Millward 2000), conflicting with the conclusions of other workers (Campbell *et al.* 2001).

Some workers have investigated the relative effects of delivering amino acids (as protein), either in a single meal (so-called pulse feeding in which 80% of the protein intake is given in a single meal) or as protein spread feeding, where the same daily intake is spread over four meals. In older women, protein pulse feeding apparently improved protein retention whereas in young women it did not, a puzzling finding (Arnal *et al.* 1999, 2000). Furthermore, feeding of a 'fast' protein (one which is digested and absorbed relatively easily, *e.g.* whey) appears to increase net protein retention in the elderly, whereas casein, a so-called 'slow' protein which results in the delivery of amino acids over a longer period, results in greater accretion in the young. In our view the dichotomy between whey and casein is a false one since most proteins are of the fast variety rather than exhibiting the characteristics of casein.

6.9 Caloric restriction

It has been known for many years that decreasing the dietary energy intake in a wide variety of animals, mostly those with a short lifespan, can increase longevity (Dirks and Leeuwenburgh 2006) (see Chapter 2, Section 2.5). The mechanisms underlying these undoubted effects are controversial but there has been much interest in a group of proteins, the sirtuins, which are induced by caloric restriction and appear to have a wide-ranging involvement in metabolism connected to energy generation (Haigis and Guarente 2006). Mammalian sirtuins, which are certainly present in the human body, seem (from animal studies) to be involved in stress resistance and adipogenesis, gluconeogenesis, and insulin and glucose homeostasis, and as such they are likely candidates for the proteins involved in regulation of cell and tissue maintenance/senescence. The obvious question is to what extent caloric restriction works in human beings. As Dirks and colleagues point out, there is almost no definitive evidence. Individuals who adopt a programme of self-denial and marked reduction of energy intake do show benefits in terms of better insulin action, reduction of risk factors for cardiovascular disease, *etc.*, but they also experience changes which may not be beneficial, such as decreased bone and muscle mass and attenuation of the hypothalamic pituitary axis. In a number of centres in the US, there are ongoing trials of individuals who have opted for a severely limited dietary intake but no long-term data are yet available.

6.10 The effects of physical activity/exercise

It is agreed that resistance exercise stimulates muscle protein synthesis in both the young and elderly. The effects of exercise on muscle protein synthesis have been reviewed by Rennie (2001). There appears to be no reason why older subjects may not increase the rate of muscle protein synthesis by exercise, with physical inactivity probably contributing to sarcopenia. Despite this, even individuals who continue to be physically active demonstrate decreases in functional ability and decreases in muscle mass (Roth *et al.* 2000). Veteran weightlifters, for example, show decreases in muscle protein mass at about the same rate as sedentary individuals, although because their peak muscle mass is so much greater they retain muscle strength for longer and suffer less disability (Pearson *et al.* 2002).

The optimal timing of nutrient intake after exercise may affect the extent of the muscle protein response and this has been shown in terms of both aerobic exercise and resistance exercise training. In both cases, the intake of protein-containing foods soon after the exercise resulted in a bigger anabolic response in muscle, one which was manifested following physical training by a greater increase in muscle cross-sectional area and muscle fibre area (Freyssenet *et al.* 1996; Esmarck *et al.* 2001; Andersen *et al.* 2005) (see Figure 6.4).

It is unlikely that physical activity increases muscle protein requirements. It is our view that there are no circumstances in which even strenuous endurance exercise, such as running, bicycling or swimming, increases protein oxidation to the extent that food eaten to cover energy requirements would not also supply sufficient protein to meet any increased requirements for amino acids used as fuel. This is not a popular view in the exercise community, but it seems to be based on good evidence (Rennie and Tipton 2000).

The UK Department of Health currently recommends that all adults, including older adults, undertake a minimum of 30 minutes of moderate activity at least five times a week, although benefit is also achieved by taking multiple shorter bouts of physical activity throughout the day, including lifestyle activities such as climbing stairs or brisk walking (see Chapter 14, Section 14.6). The latter approach often appeals to older people who may be required to limit the intensity of activities by cardiovascular and musculoskeletal problems, although a structured programme designed with these limitations in mind has the potential to develop capabilities and muscle strength. The literature is now replete with

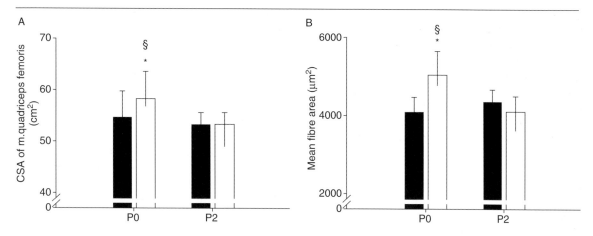

Figure 6.4: Changes in cross-sectional area (A) and mean fibre area (B) of quadriceps femoris. Baseline (filled bars) and post-training (open bars) measurements are given for both groups P0 and P2. P0 received an oral protein supplement immediately after each session of a 12-week resistance exercise programme, whereas in group P2 the supplement was withheld for two hours.
Source: Esmarck *et al.* (2001).

reports of the benefits of appropriate exercise (both resistance and endurance types) to older subjects.

6.11 Can nutraceuticals help maintain muscle mass?

In our view the evidence that secretagogues of growth hormone or so-called anabolic steroid precursors have any beneficial effect is almost non-existent. Giving individual amino acids in excess of their requirements to make protein appears to be an unlikely avenue for lean tissue maintenance since, for those amino acids which are rate-limited for protein synthesis, such as the branched chain amino acids and methionine, provision of excess simply results in their rapid transamination and catabolism. This makes sense because the branched chain amino acids are toxic in excess, as can be seen by the neurological problems observed in the diseases of amino acid metabolism such as maple syrup urine disease. Similar arguments can be applied to the aromatic amino acids. Recent rat data suggest that there is defective down-regulation of proteolysis after feeding in the elderly compared with the young and that leucine supplemented diets restored these defects (Combaret *et al.* 2005). Whether this is true for older humans remains to be seen.

The extent to which other supplements may be beneficial for muscle maintenance is difficult to confirm since most studies concerned with the use of the nutraceuticals have been aimed at lessening the effects of sepsis or inflammation. Certainly, there is some evidence that providing glutamine and arginine to patients with muscle wasting due to cancer (May *et al.* 2002) and HIV (Clark *et al.* 2000) and to older people (Hurson *et al.* 1995) may have some anabolic benefits, but it is unlikely that these translate into everyday life, in which most individuals are sufficiently supplied with glutamine and arginine from their diet.

The extent to which other nutraceutical compounds, such as α-lipoic acid, Coenzyme Q, soya derivatives (*e.g.* the emulsifier, lecithin; soya protein and oil) and polyphenols (found in tea, coffee, red fruits and in wine), have beneficial effects through their ROS scavenging activities is not known for skeletal muscle. Large prospective, randomised controlled trials of β-carotene and vitamin A have shown no benefits in lessening the progression of cancers through this scavenging mechanism (Omenn *et al.* 1996), but no data are available concerning muscle wasting. Creatine supplementation seems to have no beneficial effect on muscle wasting in old mice (Derave *et al.* 2005), but the evidence that creatine has acute effects on muscle protein metabolism in human beings, independent of its effects on muscle power, and thus on a greater propensity to train, is nonexistent (Louis *et al.* 2003a; 2003b). However, recently it was observed that creatine supplementation was able to promote the activation of satellite cells in human muscle during resistance training (Olsen *et al.* 2006). These effects may help explain the known increases in muscle mass enjoyed by strength trainers who take creatine supplements.

It seems likely that the influence of insulin resistance and obesity in development of the metabolic syndrome is substantial and therefore eating a diet which is low in saturated fatty acids and contains carbohydrate-rich foods with a low glycaemic index from an early age probably contributes to holding back the development of the metabolic syndrome and type 2 diabetes. The KANWU multi-centre study showed that switching from a diet rich in saturated fatty acids to one rich in monounsaturates for three months improved insulin sensitivity in healthy people (Vessby *et al.* 2001) but, so far as we are aware, no long-term prospective trials have taken place. There is evidence that vegetarians and vegans have better glucose tolerance (Goff *et al.* 2005; Valachovicova *et al.* 2006), something which resides in increased insulin sensitivity of muscle, but this may be associated with lifestyle in general rather than diet. In particular, there are no data on the relative success of particular diets and related lifestyle attributes in maintaining muscle mass during ageing. Many older people have low intakes and/or status of some minerals and vitamins (see Chapter 1, Section 1.6.2 and Chapter 14, Section 14.5.3) and the extent to which these deficits contribute to the decrease in the ability to maintain muscle mass is plausible but not explored in detail. There is a propensity towards zinc, magnesium, chromium, cobalamin and vitamin D deficiencies in patients with sarcopenia. Supplementation with zinc and magnesium yields improvements in muscle strength in individuals with deficiencies, but not in replete individuals. Early studies suggested chromium supplementation augments muscle hypertrophy, however further studies have now clearly refuted this (Lukaski 2000). Vitamin D supplementation, however, may well prove beneficial through IGF-1 receptor activation as described earlier (see Section 6.7.1).

6.12 Skeletal muscle spasms with progressive ageing

Skeletal muscle spasms occurring as nocturnal leg cramps are common in the elderly, regularly affecting a third of adults over 60 years of age with increasing frequency with progressive ageing (Naylor and Young 1994). These spasms are believed to result from spontaneous activation of anterior horn cells, triggering rapid contraction of motor units in the order of 300 times per second. Diuretics, beta agonists, steroids, opiates and statins (Thompson *et al.* 2003) are known precipitants in addition to a number of common medical conditions such as renal dysfunction (Tyler 1970), peripheral vascular disease (Abdulla *et al.* 1999), diabetes (Shuman 1953) and thyroid disease.

Electrolyte and hydration status, specifically calcium, magnesium and potassium depletion, can all directly cause uncontrolled muscle contraction and should be sought as explanations before exploring other treatments. Passive stretching of the calf muscles three times a day has been reported to reduce the frequency of nocturnal cramp (Daniell 1979), supporting the so called 'squatting hypothesis', *i.e.* that as use of chairs and modern toilets negate the need to squat, tendons shorten and muscles are inadequately stretched throughout the day (Sontag and Wanner 1988). However, a recent randomised controlled trial has found no benefit of stretching exercises over placebo (Coppin *et al.* 2005).

Pharmacological treatments for muscle spasms are generally poorly validated. Substantial claims have been made for quinine which reduces the motor end plate excitability (Man-Son-Hing *et al.* 1998), although side-effects are significant and include blindness, arrhythmias and death (Mandal *et al.* 1995). Small unconfirmed trials also suggest that naftidrofuryl oxalate (a vasodilator) and orphenadrine citrate (an anti-cholinergic) can reduce spasm symptoms (Butler *et al.* 2002).

6.13 Summary and recommendations

The imminent epidemic of sarcopenia will have a major effect on our ageing population with significant influence upon morbidity and mortality and subsequent knock on effects on resources needed to manage the care of the older population.

So far it is not possible to make more than general recommendations, limited to the following: take exercise, eat moderately and avoid mineral, vitamin and hormonal deficiencies. Vitamin D supplementation appears essential for at-risk populations, especially institutionalised older people who have limited exposure to natural sunlight, but studies are awaited to confirm any beneficial effect on muscle mass. Protein supplementation is not advised, as intake exceeds requirements for the majority of older individuals, but maintenance of a high protein/energy ratio makes sense; in practice this means reducing fat and carbohydrate without reducing protein intake. Regular structured exercise programmes targeted at older adults are likely to be very important in limiting sarcopenia by increasing lean tissue mass and strength and preserving function even in the tenth decade of life.

6.14 Key points

- Skeletal muscle is required for a diverse range of essential metabolic functions, in addition to the preservation of posture and mobility.
- Morbidity and mortality associated with sarcopenia affect a broad cross-section of older adults and are associated with a substantial economic cost to society. Actual prevalence and natural history are not clearly defined, but up to one quarter of the over 65 age group and more than half of the over 80 year olds are affected, with a greater incidence among women.
- Specific changes in muscle composition occur, specifically loss of type II fibres in proximal muscle groups and increase in type I collagen.
- Pro-inflammatory activation of the innate immune system, possibly triggered by mitochondrial DNA defects, has been put forward as the underlying cause of sarcopenia.

- Skeletal muscle demonstrates incipient insulin resistance with ageing even in individuals with no objective signs of glucose intolerance. There is some emerging evidence that *n*-3 polyunsaturates might have a protective effect.
- Anabolic triggers, such as protein-containing meals, are less effective in older individuals compared with young people.
- Protein requirements are not increased in older people.
- The benefits of regular (*i.e.* five times a week) exercise are not diminished in older muscle. Exercise also enables maintenance of muscle mass and function. The benefits may be maximised if followed immediately by a protein-containing meal.
- Vitamin and mineral deficiencies are associated with reduced muscle mass but supplementation *per se* is of no additional value.

6.15 Recommendations for future research

- Further information is required about the natural history of sarcopenia and the underlying pathophysiology of this condition.
- Large-scale longitudinal studies are warranted to establish the true rates of muscle wasting, with subset analysis of ethnic and socio-economic groups. Such a programme could identify further risk factors and confirm those currently hypothesised.
- Further research should clarify the cost/benefit ratios of exercise-based interventions. Supervised exercise programmes for the dependent elderly are associated with significant cost, particularly if domiciliary care is provided. However, social care resource savings, through hospital admissions avoided or shortened, and independent living, may substantially offset these costs.
- Basic molecular research is required to further elucidate the causes of reduced muscle anabolism in ageing in order to formulate alternative effective interventions.

6.16 Key references

Baumgartner R, Koehler K, Gallagher D, *et al.* (1998) Epidemiology of sarcopenia among the elderly in New Mexico. *American Journal of Epidemiology*, **147**, 755–63.

Cuthbertson D, Smith K, Babraj J, *et al.* (2005) Anabolic signaling deficits underlie amino acid resistance of wasting, aging muscle. *FASEB Journal*, **19**, 422–4.

Gallagher D, Visser M, De Meersman R, *et al.* (1997) Appendicular skeletal muscle mass: effects of age, gender, and ethnicity. *Journal of Applied Physiology*, **83**, 229–39.

Goodpaster B, Park S, Harris T, *et al.* (2006) The loss of skeletal muscle strength, mass, and quality in older adults: the health, aging and body composition study. *Journals of Gerontology Series A-Biological Sciences & Medical Sciences*, **61**, 1059–64.

Petersen K, Befroy D, Dufour S, *et al.* (2003) Mitochondrial dysfunction in the elderly: possible role in insulin resistance. *Science*, **300**, 1140–2.

7
Healthy Ageing: The Skin

7.1 Introduction

Skin is the most visible part of human anatomy and provides our barrier and defence to the outside world. It signals health and appearance to our fellow human beings and its quality and function are markedly influenced by the environment in which we live, as well as by our diet. The skin reflects to others information on our biological age and its appearance summates our lifetime exposure to sunlight. Humans are instinctively adept at recognising the features of age, colour, health and attractiveness based on skin appearance and it is possible in part to diagnose a range of nutritional deficiencies from the general condition of skin. In this chapter, we describe the structure and function of skin, including some of the *in vitro* models that may be used to study it experimentally, before describing the changes that occur in skin with ageing and response to sunlight. Finally, the chapter describes the effects of nutrition and how a modified diet can prevent and/or improve skin ageing and other aspects of skin condition.

7.2 Skin structure and function

7.2.1 Anatomy

Human skin is composed of two main tissues, a stratifying squamous epithelium called the epidermis overlying the supporting, collagen-rich dermis (Figure 7.1) (McGrath *et al.* 2004). The primary cell of the epidermis is the keratinocyte, which proliferates in the basal layer, differentiates and, as the keratinocytes mature and move towards the skin surface, gives rise to the stratified epithelium. Individual cells (squames) are shed continuously (desquamed) from the skin surface in a highly coordinated process requiring multiple protease activation in the uppermost epidermal layer, the stratum corneum (Elias 2005).

The dermis provides skin with almost all of its structural resilience. Collagens types I and III, which are the most abundant proteins by far comprising about 70% of the dermal protein dry weight, maintain the skin's structural integrity and resistance to gross mechanical force. The dermis may affect one's ageing parameters by giving skin a more youthful, firm demeanour and this can be influenced by dietary intake. Embedded in these two main skin tissues are the skin accessory structures (Figure 7.1), including hair follicles, the oil-generating sebaceous glands and thermoregulatory glands, the vascular system, nerve fibre network and specialist immune cells such as Langerhan and mast cells. The pigment-generating cells (melanocytes) are located in the basal epidermal cell layer and function by making either the dark eumelanin or reddish-yellow pheomelanin pigments. Two of the most noticeable changes as skin ages are alterations to pigment production (*e.g.* age spots) and the formation of wrinkles. Altered melanocyte function and reorganised, cross-linked highly structured collagen matrices directly drive these visible ageing changes respectively, but the primary cause of both is excessive lifetime exposure to sunlight. A layer of subcutaneous fat in which the deeper hair follicle bulbs reside is present underneath the dermis. Alterations in subcutaneous fat leading to fewer larger fat compartments give rise to the undesirable features of cellulite.

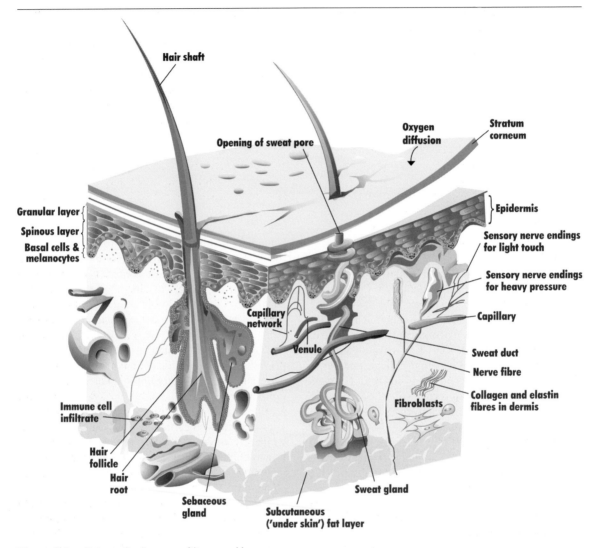

Figure 7.1:   Schematic diagram of human skin.

There is now substantial evidence that the skin contains epithelial stem cell niches located in the 'bulge' region of the hair follicle (Cotsarelis *et al.* 1990) responsible for regenerating the hair for the next hair growth cycle or after plucking, and in the epidermis in the deep rete ridges (Kaur 2006). The potential of skin-derived stem cells for autologous regenerative medicine is under investigation and initial animal studies show potential (Amoh *et al.* 2005).

7.2.2 Skin facts

The skin is generally considered the largest organ in the human body by weight (at least 3 kg for the average adult), covering an area of about 1.8 m^2. Over a lifetime, over 40 kg of squames are shed, equating to about 3–5 million squames each day. These appear eventually as grey dust in the vacuum cleaner, on the undusted shelf or the suspended flecks in a beam of sunlight. There are regional variations in skin type and quality, with the epidermis being thickest on the soles of the feet and palms of the hand, and the scalp containing the highest density of hair follicles.

7.2.3 Function

Without the barrier function of skin, animal life would be impossible on dry land. Accordingly, one of the most critical functions of the epidermis is the creation of a highly water impermeable barrier in the stratum corneum (Elias 2005). This barrier is highly effective in keeping water in to prevent desiccation and in keeping pathogens, chemical and physical materials out. The water-impermeable multi-lamellar lipids are located in the stratum corneum and are composed of three main non-polar lipid classes: fatty acids, cholesterol and ceramides (Elias 2005). Skin is unable to synthesise the longer chain *n*-6 fatty acids required for proper barrier function and desquamation, and the precursor to these, the so-called essential fatty acid (EFA) linoleic acid, must be supplied from the diet. Although human EFA deficiency is rare, in animal models it gives rise to a dry, scaly skin appearance, abnormal desquamation and a pronounced barrier defect (Bowser *et al.* 1985; Wright 1991; Elias 2005).

Components of both the adaptive and innate immune system function in skin (Clark and Kupper 2005). In the adaptive response for example, mild irritation is often accompanied by a neutrophil-rich inflammatory cell infiltrate and vasodilation as part of the cellular repair process. Allergic responses are often mediated by the activation and migration of epidermal Langerhan cells to lymph nodes. In contrast, sun exposure, specifically to the UVB component of sunlight, causes immunosuppression, perhaps to spare the skin from an overly destructive immune reaction. More recently the innate response of the immune system in skin has been better described. The skin is a source of several antimicrobial peptides which are up-regulated in response to both infection and UV irradiation. It has been suggested that the latter response may be to compensate for the down-regulation of the adaptive response to UVB. The most recent data have provided strong evidence that one antimicrobial peptide LL-37 with broad antimicrobial activity, is increased in human skin following acute UVB radiation most probably via a vitamin

D/vitamin D-receptor dependent pathway (Mallbris *et al.* 2005; Weber *et al.* 2005).

The nerve fibre network in skin (Reilly *et al.* 1997) mediates the transmission of the sensations of touch, temperature, pain, pleasure and itch to the brain. Each sensation is mediated by specific nerve fibre sub-types (see Scholz and Woolf 2002) and is integral to human experience. The nerve fibre network also mediates irritant skin reactions through the release of pro-inflammatory cytokines and the mediation of axon flare responses. Although these data are less clear-cut, dietary components may also impact the skin's inflammatory response to noxious stimuli.

7.3 Intermediate metabolism

Skin tissues engage in, and derive energy using, aerobic glycolysis. Despite the presence of oxygen there is preferential conversion of glucose to lactate via the glycolytic cycle (Krebs 1972; Philpott and Kealey 1991). This results in the production of substantial amounts of lactate, which is carried to the liver by the bloodstream and converted back to glucose (the Cori cycle). Skin tissues have a strong preference for the metabolism of glucose rather than fatty acids or ketone bodies, though alternative citric acid cycle intermediates such as glutamine are also actively utilised (Williams *et al.* 1993). Interestingly, of the relatively small amount of oxygen that is metabolised by skin the majority is supplied to the epidermis and upper dermis by diffusion from the atmosphere (Stucker *et al.* 2000).

As the majority of adenosine triphosphate (ATP) is generated by glycolysis in skin, the mitochondria may be less important for ATP generation, but they have a pivotal role in ageing effects (see Chapter 2, Section 2.3.3) (Wallace 1992). So-called common mitochondrial mutations accumulate in skin in response to repeated acute photodamage (Ray *et al.* 2000; Berneburg *et al.* 2004). Over time, the accumulation of mitochondria mutations may lead to altered cell function, including enhanced free radical leakage and aberrant signalling for apoptosis, but not necessarily non-melanoma cancers (Harbottle and Birch-Machin 2006).

7.4 Skin research models

Skin is a relatively easily sampled tissue and as a result multiple *in vitro* research models have been

Table 7.1: Examples of commonly used skin *in vitro* models suitable for human skin ageing research

Model	Cell type(s)	Ageing methods	Example measure of ageing	Example references
Single cells and co-cultures	Fibroblast Keratinocyte Melanocyte Dermal papilla Endothelial	UVA1/2; UVB radiation Oxidative stress (*e.g.* H_2O_2) including (non-physiological) atmospheric oxygen Passage number *in vitro* Age of donor Mixed young and old cells	Protein cross-links/AGE Collagen synthesis/MMP expression Growth factor receptor number Cytokine secretion Growth rate/mitogenesis DNA damage (*e.g.* 8-OHdG) Mitochondrial mutations β-Galactosidase expression Telomere shortening, telomerase Hayflick limit Cell senescence Differentiation and gain of function Loss of inductive functions	Lohwasser *et al.* (2006) Varani *et al.* (2001); Naru *et al.* (2005) Green *et al.* (1983) Ashcroft *et al.* (1997) Ashcroft *et al.* (1997) Dekker *et al.* (2005) Ray *et al.* (2000) Krishnan *et al.* (2004) Reviewed by Campisi (1998) de Magalhaes (2004) de Magalhaes (2004) Wlaschek *et al.* (2003) Alaluf *et al.*, (2000); Gharzi *et al.* (2003)
LSEs/nested collagen matrices (Grinnell *et al.* 2006)	Fibroblasts Keratinocytes Melanocytes	UVA1/2; UVB radiation Oxidative stress including (non-physiological) atmospheric oxygen Glycation of collagen	Apoptosis (TUNEL) 8-OHdG Glycation	Dekker *et al.* (2005) Dekker *et al.* (2005) Pageon and Asselineau (2005)
Organ culture and skin organoids	Tissue biopsies Hair follicles	Nutrient stress Oxidative stress including (non-physiological) atmospheric oxygen	Rate of hair growth Loss of inductive function UV radiation	Philpott *et al.* (1990) Gharzi *et al.* (2003) Corre *et al.* (2006)

AGE: advanced glycation end products; DNA: deoxyribonucleic acid; LSEs: living skin equivalents; MMP: matrix metalloproteinases; 8-OHdG: 8-hydroxy-2′deoyguanosine; TUNEL: terminal transferase-mediated dUTP nick-end labelling; UV: ultraviolet.

developed for its study and the evaluation of drugs and nutritional agents. A sample of models used for skin ageing research are summarised in Table 7.1.

7.5 Vitamin D and health

Uniquely, precursor vitamin D is made in skin, its synthesis requiring UVB radiation, most generally obtained from sun exposure. Photons from UVB radiation are absorbed by 7-dehydrocholesterol in skin converting it to previtamin D3 which is rapidly metabolised to vitamin D3. In turn, vitamin D3 is converted in the liver to 25-hydroxyvitamin D3 and in the kidney to the biologically active form 1,25-dihydroxyvitamin D3. Serum vitamin D, in the range of 33–80 ng/ml 25-hydroxyvitamin D, is considered essential for optimum health (Grant and Holick 2005) including for the prevention of rickets (Wharton and Bishop 2003), osteoporosis (see Chapter 4, Section 4.2.2.3 and Chapter 14, Section 14.3.2) and possibly a reduced risk of a range of autoimmune disease, cancers, type 1 diabetes and improved innate immune response (Holick 2004; Dixon *et al.* 2005; Grant and Holick 2005; Garland *et al.* 2006; Liu *et al.* 2006). Rickets, once thought to be a disease of the past, is reappearing (see Chapter 14, Section 14.5.3), with higher risk linked to darker, more pigmented skin tones, a more northerly latitude and lifestyles that lead to a minimal effective UVB exposure from the sun.

Recently, a vigorous debate has ensued about the merits of adequate sun exposure to make a sufficiency of vitamin D, compared to the risks arising from skin cancer from moderately increased sun exposure (Holick 2004; Grant and Holick 2005; news.bbc.co.uk/1/hi/health). For improved public health, the debate continues as to whether vitamin D is most effectively provided for population health by dietary recommendations (*e.g.* one portion of oily fish per week), fortification of staple foods such as milk and butter, dietary supplementation and/or recommendations for modest sun exposure. It has been roughly estimated that a sufficiency of vitamin D synthesis in skin can be provided by exposure of 40% of the body to 25% of the UVB MED (minimal erythemal dose) (Grant and Holick 2005). Concerns about staple food supplementation with vitamin D have centred on side-effects from excess vitamin D (hypervitaminosis). It is thought that sun exposure cannot lead to excessive vitamin D as additional sun exposure converts vitamin D_3 in skin to inactive derivatives such as lumisterol and tachysterol (Holick 2004). The reference nutrient intake (RNI) for vitamin D in the UK is stated as zero for 'a normal (outdoor) lifestyle' or $10 \, \mu g$ if 'confined indoors' (Wharton and Bishop 2003). Hence recommendations exist for dietary intake ($10 \, \mu g$/day) by older people. Similar recommendations exist for pregnant and lactating women, and a slightly lower recommendation for young children (Department of Health 1991). The latest UK evaluation of the safe upper levels for vitamins and minerals can be downloaded from the Food Standard Agency website (www.food.gov.uk/multimedia/webpage/vitandmin). Recently it has been reported that higher levels of vitamin D may be safer than originally thought (Hathcock *et al.* 2007).

Until the debate resolves on how best to improve public health through vitamin D supplementation, ensuring personal adequate dietary intake of this vitamin makes sense. Failing this, particularly in at-risk communities with more pigmented skin at higher latitudes, the benefit from the natural generation of adequate vitamin D via limited sun exposure during the midday hours has been considered by some to greatly outweigh any safety hazards (Holick 2004; Grant and Holick 2005).

7.6 Skin ageing

The skin as the outermost protective barrier of the body is exposed to numerous exogenous sources of environmental, oxidative stress. Many of these xenobiotic factors have been shown to directly induce key changes and modifications in the histological and physical properties of the skin. Factors such as ultraviolet irradiation, smoking, psychological stress, hormonal status, alcohol and caffeine consumption may all contribute to skin ageing. Hence the major structural and functional changes which occur with increasing age are usually broadly categorised as either intrinsic or extrinsic ageing (Jenkins 2002).

7.6.1 Skin ageing: clinical appearance and histology

Both sun-induced skin extrinsic ageing (photo-ageing) and intrinsic ageing are cumulative processes. Clinically, intrinsically, chronologically aged skin appears thinner and more evenly pigmented than photo-damaged skin, demonstrates fine lines and is often laxer and flaccid to touch (loss of elasticity). In comparison photo-aged skin is typically characterised by having mottled pigmentation, sallowness of colour, a rough, leathery, dry texture and coarse, deep wrinkles.

The major histological features of sun-protected, intrinsically aged skin include a thin epidermis, significant flattening of the dermal–epidermal junction (with loss of the rete pegs), thinning of the dermis and subcutaneous adipose layer and reduced numbers of keratinocytes, fibroblasts, Langerhan cells, mast cells and melanocytes. These changes impair the skin's response to environmental challenges and result in a decreased capacity to repair injury. In comparison, photo-aged skin typically has a thicker, trophic-like epidermis, flat epidermal–dermal junction, marked elastogenesis giving rise to elastosis and an increased inflammatory cell infiltrate including neutrophils and mast cells. The major structural changes in photo-aged skin giving rise to wrinkles (collagen reorganisation) and sallowness (elastosis) are largely localised in the dermal connective tissue (Scott and Green 2005). Although the histology of sun-protected and sun-exposed skin is different, many biological features are superimposed. For example, increased matrix metalloproteinase (MMP) activity and decreased collagen synthesis are typical changes which occur both in an intrinsically and extrinsically aged skin.

7.6.2 Skin ageing: mechanisms

The biological cause of intrinsic skin ageing is far less clear than that of extrinsic ageing. Numerous theories have been proposed to explain chronological ageing (see Chapter 2, Section 2.2) but one popular proposal, the free radical theory, states that reactive oxygen species are generated by oxidative metabolism and that radical mediated oxidative reactions (*e.g.* causing telomere shortening) (see Section 7.6.3) are the cause of cellular damage and progressive ageing (see Chapter 2, Section 2.3).

Upon exposure to UV radiation a primary initiator of the acute photo-damage cascade is the epidermal growth factor receptor (EGFR). Recent evidence suggests it is activated by tyrosine autophosphorylation in the absence of the EGF ligand. Autophosphorylation is stimulated by the oxidative inhibition of its cognate protein tyrosine phosphatase (Xu *et al.* 2006). Downstream events of EGFR activation include AP-1 stimulation leading to matrix metalloproteinases up-regulation, degradation of collagen and other major components of the dermal extracellular matrix. Transforming growth factor beta (TGF-β), a key regulatory cytokine, is inhibited, reducing both collagen type I and III synthesis (Massague 2000; Quan *et al.* 2005). TGF-β also inhibits the enzymes involved in the breakdown of collagen (Edward 1986). It is the accumulation of damaged, disorganised collagen and accumulated elastosis over years of exposure to ultraviolet radiation (UVR) that results in the clinical manifestations of photo-damage (Varani *et al.* 2002).

7.6.3 The role of telomeres in skin ageing

Telomeres are protein-DNA complexes at the ends of chromosomes which protect the ends from degradation and fusion and are essential for the stable maintenance of linear chromosomes (see Chapter 2, Section 2.3.2). They are central to cellular proliferative capacity and gene expression in the skin. When telomeres become critically shortened, skin cells may

enter proliferative senescence or change expression of genes in close proximity to the DNA terminus (Ning *et al.* 2003). The telomere overhang also provides a double helix loop that protects the chromosome from degradation (Griffith *et al.* 1999). Intrinsic skin ageing is strongly associated with progressive telomere shortening, the result of cumulative cell division (Sugimoto *et al.* 2006). However, in sun-exposed skin the impact of UVR exacerbates mean telomere loss (Wainwright *et al.* 1995) with significant telomere loop disruption (Li *et al.* 2003).

7.6.4 Neuroendocrine stress and skin ageing

Neuroendocrine stress resulting from everyday life occurrences has been shown to be a key driver of age-associated conditions (Bjorntorp 2002). There is evidence that the skin may be acting as a neuroendocrine organ in its own right. All the key elements controlling the activity of the hypothalamus–pituitary–adrenal (HPA) axis (the pathway responsible for the body's response to stress) are expressed in the skin (Slominski *et al.* 2000; Arck *et al.* 2006).

It is likely that not only is the skin acutely sensitive to environmental stress stimuli (such as ultraviolet irradiation), but also that the neuroendocrine components may be involved in the general control of skin function (*e.g.* pigmentation, itch, dryness, elasticity). Coupled with this, it appears likely that the 'local' HPA axis within the skin may become increasingly dysfunctional with age (Kappeler *et al.* 2003). Therefore, even in the absence of a highly stressful lifestyle, these neuroendocrinological changes will have a significant impact on skin and are likely to contribute to the typical characteristics of an aged skin appearance with time. An increased degree of stress may serve to exacerbate these responses and accelerate the rate of ageing (Wainwright *et al.* 2006).

7.6.5 Hormonal pathway interactions and skin ageing

Throughout adult life all physiological functions gradually decline. There is diminished capacity for protein synthesis, a decline in immune function, a loss of muscle mass and strength and decrease in bone mineral density. The quality of skin and hair also declines significantly. Changes in the endocrine system with age (see Chapter 13, Section 13.2), most notably involving oestrogen, testosterone, insulin/ IGF and thyroid hormone, are thought to contribute significantly to most of these events (Sator *et al.* 2004). All the cells present within the skin (keratinocytes, Langerhan cells, melanocytes, fibroblasts) are under hormonal influence.

The most dramatic and rapidly occurring change in women over 50 is the change in oestrogen levels. The effects of oestrogen on skin are well described (Hall and Phillips 2005). The fall in hormone levels at menopause induces numerous physiological changes in the skin, including a reduction in the biosynthesis of collagen and hyaluronic acid. It also affects secretion by the sebaceous glands. These changes lead to a decline in the quality of skin, leading to a loss of skin elasticity and strength and increased skin dryness (Shah and Maibach 2001). The cyclic production of oestrogen during the reproductive years is replaced by very low constant levels and results in the typical menopausal symptoms (Shah and Maibach 2001). Levels of serum total and free testosterone also gradually decline in males (Sternbach 1998).

Normal ageing is accompanied by a slight decrease in pituitary thyroid stimulating hormone (TSH) release and more importantly by a decreased peripheral degradation of the T_4 form of the thyroid hormone, which results in a gradual age-dependent decline in concentration of the T_3 form (triiodothyronine). T_3 is an important regulator of growth and development and affects virtually every system in the body, including cardiac function, bone density, weight gain and neuronal function (Leonhardt and Heymann 2002). Applied to skin, T_3 is proposed to accelerate cell proliferation and wound healing (Safer *et al.* 2005).

The adrenal secretion of dehydroepiandrosterone (DHEA) gradually decreases over time and this change has been causally related to many of the chronic diseases associated with ageing. For example, DHEA has been shown to be critically involved in wound healing and repair (Mills *et al.* 2005). Finally, the growth hormone (GH)/insulin-like-growth factor-1 (IGF-1) axis shows a gradual decline during ageing. The decrease in GH release by the pituitary gland causes a subsequent reduction in the production of IGF-1 by the liver and other organs, which has important effects on cellular growth and metabolism. Interestingly, the production of GH from the pituitary in the elderly can be restored to its youthful secretory capacity with GH-releasing peptides.

7.7 Nutritional influences on skin health

Hair follicles and the epidermis are tissues with high cell proliferation rates and require adequate amounts of protein, carbohydrate, oxygen and fats to fuel the high turnover of cells. The high dependency of skin on adequate nutrition is evidenced by the development of serious skin lesions in response to a variety of nutritional deficiencies (Roe 1986). Whilst the incidence of nutritional deficiencies is low in developed countries, unbalanced and incomplete diets, such as associated with modern lifestyles, could adversely affect health status and skin condition. Optimisation of the diet, therefore, will not only help prevent development of skin disorders but may be reasonably proposed to improve overall skin condition and skin appearance.

Information on nutrient intake in the UK may be obtained from the National Diet and Nutrition Survey for adults aged 19–64 years, with a summary available in downloadable format from the Foods Standard Agency (www.food.gov.uk). Cross-sectional studies support a relationship between human skin condition and nutrient concentrations in serum and diet (Boelsma *et al.* 2003), while the evidence for the skin bioavailability of dietary vitamin E, carotenoids, polyphenols, vitamin C, zinc and selenium has recently been comprehensively reviewed (Richelle *et al.* 2006). New insights into the relationship between food intake and skin health and ageing have been discovered (Boelsma *et al.* 2001; Cosgrove *et al.* 2007).

7.8 Vitamins essential for skin

7.8.1 Vitamin A (retinol)

Vitamin A is a member of the retinoid class of molecules and has three active forms: retinal, retinol and retinoic acid. Retinoids, including retinol and retinoic acid, are important signalling molecules in vertebrates and act to alter the transcriptional activation or repression of numerous genes (Mangelsdorf *et al.* 1994; Roos *et al.* 1998). Recognition of the importance of retinoids in dermatology dates back to the 1920s when abnormal keratinisation in vitamin A-deficient animals was described (Wolbach and Howe 1978). Retinoids exert profound pleiotropic effects in skin, affecting many aspects of cell differentiation and proliferation. In keratinocytes, retinoids induce proliferation, resulting in epidermal hyperplasia, and modulate epidermal differentiation. Dermal fibroblasts are also important target cells of retinoids and are stimulated to produce extracellular matrix proteins (Varani *et al.* 2000) and regulate MMP activation. Retinoids strongly influence pigmentation and can lighten hyper-pigmented skin in animals and humans. Certain retinoids, such as 13-cis-retinoic acid, also have a powerful sebo-suppressive effect through their effects on sebocyte differentiation. The retinoids have beneficial effects for acne, psoriasis, neoplastic processes, photo-aged skin and, most recently, reversal of extrinsically aged skin (Mayer *et al.* 1978; Griffiths *et al.* 1993; Kang *et al.* 2001a; Zouboulis 2001; Sardana and Sehgal 2003).

7.8.2 Vitamin C

Vitamin C is the predominant water-soluble antioxidant vitamin in skin and required for the correct maturation and repair of tissues. The effects of deficiency are well known partly because of its historical significance in relation to scurvy. Clinical manifestations of scurvy reflect the impaired synthesis and cross-linking of collagen. Early signs of the disease include bleeding of the gingiva and bleeding under the skin, causing tiny pinpoint bruises. The deficiency can progress to the point that it causes poor wound healing, anaemia and poor bone growth (Osler 1892; Englard and Seifter 1986). Vitamin C is important for the maintenance of connective tissues such as the dermal layer of skin and in the healing of wounds. This is primarily due to its role as a co-factor for the enzymes lysyl hydroxylase and prolyl hydroxylase, required for hydroxy lysine and hydroxy proline formation during collagen biosynthesis. Vitamin C has also been shown to promote collagen mRNA synthesis by fibroblasts (Pinnell 1985).

7.8.3 The B vitamins

The B vitamins required for optimal skin health include riboflavin (vitamin B_2), niacin (vitamin B_3) and pyridoxine (vitamin B_6).

Riboflavin is an important coenzyme in the conversion of carbohydrates, fats and proteins into energy and typically takes the form of flavin adenine dinucleotide (FAD) or flavin mononucleotide (FMN). It is important in the maintenance of the skin and mucous membranes and plays a crucial role in preventing cellular oxidative damage through its involvement in the recycling of glutathione, a key antioxidant molecule. A deficiency of riboflavin can cause skin disorders such as seborrhoeic dermatitis, characterised by red and scaling skin and dandruff on the scalp (Roe 1991; Lakshmi 1998).

Niacin (B_3) is required for energy production. Two unique forms of vitamin B_3 (NAD and NADP) are essential for conversion of the body's proteins, fats and carbohydrates into usable energy. The vitamin is needed for the maintenance of healthy skin and, like riboflavin, inhibits the oxidation of key cellular components such as DNA and cell membranes. It is essential for DNA synthesis, which is particularly important during epidermal turnover and is required for the synthesis of steroid hormones, essential for skin function. Vitamin B_3 deficiency causes the disease pellagra, characterised by severe dermatitis (inflamed cracked, scaly skin) and discoloured skin (Karthikeyan and Thappa 2002).

Pyridoxine (vitamin B_6) is needed to support cellular energy production and is involved in amino acid metabolism. DNA and phospholipid synthesis are dependent on vitamin B_6. It is an essential co-factor for cell renewal and, like riboflavin, is especially important for the healthy function of tissue that needs to regenerate itself quickly. Deficiency also adversely affects the maturation of newly formed collagen. For this reason, the skin is one of the first tissues to show problems when vitamin B_6 is deficient. Due to the abundance of pyridoxine in many foods, deficiency in the West is rare. Such deficiency when it occurs causes skin disorders including seborrhoeic dermatitis, with symptoms similar to those seen in riboflavin and niacin deficiencies (Prasad *et al.* 1983; Coburn *et al.* 2003).

Pyridoxine was originally referred to as the anti-dermatitis factor as skin inflammation (dermatitis) and eczema increased when foods with vitamin B_6 were eliminated from the diet. Topical vitamin B_6 creams are used to this day in treatment of skin inflammation, particularly to treat symptoms of seborrhoeic dermatitis.

7.8.4 Vitamin D

The role of this vitamin in skin and bone health is described in Section 7.5 and in Chapter 4, Section 4.2 and Chapter 14, Sections 14.3.2 and 14.3.5.

7.8.5 Vitamin E

Vitamin E is the predominant lipophilic antioxidant in skin, providing cellular protection against free radical damage. Given the well-recognised association between free radical damage and skin ageing, vitamin E is considered an important skin anti-ageing active and is included in many topical skin creams. It shows a characteristic concentration gradient in the skin, with levels decreasing towards the outer stratum corneum layers. Exposure of the skin to UV results in significant depletion of the vitamin (Thiele *et al.* 2005).

Deficiency of vitamin E leads to an increase in lipid peroxidation in skin, a key mediator of oxidative damage highlighting its importance as a skin antioxidant. The vitamin is most effective in conjunction with vitamin C, glutathione, selenium and niacin. Vitamin C is required to keep vitamin E in its metabolically active form; glutathione is required to keep vitamin C in its active form; and selenium and niacin (in the form of NADPH) are required to keep glutathione in its active form. This means that a diet high in vitamin E cannot have its optimal effect unless it is also rich in foods that provide these other nutrients (Packer and Valacchi 2002).

7.9 Nutrition, UV protection and skin ageing

Sun exposure, particularly acute episodes leading to sunburn, is the key cause later in life of photocarcinogenesis and photo-ageing. Accordingly, excessive sun exposure is recognised as a health issue throughout the life-course. In the US, about two-thirds of the cumulative erythemal UV dose/year occurs inadvertently, when no topical sun protection is used and not during periods of intentional sunbathing (Godar 2001; Godar *et al.* 2001). In addition, three-quarters of lifetime sun exposure is delivered during adulthood and old age (Godar *et al.* 2003). These factors argue strongly in favour of continual photo-protection throughout life. Fortunately, there is convincing evidence from *in vitro*

animal and human studies that dietary constituents can afford an important degree of endogenous photo-protection and may therefore be presumed to help reduce skin photo-ageing. Whilst the level of sun protection (measured as the sun protection factor; SPF) with an SPF 2–4 is considerably lower than that afforded by topical sun creams with an SPF of 5 → 50, over a lifetime dietary photo-protection is still expected to contribute very significantly to overall improved skin appearance.

The ability of a nutrient to provide systemic photo-protection requires it to have one or more of the following functions: prevent the absorption of UV light by skin, protect target molecules by acting as an antioxidant scavenger, induce cellular repair systems or suppress cellular responses such as inflammation. Some vitamins (*e.g.* C and E), carotenoids (see Section 7.9.1), minerals and *n*-3 polyunsaturated fatty acids have all been shown to provide photo-protective benefits and are believed to operate through one or more of the above mechanisms.

7.9.1 Carotenoids and UV protection

Carotenoids are plant pigments and function in the protection of the plant against excess light and are among the most efficient natural scavengers of singlet molecular oxygen (Stahl and Sies 1997). The major carotenoids important for human health are α-carotene, β-carotene, lycopene, phytoene and phytofluene, as well as the xanthophylls lutein, zeaxanthin and α- and β-cryptoxanthin (Khachik *et al.* 1997). All have an extended system of conjugated double bonds that is crucial for their antioxidant properties. The absolute levels of carotenoids vary among different skin sites, with the highest levels for β-carotene found in the skin at the forehead, palm of the hand and dorsal arm (Stahl *et al.* 1998).

There are now comprehensive clinical data demonstrating the photo-protective benefits of dietary carotenoids (Köpcke and Krutmann 2008). Several studies involving β-carotene supplementation at levels of between 24 mg and 180 mg per day have shown increased MED (minimal erythemal dose; the minimum UVB dose required to induce skin redness after 24 hours) or have demonstrated reduced erythema following a standard UV dose (Mathews-Roth *et al.* 1972). This benefit is only achieved, however, following 10–12 weeks of supplementation. Similar studies conducted for shorter periods of between 3–4 weeks have not resulted in any sig-nificant change (Wolf *et al.* 1988; Garmyn *et al.* 1995), indicating that the protective effect requires a significant accumulation of carotenoids in the skin. In parallel, non-invasive methods have been developed using reflectance spectroscopy or Raman spectroscopy to determine carotenoid levels in skin (Stahl *et al.* 1998; Hata *et al.* 2000; Alaluf *et al.* 2002; Darvin *et al.* 2005).

Given concerns about the safety of β-carotene when ingested in high doses (Albanes *et al.* 1996), the effect of partially replacing it with other carot-enoids for sun protection has been investigated. The photo-protective effect of β-carotene supplementa-tion alone (24 mg) was compared with that of a carotenoid mixture consisting of β-carotene, lutein and lycopene (8 mg/day each). After 12 weeks' sup-plementation, the intensity of erythema 24 hours after a standard dose of UV irradiation was dimin-ished to a similar extent in both groups.

A further study, involving 25 people, demon-strated that an antioxidant mixture of β-carotene and lycopene (6 mg/day each) with additional α-tocopherol and selenium led to increased protection against UV-induced skin damage after seven weeks, with a reduction in lipid peroxidation and number of sunburn cells (Cesarini *et al.* 2003).

Lycopene has also been investigated individually and increased consumption over several weeks is correlated with a photo-protective effect. Stahl and colleagues (2001) observed increased protection against UV erythema following a 10-week dietary intervention with tomato paste. Ten individuals consuming 40 g tomato paste and 10 g olive oil a day for 10 weeks, providing 16 mg lycopene, exhibited a 40% lower UV erythema formation than the placebo group, who received olive oil alone. At the end of the intervention, serum levels of lycopene increased from 0.4 µmol/L to around 0.7 µmol/L with total skin carotenoids also increasing significantly.

In a further study individuals were asked to consume lycopene (10.2 mg/day), a commercial tomato extract (9.8 mg lycopene/day) or the tomato extract solubilised in a drink (8.2 mg lycopene/day) for 12 weeks. All groups demonstrated a reduction in erythema formation following UV radiation, but the protective effect was more pronounced with the tomato extract in both capsule and drink formats (Aust *et al.* 2005). These and other studies indicate that the amelioration of UV-induced erythema is a property that can be broadly attributed to the carot-enoid family (Heinrich *et al.* 2003).

The photo-protective effect of lutein in isolation has not been studied in humans. However, the effec-tiveness of lutein in combination with zeaxanthin (ratio 20:1) has been demonstrated in hairless mice, with supplementation resulting in reduced epider-mal hyper-proliferation and inflammatory response following UVB irradiation (Gonzalez *et al.* 2003).

Whilst the efficacy of UV protection provided by the carotenoids is not comparable with the use of a high sun protection factor sunscreen, dietary intake provides photo-protection (Mathews-Roth *et al.* 1972; Albanes *et al.* 1996; Stahl *et al.* 2001; Cesarini *et al.* 2003; Heinrich *et al.* 2003), which may be rea-sonably effective all over the body. This will be of particular importance during inadvertent sun expo-sure, when no topical protection is used, estimated to be around two-thirds of the total erythemal dose accumulated per year.

The protective effects of carotenoids against UV-induced erythema have also been discussed in the context of skin cancer prevention. However, the evi-dence for such an effect is currently weak. Epidemi-ological studies have provided no evidence for a diminished risk of skin cancer associated with dietary intake or blood levels of β-carotene (Baron *et al.* 1998). Indeed, supplementation with carotenoids (but not supply through foods) may in fact be an enhanced risk factor in smokers.

7.9.2 Vitamins E and C and UV protection

Vitamin E (tocopherols and tocotrienols) and vitamin C (ascorbic acid) are naturally present in the skin and form part of the skin's natural defence against reactive oxygen species. The interaction between tocopherol and ascorbate is thought to be particularly important in the protection of skin against photo-oxidation. *In vitro* at least, vitamin C has been shown to regenerate tocopherol from the tocopheroxyl radical and transfers the radical load to the aqueous compartment where it is finally elimi-nated by antioxidant enzymes (Wefers and Sies 1988).

Several studies have now reported on the effec-tiveness of high doses of vitamins E and C against UV-induced erythema with significant efficacy observed only when the two vitamins are used in combination. In a study conducted over 50 days, the effectiveness of very high doses of α-tocopherol (2 g/d) and ascorbate (3 g/d) as single dietary components were compared with that of α-tocopherol and ascorbate combined (2 and 3 g/day respectively). (For comparison the recommended daily amounts for American adults are 60 mg for vitamin C and 30 mg for vitamin E; the UK RNI for vitamin C is lower at 40 mg). Protection against UV-induced erythema was significantly increased following the combination treatment with minimal erythemal dose increasing from 100 to 180 mJ/m^2 UVB. Neither vitamin when provided alone gave rise to a statistically significant increase in UV protection (Fuchs and Kern 1998). Shorter-term intervention with high doses of vitamins E and C has also been shown to afford some UV protection, although at a relatively moderate level. When ingested together for eight days at doses of 1000 IU/day α-tocopherol and 2 g ascorbic acid/day, a minor improvement in minimal erythemal dose was observed (Eberlein-Konig *et al.* 1998).

Vitamin E given orally at 400 IU/day for a period of six months affords no significant increase in UV protection (Werninghaus *et al.* 1994). Similarly, in a study with 12 volunteers, vitamin C given at 500 mg/day over eight weeks had no effect on the UV-induced erythemal response (McArdle *et al.* 2002).

Human and animal studies have also been conducted to examine the effectiveness of topically applied vitamins E and C. These have demonstrated that vitamin E (1%), and to a lesser extent vitamin C (15%), can reduce phototoxic damage when applied in this way. UV-induced erythema, sunburn cell formation, skin wrinkling, lipid peroxidation and DNA damage were reduced to some extent (Dreher *et al.* 1998; J.-Y. Lin *et al.* 2003, 2005).

7.9.3 Omega-3 fatty acids and sun protection

Following initial studies indicating that fish oils could reduce UV-induced erythema in hairless mice (Orengo *et al.* 1989), further studies have shown that high doses of dietary *n*-3 polyunsaturated fatty acids (so-called omega 3 polyunsaturates) can reduce the sunburn response in humans. In one study, 15 individuals were supplemented with 10 g fish oil containing 1.8 g eicosapentaenoic acid (EPA) and 1.2 g docosahexanenoic acid (DHA) daily for three or six months (Rhodes *et al.* 1994). After six months of supplementation, the minimal erythemal dose was

increased by around twofold. This was associated with a pronounced increase in composition of *n*-3 polyunsaturated fatty acids in skin lipids from <2% to >24% total fatty acids. The increase in minimal erythemal dose returned to baseline two months after supplementation ceased. The photo-protective effects of fish oil have also been examined in light-sensitive patients with polymorphic light eruption (PLE). PLE is a common, intermittent, sunlight or artificial UV radiation-induced eruption of non-scarring, itchy papules. After fish oil supplementation patients show a reduction in both basal and UVB-dependent prostaglandin E$_2$ levels and some improvement in the clinical threshold for PLE provocation (Rhodes *et al.* 1995).

In a further double-blind randomised study, 42 healthy subjects consumed 4 g/day of EPA or the monounsaturated fatty acid oleic acid. After three months of EPA supplementation, a significant increase in the UV-induced erythemal threshold was observed. Moreover, UV-induced p53 expression (a marker of UV-induced DNA damage) in skin was also reduced (Rhodes *et al.* 2003). These changes in sunburn sensitivity and p53 expression indicate the ability for high levels of dietary EPA to protect against UV-induced genotoxicity and highlight the potential of longer-term supplementation for protection against skin cancer in humans.

The precise mode of action by which *n*-3 polyunsaturates can reduce UV-induced erythema is unclear. However, a number of potential mechanisms have been postulated. *n*-3 polyunsaturates compete with *n*-6 polyunsaturates for metabolism by cyclooxygenase and lipooxygenase, resulting in the production of less inflammatory prostaglandins and leukotrienes (Lands 1992). These are important mediators of erythema in the human sunburn response and a reduction would be predicted to lead to reduced sunburn. In support of this, a reduction in UVB-generated prostaglandin E$_2$ levels has been demonstrated in the skin of individuals with polymorphic light eruption taking fish oil supplements (Rhodes *et al.* 1995). Similarly, a reduction in cultured keratinocytes and mice skin following *n*-3 polyunsaturated fatty acid supplementation has been reported (Henderson *et al.* 1989; Pupe *et al.* 2002). A second mode of action has been proposed, suggesting that highly unsaturated fatty acids are preferentially damaged by free radicals and may provide an oxidisable buffer, protecting more vital structures from attack (Rhodes *et al.* 1994). However, no direct data for this possibility have been provided.

7.9.4 Polyphenols and sun protection

Polyphenols are major constituents of the diet, found in many regularly consumed fruits and vegetables and are efficient antioxidants *in vitro*. The so-called green tea polyphenols have received the most attention as protective agents against UV-induced skin damage. Animal studies have demonstrated that tea polyphenols, when applied topically or orally in high doses, ameliorate adverse skin reactions following UV exposure, including skin damage, erythema and lipid peroxidation (Kim *et al.* 2001; Katiyar 2007). In addition, high-dose topical application of green tea polyphenols prior to UVB exposure protects against local and systemic immune suppression, associated with inhibition of inflammatory leukocyte infiltration (Katiyar 2003).

Feeding of green tea polyphenols has also been associated with reduction of UVB-induced skin tumours in hairless mice (Wang *et al.* 1991), possibly due to its inhibition of UV-dependent activation of AP-1, a nuclear transcription factor that alters expression of a multitude of pro-inflammatory genes (Barthelman *et al.* 1998). In a similar model, topical application of green tea polyphenols or the major constituent (-)-epigallocatechin-3-gallate, reduced UVB-dependent oxidation of lipids and proteins and depletion of antioxidant enzymes (Vayalil *et al.* 2003).

There is also evidence in topical human studies of the photo-protective effect of polyphenols. Topical application of green tea polyphenols to human subjects inhibited the UVB-induced erythema response (Katiyar *et al.* 2000), whilst analysis of the active components of green tea demonstrated that the (-)-epigallocatechin-3-gallate (EGCG) and (-)-epicatechin-3-gallate polyphenolic fraction were the most efficient in inhibiting erythema when applied topically (Elmets *et al.* 2001). Treatment resulted in a reduction of 'sunburn' cells and lowering of DNA damage following a UV challenge. In a further study, topical application of EGCG, following a controlled acute dose of UVB (four times the minimal erythemal dose, MED), was found to protect human skin against UV-induced oxidative stress, as demonstrated by a reduction in hydrogen

peroxide and nitric oxide formation, lipid peroxidation and inflammatory leukocyte infiltration (Katiyar *et al.* 2001).

Other polyphenols and flavanoids have also been investigated *in vitro* and in animal models for photo-protective and skin cancer prevention benefits. Topically applied silymarin and apigenin are both reported to be beneficial (Birt *et al.* 1997; Katiyar *et al.* 1997).

7.10 Nutrition and wound healing

Impaired wound healing in the elderly is a major clinical and economic problem and is primarily associated with concomitant patient disease rather than with simply being old. Healing occurs in three key stages; the first, or inflammatory phase, is essential for healing to begin and lasts for 4–6 days. During this stage, inflammatory cells migrate into the wound and clear necrotic tissue and bacteria from the area and secrete a variety of growth factors. The second stage, the proliferation phase, which lasts approximately two weeks, is marked by an increase in number and migration of endothelial, fibroblast and epithelial cells, responsible for the formation of granulation tissue and subsequent tissue repair. The third stage, maturation, is characterised by the destruction and remodelling of initial extracellular matrix and includes synthesis of new collagen and elastin fibres.

The processes involved in wound healing result in a significant increase in cellular activity, leading to an increased metabolic demand for nutrients. It is therefore not surprising that poor nutritional intake or lack of individual nutrients affect many aspects of wound healing. However, most deficiency states are multiple and it can be difficult to distinguish which deficiency state is responsible for impaired skin function. A lack of protein, fat, carbohydrate and specific micronutrients can all affect the efficiency of wound healing, as do arginine and the vitamins A, C and E and zinc (see below) (Williams and Barbul 2003; Lansdown 2004a, 2004b).

7.10.1 Proteins and amino acids

Proteins and amino acids form the main building blocks for tissue growth, cell renewal and repair systems following injury (Munro 1974). Amino acid supply and protein synthesis must increase at wound sites to ensure normal wound healing. In tissues with a high metabolic rate, such as skin, deficiencies in protein and specific amino acids will adversely influence homeostasis and reduce healing in wounds, leading to thin, fragile skin with reduced tensile strength (Levenson and Demetriou 1992). This is demonstrated in kwashiorkor, a condition associated with protein-calorie malnutrition, which is characterised by erythema, cracking and scaling of the skin, discolouration, inflammation and impaired wound healing.

Protein and amino acid deficiencies impair all three stages of wound healing, but their primary uses are for collagen synthesis and for use as a potential source of energy when fat and carbohydrate sources are depleted (Cartwright 2002). The supply of individual amino acids, such as proline, arginine and glutamine, become particularly important during wound healing (Kirk *et al.* 1993), while collagen synthesis is particularly sensitive to proline deficiency (Bailey 1978).

Arginine is required for normal vascular and immune function and for the activity of macrophages and other leucocytes in wound healing. It is also used in the synthesis of collagen precursors. Whilst it is a non-essential amino acid in healthy individuals, the requirement for arginine increases during periods of metabolic demand such as wound repair. It then becomes an essential amino acid that has to be provided through the diet (Efron and Barbul 1998; Basu and Liepa 2002).

Glutamine plays an indirect role in wound healing acting as an energy source, via gluconeogenesis in the liver, for proliferating dermal fibroblasts. It is also a precursor for nucleotide synthesis in dividing cells (Zetterberg and Engstrom 1981) and has a central role in stimulating the inflammatory immune response during the early phase of wound healing (Demling and DeSanti 1999). *In vitro* experiments demonstrate that glutamine is also an important fuel for hair follicle growth and maintenance (Williams *et al.* 1993) suggesting a direct role for this amino acid as a metabolic fuel supporting cell proliferation in repairing skin.

7.10.2 Carbohydrates and fats

Carbohydrates and fats are the primary sources of energy in the body and consequently in wound healing. Simple wounds have little energy impact on overall metabolism, but large, complicated wounds or burns can divert a disproportionate amount of energy to the healing wound (Barbul and Purtill 1994). Glucose is the main source of fuel used to generate cellular energy. The liver, however, triggered by the surges in catecholamines and cortisol during wounding, can initiate gluconeogenesis using amino acids from degraded muscle protein. An adequate supply of glucose is therefore important in preventing depletion of amino acids and protein and subsequent protein–calorie malnutrition.

The role of fats in wound healing has not been widely studied. Fatty acids have a key role in the synthesis of cell membranes, formation of the epidermal barrier, cell-signalling pathways, inflammatory reactions and synthesis of extracellular matrix. However, while there are few clinical reports on the influence of fatty acid deficiency in wound repair, evidence in rats suggests that it can impair the rate of wound healing (Hulsey *et al.* 1980).

Linoleic and linolenic acid must be supplied by the diet. Whilst the longer chain derivatives arachidonic acid and EPA can be produced from these essential fatty acids by the liver, the rate of synthesis is not sufficient for basic metabolic needs, particularly during periods of increased stress and major trauma when fatty acid metabolism is increased. In particular, skin lacks the desaturase enzymes required for polyunsaturated fatty acid production (Wright 1991). Given their role as constituents or precursors of phospholipids and prostaglandins, deficiencies of these lipids lead to impaired wound healing (Caldwell *et al.* 1972; Caffrey and Jonsson 1981).

The potential benefit of *n*-3 fatty acids on wound healing has also been investigated. These essential fatty acids have clear anti-inflammatory benefits in skin due to inhibition of eicosanoid production and other mediators (Kremer *et al.* 1987; Simopoulos 1991). However, in one study with rats, animals consuming diets enriched with *n*-3 fatty acids for 30 days had weaker wounds than the control group. It is suggested that this may be due to impaired orientation or cross-linking of the collagen fibres as the level of collagen was unaffected (Albina *et al.* 1993).

7.10.3 Vitamins

Among the micronutrients, vitamins A and C are most closely associated with wound healing. Vitamin

C serves several essential roles, including collagen production, calcium metabolism and as a mediator of several enzymes in skin (Ringsdorf and Cheraskin 1982). The effects of deficiency are most evident in scurvy (see above). The role of vitamin C in wound healing has also been extensively researched in the guinea pig, where collagen defects and abnormal scar tissue formation have been reported (Bourne 1944; Abercrombie *et al.* 1956). There is little evidence to suggest that high-dose supplementation with vitamin C (>1 g/day) will promote wound healing. Tissue saturation with vitamin C occurs at intakes of ~200 mg/day, so any dosage above this is probably unnecessary (Levine *et al.* 1999). In a randomised controlled trial of 88 patients receiving 500 mg of vitamin C for a period of 12 weeks, no significant improvement in wound healing was demonstrated (ter Riet *et al.* 1995). However, in cases of severe sepsis or illness, a daily intake of 300 mg/day has been suggested (Williams 2002). Hospitalised older patients seem to be at most risk of vitamin C deficiency (Selvaag *et al.* 2002).

Vitamin A is known to influence the healing process, with the mechanism thought to be correlated with both the inflammatory and maturation stages of wound healing. Vitamin A functions as an immuno-stimulant and potentially enhances healing by increasing the number of monocytes and macrophages in the wound (Barbul *et al.* 1978; Cohen *et al.* 1979). In addition, it stimulates fibroblasia, increasing collagen synthesis, and epithelialisation (Demetriou *et al.* 1985; Connor 1986). Whilst vitamin A deficiency clearly delays wound healing, supplementation of non-deficient animals with the vitamin has no obvious effect on the wound healing process (Niu *et al.* 1987).

7.10.4 Trace elements

Of the essential trace elements, zinc is the best known with regards to wound healing. Concentrations are naturally highest in tissues undergoing active proliferation, including the skin. Up to 20% of the body's zinc is located in the skin and its appendages (Molokhia and Portnoy 1969). Levels tend to be proportional to the level of mitotic activity and are therefore at least six times higher in the epidermis than the dermis in normal skin (Henzel *et al.* 1970). Following acute injury, local concentrations rise by

around 15% and remain high during all three phases of wound healing (Lansdown *et al.* 1999). Evidence of its essential role in skin was first provided in humans in the 1950s (Valle 1956). It is a co-factor for a large number of enzymes, notably those involved in nucleic acid synthesis, collagen synthesis, inflammatory reactions, immune responses and metalloproteases (Lansdown 1996). In zinc deficiency, fibroblast proliferation and collagen synthesis are reduced, leading to decreased wound strength and delayed epithelialisation. These effects are rapidly reversed following addition of zinc to adequate levels (Barbul and Purtill 1994). The current reference dietary intake for zinc is 15 mg and studies have shown no improvement in wound healing following zinc supplementation in patients who are not zinc-deficient (Hallbook and Lanner 1972). However, where zinc levels are depleted, such as in severe stress or following long-term steroid treatment, zinc supplementation has been recommended to improve wound healing (Goodson and Hunt 1988).

Iron is also an essential element for wound healing. Deficiencies of iron are diagnosed through anaemia with consequent possible wound hypoxia, hair loss, inflammatory changes in the skin, abnormal keratinisation and reduced tensile strength of skin following wound healing (Lansdown 2001).

Other trace elements that may affect healing when deficient include copper, manganese and selenium (Meyer *et al.* 1994; Gosling *et al.* 1995; Kagan and Li 2003).

Chronic wounds place a high metabolic demand on patients, so it is important that they receive adequate energy in the diet and malnutrition is prevented. For most nutrients essential to wound healing, supplementation is only beneficial in cases of deficiency. There is little evidence that supplementation to otherwise healthy individuals will benefit the wound healing process.

7.11 Dietary intake and skin conditions

A few epidemiological studies have been undertaken to examine the impact of diet on visible skin conditions. One study described correlations between actinic (sun-induced) skin damage in the sun-exposed site of 453 individuals of European descent and the types of food they consumed (Purba *et al.* 2001). Dietary intake was assessed and skin measurements taken of Greek-born subjects living in Australia, Greeks living in rural Greece, Anglo-Celtic Australians and Swedes living in Sweden. After controlling for age and smoking, less actinic damage was associated with higher intake of vegetables, olive oil, fish and legumes. More actinic damage was associated with higher intakes of dairy foods, butter, margarine and sugar products. Among the Anglo-Celtic Australians, dried fruit, apples and tea accounted for 34% of the variance. An intervention study would, however, be needed to determine whether visible cutaneous actinic damage could be prevented in part with higher intakes of the apparently beneficial foods outlined above.

In the West, acne vulgaris is a skin disease afflicting 79–95% of the adolescent population. Epidemiological evidence suggests that acne incidence rates are considerably lower in non-westernised societies. An examination of populations aged 15–25 years in Papua New Guinea and in Paraguay reported no cases of acne. It is unlikely that these dramatic differences can be attributed solely to genetic differences but may result from a combination of environmental factors, including diet and lifestyle (Cordain *et al.* 2002).

7.12 Gene–nutrient interactions and skin

It has been known for many years that certain nutritional ingredients can regulate cellular physiology by directly activating gene expression. The nuclear hormone receptors, including steroid hormones and vitamin D receptors, are a family of intracellular receptors that allow cells to respond to extracellular signals through the binding of their relevant ligands. In many cases these ligands are nutritional molecules and their ability to activate such cellular receptors provides a mechanism by which dietary ingredients can activate gene expression and metabolic pathways in a highly specific manner. A number of these receptors are expressed in skin and mediate nutrient effects on skin function.

7.12.1 Vitamin A

Retinoids (see also Sections 7.8.1 and 7.10.3) exert their effects on target cells, including those in the skin, by binding and activating nuclear retinoid receptors. Specifically, there are retinoic acid receptors (RARs) that bind all-trans-retinoic acid and 9-cis-retinoic acid and retinoid X receptors (RXRs) that bind only 9-cis retinoic acid, which act via polymorphic *cis*-acting responsive elements, the RA responsive elements (RAREs), and retinoid X responsive elements (RXREs), present in the promoters of retinoid-responsive genes (Giguere 1994; Gronemeyer and Laudet 1995; Mangelsdorf *et al.* 1995). Topical retinoids have been used successfully to treat many dermatological conditions, including psoriasis, acne, rosacea and photo-ageing (Kang *et al.* 2001; Zouboulis 2001b). The benefit of oral retinoid treatment has also been reported, with isotretinoin (13-cis-retinoic acid) being the first oral drug described for treatment of severe acne (Chivot 2005). However, the effectiveness of oral vitamin A or β-carotene for the treatment of dermatological conditions has not been described.

7.12.2 Vitamin D

The active form of vitamin D also exerts its action through a specific intracellular receptor. In common with the other steroid hormone receptors, the vitamin D receptor (VDR) has both a ligand/hormone-binding and DNA-binding domain. The vitamin D receptor forms a complex with the retinoid-X receptor, and the heterodimer is then able to bind to DNA and modify gene expression. The vitamin D receptor binds several forms of cholecalciferol, but its affinity for 1,25-dihydroxycholecalciferol is roughly 1000 times that for 25-hydroxycholecalciferol, which explains their relative biological potencies.

7.12.3 Peroxisome proliferator-activated receptors (PPARs)

More recently, the importance of peroxisome proliferator-activated receptors (PPARs) in skin function has been described. These are also members of the nuclear receptor super-family and, in common with other members of the family, function as ligand-dependent transcription factors which activate genes that contain PPAR responsive elements in their promoter region (Issemann and Green 1990). Natural activators of these receptors include polyunsaturated fatty acids, including DHA, EPA, linoleic, linolenic and arachidonic acids, albeit with differing affinities (Xu *et al.* 1999). They play a crucial role in many aspects of mammalian physiology, including a significant role in skin homeostasis (Friedmann *et al.* 2005). PPAR involvement in both epidermal maturation and skin wound repair has been reported (Hanley *et al.* 1999; Komuves *et al.* 2000; Michalik and Wahli 2006).

There are three distinct PPAR isoforms; namely α, β/δ and γ. Each is encoded by a separate gene and plays a distinct role with differing tissue distribution, but all are expressed in skin. Whilst all influence keratinocyte differentiation, PPARα is primarily associated with lipid metabolism and inflammation, whilst PPARβ plays a greater role in cell migration and tissue remodelling during wound healing. PPARγ regulates both lipid storage and inflammation (Desvergne and Wahli 1999; Rosen and Spiegelman 2001; Westergaard *et al.* 2001; Grose and Werner 2002). The health benefits attributable to activation of PPARs through consumption of polyunsaturated fatty acids have been widely reported, but dietary benefits on skin function have yet to be described. Recently the PPARα activating lipids conjugated linoleic acid and petroselinic acid have been clinically demonstrated to be effective topical treatments for photo-damaged skin. These lipids show promise as a class of actives, to join retinoids and estrogenic molecules as effective treatments of photo-aged skin (Santhanam *et al.* 2005; Feinberg *et al.* 2006).

7.12.4 Oestrogens and phytoestrogens

Oestrogen (see Section 7.6.5) also exerts its biological action through activation of a steroid hormone receptor. The oestrogen receptor functions as a homodimer and when activated by its ligand binds to specific sequences within the promoter of target genes to activate gene transcription. It exists as two subtypes, ERα (Brzozowski *et al.* 1997) and ERβ (Kuiper *et al.* 1998), which differ in tissue distribution and ligand binding affinities (Kuiper *et al.* 1997; Petersen *et al.* 1998). ERα is poorly expressed in skin, being restricted to sebocytes, whilst ERβ is highly expressed in the epidermis, sebaceous glands (basal cells and seboocytes), eccrine sweat glands and the hair follicle (Pelletier and Ren 2004).

Whilst oestrogen is a mammalian hormone and not found as a dietary source, plant constituents have been found with estrogenic activity and are referred to as phytoestrogens. The isoflavones genistein and daidzein are members of the flavonoid family, found primarily in soy, and are considered typical phytoestrogens. The structure of an isoflavone has similarities to that of oestrogen and binds weakly to the oestrogen receptor mimicking oestrogen activation (Zava and Duwe 1997) (see Chapter 13, Section 13.4.4).

Both oral and topical application of isoflavones may have beneficial effects in skin. There is evidence that isoflavones, particularly genistein, can be photoprotective. Both topical and oral application have been shown to inhibit UVB induced photo-carcinogenesis and photo-ageing in mice, whilst topical application of genistein 5 μmol/cm^2 to six male subjects blocked UVB-induced erythema (Wei *et al.* 2003; Kim *et al.* 2004) and topical genistein inhibited UVR induction of *c-jun* and collagenase in human skin *in vivo* (S. Kang *et al.* 2003).

There are numerous reports describing the effect of falling oestrogen levels on skin quality around the menopause, and some evidence of the benefit provided by oestrogen replacement therapy, including increased collagen content and skin thickness and improved skin moisture (Verdier-Sevrain *et al.* 2006). However, there are few reports of the beneficial impact of isoflavone supplementation on skin of postmenopausal women. In one double-blind placebo-controlled trial of 94 postmenopausal women fed soy supplements containing 118 mg isoflavones, there was a significant improvement in skin dryness (Kotsopoulos *et al.* 2000) while a soy extract containing commercial product has also been reported to improve skin ageing in postmenopausal women (Lange Skovgaard *et al.* 2006).

Despite the claims surrounding the potential value of phytoestrogens in the prevention and treatment of skin ageing, extensive supporting clinical data are lacking.

7.13 Skin nutrition: topical or dietary?

Even though the skin is accessible to topical products, skin nutrients are nearly always best delivered systemically via the diet. However, certain skin conditions may be best treated topically, for example dry skin or localised skin problems such as itchy, inflamed, hyper-pigmented or aged skin and superficial skin infections.

7.14 Key points

- Skin signals health, appearance and attractiveness to our fellow human beings. It is composed of two main tissues, the outer epidermis and the deeper, collagen-rich dermis.
- The skin functions to maintain a robust barrier to the outside world and to prevent desiccation of our bodies.
- Skin is relatively easily sampled and multiple, valuable *in vitro* cell research models have been developed and are available to study and investigate its properties.
- The skin ages in very characteristic ways, giving rise to visible unattractive features such as wrinkling, uneven pigmentation and sagging. For this reason maintaining a 'youthful' appearance is a major interest for consumers, and the cosmetic and food industries.
- Several biological ageing mechanisms have been proposed (*e.g.* photo-damage, oxidative damage, telomere shortening, neurological and physical stress, hormonal interactions) and each mechanism is currently the subject of many research investigations.
- Despite the very large number of supplement preparations that claim skin benefits, there are very few published placebo-controlled clinical trials using the products to test the claims (Lassus *et al.* 1991; Eskelinen and Santalahti 1992; Brown *et al.* 2004; Segger and Schonlau 2004; Lange Skovgaard *et al.* 2006). Many more placebo-controlled human studies are required to support food and supplement product claims.
- While the sun protection efficacy of dietary supplementation with β-carotene (>20 mg/day) and possibly other carotenoids is supported (see Section 7.9.1), the safety of higher doses of

β-carotene (30 mg/day) in smokers is unacceptable (Albanes *et al.* 1996; Goodman *et al.* 2004). It seems likely that modest sun protection is provided by ingestion of combinations of ingredients such as carotenoids, *n*-3 fatty acids and vitamins C and E (summarised in Section 7.9). However, whether dietary sun protection will give rise to measurable effects on skin ageing or other skin benefits remains to be tested in longer term (>12-week) clinical studies.
- There are few human studies investigating the dietary effects of (non-vitamin) plant-derived ingredients on skin (Section 7.7). Two non-carotenoid ingredient classes with potential are polyphenols, including green tea extracts containing (-)-epigallocatechin-3-gallate, where animal studies suggest skin anti-cancer, anti-inflammatory and photo-protection benefits, and isoflavones with potential for sun protection and skin ageing benefits. There is great scope to explore the potential of plant ingredients to positively influence skin properties and appearance.
- Poor nutrition has an adverse impact on wound healing. Therefore, it is not surprising that a balanced diet is recommended for optimal wound repair.
- Severe nutritional deficiencies (*e.g.* scurvy from vitamin C deficiency and pellagra from niacin deficiencies) that noticeably affect skin condition and skin ageing are now very rare in the developed world. However, the refinement of public health advice for optimal vitamin D bio-availability, either from balancing sun exposure with risk of photo-ageing and skin cancer (see Section 7.5) or from fortified foods and supplements, requires more debate.

7.15 Recommendations for future research

- Further double-blind, placebo-controlled, clinical studies are required to investigate the ability of nutritional supplements and drinks to provide benefits for skin. Currently skin ageing benefits are best supported in the literature,

but many other unsubstantiated claims are made.
- Several biological research areas show promise in elucidating the mechanisms of skin ageing and poor skin condition but require further

Continued

investigation. Areas of current high interest in improving skin functioning include the role of mitochondria, biological effects of UV radiation, the skin's innate immune system, the ligand-activated nuclear hormone receptor classes including PPARα activation, and the recent discoveries that the neuroendocrine, stress and steroidogenesis pathways operate in skin.

• Genome-wide association studies have recently become feasible, following the sequencing of the human genome. It is now feasible to use such technologies to identify the gene(s) that associate with complex human traits that have a genetic background; for example, pigmentation (Stokowski *et al.* 2007). Future research will depend more on the collection of DNA samples from high-quality clinical cohorts. A recent example of this approach has been the discovery that the filaggrin gene is linked to atopic dermatitis and ichthyosis vulgaris.

7.16 Key references

Boelsma E, Hendriks HF and Roza L (2001) Nutritional skin care: health effects of micronutrients and fatty acids. *American Journal of Clinical Nutrition*, **73**, 853–64.

Heinrich U, Gartner C, Wiesbusch M, *et al.* (2003) Supplementation with beta-carotene or a similar amount of mixed carotenoids protects humans from UV-induced erythema. *Journal of Nutrition*, **133**, 98–101.

Holick MF (2004) Sunlight and vitamin D for bone health and prevention of autoimmune diseases, cancers, and cardiovascular disease. *American Journal of Clinical Nutrition*, **80**, 1678S–88S.

McGrath JA, Eady RAJ and Pope FM (2004) Anatomy and organization of human skin. *Rook's Textbook of Dermatology*. Ed. T Burns, S Breathnach, N Cox and C Griffiths. Oxford, Blackwell.

Rhodes LE, Durham BH, Fraser WD and Friedmann PS (1995) Dietary fish oil reduces basal and ultraviolet B-generated PGE2 levels in skin and increases the threshold to provocation of polymorphic light eruption. *Journal of Investigative Dermatology*, **105**, 532–5.

8
Healthy Ageing: The Brain

8.1 Introduction

Stroke, dementia, Parkinson's disease and depression are common diseases affecting the brain in older people and account for most cases of disability requiring nursing care in this age group. The incidence of these diseases increases exponentially with increasing age. Consequently, improvements in life expectancy have resulted in a substantial increase in the absolute number of individuals suffering from these diseases in old age (Lang and Lozano 1998; Cummings 2004). Moreover, affected individuals are likely to suffer disability for a longer period. Stroke is the third most common cause of death in older people and the age-specific stroke rates in older people are higher in women than in men (Rothwell *et al.* 2005). Dementia affects about 1 in 20 people aged 65 years and over and affects more women than men (Matthews and Brayne 2005). Stroke and dementia are the two most frequent reasons for admission to long-term institutional care in older people. A stroke is the brain equivalent of a heart attack. Blood must flow to and through the brain for it to function. If blood flow is obstructed by a blood clot moving to the brain, or by narrowing or bursting of blood vessels, the brain loses its energy supply, causing damage to tissues resulting in a stroke. Stroke may result from either a blockage or bleeding from a large blood vessel supplying the brain, causing focal or global loss of brain function. Cognitive impairment or dementia may result from stroke or occlusive vascular disease affecting smaller blood vessels supplying different areas of the brain.

Depression is one of the most prevalent and costly of all mental disorders and a leading cause of disability, affecting one in four people over their lifetime. Many of the established risk factors for stroke are also believed to be relevant to dementia, Parkinson's disease and depression (Cummings 2004). Identification of the importance of particular nutrients for risk of dementia, Parkinson's disease and depression is a challenge for scientists, as it is difficult to distinguish the effects of diet from confounding due to other aspects of lifestyle and to eliminate the effects of bias due to established disease from associations that are causal (referred to as 'reverse causality'). However, the results of observational epidemiological studies have prompted large-scale trials assessing the effects of vascular risk modification or nutritional supplements in people at high risk of suffering from these diseases. This chapter examines the relevance of lifestyle modification and nutrition for risk of stroke, dementia, Parkinson's disease and depression. The nutritional factors described include sodium, antioxidant vitamins (vitamins E and C and β-carotene), B vitamins (folate and vitamin B_{12}), alcohol, fatty acids and trace elements.

8.2 Stroke

Annually, 15 million people worldwide suffer from stroke, of whom five million die and five million are left permanently disabled. Stroke (or cerebrovascular disease) is the third most common cause of death after heart disease and cancer and is a major cause of disability in older people. Most strokes (~75%) occur in people aged 65 years or greater. The age-specific incidence rates for stroke in old age in the UK increase from 5/1000/year at age 65–74 years to

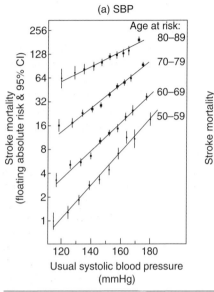

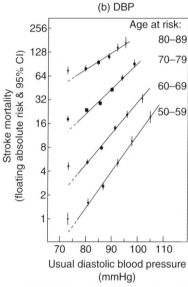

Figure 8.1: Stroke mortality rate in each decade of age vs. (a) usual systolic blood pressure (SBP) and (b) usual diastolic blood pressure (DBP) at the start of that decade.
Source: Prospective Studies Collaboration (2002). Reproduced by permission of Elsevier.

25/1000/year at age 85 years or greater (Rothwell *et al.* 2005). Strokes may result from either a blockage of (ischaemic stroke) or bleeding from (haemorrhagic stroke) a blood vessel supplying the brain. About 80% of strokes are ischaemic and 15% are haemorrhagic and 5% due to subarachnoid haemorrhage. Strokes are believed to arise from the effects of high blood pressure, smoking, tobacco use, unhealthy diet, lack of physical activity and obesity. The effects of obesity are almost entirely explained by the effects of being overweight on blood pressure, blood lipids and diabetes mellitus. The age-specific incidence rates of stroke are declining in many developed countries, largely as a result of better control of high blood pressure and reduced levels of smoking (Rothwell *et al.* 2005). However, the absolute number of strokes continues to increase because of the ageing population (see Chapter 1, Section 1.1). Strokes carry a high risk of death in the immediate aftermath of the acute event. Survivors can experience loss of vision or speech and have paralysis and confusion. About 60% of people experiencing a stroke die or become dependent and many require long-term institutional care.

8.2.1 Blood pressure and risk of stroke

Elevated blood pressure is the most important risk factor for stroke in the older population. The most reliable evidence for the importance of blood pressure for risk of stroke and other vascular causes of death has been provided by the Prospective Studies Collaboration (2002), involving individual participant data from one million adults with no previous vascular disease recorded at baseline from 61 prospective observational studies. This meta-analysis related mortality during each decade of age at death to the estimated usual blood pressure at the start of that decade (Figure 8.1). There was a linear and graded relationship of blood pressure with death from stroke, with no threshold below which a lower value was not associated with a lower risk, at least down to about 115 mmHg usual systolic blood pressure (SBP) and 75 mmHg usual diastolic blood pressure (DBP). At ages 40–69 years, each difference of 20 mmHg usual SBP (or, approximately equivalently, 10 mmHg usual DBP) was associated with more than a twofold difference in the stroke death rate, and with twofold differences in the death rates from ischaemic heart disease (IHD) and from other vascular causes of death (see Chapter 10 for more information on heart disease). All of these proportional differences in vascular mortality were about half as extreme at ages 80–89 years as at ages 40–49 years, but the annual absolute differences in risk are greater in old age. The age-specific associations of blood pressure with stroke mortality were similar for men and women, and for cerebral haemorrhage and cerebral ischaemia.

8.2.2 Dietary determinants of blood pressure

Sodium, fatty acids, energy and alcohol consumption are the most important dietary determinants of blood pressure (see Chapter 10, Section 10.7.6.1). Sodium intake is the major dietary determinant of blood pressure in the population and a determinant of the change in blood pressure with increasing age. Among the total intake of dietary sodium, about 70% comes from manufactured food, 15% from naturally occurring sodium and 15% from discretionary sources. The importance of dietary salt (the major source of dietary sodium) for blood pressure was quantified by the INTERSALT study, which examined blood pressure levels in relation to urinary sodium excretion in an ecological study of 26 countries (Intersalt Cooperative Research Group 1988; Elliott *et al.* 1996). The study showed that differences in blood pressure levels were correlated with differences in salt intake. The most reliable evidence for the importance of sodium was provided by the Dietary Approaches to Stop Hypertension (DASH) trial, which randomised people to an experimental diet low in total fat and in saturated fatty acids and high in fruit and vegetables compared with a standard American diet, and the intervention was associated with reductions in blood pressure of 5.5/3.0 mmHg (Appel *et al.* 1997). The follow-on DASH-sodium trial examined the effect of the combined DASH trial with reduced sodium intake and the latter achieved additional reductions in blood pressure of 2.5/1.2 mmHg (Sacks *et al.* 2001). However, dietary advice to lower blood pressure is not very effective and a population approach is required to achieve a sustained reduction in salt intake. With the current cooperation of the food industry to lower salt levels in processed food, a gradual lowering in salt intake in the population may be achieved over time (MacGregor and He 2002).

Alcohol intake is an independent risk factor for hypertension with an increase in blood pressure occurring with an alcohol intake in excess of two drinks a day (Marmot *et al.* 1994). Randomised trials assessing the effects on blood pressure of reductions in intake of alcohol have shown highly significant dose-dependent reductions in blood pressure with reductions in intake of alcohol. The average consumption of alcohol has increased in recent years and this may also contribute to obesity. Sensible limits for weekly alcohol intake (21 units for men and 14 units for women) may not apply to older people because of age-related changes in metabolism, advancing ill health and increased sensitivity to the effects of alcohol. Limits appropriate to age have not been established for older people elsewhere but are likely to be lower than those for younger people.

Blood pressure levels in the population are also related to bodyweight and fatness. On average, a 5 unit increase in body mass index (*e.g.* 30 vs. 25 kg/m^2) is associated with a 5 mmHg higher level of systolic blood pressure. The average body mass index of most developed populations has increased in recent years and this has had a major effect on both coronary heart disease and stroke. It is likely that the effects of obesity on vascular disease risk are explained by its effect on blood pressure, blood lipids and diabetes mellitus. Conversely, weight reduction is associated with reductions in blood pressure and blood lipids and risk of diabetes mellitus. Hence increased physical activity and the associated weight loss are associated with reductions in systolic and diastolic blood pressure. In particular, aerobic exercise has been associated with a significant reduction in mean systolic blood pressure. Public health strategies to reduce blood pressure should include increasing physical activity and reduction in alcohol consumption, in addition to a reduction in dietary salt (the recommended level being 6 g/day, equivalent to 2.5 g sodium/day). (See Chapter 14 for information about public health strategies.)

8.2.3 Homocysteine and risk of stroke

Homocysteine is a sulphur-containing amino acid that is present in all cells (see Chapter 10, Section 10.4.2.2). Elevated plasma concentrations of total homocysteine reflect impaired status of folate and of vitamin B_{12}. Dietary intake of folate is one major determinant of blood homocysteine concentrations, but in the general population vitamin B_{12} deficiency is a more important cause of elevated homocysteine concentrations in older people. Elevated homocysteine concentrations have been suggested as a modifiable risk factor for stroke (McCully 1969; Clarke *et al.* 1991). The occurrence of premature stroke and other vascular events in individuals with the rare genetic disorder homocystinuria which is associated with greatly elevated plasma homocysteine concentrations has prompted the homocysteine hypothesis that higher blood concentrations of homocysteine (mostly within the 'normal' range) may be relevant to stroke in the general population (McCully 1969). Untreated individuals with homocystinuria suffer from strokes and other vascular events in their second and third decades and have mental retardation. Individuals with homocystinuria have about 10-fold higher absolute mean plasma homocysteine concentrations (*i.e.* 100–300 µmol/L) compared with levels among middle-aged individuals in the general population (*i.e.* normal range of 10–15 µmol/L). Supplementation of affected individuals with homocystinuria with vitamin B_6, folic acid, vitamin B_{12} and betaine reduces the risk of the vascular and other complications in affected children (Clarke 2005a).

Many observational epidemiological studies have reported that people with coronary heart disease (CHD) or stroke have higher homocysteine concentrations compared with age- and sex-matched controls. These include prospective studies where the blood sample for homocysteine determination was taken before the onset of vascular disease, limiting the effect of established disease on plasma homocysteine concentrations. In 2002, the Homocysteine Studies Collaborative Group reported the results of an individual patient data meta-analysis of 30 studies relating homocysteine to risk of CHD and stroke, involving 1855 CHD events and 435 stroke events in prospective studies. Among these prospective studies, after adjustment for established CHD risk factors, a 25% (typically a 3 µmol/L) lower blood homocysteine concentration was associated with 11% (95% CI: 4–17) lower risk of CHD and 19% (95% CI: 5–31) lower risk of stroke. However, there is substantial uncertainty about whether the associations of elevated homocysteine concentrations with stroke and other vascular events are causal. A common polymorphism exists for the gene encoding a key enzyme involved in homocysteine metabolism that is associated with elevated homocysteine concentrations. The 677C→T polymorphism for the gene encoding methylene-tetrahydrofolate reductase (*MTHFR*) affects about 10% of Northern European populations. The TT genotype for MTHFR is asso-

ciated with reduced production of 5-methyltetrahydrofolate and with 20–25% (*i.e.* about 2–2.5 µmol/L) higher plasma homocysteine concentrations than the CC genotype. This polymorphism provides a natural randomisation experiment, whereby people are allocated during the very early stages of life to either the TT genotype (and these have higher homocysteine) or the CC genotype (and these have lower homocysteine levels throughout life). Since the polymorphism is distributed at random during meiosis (the cellular process that results in the number of chromosomes in gamete-producing cells being reduced to one half), the groups should not differ systematically in any other way. It should be possible to compare the disease risks among those with TT with those with CC. However, since the effect of 677C→T on disease is modest, epidemiological studies assessing the effects of this polymorphism on risk of disease require a large number of participants to identify or exclude a modest difference in disease outcomes among those with or without the TT mutation.

Casas and colleagues carried out a meta-analysis of 30 studies of 677C→T polymorphism of MTHFR and risk of stroke involving 3472 cases and 42,111 controls (Casas *et al.* 2005). This meta-analysis concluded that individuals who had the TT genotype had a 26% higher risk of stroke compared with those with the CC genotype for MTHFR (odds ratio: 1.26 [95% CI: 1.14–1.40]). The relative risk of stroke for TT vs. CC genotype was consistent with the difference in risk of stroke of 1.20 (1.10–1.30) for a corresponding difference in homocysteine concentrations between TT and CC, predicted from the observational non-genetic studies, and thus provided some support for causality.

8.2.4 Randomised trials of B vitamin supplementation to prevent stroke and CHD

While elevated plasma homocysteine concentrations can be easily lowered by dietary supplementation with folic acid, it is unclear if lowering homocysteine concentrations can lower the risk of CHD or stroke. The Homocysteine-Lowering Trialists' Collaboration (2005) provided individual data on 2596 participants from 25 randomised trials assessing the effects on plasma homocysteine concentrations of folic acid supplements with or without the addition of vitamin

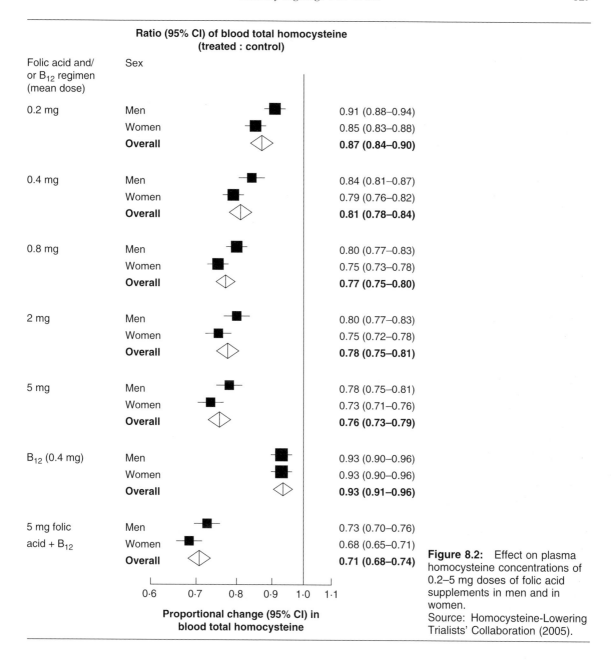

Figure 8.2: Effect on plasma homocysteine concentrations of 0.2–5 mg doses of folic acid supplements in men and in women.
Source: Homocysteine-Lowering Trialists' Collaboration (2005).

B_{12} or vitamin B_6. The aim of the meta-analysis was to determine the size of the reduction in homocysteine concentrations achieved with different oral doses of folic acid and with the addition of vitamin B_{12} or B_6. The meta-analysis reported that the proportional reductions in plasma homocysteine concentrations produced by folic acid were greater with higher pre-treated and lower pre-treatment folate concentrations. The proportional effects on homocysteine concentrations of folic acid were greater in women compared with men. Figure 8.2 shows that, after standardisation for sex, at pre-treatment homocysteine concentrations of 12 µmol/L and pre-treatment folate concentrations of 12 nmol/L, daily doses

Table 8.1: Characteristics of the homocysteine-lowering trials for prevention of cardiovascular disease

Trial	Folate fortified population	Prior disease	Number randomised (planned or actual)	Scheduled duration of treatment (y)	Folic acid (mg)	B_{12} (mg)	B_6 (mg)	Observed/estimated difference in plasma homocysteine (%)
CHAOS-2	–	CHD	1880	2	5.0	–	–	13
SU·FOL·OM3	–	CHD	2000	5	0.5	0.02	3	25
WENBIT	–	CHD	3000	3	0.8	0.4	40	25
NORVIT	–	CHD	3750	3	0.8	0.4	40	25
SEARCH	–	CHD	12064	7	2.0	1.0	–	25
HOPE-2	+/–	CHD	5522	5	2.5	1.0	50	20
WACS	+	CHD	5442	7.4	2.5	1.0	50	20
SU·FOL·OM3	–	Stroke	1000	5	0.5	0.02	3	25
VITATOPS	–	Stroke	(8000)	3	2.0	0.5	25	25
VISP	+	Stroke	3680	2	2.5	0.4	25	15
FAVORIT	+	Renal	4000	5	2.5	0.4	20	33
HOST	+	Renal	2056	5	40.0	2.0	100	33

of 0.2 mg, 0.4 mg, 0.8 mg, 2 mg and 5 mg of folic acid were associated with reductions in homocysteine of 13% (95% CI: 10–16), 20% (95% CI: 17–22), 23% (95% CI: 21–26), 23% (95% CI: 20–26) and 25% (95% CI: 22–28), respectively. Vitamin B_{12} produced a 7% (95% CI: 4–9) further reduction in plasma homocysteine concentrations, but vitamin B_6 had no significant effect on homocysteine concentrations. The mean duration of treatment in these trials was eight (SD six) weeks, ranging from 3 to 24 weeks. The lowest dose of folic acid associated with the maximum reduction in homocysteine concentrations was 0.8 mg folic acid and doses of 0.2 mg and 0.4 mg of folic acid were associated with about 60% and 90% of this maximal effect, respectively. Concomitant treatment of folic acid (5 mg) and vitamin B_{12} (0.4 mg) was associated with reductions in plasma homocysteine concentrations of 30% (95% CI: 27–33). This meta-analysis of short-term trials cannot assess the efficacy of lower folic acid doses administered for longer than 12–24 weeks, but there was no significant heterogeneity in the effects of folic acid by duration of therapy in the individual trials.

In the late 1990s, several large randomised trials in people at high-risk of cardiovascular disease were initiated to test the hypothesis that homocysteine-lowering with folic acid (and other B vitamins) could reduce the risk of recurrent cardiovascular disease (B-Vitamin Treatment Trialists' Collaboration 2006). These trials were designed at a time when the association of homocysteine with risk of vascular disease was believed to be somewhat stronger than is currently the case.

In the light of the more modest effects of homocysteine on risk of vascular disease in the observational studies, the principal investigators of these trials agreed to pool data for the B-Vitamin Treatment Trialists' Collaboration (2006), a prospective meta-analysis of all the large-scale trials of B vitamins for the prevention of CHD and stroke. This collaboration reviewed the statistical power of these large-scale trials to assess their ability to detect a 10–20% reduction in risk of CHD and stroke. Table 8.1 shows a summary of trials, involving more than 1000 participants treated with homocysteine-lowering B vitamins for at least one year to prevent cardiovascular events. Among these 12 large randomised trials, seven are being conducted in populations without mandatory folic acid fortification (five involving participants with prior CHD and two with prior stroke) and five in populations with fortification (two with prior CHD, two with renal disease and one with prior stroke). Table 8.1 shows the observed homocysteine difference by allocated treatment, together with the estimated duration of treatment for each trial. In the US and Canada, folic acid fortification began in 1996, although it was officially mandated in 1998 for the prevention of neural tube defects, and this attenuated the effects of B vitamin supplementation on plasma homocysteine concentrations in the general population but not in renal disease. In order to estimate and compare the statis-

Table 8.2: Estimated power of the individual trials and combination of the large trials in people with prior CHD, prior stroke or renal disease to detect differences in risk of 10% or 20% for major coronary events (MCE), stroke and major vascular events (MVE)

Population/Trial	N	Estimated no. of events			10% Reduction in risk Approx power at 2P < 0.05			20% Reduction in risk Approx power at 2P < 0.05		
		MCE[†]	Stroke[§]	MVE[‡]	MCE[†]	Stroke[§]	MVE[‡]	MCE[†]	Stroke[§]	MVE[‡]
CHD										
CHAOS-2	1882	87	32	226	5	4	7	9	6	17
SU·FOL·OM3	2000	190	190	626	12	12	36	36	36	92
WENBIT	3000	209	77	563	12	7	28	38	17	83
NORVIT	3749	606	94	1575	29	7	79	85	19	99
SEARCH	12064	1400	373	2800	55	18	89	99	59	99
HOPE-2	5522	718	276	1795	22	11	58	70	32	99
WACS	5442	268	134	850	10	7	26	31	17	79
All CHD	11022	3478	1177	8434	86	39	99	99	94	99
STROKE										
SU·FOL·OM3	1000	95	95	358	8	8	24	21	21	75
VITATOPS	8000	321	951	1690	16	41	68	53	95	99
VISP	3680	221	288	504	7	8	11	16	20	34
All stroke	12680	637	1334	2552	21	46	78	69	97	99
RENAL										
FAVORIT	4000	480	220	1000	37	18	72	94	63	99
HOST	2056	247	113	514	21	12	45	71	37	97
All renal	6056	727	333	1514	52	26	88	99	80	99

[†]MCE: Major coronary events (Non-fatal MI + fatal CHD).
[§]Stroke: Non-fatal or fatal stroke.
[‡]MVE: Major vascular events (Non-fatal MI + Fatal CHD + non-fatal stroke + revascularisation).

tical power to detect a difference in vascular disease in each trial, major coronary events were defined as the first occurrence of non-fatal myocardial infarction (MI) or coronary death (including death from heart failure and sudden or unexpected deaths believed to be coronary in origin); stroke was defined as fatal or non-fatal stroke (but not including transient cerebral ischaemic attacks); major vascular events were defined by any major coronary event, any stroke or any coronary or non-coronary revascularisation. Table 8.2 shows the estimated number of vascular events (major coronary events, stroke and major vascular events) and the power for each trial to detect a 10–20% reduction in risk of CHD, stroke or major vascular events. As is apparent, few trials have sufficient power on their own to detect a 10% reduction in the risk of CHD. But, taken together, these 12 trials involve about 52,000 participants: 32,000 with prior vascular disease in unfortified populations; 14,000 with vascular disease; and

6,000 with renal disease. People with renal disease typically have plasma homocysteine concentrations that are more than double those found in the general population and have a particularly high risk of vascular disease. Hence a combined analysis of these trials should have sufficient power (about 99%) to determine whether lowering homocysteine by about 25% reduces the risk of CHD by about 10% within just a few years.

Results from the four trials (Baker *et al.* 2002; Toole *et al.* 2004; Bonaa *et al.* 2006; Lonn *et al.* 2006) are shown in Table 8.3. These results involve about 14,000 participants with follow-up varying from 1.7 to 5 years. The odds ratios and 95% confidence intervals for the effects of homocysteine-lowering treatment are shown for each trial, together with a summary estimate for all trials for each of the three main outcomes. For each outcome, summary estimates of the odds ratios from all studies were obtained by combining the separate estimates of the

Table 8.3: Effects of B-vitamin supplementation on CHD, stroke and cardiovascular disease events in the large homocysteine-lowering trials reported before September 2006

Outcome	Trial	Active treatment Events/Allocated	Placebo or control			
			Events/Allocated	Overall event rate (%)	Annual event rate (%)	Odds ratio (95% CI)
CHD[†]	CHAOS-2	12/942	23/940	1.9	0.9	0.53 (0.27–1.03)
	VISP	114/1827	123/1853	6.4	3.2	0.94 (0.72–1.22)
	HOPE-2	341/2758	349/2764	12.5	2.5	0.98 (0.83–1.15)
	NORVIT	329/1872	153/943	17.1	5.7	1.10 (0.89–1.35)
	All	**796/7397**	**648/6502**			**0.99 (0.88–1.10)**
Stroke[§]	VISP	152/1827	148/1853	8.1	4.1	1.05 (0.83–1.32)
	HOPE-2	111/2758	147/2764	4.7	0.9	0.75 (0.58–0.96)
	NORVIT	49/1872	27/943	2.7	0.9	0.91 (0.56–1.48)
	All	**312/6457**	**322/5560**			**0.89 (0.76–1.05)**
Cardiovascular Disease[‡]	VISP	249/1827	257/1853	13.7	6.9	0.98 (0.81–1.18)
	HOPE-2	519/2758	547/2764	19.3	3.9	0.94 (0.82–1.07)
	NORVIT	369/1872	172/943	19.2	6.4	1.10 (0.90–1.34)
	All	**1137/6457**	**976/5560**			**0.98 (0.90–1.08)**

[†]CHD: Non-fatal myocardial infarction or death from CHD (revascularisation events are not included).
[§]Stroke: Non-fatal or fatal stroke.
[‡]Cardiovascular disease: Death from cardiovascular causes, MI or stroke (revascularisation events are not included).

inverse-variance weighted log odds ratios of the individual studies. There is no clear evidence for benefit of B vitamin supplementation on the risk of vascular events in these trials, with a summary odds ratio 0.89 (95% CI: 0.76–1.05) for stroke in this meta-analysis. However, the confidence intervals around the odds ratios are wide and cannot exclude a 10% difference in risk for CHD or a 20% difference for stroke associated with a 25% difference in homocysteine as predicted by the prospective cohort studies and genetic epidemiologic studies over the longer term.

As is apparent from the estimates for power provided in Table 8.2, even the combined results of these four trials have very limited statistical power to detect a 10% difference in the risk of CHD. The combined results of the ongoing and completed trials could guide national public health policy about benefits or hazards of increasing population mean plasma folate concentrations by folic acid fortification for the prevention of cardiovascular disease. Hence, it is important to defer judgement on this question (and recommendations on the use of folic acid and vitamin B_{12}) until more evidence emerges from the ongoing homocysteine-lowering trials. While absent evidence does not constitute evidence

of no effect of B vitamins for prevention of stroke, it is clear that the magnitude of the effects of blood pressure and smoking are much greater than those associated with differences in homocysteine levels.

8.2.5 Cholesterol and risk of stroke

Observational epidemiological studies of the associations of total cholesterol with total stroke have reported conflicting results, as total cholesterol is positively associated with ischaemic stroke and inversely associated with haemorrhagic stroke (Prospective Studies Collaboration 1995; Asia Pacific Cohort Studies Collaboration 2003), but the reasons for the discrepant findings remain unclear. In contrast to the observational epidemiology, a meta-analysis of the randomised trials of a few years of drug treatment with statins, which greatly reduce the number of circulating LDL particles, has shown that regimens that reduce both LDL cholesterol and total cholesterol by about 1.5 mmol/L also reduce the incidence of coronary artery disease and of ischaemic stroke by about one third, approximately independently of age or blood pressure (and of baseline blood lipid levels), and do not appear to increase the incidence of haemorrhagic stroke (Cholesterol

Treatment Trialists' Collaboration 2005). Reducing the intake of saturated fat, *trans* fatty acids and dietary cholesterol and replacing such LDL-raising fats, partly by monounsaturated fat and by polyunsaturated fat, can achieve substantial improvements in total/HDL-cholesterol ratio that would be expected to lower both CHD and stroke risk (Clarke *et al.* 1997).

8.2.6 Antioxidants and risk of stroke

Several large-scale observational studies have shown that reduced intake of antioxidant vitamins or reduced blood levels of antioxidant vitamins were associated with higher risks of stroke. However, the results of large-scale trials administering antioxidant vitamins have failed to demonstrate any beneficial effects of antioxidant vitamins on the risk of stroke or any other vascular events. The HOPE trial showed that dietary supplementation of 9541 people aged 55 years or older at high risk of cardiovascular events, for 4.5 years of treatment had no effect on the risk of stroke (Heart Outcomes Prevention Evaluation (HOPE) Study Investigators 2000). The Heart Protection Study examined the effects of dietary supplementation of 20,536 men and women at high risk of cardiovascular events with a cocktail of antioxidant vitamins (vitamins E and C and β-carotene) (Heart Protection Study 2002) and reported no protective effect on risk of stroke or other vascular end-points.

8.2.7 *n*-3 and *n*-6 fatty acids and risk of stroke

An inverse association between fish intake and risk of stroke has been reported in several, but not all prospective studies. Some studies have shown that higher consumption of fish and fish oil, rich in the long chain *n*-3 fatty acids eicosapentaenoic acid (EPA) and docosahexaenoic acid (DHA) was associated with a reduced risk of thrombotic cerebral infarction, but was unrelated to haemorrhagic stroke. *n*-3 fatty acids are long-chained polyunsaturated fatty acids with more than one double bond, with the first occurring between the 3rd and 4th carbon from the methyl end. Observational epidemiological studies have reported that people who eat fish several times a week, compared with those who do not, have a significantly lower risk of stroke (He *et al.* 2002), but the results are not entirely concordant (C. Wang

et al. 2006). Increasing the intake of *n*-3 fatty acids also produces a modest reduction in systolic blood pressure of about 3 mmHg (Geleijnse *et al.* 2002), but *n*-3 fatty acids may affect the risk of stroke independently of their effects on blood pressure. Large-scale trials of *n*-3 fatty acids for the prevention of vascular disease are currently underway which should clarify the relevance of *n*-3 fatty acids for prevention of stroke and CHD. For example, the ASCEND (A Study of Cardiovascular Events in Diabetes) trial in the UK should provide the reliable evidence about the effects of aspirin and of *n*-3 fatty acids in diabetes (see www.ctsu.ox.ac.uk/ascend/ for further details). The ASCEND trial aims to recruit at least 10,000 people with diabetes (either type 1 or type 2) who do not have known vascular disease. In ASCEND, participants will be randomly allocated to take 100 mg aspirin daily or placebo and 1 g capsules containing naturally occurring *n*-3 fatty acids or placebo capsules containing olive oil.

8.3 Dementia

Dementia is characterised by an insidious, slowly progressive memory loss with alteration of higher intellectual function and cognitive abilities. Dementia is defined as a syndrome consisting of a progressive impairment of memory and at least one other cognitive deficit (aphasia, apraxia, agnosia or disturbance in executive function) in the absence of another explanatory disorder of the brain (Cummings 2004). Different types of dementia are now distinguished, including Alzheimer's disease, vascular dementia and dementia with Lewy bodies. Alzheimer's disease is the most common cause of dementia. Alzheimer's disease and vascular dementia have distinct pathological features, but these two disorders frequently coexist and the combination is associated with a greater severity of cognitive impairment. While clinicians have placed much emphasis on the distinction between dementia and cognitive impairment, the distinction between these may be viewed as arbitrary. Cognitive impairment is a quantitative disorder and its distribution in the population shows a continuum of severity with dementia at the tail of the distribution. The fact that cognitive impairment is common in the population does not imply that it is intrinsic to ageing. The distribution of cognitive impairment is shifted downwards with increasing age, such that the mean scores decrease

134   *Healthy Ageing*

and the prevalence of cognitive impairment increases.

While the aetiology of Alzheimer's disease is unknown, some experts have speculated that the accumulation of β-amyloid peptide in the brain is central to the pathogenesis of Alzheimer's disease (Cummings 2004). Mutations in the amyloid precursor proteins leading to pre-senile dementia, over-expression of β-amyloid protein in Down's syndrome and mouse knock-out models have provided support for this hypothesis. Alternative hypotheses for the aetiology of Alzheimer's disease have placed greater emphasis on the role of vascular factors and neuronal cell death. Dementia with Lewy bodies is characterised by Parkinsonism, visual hallucinations and fluctuating confusion.

The age-specific incidence rates for dementia in the UK increase exponentially from 7/1000/year at age 65 to 85/1000/year at age 85 years or more (Matthews and Brayne 2005). In addition, many more individuals suffer from mild cognitive impairment without progressing to frank dementia. The onset of dementia is insidious and the underlying disease is believed to begin many years before manifestation of symptoms of dementia.

8.3.1 Vitamin B₁₂ and folate and risk of cognitive impairment and dementia

The hypothesis that elevated serum total homocysteine may also be a risk factor for Alzheimer's disease was prompted by the observation in a retrospective case-control study that patients with histologically confirmed Alzheimer's disease had higher concentrations of homocysteine in blood samples collected before death than age-matched controls (Clarke *et al.* 1998) (see Figure 8.3). This longitudinal study compared homocysteine levels taken during life from 76 cases with a histological diagnosis of 'Alzheimer's disease' made at post-mortem with 108 controls without cognitive impairment. Clarke *et al.* (1998) reported a 4.5-fold (95% CI: 2.2–9.2) risk for histologically confirmed Alzheimer's disease associated with homocysteine levels in the upper, compared with the lower, third after controlling for age, sex, smoking, social class and apolipoprotein E (ApoE) genotype. The homocysteine measurements were taken on blood samples that had been collected yearly for three successive years and were stable over this period and independent of the duration and severity of symptoms of dementia prior to enrolment.

Since then, several studies have confirmed these findings, but a few studies have been unable to do so. The most reliable evidence for the relevance of homocysteine with risk of dementia comes from an eight-year follow-up prospective study of 1092 dementia-free older individuals which reported that elevated homocysteine levels were associated with a twofold higher risk of dementia and of Alzheimer's disease (see Figure 8.4) (Seshadri *et al.* 2002). After adjustment for age, sex, apolipoprotein-E genotype, and vascular risk factors other than homocysteine and plasma levels of folate, vitamins B₁₂ and B₆, the relative risk for dementia was 1.4 (95% CI: 1.1–1.8) for a one standard deviation increase in plasma homocysteine concentrations.

Several prospective studies in non-demented individuals reported an association between baseline homocysteine and subsequent cognitive decline in non-demented individuals. For example, the MacArthur Study of Successful Aging involving 499 men aged 70–79 years reported that elevated homocysteine and low folate, vitamin B₁₂ or B₆ status were

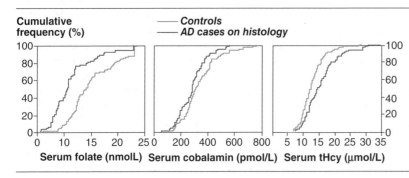

Figure 8.3: Cumulative frequency of serum folate, cobalamin and homocysteine (tHcy) in patients with a histological diagnosis of Alzheimer's disease (AD) and in controls.
Source: Clarke *et al.* (1998). © American Medical Association, 1998. All rights reserved.

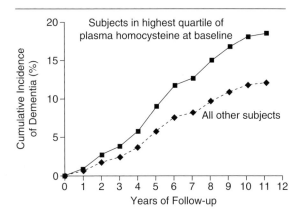

Figure 8.4: Risk of dementia in relation to homocysteine concentrations.
Source: Seshadri *et al.* (2002). © Massachusetts Medical Society, 2002. All rights reserved.

each associated with poor cognitive function (Kado *et al.* 2005). Brain imaging studies have provided important information on the associations of homocysteine with cognitive impairment and with the underlying cerebrovascular and neurodegenerative changes. The initial case-control study (Clarke *et al.* 1998) of homocysteine and Alzheimer's disease showed that atrophy of the medial temporal lobe on CT scan of the brain of cases with Alzheimer's disease was more rapid in individuals with elevated homocysteine concentrations. In the Rotterdam Brain Scan Study of 1077 men and women aged 60–90 years, plasma homocysteine concentrations were associated with increased risk of severe deep and periventricular white matter lesions and of silent brain infarcts in a cross-sectional analysis of MRI scans (Vermeer *et al.* 2002). These MRI lesions were three times more common in individuals in the top quintile of homocysteine values compared with the bottom four quintiles. The severity of the white matter lesions increased with increasing homocysteine levels and the association remained significant even after adjustment for atherosclerotic disease and the presence of silent infarcts (Vermeer *et al.* 2002). A subsequent analysis from the same study reported that atrophy in the cerebral cortex and hippocampus was associated with elevated homocysteine levels (den Heijer *et al.* 2003). More recent evidence from a UK cross-sectional study of 1000 older people in Banbury has demonstrated an association of cogni-

tive impairment with low plasma levels of holotranscobalamin (the active fraction of vitamin B_{12}) and with high levels of methylmalonic acid (a metabolic marker of vitamin B_{12} deficiency) in addition to elevated homocysteine concentrations (Hin *et al.* 2006). It is possible that low vitamin B_{12} may have an effect on risk of dementia that is independent of differences in plasma homocysteine. Many of the homocysteine-lowering trials designed for the prevention of CHD and stroke will include some assessment of cognitive function and may provide evidence about whether lowering homocysteine concentrations (and administration of high-dose vitamin B_{12}) could slow the rate of cognitive decline (Clarke 2006).

8.3.2 Possible hazards of folic acid

While folic acid is widely used to treat anaemia, the hazards of inappropriate use of folic acid treatment in people with vitamin B_{12} deficiency at folic acid dose levels above 1–2 mg have long been appreciated (Ross *et al.* 1947; Food and Nutrition Board. Institute of Medicine 2002). There have been case reports that folic acid treated patients with pernicious anaemia had an accelerated decline in neurological function (Lindenbaum *et al.* 1988; Food and Nutrition Board. Institute of Medicine 2002). Consequently, the amount of folic acid is routinely limited to a maximum of 1000 µg/day because of concerns about the adverse effects of high-dose folic acid in people with vitamin B_{12} deficiency. In 1998, the US introduced mandatory folic acid fortification of all grain products at a dose of folic acid of 140 µg per 100 g of grain. It was believed that this would increase the average daily intake by 100 µg/day. The prevalence of low serum folate has decreased from 16%–22% pre-fortification to 0.5%–1.7% post-fortification (Pfeiffer *et al.* 2005). Folic acid fortification has been very successful in lowering the risk of neural tube defects (S. Liu *et al.* 2004; Mills and Signore 2004). The required level of fortification was considered generally safe. However, concern persists about the safety of folic acid fortification in older people with vitamin B_{12} deficiency. In the US, introduction of folic acid fortification has resulted in 200–300% increases in serum folate concentrations and voluntary fortification in the UK has also resulted in a substantial increase in folate status.

Elevated homocysteine levels in older people may reflect impaired status of either vitamin B_{12} or folate

Table 8.4: Completed trials of B-vitamin supplementation for prevention of cognitive impairment and dementia

Name and year of publication	No. of participants	Folic acid	B_{12}	Treatment duration (months)	Outcome measures*
Seal et al. (2002)	31		+	1	MMSE/ADAS
de la Fournierre et al. (1997)	11		+	5	ADAS
Bryan et al. (2002)	40	+		1.5	Battery
Fioravanti et al. (1997)	30	+		2	Battery
Sommer et al. (2003)	–	+		–	Battery
Clarke, Harrison et al. (2003)	149	+	+	3	MMSE/ADAS
Stott et al. (2005)	200	+	+	3	TICS-M
Lewerin et al. (2005)	209	+	+	3	Battery
Durga et al. (2007)	728	+		36	Battery
McMahon et al. (2006)	276	+	+	24	Battery
Eussen et al. (2006)	193	+	+	6	Battery
Schirmer (unpublished)	780	+	+	40	MMSE
HOPE-2 (unpublished)	1000	+	+	60	MMSE

*ADAS: Alzheimer's disease assessment scale; MMSE: mini-mental state examination scores.
+Folic acid or vitamin B_{12} allocated treatment.

or a combination. However, the relative importance of vitamin B_{12} deficiency as a determinant of homocysteine concentrations and cognitive impairment is probably greater than that for folate deficiency in older people. Cross-sectional studies of older people have shown that a high proportion of older people have biochemical evidence of low vitamin B_{12} status, and the prevalence of low vitamin B_{12} status increases from 5% at age 65 to 20% at age 80 years (Clarke, Refsum et al. 2003). It is unclear the extent to which the associations of low vitamin B_{12} status with risk of dementia, depression and stroke are causal. Moreover, low vitamin B_{12} status may be more relevant in the setting of mandatory folic acid fortification. Consequently, there is some concern, particularly in countries with mandatory folic acid fortification, that individuals with low vitamin B_{12} status may have more rapid deterioration of neurological function in the context of a high intake of folate (Morris et al. 2005). In a recent cross-sectional study of 1459 older people in the US carried out after the introduction of mandatory fortification, Morris et al. (2007) reported that low vitamin B_{12} (vitamin B_{12} <150 pmol/L) and high serum folate (serum folate >60 nmol/L) was associated with a fivefold increased risk of cognitive impairment compared with those with normal levels, providing some evidence of a possible hazard of high levels of folic acid fortification.

It is important to ascertain the relevance, if any, of vitamin B_{12} for risk of brain disease in older people by carrying out randomised trials of vitamin B_{12} supplements in older people. There are several ongoing randomised trials assessing the effects of homocysteine-lowering vitamin supplements on cognitive function, but it is unclear if any of these trials will be able to determine the independent relevance of vitamin B_{12} on folic acid use for prevention of cognitive impairment (see Table 8.4). Further trials of vitamin B_{12} supplementation or placebo involving a large number of high-risk older participants are required to assess the relevance of vitamin B_{12} supplements or placebo for the prevention of cognitive impairment and dementia. In the FACIT trial, 818 healthy middle-aged adults (age 60 years) were randomised to folic acid (0.8 mg) for three years, resulting in 26% lowering in homocysteine concentration and a modest improvement in some domains of cognitive function (Durga et al. 2007). A systematic review of 14 randomised trials of vitamin B_6 or vitamin B_{12} or folic acid supplementation and cognitive function concluded that there was insufficient evidence of beneficial effects of these vitamins on cognitive function.

The results of these ongoing trials of B vitamins are required before recommending B vitamin supplementation for the prevention of dementia. Nevertheless, the evidence suggests that the benefits of folic acid fortification for prevention of neural tube defects are likely to outweigh any possible hazards of folic acid fortification for older people provided public health strategies avoid an excessive intake of folic acid in older people with vitamin B_{12} deficiency.

Thus, if mandatory fortification with folic acid is introduced in the UK, it will be important to control voluntary fortification of breakfast cereals and spreads (which have already had a substantial effect on increasing the population mean folate levels) to avoid any potential hazard in older people due to excessive intakes of folic acid in the setting of vitamin B_{12} deficiency.

8.3.3 Oxidative stress and Alzheimer's disease

A growing body of evidence suggests that oxidative processes may be involved in the aetiology of Alzheimer's disease. Accumulated damage by reactive oxygen species to lipid membranes and DNA is thought to disrupt normal cell functioning and lead to neuronal death. The antioxidant nutrients have been shown to decrease lipid peroxidation and oxidative proteins and prevent mitochondrial dysfunction and neurotoxicity and neuronal death. Several prospective studies have examined the association between dietary intake of antioxidants and Alzheimer's disease. Three prospective studies have reported on the association of vitamin E and vitamin C supplement use and Alzheimer's disease, but the results have been conflicting. The results of randomised trials of supplementation with antioxidant vitamins on cognitive function have been disappointing. The Heart Protection study involving 20,536 men and women at high risk of cardiovascular events treated with a cocktail of antioxidant vitamins (vitamins E and C and β-carotene) or placebo reported that the antioxidant vitamins had no protective effect on cognitive function or risk of dementia (Heart Protection Study 2002). Composite dietary patterns, such as the Mediterranean diet, have been linked with lower risk of Alzheimer's disease (Scarmeas *et al.* 2006), but such studies are difficult to interpret because of clustering of differences in antioxidants, fatty acids and flavonoids in the Mediterranean diet.

8.3.4 Dietary fat and dementia

In a four-year follow-up of a cohort of 815 older people in the Chicago Health and Aging Study, intakes of saturated fat and *trans* unsaturated fatty acids were associated with an increased risk of Alzheimer's disease, whereas intakes of polyunsaturated and monounsaturated fatty acids were associ-

ated with reduced risk of Alzheimer's disease (Morris *et al.* 2003). The strongest effect was observed for *trans* fatty acids; the top 80% in *trans* fatty acid consumption had, on average, four times the risk of developing Alzheimer's disease (after adjusting for the effects of the other fats) than the 20% with the lowest *trans* fat consumption. In the case of saturated fat, there were similar but weaker associations, the top 80% of saturated fat consumption was associated with a 2.5 times higher risk compared with those in the bottom 20% consumption category. Similar, but inverse associations were found for intake of polyunsaturated and monounsaturated fatty acids (Morris *et al.* 2003).

Observational studies suggest possible benefits of *n*-3 fatty acid consumption for prevention of dementia. In a seven-year follow-up of the PAQUID study of 1674 free-living older French people, eating fish at least once a week compared with not doing so was associated with a reduction in the risk of dementia by a third (hazard ratio: 0.66; 95% CI: 0.47–0.93). A recent randomised double-blind placebo-controlled trial of 174 older patients with mild to moderate Alzheimer's disease in Sweden reported no difference in cognitive function between a group supplemented with daily intake of 1.7 g of DHA and 0.6 g of EPA for six months and the control group (Freund-Levi *et al.* 2006). However, they found a significant delay in the rate of cognitive decline in a small sub-group ($n = 32$) with very mild cognitive dysfunction. In the UK, the Older People and *n*-3 Long-chain (OPAL) polyunsaturated fatty acids study is currently assessing the effects of daily supplementation with 0.7 g for two years of *n*-3 long-chain fatty acids or placebo on the rate of cognitive decline in 798 older people.

8.3.5 Blood pressure and risk of dementia

Elevated blood pressure in mid-life is strongly related to risk of developing dementia in old age. The importance of lowering blood pressure for reduction in the risk of dementia was highlighted by the Systolic Blood Pressure in the Elderly Trial (Syst-Eur) (Forette *et al.* 1998). In this trial examining older patients with isolated systolic hypertension, treatment with a calcium channel blocker reduced the incidence of dementia by 50% in a two-year follow-up. The trial was too small to provide definitive evidence about the relevance of blood pressure-lowering therapy for the prevention of dementia. The Hypertension in the Very Elderly Trial (HYVET) provided randomised evidence for the effects of blood pressure-lowering therapy on cognitive function in almost 4000 people aged 80 years or greater (Peters *et al.* 2008).

8.3.6 Aluminium and Alzheimer's disease

While there was circumstantial evidence linking aluminium to risk of Alzheimer's disease, most experts now believe that any such association is unlikely to be causal (Rondeau 2002). The hypothesis was put forward after finding aluminium in plaques and tangles in the brain (Perl and Brody 1980), but these associations are likely to be a consequence of the disease rather than a cause. There is no evidence that use of aluminium containers for storage or cooking of food is related to an increased risk of developing dementia.

8.3.7 Caffeine, alcohol and cognitive decline

A positive relationship has been demonstrated between habitual coffee consumption and cognitive function in older people (Jarvis 1993; Johnson-Kozlow *et al.* 2002; Rogers 2007). Although caffeine increases blood pressure, which should increase risk of cognitive impairment later in life, it appears to have additional effects which may offset an adverse effect on blood pressure (Rogers 2007). For example, caffeine consumption may lower the risk of type 2 diabetes and ischaemic brain damage. Some studies have reported that people who drink coffee have a reduced risk of Alzheimer's disease in later life (de Mendonca and Maia 2002), but large prospective studies of caffeine intake and Alzheimer's disease are needed to confirm or refute this hypothesis.

Excessive alcohol consumption, and particularly binge drinking, has been associated with increased risk of cognitive impairment and dementia in later life (Hulse *et al.* 2005). However, there is some evidence that moderate or light drinking may reduce cognitive decline in older people. For example, a Finnish study of 1341 men and women followed up for a period of 21 years at ages 65–79 years reported that moderate alcohol consumption in middle and old age was favourably related to several measures of cognitive function (episodic memory, psychomo-

tor speed and executive function) in later life (Ngandu *et al.* 2006). Whether this association is causal is uncertain and the mechanism involved remains to be elucidated.

8.3.8 Physical activity and dementia

There is some evidence from cohort studies that regular physical activity in old age is associated with reduced cognitive decline in later life (Lautenschlager and Almeida 2006). Larson and colleagues (2006) reported, in a six-year follow-up of a cohort study of 1740 people aged over 65 years, an age- and sex-adjusted hazard ratio for incident dementia of 0.62 (95% CI: 0.44–0.86) for those who exercised more than three times a week compared with those who did not exercise regularly. The suggested benefits have not yet, however, been adequately supported by data from randomised clinical trials.

8.4 Depression

Depression is a condition in which sadness, hopelessness and lack of energy dominate the lives of affected individuals limiting their ability to cope with their everyday activities. Depression affects people in different ways and to different degrees. It is a clinical syndrome that is diagnosed based on clinical criteria. Depression is commonly described as unipolar depressive disorder and has various subtypes according to the severity of symptoms (mild, moderate and severe) and the presence of other psychiatric symptoms. Depressive symptoms may also be seen in bipolar affective disorder, a condition characterised alternately by mania and depression. Both types of depression have a prevailing feeling of sadness and emotional and social withdrawal and may involve disturbed sleep, appetite and energy and additional 'physical' symptoms. Depression is associated with a disturbance in biogenic amines, such as noradrenaline and serotonin, but the aetiology is not understood. Risk factors that predispose an individual to depression include a personal or family history of depression or substance abuse, serious medical illness, lack of social support, history of early childhood trauma or neglect, divorce, death or illness in a family member, low socio-economic status or stressful work. Major depressive symptoms last at least several weeks and are characterised by depressed mood and loss of interest or pleasure in nearly all activities. Depression in the elderly is closely related to poor physical health. Most cases of depression in older people have been overlooked because of concomitant chronic disease. Many patients with depression attribute their symptoms to a physical problem. Major depression is commonly associated with heart disease, stroke and cancer. Recent research has focused on the role of vascular factors and nutrition in risk of depression.

Low serum cobalamin (an indicator of vitamin B_{12} status) and elevated levels of homocysteine and methylmalonic acid (metabolites that are elevated in the setting of vitamin B_{12} deficiency) have been associated with risk of depression in old age and are correlated inversely with a variety of measures of wellbeing. There have been many reports of an association between folate deficiency and depression. The response to antidepressant drug treatment is often poorer in patients with low folate status and it has been reported that improved clinical responses can be obtained by combining drug treatment with folic acid treatment (Coppen and Bailey 2000). There is no clear randomised evidence that dietary supplementation with *n*-3 fatty acids may be protective for depression. The results of ongoing trials of *n*-3 supplementation assessing effects on cognition and mood are awaited.

Selenium supplementation has also been recommended for patients with depression. Selenium status has been shown to be associated with mood changes, with deficiency resulting in poorer mood and hostile activity (Hawkes and Hornbostel 1996; Benton 2002). A few small studies have suggested supplementation to decrease anxiety, depression and tiredness (Benton and Cook 1991), with improvements greatest in those whose diets were lowest in selenium. However, a larger double-blind placebo-controlled intervention of 501 subjects aged 60–74, randomly allocated to receive 100, 200 or 300 μg of selenium a day for six months, found no evidence of any beneficial effect on mood or quality of life (Rayman *et al.* 2006). (The UK reference nutrient intake for selenium is 75 and 60 μg/day for adult males and females respectively.)

8.5 Parkinson's disease

Parkinson's disease is characterised by tremor, rigidity and akinesia (an absence or lack of movement) and the diagnosis is made on the basis of clinical criteria. The clinical features first described by James Parkinson in 1817 continue to apply today. These include tremor in the hands, arms and elsewhere, rigidity and slowness of movement, and impaired balance and coordination (Lang and Lozano 1998). The combination of asymmetry of symptoms and signs, the presence of resting tremor and a good response to the drug levodopa help to distinguish idiopathic Parkinson's disease from atypical Parkinsonism due to other causes (*e.g.* dementia with Lewy bodies, progressive supranuclear palsy that have a much more adverse prognosis). The prevalence of idiopathic Parkinson's disease increases exponentially with age, affecting about 3% of the population aged 65 years or greater. The aetiology of Parkinson's disease is unknown, but neuropathological features involve progressive death of the dopaminergic neurons of the substantia nigra in the basal ganglia region of the brain that controls movement and coordination. The death of these neurons is closely associated with accumulation of clumps of proteins in the brain stem called Lewy bodies. Like Alzheimer's disease, there is considerable debate about whether the deposition of protein is a cause of the disease or a consequence of the disease. Lewy bodies are not specific to Parkinson's disease and may represent neurons that have sequestered toxic proteins and provided a defence against neurodegenerative process. An alternative view is that the formation of Lewy bodies from neurofilaments alters the critical function of neurons. Dementia is increasingly recognised as an important feature of Parkinson's disease in the elderly and is more common in individuals with Parkinsonism than in age-matched older controls; most cases of Parkinson's disease ultimately develop dementia. It is likely that many of the risk factors associated with dementia may also be associated with Parkinson's disease.

8.5.1 Diet and Parkinson's disease

A number of foods and nutrients have been implicated in the risk of Parkinson's disease and plausible biological hypotheses have been proposed (*e.g.* via the influence of dietary factors on oxidative stress and neurodegeneration). Although several case-control studies have investigated the link between diet and Parkinson's disease, there have been relatively few cohort studies. A recent systematic review concluded that there is insufficient evidence of significant associations for most foods or nutrients (Ishihara and Brayne 2005). The strongest evidence suggests an inverse association with caffeine and alcohol intake, but findings have not been entirely consistent. In the Rotterdam Study, a prospective, population-based cohort study of people aged 55 years and older, the authors evaluated the association between dietary intake of folate, vitamin B_{12} and vitamin B_6 and the risk of incident Parkinson's disease among 5289 participants who were free of dementia and parkinsonism and underwent complete dietary assessment at baseline (de Lau *et al.* 2006). Parkinson's disease was assessed through repeated in-person examination and continuous monitoring by computer linkage to medical records. After a mean follow-up of 9.7 years, the authors identified 72 participants with incident Parkinson's disease. Higher dietary intake of vitamin B_6 was associated with a significantly decreased risk of Parkinson's disease (hazard ratio per SD, 0.69 [95% CI: 0.50–0.96]; for highest versus lowest tertile, 0.46 [0.22–0.96]). Stratified analyses showed that this association was restricted to smokers. No association was observed for dietary folate and vitamin B. Further research is needed to elucidate the role of diet in the risk of Parkinson's disease and to study possible gene–nutrient interactions.

8.6 Implications for research and public health

Additional observational studies involving a larger number of participants are required to assess the effects of lifestyle and nutritional exposures for common brain diseases in older people using standardised instruments to assess nutrition and lifestyle. The UK Biobank commenced recruitment in 2006 and it will take the form of a very large cohort study of 500,000 middle-aged volunteers who will be followed up for several decades. Participants will be asked to provide information on medical history, lifestyle and aspects of diet, and a blood sample for assessment of DNA and other biomarkers. The study will assess the combined effects of genotypes and nutrition on risk of brain diseases in older people, including stroke, Parkinson's disease and dementia in due course.

Ongoing large-scale trials assessing the effects of blood pressure therapy or supplementation with B

vitamins on the risk of stroke and cognitive function (see Section 8.2.4) are likely to be informative (B-Vitamin Treatment Trialists' Collaboration 2006). Further trials assessing the effects of dietary supplementation with *n*-3 fatty acids on risk of vascular disease and cognitive function are currently underway. Since the absolute risk of dementia and stroke increases among people aged 75 years or older, primary prevention trials are now required in high-risk older people to assess the combined effects of vitamin B_{12} supplementation and other cardioprotective therapy on risk of brain diseases in older people. In 1998, the US Department of Agriculture introduced mandatory folic acid fortification of all grain products at a dose of folic acid of 140 µg per 100 g of grain (Pfeiffer *et al.* 2005). The prevalence of low serum folate has decreased from 16%–22% pre-fortification to 0.5%–1.7% post-fortification and the actual level of fortification is about double that which was intended (Pfeiffer *et al.* 2005). Concern has been expressed about the safety of folic acid fortification in older people with vitamin B_{12} deficiency, where individuals with low vitamin B_{12} status appear to have a more rapid deterioration of cognitive function in the setting of high intakes of folate (Morris *et al.* 2005). Concern about the possible adverse effects of high intakes of folic acid on neurological function in people with vitamin B_{12} deficiency has delayed the introduction of mandatory folic acid fortification in the UK. Vitamin B_{12} deficiency is common in older people and the prevalence increases from about 5% at age 65 to 20% at age 80 years (Clarke *et al.* 2004). Vitamin B_{12} is a more important determinant of elevated homocysteine concentrations in older people than folate (Clarke *et al.* 2004). Studies of older people indicate that only a small proportion of those identified with biochemical evidence of vitamin B_{12} deficiency have anaemia or neuropathy or cognitive impairment (Hin *et al.* 2006).

The UK Scientific Advisory Committee on Nutrition (2006) recognised that vitamin B_{12} deficiency is an important public health issue for older people and that a management strategy should be assessed irrespective of whether mandatory folic acid fortification is introduced. Yet, none of the large homocysteine-lowering trials for the prevention of cardiovascular events (B-Vitamin Treatment Trialists' Collaboration 2006) can distinguish the independent effects of vitamin B_{12} from that of folic acid. To address the management of the older population with biochemical evidence of vitamin B_{12} deficiency in the absence of symptoms, additional randomised evidence should be sought for the effects of daily oral dietary supplements of vitamin B_{12} in individuals aged 70 years or more in the absence of prior vascular disease, anaemia or cogni-tive impairment. In addition to testing the relevance of vitamin B_{12} for the maintenance of cognitive function in a high-risk older population, trials adopting a factorial design could simultaneously assess the efficacy of other practicable treatments for the prevention of dementia and inform strategies for healthy ageing.

8.7 Key points

- Stroke, dementia, Parkinson's disease and depression are common diseases affecting the brain in older people and account for most cases of disability in this age group. The incidence of these diseases increases exponentially with increasing age.
- Since the brain is dependent on a constant supply of oxygen and nutrients for optimum function, it is not surprising that these diseases have been linked with poor nutrition and with derangements in the blood supply to the brain.
- Observational studies have suggested that atherosclerotic vascular disease and nutritional factors may be relevant to the aetiology of cognitive impairment, dementia, Parkinson's disease and depression.
- Elucidation of the role of lifestyle modification and of nutrition for the prevention of dementia, Parkinson's disease or depression is complicated by the difficulty of distinguishing causal relationships associated with diet, or other aspects of lifestyle, from the consequences of having these diseases.

- Randomised trials of vascular risk factor modification or vitamin supplementation are required to assess if such treatment can prevent these diseases. These trials should initiate therapy before the onset of disease and include a sufficient number of participants to have adequate power to assess the effects of treatment.
- Randomised evidence for the effects on cognitive function of B vitamins should be available on about 20,000 of the 50,000 participants in the 12 large ongoing homocysteine-lowering trials for the prevention of cardiovascular events.
- Randomised trials assessing the effects of *n*-3 fatty acids on stroke, cognitive function and depression should be available in the next few years. Results are likely to confirm or refute the findings suggested in observational studies.
- Physical inactivity is a risk factor for cardiovascular disease. Cohort studies have also shown physical activity to be associated with better cognitive function and less cognitive decline in later life but there is little data available from randomised trials.

8.8 Recommendations for future research

- Large-scale epidemiological evidence from prospective studies is required to assess the effects of specific dietary patterns, and blood lipid and fatty acid profiles on risk of brain diseases, such as stroke, dementia, depression and Parkinsonism.
- Research is needed to evaluate brief diagnostic instruments for the assessment of cognitive function, depression and Parkinson's disease that would be feasible to use in large-scale studies.
- Large trials (and a meta-analysis of such trials) should be conducted to clarify the role of long chain *n*-3 fatty acids and α-linolenic acid in the prevention of cardiovascular disease and cognitive impairment.

Continued

- Large-scale trials (and meta-analysis of such trials) of B vitamins are required in people with prior cardiovascular disease to assess whether lowering homocysteine levels reduces the risk of cardiovascular disease and cognitive impairment. There is a need for further trials of vitamin B_{12} supplementation alone in older people.

8.9 Key references

B-Vitamin Treatment Trialists' Collaboration (2006) Homocysteine-lowering trials for prevention of cardiovascular events: a review of the design and power of the large randomized trials. *American Heart Journal*, **151**, 282–7.

Cholesterol Treatment Trialists' (CTT) Collaboration (2005) Efficacy and safety of cholesterol-lowering treatment: prospective meta-analysis of data from 90,056 participants in 14 randomised trials of statins. *Lancet*, **366**, 1267–78.

Clarke R, Smith AD, Jobst KA, *et al.* (1998) Folate, vitamin B12, and serum total homocysteine levels in confirmed Alzheimer disease. *Archives of Neurology*, **55**, 1449–55.

Homocysteine Studies Collaboration (2002) Homocysteine and risk of ischemic heart disease and stroke: a meta-analysis. *Journal of the American Medical Association*, **288**, 2015–22.

Prospective Studies Collaboration (2002) Age-specific relevance of usual blood pressure to vascular mortality: a meta-analysis of individual data for one million adults in 61 prospective studies. *Lancet*, **360,** 1903–13.

9
Healthy Ageing: The Eye

9.1 Introduction

The prevalence of vision impairment rises steeply from around 60 years of age. Distance visual acuity is the basis for categorising vision impairment in the World Health Organization's International Classification of Diseases (ICD) and is usually measured using an illuminated Snellen chart. In the UK a large study of health screening in the over-75s reported an overall prevalence of binocular visual acuity <6/18 (equivalent to severe visual impairment) of 12.4% overall; 10.3% were categorised as having low vision (binocular acuity <6/18 to 3/60) and 2.1% were blind (binocular acuity <3/60) (Evans *et al.* 2002) (Figure 9.1). These overall figures conceal the dramatic increase in the prevalence with advancing age, with one in four of those aged 85 years and over being visually impaired compared to 8% of those aged 75–79 years. Using a higher cut point for visual impairment of visual acuity <6/12 (equivalent to the visual standard required for driving in most countries) the figures were 19% and 46% respectively.

Studies of how vision impairment affects people have found that common functional problems reported include mobility (walking, using public transport, car driving), recognising people (near and distance), reading, watching television and light-related difficulties such as glare, and difficulties with night driving (Frost, Sparrow *et al.* 1998; Mangione *et al.* 1998). Psychosocial problems include low self-esteem, depression, difficulty with social relations and financial worries. The type and severity of these problems depend not only on the severity of vision loss but also the prognosis of the eye condition.

The major causes of visual impairment in the older population are refractive errors, cataracts and age-related macular degeneration (AMD) (Reidy *et al.* 1998; Congdon, O'Colmain *et al.* 2004; Evans *et al.* 2004). The relative contribution of these conditions varies according to the levels of visual acuity and age group. Refractive errors and cataracts are the major remediable causes, ranging from 70% to 50% as a proportion of all visual impairment. With increasing age or worse level of vision impairment, the proportion of treatable vision impairment declines as AMD becomes more prevalent. Diabetic retinopathy and glaucoma account for less than 10% of vision impairment in the older population in the UK (Evans *et al.* 2004) but a higher proportion of blindness due to their progressive nature. An analysis of blindness registrations in England and Wales found that the main cause was 'degeneration of the macula and posterior pole' (48.5%) followed by glaucoma (11.7%), diabetic retinopathy (3.4%), optic atrophy (3.4%), cataract (3.3%) and other conditions (20.0%) (Evans *et al.* 1996).

9.1.1 Refractive errors

Refractive errors are due to problems with accommodation (light focusing on the back of the eye) and are corrected by spectacles or contact lenses. The most common refractive errors are myopia (short sight) and hyperopia (long sight) and both result in blurred vision. There is a strong association with age for both conditions but in the opposite direction. Myopia decreases with age while hyperopia increases. For example, in a meta-analysis of data from a number of population-based studies in western countries, refractive errors due to myopia decreased from 36% at ages 40–49 to around 15% at ages 70

A

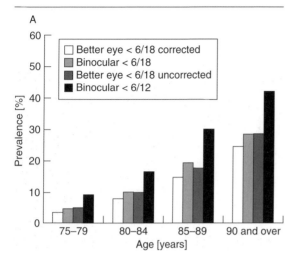

B

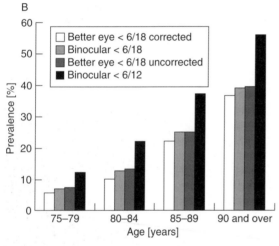

A: men; B: women

Figure 9.1: Prevalence of vision impairment by age and gender in people aged 75 years and over according to different criteria for visual acuity. Source: Evans *et al.* (2002). Reproduced by permission of BMJ Publishing Group.

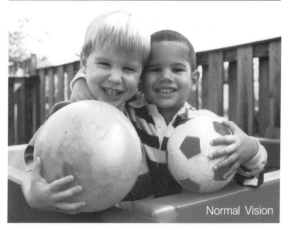

Normal Vision

Figure 9.2: Scene viewed with normal vision. Credit: National Eye Institute, National Institutes of Health.

and over, while for hyperopia the figures were 3.6% at the younger ages and over 20% in the over seventies (Kempen *et al.* 2004). It is thought that these age changes are due to loss of elasticity in the lens and ciliary muscles with ageing. The effects of increasing hyperopia at older ages lead to difficulties with near vision activities, such as reading or sewing. Regular optometry checks with provision of spectacles as appropriate is the main service for refractive errors, but the high levels of vision impairment due to refractive errors in the older population suggest that there are substantial barriers (social or economic) to the uptake of these services.

9.1.2 Cataract

Cataract is the term usually given to opacification of the lens which interferes with vision. In developed countries, studies show that lens opacification starts around middle age and with advancing age progressively becomes more widespread and dense. The first symptoms are often night-time glare and people may discontinue driving at night. With progressive lens opacification daytime vision becomes blurred. Figure 9.2 shows a scene viewed with normal vision, and Figure 9.3, the same scene as viewed by a person with cataract.

Fortunately the loss of vision due to lens opacification is easily restored through removal of the lens and replacement by an artificial lens. The prevalence of cataract and lens opacities is influenced by the availability of, and criteria for, cataract surgery. A pooled analysis of the major population-based studies in developed country settings (mainly US) described prevalence rates of unoperated significant lens opacities ranging from around 2% at ages 40–49, 15% at ages 60–64 to >50% of those aged 75 (Congdon, Vingerling *et al.* 2004). Cataract surgery represents a substantial proportion of health care costs in all western countries.

9.1.3 Age-related macular degeneration (AMD)

AMD is considered to represent the late stage of a constellation of morphological changes in the retina that occur in the ageing eye and are collectively called age-related maculopathy (ARM) (International ARM Epidemiological Study Group 1995). These early changes, especially yellowish deposits (drusen), along with abnormalities of pigmentation and patchy atrophy of the retinal pigment epithelium, are found in the older population but are not usually associated with vision loss. Results from the seven-country EUREYE study show that by age 65–69, 47% of men and women in the population have drusen and/or pigmentary irregularities (Augood *et al.* 2006). Similar findings have been reported in other studies (Klein *et al.* 1992; Vingerling *et al.* 1995). Longitudinal studies have shown that these features are a risk factor for the development of AMD, although the proportion who develop AMD is relatively small and dependent on the type of AMD studied, morphology, age and length of follow-up (Klein *et al.* 1997; van Leeuwen, C.C.W. Klaver *et al.* 2003; Wang *et al.* 2003). In the Rotterdam study the five-year incidence of AMD was highest in those aged 80 and over, especially in those with large drusen and pigment abnormalities (42%) compared to those in the same age group with small, soft drusen (2.4%) (van Leeuwen, C.C.W. Klaver *et al.* 2003). In studies from Europe, the US and Australia, the prevalence of AMD is of the order of 3–5% in the population aged over 65 years, rising with age to around 20% in people aged 85 years and over (Congdon, O'Colmain *et al.* 2004; Augood *et al.* 2006).

There are two main types of late disease. Neovascular AMD (NV-AMD), also referred to as exudative or 'wet' AMD, is characterised by invasion by neovascular complexes known as choroidal neovascularisation (CNV). The other form of late disease is characterised by extensive loss of the choriocapillaris (see Section 9.4) and the overlying retinal pigment epithelium, resulting in geographic atrophy (GA-AMD) or 'dry' AMD. NV-AMD accounts for around two-thirds of all end-stage disease, with GA-AMD accounting for the remainder. While vision loss in both can be extensive, NV-AMD accounts

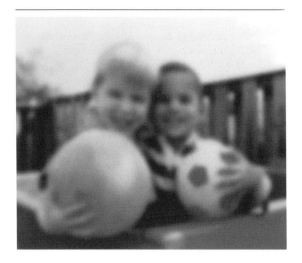

Figure 9.3: Scene viewed with cataract.
Credit: National Eye Institute, National Institutes of Health.

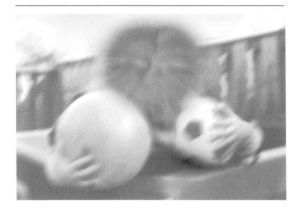

Figure 9.4: Scene viewed with age-related macular degeneration.
Credit: National Eye Institute, National Institutes of Health.

for 90% of all subjects registered as blind due to AMD. Characteristically, the condition leads to loss or impairment of central vision while the peripheral vision is, to some extent, retained (Figure 9.4).

Currently, there are no effective therapies to restore vision or prevent progression in GA-AMD. Established therapies for NV-AMD are based on suppressing the neovascular response or inducing thrombosis within the new vessels. Therefore, none

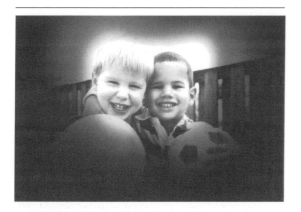

Figure 9.5:   Scene viewed with glaucoma.
Credit: National Eye Institute, National Institutes of
Health.

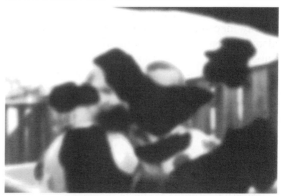

Figure 9.6:   Scene viewed with diabetic retinopathy.
Credit: National Eye Institute, National Institutes of
Health.

of the treatments is effective in restoring vision, but they do prevent or slow reductions in sight.

A review of the structure and function of lens and retina and the role of nutritional factors in cataract and AMD is presented later in this chapter.

9.1.4 Glaucoma

There are different types of glaucoma, but all are characterised by optic nerve damage (Figure 9.5). This may occur with or without an increase in intra-ocular pressure (IOP). Primary open angle glaucoma (POAG) is the most common form of glaucoma in western populations of European origin, while primary angle closure is more common in Asian Chinese people (N. Wang *et al.* 2002). POAG is relatively rare before mid-life but thereafter the prevalence rises with increasing age with estimates of around 1% at 55–59 rising to 6% over the age of 80 years (Coffey *et al.* 1993; Friedman, Wolfs *et al.* 2004). In the US, African Americans had rates of POAG nearly three times that of the white population. A raised IOP (usually defined as IOP>22 mmHg) is present in around a half of those with POAG and is a risk factor for the incidence and progression of POAG (Friedman, Wilson *et al.* 2004).

Few studies examining the role of nutrition in glaucoma (incidence or management) have been undertaken. No association with dietary antioxidants and the incidence of POAG was found in the Nurses' and Health Professionals' cohorts (Kang,

Pasquale, Rosner *et al.* 2003) nor with major fats or subtypes, but a high *n*-3/*n*-6 ratio was associated with increased POAG risk (relative risk (RR) of 1.49, 95% confidence interval (CI) 1.11–2.01) which was stronger for high tension POAG (RR = 1.68, 95% CI: 1.18–2.39) (Kang *et al.* 2004). The postulated mechanism is through influencing endogenous prostaglandin $F_{2\alpha}$ concentrations and hence IOP since prostaglandin $F_{2\alpha}$ analogues are used in the treatment of glaucoma to reduce IOP. However, further studies are required and as yet the effect of fatty acids remains equivocal. Alcohol consumption has been reported to be associated with raised IOP (Wu and Leske 1997) but not with POAG (Leske, Connell *et al.* 1995) in the Barbados Eye Study, while smoking does not appear to be a risk factor in several studies (Leske, Connell *et al.* 1995; Kang, Pasquale, Willett *et al.* 2003).

9.1.5 Diabetic retinopathy

Diabetes is a risk factor for cataract and AMD but the highest risk of visual loss for people with diabetes is due to diabetic retinopathy (Figure 9.6). Early retinal changes in diabetic patients result from the degeneration and weakening of the retinal capillaries leading to extensive haemorrhages and retinal ischaemia. Advanced retinopathy is characterised by neovascularisation, haemorrhages and scarring. Retinal detachment and total sight loss are the most severe consequences of diabetic retinopathy.

The prevalence of diabetic retinopathy in a community depends on the prevalence of diabetes, identification of people with diabetes and, most importantly, on good management and control of diabetes and associated problems. In the US the prevalence of any diabetic retinopathy in the population aged 40 and over was estimated at 3.4% and 0.75% for sight-threatening diabetic retinopathy (Kempen *et al.* 2004). Among diabetics the corresponding figures were 40% and 8%, with increasing prevalence with increasing age. These estimates were derived from population-based studies in western countries and are likely to be of the same order of magnitude in the UK.

Glycaemic and blood pressure control are the main factors reducing the risk of diabetic retinopathy (Stratton *et al.* 2001; Matthews *et al.* 2004; Leske *et al.* 2005). The role of other dietary factors, including weight control in the management of diabetes, are discussed in Chapter 13, Section 13.4.1.2. The role of oxidative stress in diabetes and animal studies (Bursell and King 1999; Scott and King 2004) gives some support to the notion that antioxidant-rich diets or supplements may reduce the risk of diabetic retinopathy in patients with diabetes. There is generally negative evidence from studies of people (either observational or clinical trials) with diabetes of a protective effect of antioxidants on the risk of complications (Rosen *et al.* 2001). There are few studies of people with diabetic retinopathy. In two population-based studies of people with diabetic retinopathy no protective effect was observed between antioxidant nutrients (vitamin E and C and β-carotene) and diabetic retinopathy with a possible adverse effect at high levels (Mayer-Davis *et al.* 1998; Millen *et al.* 2003). These effects appeared to be mainly observed in supplement users or those with high insulin, suggesting that people at highest risk of diabetic retinopathy may have changed their diets or used supplements. A study with more long-term data found no association between dietary intakes and diabetic retinopathy but supplement use for over three years, either with multivitamins, or with vitamin C or E, was associated with around a 50% reduction in diabetic retinopathy. Randomised trials in patients with early retinal changes are required to investigate fully the effects of dietary supplements in diabetic retinopathy risk.

9.1.6 Vision impairment in ethnic groups

There are very few data on vision impairment in different ethnic groups in the UK population. Diabetic retinopathy is likely to be more common in people of South Asian origin reflecting their greater susceptibility to diabetes. Two small studies attempted to examine ethnic differences (South Asian) in the prevalence of registerable blindness/partial sight (Hayward *et al.* 2002) or cataracts (Das *et al.* 1990). These studies suggested that rates might be higher in Asian groups. At present the UK data are too sparse and unreliable to comment on the prevalence of visual impairment or specific types of eye disease in different ethnic groups. Studies in the US have found that the prevalence of these conditions is higher in other ethnic groups compared to people of European origin. For example, the proportion of visual acuity <6/12 after excluding refractive errors due to glaucoma was 26% in US African Americans and in US Hispanics (Congdon, O'Colmain *et al.* 2004) and the prevalence of POAG has been reported as three times that of white groups (Friedman, Wolfs *et al.* 2004). Primary angle closure glaucoma is the most common type of glaucoma in populations of Chinese ancestry (China, Mongolia, Singapore) but there are no data on the prevalence of glaucoma in people of Chinese descent in the UK.

9.2 AMD and cataract: classic conditions of ageing?

AMD and cataract may be considered as classic age-related conditions. The prevalence is very low in middle age but rises exponentially with advancing age; these conditions are not found at younger ages (other than for rare genetic types or due to environmental insults such as trauma or extreme light exposure). Earlier, usually asymptomatic, signs of the conditions are, however, found in middle age or early in late life and both the prevalence of these earlier signs and their severity appear to increase with advancing age. The aetiology of both conditions is thought to fit with the general model of the 'free radical theory of ageing', *i.e.* cumulative exposure to oxidative stress (both endogenous and exogenous) along with reduced antioxidant capacity.

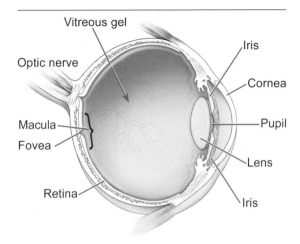

Figure 9.7: Anatomy of the eye.

Endogenous oxidative stress arises from mitochondrial respiration and will not be discussed in this chapter. A major source of external oxidative stress is light.

The eye, by virtue of its physiological function as the 'seeing' organ of the body, is particularly vulnerable to the damaging effects of light (Figure 9.7). Visible light (*i.e.* solar radiation that humans can see) consists of wavelengths of 400–700 nanometres (nm), corresponding to colour ranges from violet/blue light (shortest wavelengths) through to orange and red. Ultraviolet light (UVR), not visible to the human eye, covers a range of shorter wavelengths beyond 400 nm, and has three components, UVA (315–400 nm), UVB (280–315 nm) and UVC (<280 nm). All UVC and around 90% of UVB light is absorbed by the ozone layer. The shorter wavelengths of light have the highest energy compared to longer wavelengths and hence the greatest potential for adverse effects, *e.g.* through free radical generation. The retina is protected against UVR by the cornea and the lens, which absorbs wavelengths below 370 nm, increasing to up to 470 nm as the lens yellows with age and opacities, especially nuclear opacities, are formed (Oliva and Taylor 2005). Melanin in the retinal pigment epithelium (RPE) and choroid absorb up to a third of the shorter wavelength light.

9.3 Brief review of structure and function of the lens

In addition to absorption of UVR, the main function of the lens is to transmit and focus light onto the retina. The lens is made up of 'fibres' which are post-mitotic epithelial cells (*i.e.* they contain no organelles or nuclei), and are mainly composed of water-soluble proteins or crystallins (alpha, beta or gamma) with a high refractive index. Alpha crystallins act also as chaperones that bind to denatured proteins, keep them in solution and thereby maintain the translucency of the lens. New cells grow constantly throughout life from a single layer of epithelial cells on the lens periphery but the old fibres are not shed and are compressed with time into the nuclear region of the lens while the new cells arise in the outer region or cortex. The lens fibres are hexagonal in shape, which permits them to be closely packed with minimum intracellular spaces. This structure provides little variation in the refraction indices and maximum light transparency. Lens membranes contain large amounts of phospholipids and cholesterol. The lens has no blood supply and nutrients and waste products are obtained from the surrounding aqueous through the lens capsule. Energy production (ATP) through glucose metabolism is therefore mainly anaerobic. Nonetheless a significant proportion of ATP is mitochondrial and a major source of free radicals.

UV absorption in the lens is through a number of fluorescent biochemical compounds (filters) (Dillon 1994). One of the most important filters is O-beta glucoside of 3-hydroxykynurenine (3OHKG) formed in the lens cortex from tryptophan. 3OHKG diffuses into the nucleus and undergoes deamination into an intermediate form (α, β ketoalkene). With ageing 3OHKG and other filters decrease substantially in the lens and cortex while the adduct GSH-3OHKG increases, especially in the nucleus, suggesting that glutathione performs a scavenging role to prevent α, β ketoalkene binding to crystallins (Bova *et al.* 2001) (see Section 9.3.2). The increasing yellowing of the lens with age is mainly due to the accumulation of 3OHKG bound to protein.

The pathways through which UVR adversely damages the lens are not well understood. Studies suggest that UVR interacts with epithelial proteins, especially tryptophan residues, resulting in damage to epithelial cell membranes and ion channels leading to loss of epithelial cell glutathione, increased calcium ions and perturbation of crystallins (Hightower 1994; 1995). In addition, free radical and singlet oxygen generation occurs as a result of photo-oxidation of chromaphores.

9.3.1 Opacification of the lens

The loss of transparency of the lens arises in a number of ways, principally by increasing insolubility and unfolding of the crystalline protein leading to cross-linking and aggregation of adjacent molecules; and increases in water content increasing the distance between fibre cells. These changes disrupt the refractive index, light scattering and loss of transparency.

Advanced glycation end products (AGEs) also have adverse effects on lens protein and membranes leading to precipitation of crystallins and loss of chaperone activity. AGEs are more common in ageing cells such as the nuclear fibres in people with diabetes and in smokers (Stitt 2005). The way that opacification occurs depends in large part on the position of the lens fibres in the eye. Nuclear opacities are typified by nuclear brunescence (browning) and light scattering. Cortical opacities show disturbance of regularity of the fibres and accumulation of water and waste in the gaps between cells. Posterior subcapsular opacities which occur in swollen cells at the back of the lens and under the lens capsule cause greater interference because they lie more directly in the line of vision. Posterior subcapsular cataract is also associated with abnormal migration of epithelial cells and the production of extra-granular material. Early lens opacities are of one type only, usually nuclear opacities, but with ageing mixed opacities are seen (see Section 9.5). Although it is asserted that different types of opacities may have different risk factors, the evidence is limited by the fact that most opacities are mixed.

9.3.2 The antioxidant defence system of the lens

Glutathione is the major antioxidant in the lens (Reddy 1990) and is synthesised in the lens epithelial cells and additionally transported from the aqueous. The oxidised form can be regenerated by glutathione reductase which uses a co-factor derived from riboflavin. Other antioxidant enzymes, glutathione peroxidase and catalase, react with hydrogen peroxide

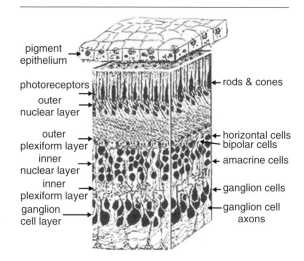

Figure 9.8: Structure of the retina.
Source: Reproduced with permission from the University of Utah.

formed from the reduction of a superoxide radical by superoxide dismutase. Selenium is an essential component of glutathione peroxidase. Superoxide dismutase is found in epithelial cells and cortical fibres but not in the nuclear fibres. Vitamin C (ascorbate) is the most important antioxidant vitamin in the eye, and found in the aqueous at concentrations of 30–50-fold that of the plasma (Varma 1987). Vitamin E is found in the lens but at similar levels as the plasma. Vitamin C acts synergistically with vitamin E, and both vitamins maintain the antioxidant activity of glutathione (Shang *et al.* 2003). Lutein and zeaxanthein are the main carotenoids; very little β-carotene is present (Taylor and Hobbs 2001). Glutathione and ascorbate in the lens decrease with age, possibly as a result of damage to cell membranes and osmosis (Taylor and Hobbs 2001).

9.4 Brief overview of retinal structure and function

The retina is made up of 10 layers of neuronal cells, predominantly photoreceptors (rods and cones) and ganglion cells (Figure 9.8). Rods outnumber cones in the ratio 20:1, except in the macula. The macula (yellow spot) is the central region of the retina and at its centre lies a small depression (fovea) within which is the foveola, an area rich in cones which provide fine acuity (Curcio *et al.* 2000; Jackson *et al.* 2002). Like all central nervous system tissue, rods and cones do not replicate themselves and are therefore susceptible to cumulative damage. The outer segments of the photoreceptors consist of a stack of discs, the membranes of which are rich in proteins (pigment molecules such as rhodopsin) and long chain polyunsaturated fatty acids (PUFAs), especially docosahexaenoic acid (DHA). Although the exact role of DHA in the retina is not well understood, it is thought to act in a number of ways, stabilising photoreceptor cell membranes, modulating membrane transport systems and acting as a precursor for other biologically active molecules (Hodge *et al.* 2005; San Giovanni and Chew 2005).

The outer segments of the photoreceptors are constantly shed (around a 10-day cycle) with synthesis of new membranes. The retinal pigment epithelium (RPE) lies posterior to the photoreceptors, each RPE cell connecting to the adjacent photoreceptors through microvilli. The RPE performs a number of critical functions; it phagocytoses the waste products from shed membranes, stores retinol (the precursor to regeneration of photo-pigments), synthesises glycosaminoglycans, transports nutrients from the choroid and removes waste products of photoreceptor metabolism to be cleared by the choroid. The choroid capillaries (choriocapillaris) lie external to the RPE, separated by a thin membrane mainly made up of collagen (Bruch's membrane). The choroid is particularly thick in the central area of the retina and has one of the fastest blood flows in the body, which is thought to be related to absorption of excess heat.

With ageing the number of rods decreases with 30% lost by the ninth decade (Curcio *et al.* 2000). The greatest loss occurs close to the fovea. The number of cones remains stable. Rod degeneration with ageing leads to reduced light sensitivity and a slowing of dark adaptation. The exact mechanism of the reduction in rod sensitivity with ageing is unknown. Local retinoid deficiency (*e.g.* due to reduced transfer of retinol from the blood or to vitamin A depletion with ageing) (Curcio *et al.* 2000) has been suggested as one possible mechanism while long chain PUFAs may also play a role. The practical implications of the effects of rod degeneration are to ensure good home lighting, but the nutritional implications are as yet untested, although one ongoing randomised trial is evaluating the effects of fish oil supplements on photoreceptor response

in people over 70 years (www.lshtm.ac.uk/nphiru/research/n3pufas.html).

9.4.1 Light and the retina

Primate and laboratory studies have shown that blue light, especially in high oxygen environments, causes retinal damage in a number of ways (Winkler *et al.* 1999; Beatty *et al.* 2000; Zarbin 2004) resulting directly from the generation of reactive oxygen species (ROS) (both free radicals and highly reactive species such as singlet oxygen) and through activation of other compounds. When light strikes the membranes of the outer segments of photoreceptor cells, it interacts with pigment molecules, such as rhodopsin, causing a biochemical cascade, including sodium conductance and hyperpolarisation of the photoreceptor and release of all-trans-retinal. A cycle of reactions ('the visual cycle') follows, which leads to the replenishment of the pigment (reduction of all-trans-retinal to all-trans-retinol, transported into RPE cells where it is esterified into long chain fatty acids and converted to 11 cis retinol, oxidised to 11 cis retinal and transported back to the photoreceptors to be combined with opsin to form rhodopsin). Light-induced damage occurs from free all-trans-retinal which is thought to be the precursor of lipophilic retinoids formed in rod outer segments – retinal A2E and its isomer iso-A2E. While full understanding of the role played by these retinoids is incomplete, A2E has been shown to increase oxidative stress through targeting cytochrome oxidase leading to mitochondrial apoptosis in both RPE and photoreceptor cells (Sparrow *et al.* 2000; Shaban and Richter 2002), to cause loss of lysosomal integrity and inhibit RPE phagocytosis (Zarbin 2004). The light environment of the retina means that a number of other reactions leading to ROS formation occur outside the main visual cycle, for example from oxidation of PUFAs in cell membranes, lipofuscin and singlet oxygen from porphyric photosensitisers in the choroidal blood.

9.4.2 The antioxidant defence system in the retina

Not surprisingly in the retinal environment of high oxygen tension and light exposure, the cells contain a number of potent antioxidants, some at very high concentrations compared to elsewhere in the body. These include enzymes, principally superoxide dismutase, catalase, glutathione and glutathione peroxidase; and antioxidant vitamins C and E and the carotenoids (Winkler *et al.* 1999). The antioxidant enzymes are the first-line defence system supported by the antioxidant vitamins. The only carotenoids found in the retina are lutein and zeaxanthein, which are present in very high concentrations in the macula (as seen by the yellow spot). They scavenge singlet oxygen (one of the most damaging ROS) and also protect the cell membranes from lipid oxidation. In addition, they filter blue light with a peak absorption at 460 nm (Beatty *et al.* 1999). Zinc is found in high concentrations in photoreceptors and RPE cells. Its primary function may be to react with vitamin A to form photoreceptor pigments.

9.5 The role of diet: evidence from epidemiological studies

Studies in human populations present a number of challenges, many familiar but others related to the specific context of the retina or lens.

Defining and quantifying 'disease' status has differed among studies making comparisons difficult especially in earlier studies. Grading systems, such as the Lens Opacities Classification System (LOCS) (Chylack *et al.* 1989) and the Wisconsin Age Related Maculopathy Grading System (Klein *et al.* 1991), which became the basis for a standardised classification (International ARM Epidemiological Study Group 1995), have provided a common framework and terminology.

Antioxidant vitamin levels in studies have been assessed in a variety of ways: reported dietary intakes and vitamin supplement consumption and collection of blood samples. Recall error is a problem for dietary intake methods, while both blood levels and dietary methods may not reflect habitual levels. Supplement users tend to have healthier lifestyles in many ways which need to be included in the analyses to control for confounding. Measurements in the plasma may not reflect levels in the retina; for example, there are some differences between plasma and macula carotenoids, mainly for zeaxanthein which exists in three different stereoisomers in the macula but only one in the plasma. Most studies have looked at the effects of individual antioxidants, although it is likely that the antioxidant levels of several key antioxidants in combination may be more appropriate. Collinearity of certain antioxidants, such as lutein and zeaxanthein, and low power to detect interactions are some of the methodological difficulties in assessing the effects of antioxidants in combination.

Assessing lifetime exposure to light needs to take account of time spent outdoors at different periods of the day (*e.g.* in the middle of the day when solar radiation is highest), the reflectance of different surfaces, and use of ocular protection such as hats, contact lenses and glasses. Data on lifetime residence are also required for mapping to meteorological data on ambient light exposures taking account of factors such as cloud cover and altitude.

Study design limitations include difficulties in establishing temporality in concurrent measurements of nutrition and outcome (lens or fundus status) in cross-sectional or case-control studies (*e.g.* diet and blood levels may be affected either by the disease itself [reverse causation] or by recent changes in diet due to knowledge of disease status). Prospective cohort studies avoid these problems but may be limited by the difficulties and resources required to ascertain lens or fundus status over time. Case-control studies may be flawed by selection biases in cases and controls (especially controls). Randomised trials of supplementation minimise the probability of uncontrolled confounding, but have a number of other problems: choice of single or multiple supplements, appropriate dose (possible toxicity against maximum effectiveness) and, most importantly, length of follow-up.

Much of the observational evidence is derived from a few key population-based studies in western settings (Beaver Dam Eye Study and Salisbury Eye Study in the US, the Australian Blue Mountains Eye Study, the POLA study in southern France). A limitation of these studies is that they are single-centre studies with less heterogeneity in diet. The EUREYE study was specifically designed to maximise differences in diet and sunlight exposure. Seven study centres drawn from north to south Europe followed a common protocol and fundus images and blood biochemistry were assessed independently (Augood *et al.* 2004). The earlier cross-sectional studies (Beaver Dam, Blue Mountains, POLA) also have a longitudinal component which permits investigation of incidence and progression of disease but are restricted by relatively few end-points over short durations of follow-up and hence low power. Large prospective cohorts, such as the Nurses' Health Study and Health Professionals' Study, have high power but have been limited by reliance on questionnaire data and self-reported outcomes. However, sub-studies within these large cohort studies with more detailed quantification of lens and fundus status and biological measurement of nutritional variables are now available (*e.g.* Nutrition and Vision Project, a sub-study of the Nurses' Health Study).

9.5.1 Epidemiological evidence on external oxidative stress

Relatively few studies have investigated associations of light exposure and lens opacities or ARM/AMD in human populations. In the general population, exposure to sunlight has been related to cortical cataracts in some studies but not observed in all, or observed in men but not in women (McCarty and Taylor 2002). There has been even less work on the possible risks of solar radiation and macular degeneration. A study of fishermen found an association with lifetime exposure to blue light and risk of geographic atrophy (Taylor *et al.* 1992), while the POLA study in southern France found no association with estimates of ambient annual solar radiation (all wavelengths) and late AMD and a possible protective effect of higher exposures on early ARM (Delcourt, Carriere *et al.* 2001); and the Beaver Dam study found no association with UVB but an increased association of outdoor exposure with both the prevalence and incidence of early ARM (Cruickshanks *et al.* 1993, 2001). Other studies had no meteorological measurements and results were therefore limited to descriptors of time spent outdoors (Eye Disease Case-Control Study Group 1992; Darzins *et al.* 1997). These studies found no association with AMD.

Smoking has been consistently identified as a risk factor for lens opacities and AMD (DeBlack 2003; S.P. Kelly *et al.* 2004). That the association is likely to be causal is suggested by the consistency of the association across different study designs and populations, a dose–response relationship and a reduction in risk with length of cessation. Diabetes, a condition associated with high levels of oxidative stress, is also consistently found as a risk factor for both conditions (Taylor 1999; van Leeuwen, C.C. Kiaver *et al.* 2003).

9.5.2 Antioxidants and lens opacities

Because of their concentrations and antioxidant activities in the lens, most studies have focused on vitamins C and E and the carotenoids β-carotene and, more recently, lutein and zeaxanthein. Difficulties in assessing the evidence are compounded by variations in reporting, for example, by types of opacity (pure or mixed or any cataract), information on nutritional levels and comparator groups (*e.g.* median, quartile, tertile) and sub-group analyses (mainly age and sex, other risk factors). A number of reviews are available (Sarma *et al.* 1994; Christen 1999; Congdon and West 1999; Taylor and Hobbs 2001; Mitchell *et al.* 2003; Meyer and Sekundo 2005).

Cross-sectional or case-control studies have found a protective association between vitamin C measured by dietary intake and cataract (Jacques *et al.* 1988), or with cortical, nuclear and mixed cataract (Leske *et al.* 1991). A protective effect on incident nuclear cataract was found in the Beaver Dam study but only in those with other risk factors, such as hypertension (Lyle *et al.* 1999a). Conversely, the Salisbury Eye Study (Vitale *et al.* 1993), a case-control study in Italy (Tavani and La Vecchia 1999) and the prospective Nurses' Health Study (Hankinson *et al.* 1992) found no association. Protective associations have been reported for vitamin C measured in plasma with nuclear and posterior subcapsular opacities in two case-control studies in Mediterranean countries (Gale *et al.* 2001; Valero *et al.* 2002; Ferrigno *et al.* 2005) but not found in other case-control studies (Jacques and Chylack 1991; Vitale *et al.* 1993; Gale *et al.* 2001), although in one of these, a small study, an 11-fold risk of posterior sub-capsular cataract with low plasma vitamin C was described but was not significant (Jacques and Chylack 1991). The NHANES II cross-sectional study (Simon and Hudes 1999) found a strong inverse association between serum ascorbic acid and self-reported cataract extraction. Long-term (>10 years) use of vitamin C supplements has been associated with decreased risk of incident nuclear opacities in the Nutrition and Vision project (A. Taylor *et al.* 2002). No effect of vitamin C supplement was observed in the Health Physicians' or Nurses' Health Studies (Seddon, Christen *et al.* 1994; Chasan-Taber *et al.* 1999a) or in the Age-Related Eye Disease Study (Age-Related Eye Disease Study 2001).

Only one study (a case-control study) found a protective effect of increased dietary intakes of vitamin E with cortical, nuclear and mixed cataract (Leske *et al.* 1991), whereas no association was found in the Nurses' Health Study (Hankinson *et al.* 1992). The evidence for a protective effect of vitamin E measured in the serum is stronger, with inverse associations reported for incident cataract in the Beaver Dam Eye Study (Lyle *et al.* 1999b), with prevalent nuclear but not cortical cataract in the Salisbury Eye Study (Vitale *et al.* 1993), with both prevalent and incident nuclear cataract in the US-based Lens Opacities Case Control Study (Leske, Wu *et al.* 1995, 1998), and in two studies in Finland – a nested case-control study of cataract (Knekt *et al.* 1992) and with progression of cortical, but not nuclear lens opacities in hypercholesteroaemic men (Rouhiainen *et al.* 1996). Other studies have reported no association (C.R. Gale *et al.* 2001; Valero *et al.* 2002) or have reported an increased risk with high serum vitamin E (Ferrigno *et al.* 2005). Vitamin E supplements were associated with reduced incidence or progression of nuclear opacities (Leske *et al.* 1998; Jacques *et al.* 2005) but not with prevalence of opacities (Mares-Perlman *et al.* 1994), self-reported cataract (Simon and Hudes 1999) or cataract extraction (Chasan-Taber *et al.* 1999a). Long-term use of supplements containing either vitamin C or/and vitamin E reduced the incidence of cortical or nuclear cataracts in the Beaver Dam Study (Mares-Perlman *et al.* 2000).

High intakes of dietary carotene were associated with lower risk of cataract extraction in the Nurses' Health Study (Hankinson *et al.* 1992), in the Lens Opacities Case-Control Study (Leske *et al.* 1991) and in the Nutrition and Vision project for carotenoids and risk of posterior subcapsular cataracts in never smokers (A. Taylor *et al.* 2002). A number of studies have not found any association with dietary or plasma α- or β-carotene (Brown, Rimm *et al.* 1999; Lyle *et al.* 1999b). Plasma β-carotene was associated with reduced nuclear opacities in two studies in northern Europe (Knekt *et al.* 1992; C.R. Gale *et al.* 2001) but not in several others in diverse countries (Vitale *et al.* 1993; Valero *et al.* 2002; Ferrigno *et al.* 2005). In both the Nurses' Health Study and the Health Professionals' Study there were weak reduced associations with dietary carotenoids and cataract extraction, which were mainly due to lutein and zeaxanthein (Brown, Rimm *et al.* 1999; Chasan-Taber *et al.* 1999b). Further investigations of frequency of foods high in carotenoids, especially lutein (spinach and dark leafy green vegetables), also showed protective asso-

ciations with higher consumption (Brown *et al.* 1999; Chasan-Taber *et al.* 1999). High intakes of lutein at baseline were associated with reduced incidence of nuclear cataracts in the Beaver Dam Study (Lyle *et al.* 1999a); however the results for serum levels were inconsistent with the dietary data. The results for serum carotenoids indicated no association and differed in a number of subgroup analyses, for example significantly increased associations with high serum lutein were observed for cortical opacities and also for women for nuclear opacities (Mares-Perlman, Brady, B.E. Klein *et al.* 1995). Other studies have reported associations with serum levels of lutein and posterior subcapsular cataract (C.R. Gale *et al.* 2001), serum zeaxanthein and cataract (Delcourt *et al.* 2006) or no association with any type of cataract (Valero *et al.* 2002). A recent substantive review by the US FDA concluded that there was insufficient evidence to support a benefit from lutein or zeaxanthein on risk of cataract (Trumbo and Ellwood 2006).

The evidence from case-control or cohort studies does not overwhelmingly support a protective role for vitamin A. The Blue Mountains Study and POLA study reported protective associations for dietary (Cumming *et al.* 2000) or plasma vitamin A (Delcourt *et al.* 2000) but many studies have reported either no association (Jacques *et al.* 1988; Leske *et al.* 1991; Knekt *et al.* 1992; Vitale *et al.* 1993; Brown, Rimm *et al.* 1999; Chasan-Taber *et al.* 1999a, b) or a U-shaped relationship with plasma retinol (Vitale *et al.* 1993; Valero *et al.* 2002). Other potentially important micronutrients have received less attention. Serum selenium was not associated with risk of opacities in two studies that reported investigating this mineral (Knekt *et al.* 1992; Leske, Wu *et al.* 1995), while a non-significant protective effect was observed with dietary selenium (Valero *et al.* 2002). The evidence for riboflavin is mixed, with protective effects reported in some (Leske, Wu *et al.* 1991, 1995; Cumming *et al.* 2000; Jacques *et al.* 2005) but not all studies (Hankinson *et al.* 1992; Jacques *et al.* 2001). The few studies that have measured antioxidant enzymes or attempted to construct an overall antioxidant index have found inverse associations supporting the overall antioxidant hypothesis (Italian-American Cataract Study Group 1991; Delcourt, Cristol, Leger *et al.* 1999; Delcourt *et al.* 2003). Although studies have been conducted in populations which are not protein-deficient, associations have been observed with opacities and low levels of protein intake or markers of low protein status (Leske, Wu *et al.* 1995; Cumming *et al.* 2000; Delcourt *et al.* 2005).

The association of overall diet quality to risk of nuclear opacities was investigated in a subset of the Nurses' Health Study with lens measurements (Moeller *et al.* 2004). A Healthy Eating Index (HEI) was constructed based on adherence to recommended dietary guidelines for five food groups: grains, vegetables, fruit and fruit juice, milk and milk products and meat (including fish, nuts and dry beans). Women in the highest two quartiles of HEI had a 50% reduction in risk of lens opacities with no difference in effect between the third and top quartiles; the effect was even stronger in non-users of vitamin C supplements (around a 70% reduction in risk). Examination of the components of the HEI in non-supplement users found milk, fruit and variety (but not vegetable intake) made the strongest contribution to reduced risk. In this study the main vegetables consumed were tomatoes and iceberg lettuce, and therefore the effects of vegetables such as spinach and broccoli found in other studies to be protective could not be examined.

9.5.3 Body fat and lens opacities

Independent of the association with diabetes, studies have shown that body mass index or other measures of adiposity such as waist:hip ratio are predictive of cataract (Glynn *et al.* 1995; Schaumberg *et al.* 2000; Jacques *et al.* 2003).

9.5.4 Antioxidants and AMD

In comparison with epidemiological research on micronutrients and cataracts there has been far less epidemiological research on age-related macular degeneration. A number of reviews are available (Sarma *et al.* 1994; Christen 1999; van Leeuwen, C.C. Klaver *et al.* 2003; Hogg and Chakravarthy 2004).

As described earlier, vitamin C, and the carotenoids, lutein and zeaxanthein, play a key antioxidant role in the retina. Neither vitamin C nor the carotenoids are synthesised in the body and must be provided through the diet, suggesting that people with low intakes might be at particular risk of AMD. For vitamin C the evidence from observational studies is not supportive. Plasma vitamin C showed no association with AMD in three studies (Eye Disease Case-Control Study Group 1993; West *et al.* 1994; Delcourt, Cristol, Tessier *et al.* 1999), two of which were cross-sectional population studies (West *et al.* 1994; Delcourt *et al.* 1999) and one was a hospital-based case-control study of neovascular AMD (Eye Disease Case-Control Study Group 1993). Dietary intakes of vitamin C were also not associated with incidence (Mares-Perlman *et al.* 1996) or prevalence of AMD (Goldberg *et al.* 1988), although a high frequency of consumption of fruits and vegetables rich in vitamin C was protective.

The evidence for an association of dietary vitamin C with the earlier signs of ARM is also negative both for prevalent (Mares-Perlman *et al.* 1996) and incident early ARM (VandenLangenberg *et al.* 1998), while in the Blue Mountains Study a significant adverse effect was found for high dietary intake plus vitamin C supplement use (Flood *et al.* 2002). In the Physicians' Health Study, use of vitamin C supplements was not protective against early ARM or AMD (Christen *et al.* 1999).

There is some evidence that macular pigment density increases after supplementation with foods rich in lutein and zeaxanthein, although it appears that the response is very variable (Moeller and Blumberg 2000; Mozaffarieh *et al.* 2003). The evidence from epidemiological studies is based on measurements in the serum or from dietary data (until quite recently the food composition tables for lutein and zeaxanthein were very limited). The Eye Disease Case-Control Study found decreased risks of neovascular AMD with increasing levels of an overall measure of blood carotenoids (including α- and β-carotene cryptoxanthin and lycopene) (Eye Disease Case-Control Study Group 1993), with higher lutein/zeaxanthein concentrations (≥0.67 compared with ≤0.25 μmol/l) (Eye Disease Case-Control Study Group 1993) and with high intakes of dietary carotenoids, in particular lutein (Seddon, Adajni *et al.* 1994). A twofold increased risk of AMD was found for the lowest tertile of plasma zeaxanthein in a small study in the UK (Gale *et al.* 2003), while higher levels of plasma lutein and zeaxanthein were protective for all ARM (early and late combined) in the POLA study (Delcourt *et al.* 2006). Higher dietary intakes of lutein and zeaxanthein were also associated with early ARM and AMD in the NHANES III study (Mares-Perlman *et al.* 2001). In contrast, a number of studies have found no association. The Beaver Dam Eye study found no association between dietary intakes (retrospectively assessed) of lutein and zeaxanthein and early ARM or AMD (Mares-Perlman *et al.* 1996), and in a follow-up of the Beaver Dam cohort no association was found prospectively between dietary levels of these carotenoids and the development of early ARM (VandenLangenberg *et al.* 1998). Similarly negative findings for a number of antioxidants, including the individual carotenoids, were reported from the Blue Mountains Eye Study for the incidence of early ARM (Flood *et al.* 2002). A recent review by the US FDA concluded that there was no credible evidence to support a protective role for lutein or zeaxanthein on risk of AMD (Trumbo and Ellwood 2006).

Other micronutrients which play an antioxidant role in the retina have also been investigated in observational studies. Associations of serum α-tocopherol or dietary vitamin E with AMD have been reported in some (West *et al.* 1994; Delcourt, Cristol, Tessier *et al.* 1999) but not all studies (Eye Disease Case-Control Study Group 1993; Mares-Perlman, Brady, R. Klein *et al.* 1995a, 1996; Smith *et al.* 1997). Associations with prevalent early ARM and serum α-tocopherol ratio were found only for the POLA study (Eye Disease Case-Control Study Group 1993) but not observed with diet or serum in the Blue Mountains Study or Beaver Dam Study (Mares-Perlman, Brady, B.E. Klein *et al.* 1995; Mares-Perlman *et al.* 1996; Smith *et al.* 1997, 1999). The longitudinal follow-up of the Beaver Dam Study reported an association with dietary vitamin E and the incidence of early ARM (VandenLangenberg *et al.* 1998), but this was not found in the longitudinal follow-up of the Beaver Dam Study (Mares-Perlman *et al.* 1996). Use of vitamin E supplements was not associated with incident early ARM or AMD (Seddon, Adajni *et al.* 1994; VandenLangenberg *et al.* 1998; Christen *et al.* 1999). Neither serum retinol nor dietary vitamin A has been associated with AMD or early ARM in any study (Goldberg *et al.* 1988; West *et al.* 1994; Delcourt, Cristol, Tessier *et al.* 1999; Flood *et al.* 2002). Other antioxidants, primarily β-carotene but also β-cryptoxanthin, have not been found to be associated with either prevalent or incident ARM or AMD in any of the studies which have investigated these (West *et al.* 1994; Mares-Perlman, Brady, R. Klein *et al.* (1995b); Mares-Perlman *et al.* 1996; Smith *et al.* 1997; Flood

et al. 2002). Higher zinc intakes were found to be protective for prevalent and incident ARM in the Beaver Dam cohort (Mares-Perlman *et al.* 1996; VandenLangenberg *et al.* 1998) but there was no association observed in the prospective Health Professionals' Study (Cho *et al.* 2001) or the Eye Disease Case-Control Study (1992). In the Eye Disease Case-Control Study, increasing levels of an antioxidant index combining vitamins C and E, selenium and carotenoids was associated with reduced risk of neovascular AMD (Eye Disease Case-Control Study Group 1993). The POLA study investigated antioxidant enzymes and found that higher levels of plasma glutathione peroxidase but not superoxide dismutase (SOD) were significantly associated with a nine-fold increase in late AMD prevalence (Delcourt, Cristol, Tessier *et al.* 1999).

Studies have also examined associations between specific food items or patterns of diet. The Eye Disease Case-Control Study reported a higher frequency of intake of spinach or collard greens was associated with a substantially lower risk for neovascular AMD (Seddon *et al.* 1994); conversely fruit intake but not vegetables or carotenoids was inversely associated with the risk of neovascular AMD in the Health Professionals' and Nurses' Health Studies (Cho, Seddon *et al.* 2004).

Evidence is beginning to emerge on possible associations of long chain PUFAs and AMD (San Giovanni and Chew 2005). In the Health Professionals' and Nurses' Health Study, total fat intake and, unexpectedly, higher α-linolenic acid (an *n*-3 PUFA) were positively associated with risk of AMD (Cho *et al.* 2001). Three studies reported an inverse association with fish consumption and risk of AMD (Smith *et al.* 2000; Cho *et al.* 2001; Seddon *et al.* 2001). A large randomised controlled trial (AREDS 2) investigating supplementation with 1 g/day of long chain *n*-3 fatty acids (DHA and EPA) or lutein (10 mg) plus zeaxanthein (2 mg) supplements or both is currently underway (www.nei.nih.gov/neitrials/viewStudyWeb.aspx?id=120, accessed 31 January 2007).

9.5.5 AMD and dietary fat

If AMD shares common pathways with coronary heart disease, similar associations might be expected for the associations with dietary fat. To date only a few studies have investigated this. In the Beaver

Dam Eye Study a high intake of saturated fatty acids and cholesterol was associated with increased risk for early ARM (Mares-Perlman, Brady, R. Klein *et al.* 1995a). In contrast, no association was found for either early or late ARM in the US NHANES Study with dietary fat or with specific types of fatty acids as a proportion of total fat intake (Heuberger *et al.* 2001) or in a small UK-based study (Sanders *et al.* 1993). The Rotterdam Study found no association with either total or specific types of dietary fat and incidence of early ARM (van Leeuwen 2003). In the Eye Disease Case-Control Study there was some suggestion that high intakes of vegetable, monounsaturated and polyunsaturated fatty acids and linoleic acid (an *n*-6 PUFA) were associated with a greater risk for neovascular AMD (Seddon *et al.* 2001) but the results were not clear-cut.

9.5.6 Body fat and AMD

A high BMI has been positively associated with either early ARM (Smith *et al.* 1998; AREDS 2000; Delcourt, Michel *et al.* 2001) or progression to advanced AMD (Seddon *et al.* 2003; Clemons *et al.* 2005).

9.6 Role of diet: evidence from randomised trials

9.6.1 Age-related macular degeneration

A few small trials of short duration are not considered here because of the limitations of their study design; however, two systematic reviews have been published which include full details of these smaller trials (Evans 2002). Of the large studies only the Age-Related Eye Disease Study (AREDS) (Age-Related Eye Disease Study Research Group 2001) was specifically designed to investigate the effects of vitamin supplementation on AMD. The Vitamin E, Cataract and Age-related Maculopathy Trial (VECAT) was powered on cataract outcomes although data on AMD were also collected (H.R. Taylor *et al.* 2002). One other large study investigating the effects of vitamin supplements on cancer (the ATBC trial) also collected data on the occurrence of AMD (Teikari, Laatikainen *et al.* 1998).

The AREDS trial recruited 4757 participants aged 55–80 years, who were assigned to one of four

categories: no or minimal ARM signs (23%), minor ARM signs (22%), intermediate ARM (34%) and advanced AMD (20%). Over the seven years of follow-up the number of participants in the first two categories at baseline who progressed to intermediate ARM or advanced AMD was small and they were therefore excluded from analysis. The results of the trial were therefore based on 2577 participants (median age 69 years) with intermediate ARM or late AMD at baseline, and demonstrated that supplementation with either antioxidants or zinc or both resulted in a significant reduction in the rate of progression to AMD. The effect was slightly greater for the combination therapy. There were also benefits on outcomes likely to be noticed by patients (loss of lines of sight). The VECAT trial was smaller and participants tended to have minimal or no signs of early ARM. There was no evidence of a benefit from supplementation but the number of cases progressing was small. In the ATBC trial a sub-sample of those aged over 65 years underwent an eye examination at the end of the follow-up to ascertain whether they had signs of ARM or AMD. No effect of supplementation was observed.

9.6.2 Cataracts

Only three trials to date have been specifically designed to evaluate the effects of supplementation on cataracts. Participants in the AREDS trial who had no history of cataract extraction were also assessed for the development and progression of lens opacities over the follow-up period. No benefit was observed for antioxidant supplements in these outcomes or by type of lens opacity (Age-Related Eye Disease Study 2001). The VECAT study found no reduction in incidence or progression of any type of cataract with high-dose vitamin E (McNeil *et al.* 2004). The only trial to demonstrate a benefit, the REACT study, found a significant effect which was observed mainly in the US centres. It is possible that the methods used to determine cataract progression in this trial had greater sensitivity than the other trials (Chylack *et al.* 2002). Three of the other large supplementation trials in western populations designed for cancer or cardiovascular outcomes also examined cataracts and found no differences between those taking supplements or those taking placebo. A sub-group analysis in the Physicians' Health Study found a 26% reduced risk of cataract in smokers taking β-carotene, but no effect in non-smokers (Christen *et al.* 2003). This may have been a chance finding as it was not observed in the ATBC trial, which specifically recruited smokers (Teikari, Rautalahti *et al.* 1998). No effect of β-carotene was observed in the Women's Health Study (Christen *et al.* 2004). The Heart Protection Study also reported no differences in the prevalence of self-reported cataract extractions (Heart Protection Study 2002). Two linked trials of supplementation in a Chinese population, at high risk of oesophogeal cancer, found a 36% or 44% reduction in the prevalence of nuclear cataract for persons who received multivitamin or riboflavin/niacin supplements (Sperduto *et al.* 1993). The benefit was limited to those aged 65–74 years and in a population with many dietary deficiencies. No treatment effect was noted for cortical cataract in either trial. Although the number of posterior subcapsular cataracts was very small, there was a statistically significant deleterious effect of treatment with riboflavin/niacin.

To date, no trial has been able to investigate whether vitamin supplementation can prevent the onset of age-related eye disease. Such trials require very large numbers of participants and a long period of follow-up because of the relatively slow development and progression of age-related eye diseases. A limitation of the cancer and cardiovascular trials that also collected end-of-trial data on eye disease is that they had no baseline measures and it is therefore not possible to ascertain whether there were any differences in the rate of progression. The only trial that recruited sufficient people with intermediate ARM or advanced AMD at baseline did demonstrate a reduction in the rate of progression with a multivitamin and zinc supplement. Unlike the other trials which found no effect of supplementation with vitamin E or β-carotene, the AREDS trial used zinc and a high dose of vitamin C (nearly 10 times the recommended daily allowance or RDA). There was, however, no effect on cataracts of this supplement although the observational evidence for an association with vitamin C is, if anything, more persuasive for cataract than AMD. A number of trials in cancer and cardiovascular disease which are ongoing are also collecting data on these eye diseases.

9.7 Key points

- Good vision is essential to maintain quality of life and functional independence as people grow older. Refractive errors, cataracts, age-related macular degeneration, diabetic retinopathy and glaucoma are major problems resulting in loss of vision which are progressively more common with ageing. For patients with diabetes the threat of vision loss through diabetic retinopathy is an added burden.

- Studies in the older population have consistently shown that about 50% of visual impairment is due to treatable conditions (cataract and refractive error). Refractive errors can be resolved by appropriate spectacle correction and cataract by a replacement lens. For other eye conditions treatment is not curative and in the case of macular degeneration has very limited effectiveness.

- Smoking is a major risk factor for cataract and macular degeneration. Older people who continue to smoke should be advised of the risk to their eyes. Smokers with early stages of AMD, or intermediate AMD or advanced AMD in one eye, are at high risk of disease progression. There is moderate evidence that high exposures to sunlight are associated with increased risk of cataracts and AMD. It would be prudent to recommend ocular protection (sunglasses, wide-brimmed hats) when outdoors in the middle of the day.

- Laboratory and animal studies have demonstrated the important role of antioxidants in the lens and retina. Epidemiological studies also provide evidence that high intakes of antioxidants are protective against AMD and cataracts. Although there is less consistency for individual antioxidants, the data from both animal and human studies suggest that vitamin C and the carotenoids lutein and zeaxanthein play a critical role.

- Overall the evidence supports general dietary recommendations in older people especially for consumption of fruit and vegetables including:

Continued

- at least five portions of fruit a day, especially those high in vitamin C such as citrus fruits, and
- at least five portions of vegetables a day, especially those high in lutein and zeaxanthein such as spinach, kale, broccoli, red and orange peppers.
- Although the evidence is less robust, it is likely that consuming at least one portion of oily fish per week will reduce the risk of AMD.
- Vitamin supplements are of no proven benefit in the prevention of age-related eye disease. High-dose multivitamin supplements with zinc are recommended for people with intermediate AMD in one or both eyes or advanced AMD in one eye.

- Along with many anti-ageing preparations, extravagant claims have been made for a range of products/supplements. Popular among these are bilberries and gingko biloba. Although the chemical properties of these compounds are consistent with a possible beneficial effect on physiological parameters, there is minimal evidence (if any) for benefit in humans.
- Overweight should be avoided, especially high abdominal adiposity or high waist:hip ratio.
- Recommendations apply to the majority of the older population. In sub-groups, such as by ethnicity or frailty, additional recommendations may be required if diets are low in key nutrients.

9.8 Recommendations for future research

- There are few or no data on the prevalence of the major conditions leading to visual loss in ethnic minorities in the UK. Studies are required, especially in those groups expected to be at high risk for certain eye conditions, such as myopia and glaucoma in people of Chinese origin, glaucoma in people of African origin and cataracts in people of south Asian origin.
- The association of diet and eye disease should be investigated for specific ethnic groups where patterns and types of food consumption differ from those of the majority of the population.
- In the light of important recent discoveries of the role of genetic factors in age-related eye conditions, especially AMD, further research is

required to examine the effect of genetic variation on the association between diet and eye diseases (nutrigenetics).
- Further research is also required on other environment–nutrient interactions, for example the levels of antioxidants to protect the retina may depend on the levels of oxidative stress from sunlight exposure.
- Investigation of the role (if any) of dietary factors in the onset and progression of glaucoma.
- Further research is required to identify the effect of dietary intake of fatty acids, especially saturates and *trans* fatty acids, on risk of AMD and cataracts.

9.9 Key references

Age-Related Eye Disease Study Research Group (AREDS) (2001) A randomized, placebo-controlled, clinical trial of high-dose supplementation with vitamins C and E, beta carotene, and zinc for age-related macular degeneration and vision loss: AREDS report no. 8. *Archives of Ophthalmology*, **119**, 1417–36.

Beatty S, Koh H, Phil M, *et al.* (2000) The role of oxidative

stress in the pathogenesis of age-related macular degeneration. *Survey of Ophthalmology*, **45**, 115–34.

Mares JA, La Rowe TL and Blodi BA (2004) Doctor, what vitamins should I take for my eyes? *Archives of Ophthalmology*, **122**: 628–35.

Taylor A and Hobbs M (2001) Assessment of nutritional influences on risk for cataract. *Nutrition*, **17**, 845–57.

10
Healthy Ageing:
The Cardiovascular System

10.1 Pathophysiology

Cardiovascular disease (CVD) chiefly includes coronary heart disease (CHD) and stroke and also congestive heart failure and peripheral vascular disease. These diseases share a common pathophysiology involving atherosclerosis and thrombosis (or clotting). Atherosclerosis occurs as a result of thickening of the inner lining of the arteries, resulting in the development of lesions (or plaques) in the arterial wall. Atherosclerosis begins early in life and progresses with age (Figure 10.1). When plaques develop in the arteries supplying the heart, they may restrict the blood supply, causing chest pain (angina) or breathlessness on exertion. More seriously, if the cap covering a plaque ruptures, exposing the contents to the circulation, the blood may clot and obstruct the blood flow completely, resulting in a myocardial infarction (heart attack). Atherosclerosis can also cause narrowing of the arteries in the legs which presents as intermittent claudication (cramp-like pain in the calf muscles) on exertion. Interruption of the blood supply to the brain causes ischaemic stroke (the most common type of stroke in western countries), although stroke can also arise from bleeding into the brain (haemorrhagic stroke).

10.2 The scale of the problem

Cardiovascular diseases account for about 30% of all deaths worldwide and the World Health Organization (2004a) estimates in 2002 indicated that 16.7 million people die from cardiovascular diseases each year. Age has a profound impact on the occurrence, severity and prognosis of CVD. Indeed CHD and stroke are the two leading causes of death in adults aged over 60 years (World Health Organization 2003b). The situation is therefore expected to worsen as the world population ages (see Chapter 1), with the number of CVD deaths projected to increase to about 20 million a year by 2020 and to more than 24 million a year by 2030 (World Health Organization 2004a).

In the UK, around 30% of deaths occurring before the age of 75 years and 40% of deaths over the age of 75 years are due to CVD (British Heart Foundation 2006). In addition, CVD is a major cause of disability, particularly in older people. Overall around 2.6 million people in the UK have angina or have survived a heart attack, with around 25% of men and 20% of women aged 75 years having the condition (British Heart Foundation 2006). The economic burden is substantial, with an estimated cost to the UK of almost £26 billion per year.

During recent years, an increase in mortality and morbidity rates due to CVD occurred in developing countries (World Health Organization 2003b), in addition to some countries of Eastern and Central Europe (World Health Organization 2003b; British Heart Foundation 2006). However, in most other European countries, including the UK, death rates have declined since the 1960s and 1970s, as have those in North America and Australia/New Zealand (British Heart Foundation 2006). This decline has also been seen in the older age groups, suggesting that CVD is not an inevitable or unmodifiable consequence of ageing. Accurate morbidity data are difficult to obtain and are complicated by reporting bias. Nevertheless, in the UK it appears that the amount of self-reported morbidity associated with heart and circulatory disease has not fallen, and

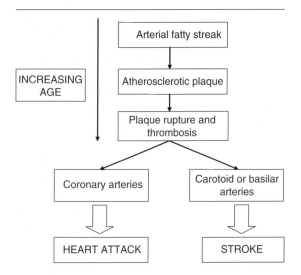

Figure 10.1: The pathology of CVD.
CVD is a consequence of two interrelated pathological processes: atherosclerosis (hardening and narrowing of blood vessels); and thrombosis (blood clotting). Atherosclerosis is characterised by the accumulation of lipids in the blood vessel walls over a long period. This can lead to impaired flow of blood (and therefore oxygen) to the heart, and angina pectoris (chest pain). A heart attack is usually precipitated by a blockage in the coronary artery following the rupture of an atherosclerotic plaque in the arterial lumen. A stroke occurs when a blockage disrupts the blood flow to the brain.
Source: Lunn J & Theobald H (2006) The health effects of dietary unsaturated fatty acids. *Nutrition Bulletin*, **31**, 178–224, with permission from Wiley-Blackwell Publishing Ltd (Lunn and Theobald 2006).

increases have been noted among older people (British Heart Foundation 2006) (Figure 10.2).

10.3 Ageing and CVD risk

CVD is a lifelong process, with atherosclerosis developing over many years (Figure 10.1). The incidence of CHD, hypertension, congestive heart failure and stroke rises steeply with advancing age in both men and women in western societies (Figure 10.3). Figure 10.4 shows the 10-year absolute risk of CHD charts that are widely used in clinical practice to estimate individual risk (see Figure 10.4 for an example). These charts show the increase in absolute risk with advancing age.

In the UK, over 60% of all cardiovascular deaths in men and 80% in women occur after the age of 75 (British Heart Foundation 2006). Age has a particular impact on risk of CHD among women, who tend to lose some of their advantage over men as they undergo the menopause. Men are about four times more likely to die from heart disease than women before the age of 65 but the gap between the sexes narrows with advancing age. The risk in women increases rapidly from around 55 years and by the age of around 70 their risk matches that of men (British Heart Foundation 2006).

In part, the rise in risk of CVD with age is due to the increased years of life providing a longer period of exposure to the major risk factors (see Section 10.4), and for the passing of time to allow for vascular damage to take effect. Atherosclerosis takes a

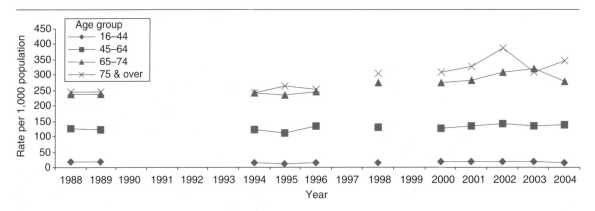

Figure 10.2: Rate of reporting longstanding cardiovascular disease by age, 1988–2004, Great Britain (British Heart Foundation 2006).
Source: Office for National Statistics (www.heartstats.org).

(a) Incidence of CHD by age and sex

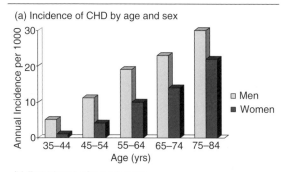

(b) Prevalence of hypertension

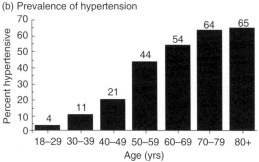

Based on NHANES III survey:1988-1991
RTN defined by BP >140,90 of treated

(c) Prevalence of heart failure by age in Framingham

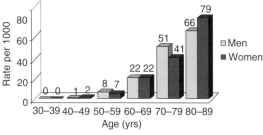

(d) Incidence of atherothrombotic stroke by age in Framingham

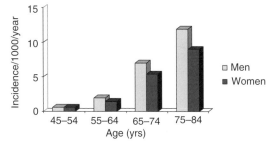

Figure 10.3: Variation of CVD with age in the adult US population.
Source: Lakatta (2002) Age-associated cardiovascular changes in health: impact on cardiovascular disease in older persons. *Heart Failure Reviews*, **7**, 29–49 with kind permission from Springer Science and Business Media.

long time to develop and, despite the fact that it can start early in life, people are usually middle-aged or older by the time it is sufficiently advanced to produce symptoms. In normal ageing, the heart undergoes changes in structure and function. Studies, such as the Baltimore Longitudinal Study (Lakatta 2002), which examined interactions between lifestyle and CVD in ageing, have demonstrated intima media wall thickening of the carotid arteries, dilation and stiffening of the arteries, endothelial dysfunction and increases in arterial pressure with age, causing arteries to become less elastic and increasing systolic blood pressure and risk of CVD. The effect of age-associated changes in hormonal status (*e.g.* levels of oestrogen and testosterone) in relation to CVD risk is discussed in Chapter 13, Sections 13.2.3 and 13.3.2.

Age is also an independent risk factor for the severity and prognosis of CVD. Fatality rates increase markedly with advanced age. This has been attributed to increased incidence of co-morbid conditions, more extensive CVD and a lesser use of beneficial therapies in older patients (*e.g.* aspirin, β-blocking drugs and angiotensin-converting enzyme [ACE] inhibitors) and procedures (*e.g.* coronary thrombolysis and angioplasty) shown to improve survival (Weaver 1991; Williams *et al.* 2002). The risk of additional cardiovascular events following a heart attack, including recurrent heart attacks, is higher in older people compared to younger people.

10.4 Risk factors for CVD in the general population

10.4.1 'Classic' risk factors

Observational epidemiological studies such as the Seven Countries Study, the Multiple Risk Factor Intervention Trial (MRFIT) and the Framingham Heart Study have established the classic risk factors for CVD. Table 10.1 shows a list of cardiovascular risk factors that are modifiable by diet and other aspects of lifestyle.

Smoking is a powerful risk factor for CVD, increasing in relation to the number of cigarettes smoked daily. Parish *et al.* (1995) demonstrated a 2–3-fold higher risk of death from heart disease among smokers compared to non-smokers in middle-aged and older men (Figure 10.5). Smoking

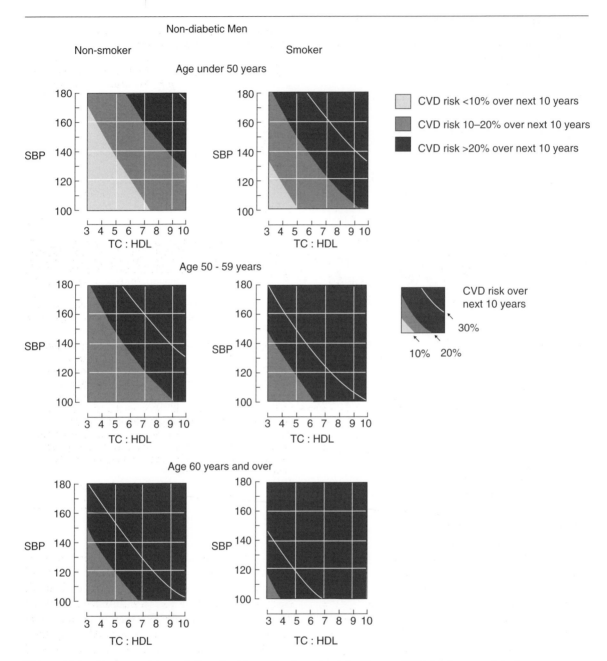

Figure 10.4: Coronary risk prediction chart for estimating absolute 10 year CHD risk for non-diabetic men without symptoms of heart disease.
SBP: systolic blood pressure mmHg; TC:HDL: serum total cholesterol to HDL-cholesterol ratio.
Source: Joint British Societies Coronary Risk Prediction Chart: Copyright the University of Manchester.

Table 10.1: Classic and emerging risk factors for CVD

Established risk factors

Smoking

Elevated blood pressure

Dyslipidaemia (*e.g.* elevated total and LDL-cholesterol, decreased HDL-cholesterol)

Diabetes mellitus

Excess weight and obesity (particularly central obesity)

Low socio-economic status

Other possible risk factors

Elevated triglyceride levels and small dense LDL particles

Elevated homocysteine

Haemostatic factors (*e.g.* fibrinogen, plasminogen-activator inhibitor-1)

Markers of inflammation (*e.g.* C-reactive protein)

Vascular (endothelial) dysfunction

Markers of oxidative stress

Maternal and/or fetal under-nutrition (low birthweight)

LDL: low-density lipoprotein.

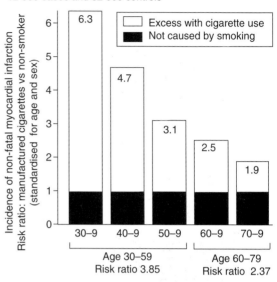

Myocardial infarction and cigarette smoking: 12 000 cases and 32 000 controls

Figure 10.5: Risk ratios of cigarette smoking and non-fatal myocardial infarction at various ages. Results in people with no previous history of major neoplastic or vascular disease. Each risk ratio is standardised for sex and for quinquennium of age, and compares those using manufactured cigarettes only with those who were not currently using any tobacco and had not been regular cigarette smokers at any time in the past 10 years. Risk ratio is given within each column. (All cases recruited from ISIS-4 were cigarette smokers.)
Source: Parish *et al.* (1995). Reproduced with permission from the BMJ Publishing Group.

cessation is associated within 3–4 years with a significant reduction in cardiovascular risk.

A positive, linear graded association exists between blood pressure and risk of CHD, stroke and other vascular causes of death (Keil 2000; Prospective Studies Collaboration 2002) (Figure 10.6) and antihypertensive treatment has been shown to reduce risk of CVD, including in those aged over 60 years (see Staessen *et al.* 1999).

High blood levels of total cholesterol and low-density lipoprotein (LDL) cholesterol are a major risk factor for CHD. There is an independent, continuous and graded positive association between total and LDL-cholesterol levels and risk of heart disease. Randomised controlled trials have shown that lowering cholesterol levels with statin therapy is associated with reductions in CHD events (Baigent *et al.* 2005). While cholesterol levels are not predictive for stroke, lowering LDL-cholesterol is also associated with reductions in the risk of stroke and other non-CHD causes of vascular disease.

Obesity is associated with an increase in cardiovascular mortality, with a particularly high risk for subjects with central obesity. Type 2 diabetes also increases CVD risk, and the relative risks associated with diabetes are more extreme in women than men (Huxley *et al.* 2006). Several studies have shown that good metabolic control and multifactorial risk factor reduction significantly lowers the coronary risk in these patients. Studies suggest that sedentary or physically inactive people are at twice the risk of developing CVD compared to active individuals (Department of Health 2004a). Risk reductions are observed with as little as 30 minutes of moderate-intensity activity a day (see Section 10.8). Together, the classic risk factors account for most cases of CVD. As they are widely distributed in most populations, even small reductions could be worthwhile. Interventions to reduce the conventional risk factors across the life-course are therefore key to lowering the burden of CVD in the general population (see Section 10.10).

In addition to age, there are a number of well-established non-modifiable risk factors including

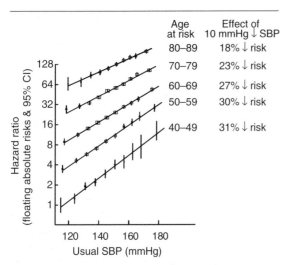

Age at risk	Effect of 10 mmHg ↓ SBP
80–89	18% ↓ risk
70–79	23% ↓ risk
60–69	27% ↓ risk
50–59	30% ↓ risk
40–49	31% ↓ risk

Data from the Prospective Studies Collaboration involving one million adults in 61 prospective studies. Data based on 33,000 IHD deaths.
BP: blood pressure; CI: confidence interval; SBP: systolic blood pressure

Figure 10.6: Age-specific risk of usual systolic blood pressure to vascular mortality at ages 40–89 years. Source: Prospective Studies Collaboration (2002). Reproduced by permission of Elsevier.

male sex, existing CVD and family history (Table 10.1). Ethnicity is also linked with CVD risk; in the UK, for example, African-Caribbeans are around 40% less likely and South Asians about 50% more likely to die of heart disease than the 'native'-born population (Wild and McKeigue 1997). CVD preferentially affects those in the lower social levels; poor housing and little education are strong indicators of high coronary mortality. Psychosocial factors, such as depression and social isolation, have been associated with an increased risk of CHD (Kuper *et al.* 2002) and may be important risk factors in the older population, although it is not clear whether this relationship is causal.

10.4.2 'Emerging' risk factors

Recent research has identified several novel risk factors that have been implicated as independent predictors of CHD (Stanner 2005). There include markers of maternal under-nutrition, inflammation, oxidative stress, endothelial damage, infectious agents and increased levels of fibrinogen, homocysteine and lipoprotein (a) (Table 10.1).

10.4.2.1 Lipid-related factors

There has been increasing interest in the ability of a number of other lipid-related factors, besides blood cholesterol and triglycerides, that might predict CVD risk including: high levels of lipoprotein (a), remnant lipoproteins and small dense LDL particles. Small dense LDL particles are likely to be the most atherogenic lipid risk factors and are clearly regulated by diet (*e.g.* the amount and type of dietary fat) but at present the methods by which they can be quantified are complicated, expensive and not for routine clinical use (Karpe 2005).

10.4.2.2 Homocysteine

Elevated plasma homocysteine level has been proposed as an independent risk factor for CHD and stroke (Clarke *et al.* 1991). This hypothesis has attracted considerable interest because homocysteine levels are easily lowered with folic acid and vitamin B_{12} (Homocysteine-Lowering Trialists' Collaboration 2005). Meta-analyses of observational studies have suggested that a 25% lower homocysteine is associated with about 10% lower risk of CHD and about 20% lower risk of stroke (Homocysteine Studies Collaboration 2002) (see Chapter 8, Section 8.2.3). Studies of CHD and stroke risk in relation to a common variant in the gene encoding the 5,10 methylene-tetrahydrofolate reductase enzyme that is associated with lifelong increased homocysteine concentrations have reported associations of this polymorphism with vascular risk, providing support for causality (Wald *et al.* 2006). Several large-scale trials are currently assessing whether lowering homocysteine concentrations can reduce the risk of CHD or stroke (B-Vitamin Treatment Trialists' Collaboration 2006) (see Section 10.7.6.4 and Chapter 8, Section 8.2.4).

10.4.2.3 Endothelial dysfunction

The vascular endothelium regulates normal functioning of blood vessels by generating several substances, such as nitric oxide, that modulate vascular smooth muscle tone, as well as platelet function. The loss of normal functioning of the endothelium, known as endothelial dysfunction, appears to be an initial step in the development of atherosclerosis. However, as all known established and novel risk factor pathways can contribute to endothelial dysfunction and strategies that improve endothelial function also reduce several other risk factors associated with vascular disease, an independent association is difficult to establish (Sattar and Ferns 2005).

10.4.2.4 Markers of blood clotting

Evidence is accumulating that some clotting factors (*e.g.* fibrinogen, factor VII, von Willebrand factor) and fibrinolytic factors (*e.g.* t-PA and plasminogen activator inhibitor type-1) are associated with an increased risk of both CHD and stroke, although further research is needed to strengthen the case for causal associations (Miller and Bruckdorfer 2005).

10.4.2.5 Oxidative stress

Reactive oxygen and nitrogen species precipitate changes that result in oxidative damage to lipid, protein and DNA biomolecules, and in this way oxidative stress is implicated in the development of CHD and stroke. Several methods are available for the measurement of the oxidation of proteins, lipids and nucleic acids, and changes in these measures have been associated with CHD and stroke or with conditions that predispose to it. Diets that are rich in antioxidant nutrients (*e.g.* vitamins C and E and β-carotene) or supplements of antioxidants can change these indicators, usually in a beneficial manner but this cannot be assumed to automatically parallel a decrease in CHD and stroke, as the major intervention studies have not shown a beneficial effect of antioxidant supplements on cardiovascular events (see Section 10.7.6.2 and Chapter 8, Section 8.2.6).

10.4.2.6 Inflammation-related factors

The role of the immune system and inflammatory pathways in the development of CHD and stroke is well established. Elevated levels of systemic markers of inflammation, including circulating concentrations of inflammatory cytokines, soluble adhesion molecules and acute phase reactants, such as C-reactive protein (CRP) and fibrinogen, in healthy middle-aged individuals, have been associated with higher risk of CHD in later life (Ridker 2001; Yaqoob and Ferns 2005). CRP, one of the proteins produced and released in response to injury and infection, has

been the most frequently studied inflammatory marker in epidemiological studies, with high levels estimated to increase risk of CHD by around 50% (Danesh *et al.* 2004). However, whether such markers of inflammation add anything of value over conventional markers of heart disease remains to be established. It is also unclear if the associations between inflammation and CHD are affected by age at measurement (see Section 10.6.5).

10.4.2.7 Chronic infections

A number of studies have reported positive associations between CHD and chronic infection with various organisms, such as *Chlamydia pneumoniae* and *Helicobacter pylori*. Infection leads to a rise in circulating levels of acute phase reactants such as fibrinogen, as well as white cell count and CRP levels, which might increase vascular risk.

10.4.2.8 Adipose tissue-derived factors

Adipose tissue secretes a diverse number of substances (termed adipokines) including enzymes, growth factors, cytokines and several other hormones involved in fatty acid and glucose metabolism (*e.g.* angiotensinogen, adipoectin, resistin, leptin, TNF-α, interleukin-6). Several adipokines are increased in the obese state and have been implicated in many processes that contribute to the development of CHD, including chronic inflammation (see Chapter 11, Section 11.2.7), insulin resistance, dyslipidaemia, hypertension and endothelial dysfunction, perhaps contributing directly to increased cardiovascular risk (Guerre-Millo 2004; Mohamed-Ali and Coppack 2005).

10.4.2.9 Early growth

Low birthweight and low weight gain during infancy are associated with an increased risk of adult CHD and stroke, hypertension, type 2 diabetes and metabolic syndrome (see Section 10.4.3) (Barker 1998). This has led to the development of the 'fetal origins hypothesis' (see Section 10.9.1).

10.4.3 Risk factor clustering

Many studies have demonstrated a clustering of cardiovascular risk factors. For example, people with diabetes are far more likely to have hypertension and/or dyslipidaemia than the general population (Bowman and Armitage 2002). The presence of more than one risk factor has a multiplicative impact on the risk of CHD. For example, the hazard of any level of blood pressure elevation is increased when there is concomitant smoking, dyslipidaemia, diabetes or existing CHD (Chobanian *et al.* 2003). The clustering of several vascular risk factors, including obesity (particularly abdominal obesity), dyslipidaemia, impaired glucose metabolism and hypertension is called the metabolic syndrome (also known as insulin resistance syndrome or Syndrome X). This is extremely concerning as the presence of this syndrome often precedes the onset of diabetes and substantially increases risk of CHD mortality and morbidity (Coppack *et al.* 2005).

10.5 Age trends in CVD risk factors

With the exception of smoking which declines steadily with advancing age, the prevalence of most of the classical modifiable cardiovascular risk factors has been shown to rise among older people. For example, data from the US Framingham Study (see Figure 10.3b) and national UK surveys (Figure 10.7) have shown the prevalence of hypertension to increase steeply with age in both sexes (Department of Health 2003; Ruston *et al.* 2004). In those aged 75 years and over, at least two-thirds of men and women in England have high blood pressure (Department of Health 2003).

Body mass index (BMI) increases until 65 years of age and then declines in both sexes, but central obesity rises further into old age, particularly among women (Department of Health 2003) (Figure 10.8). Older people are also the most physically inactive, with well over half of those aged 65 and over achieving less than 30 minutes a week and two-thirds of those aged over 75 considered inactive (Department of Health 2004a) (Figure 10.9). The prevalence of type 2 diabetes also rises with age, probably because of the increased abdominal obesity in older age groups. By age 65, around 8% of women and 12% of men in England have been diagnosed with diabetes (Figure 10.10). Age also increases the risk of metabolic syndrome (Lawlor *et al.* 2004). Among participants of the Cardiovascular Health Study in the US, a prospective multi-centre study of men and women 65 years of age or older who were free of CVD at baseline, the prevalence of the syndrome was 21–28% depending on the criteria used for its definition (Scuteri *et al.* 2005).

Cholesterol levels also tend to rise with age, although there may be a moderate decrease in the oldest age groups. The most recent National Diet and Nutrition Survey of adults in the UK found average plasma total and LDL-cholesterol levels, and the proportion of individuals with raised levels (>5.2 mmol/L and >3.4 mmol/L respectively), to increase with age, although LDL-cholesterol levels in men fell after the age of 75. The effect of ageing on high-density lipoprotein (HDL)-cholesterol levels is more inconsistent, but appears to be less than that

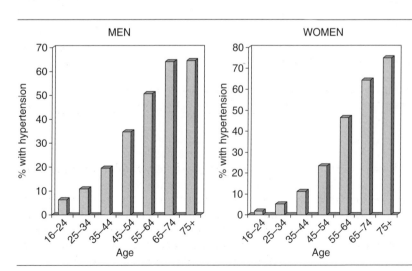

Figure 10.7: Prevalence of hypertension by age, England 2003 (Health Survey for England 2003 data; www.dh.gov.uk). *Hypertension is defined as those with a systolic blood pressure of 140 mmHg or more, a diastolic blood pressure of 90 mmHg or more, or taking drugs for high blood pressure. Source: Department of Health (2003). Reproduced under the terms of the Click-Use Licence.

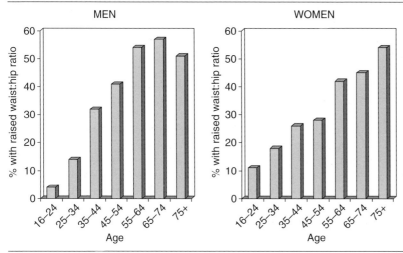

Figure 10.8: Prevalence of raised waist:hip ratio, a marker of central obesity, by age, England 2003.
Source: Department of Health (2003). Reproduced under the terms of the Click Use Licence.

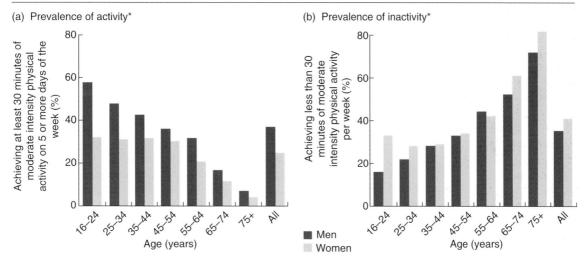

*Active is defined as achieving at least 30 minutes of moderate intensity physical activity on 5 or more days per week. Inactive is defined as achieving less than 30 minutes of moderate intensity activity per week.

Figure 10.9: Prevalence of activity and inactivity among adults, by sex and age, England, 1998.
Source: Department of Health (2004a). Reproduced under the terms of the Click-Use Licence.

on LDL- or total cholesterol (Scientific Advisory Committee on Nutrition 2005b).

Ageing has also been shown to have an adverse impact on homocysteine levels and other novel CVD risk factors. For example, fibrinogen and other haemostatic factors tend to increase with age. Plasma levels of C-reactive protein (see Section 10.4.2.6)

also show a gradual increase with age (Department of Health 2003).

The rise in prevalence of the major risk factors with advancing age is not inevitable and has been shown to be correctable. It imposes a high level of vulnerability in the older population but also opportunities for prevention (see Section 10.10).

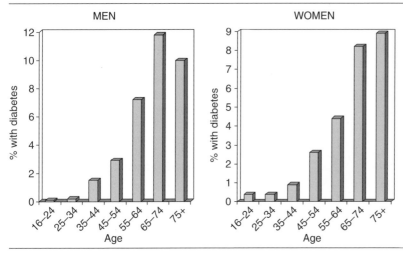

Figure 10.10: Prevalence of type 2 diabetes by age, England 2003.
Source: Department of Health (2003). Reproduced under the terms of the Click-Use Licence.

10.6 Relevance of CVD risk factors after the age of 65 years

Studies of CVD in older people suggest that the risk factors applicable in middle age (Section 10.4) remain relevant in the elderly (those 65 years of age and older) (Kannel 2002). However, changes in the magnitude of the association between CVD and some risk factors appear to occur with advancing age, and in extreme ages the predictive role of the classical risk factors is less clear. For example, based on repeated risk factor measurements, the Honolulu Heart Program showed that Japanese men aged 45–93 years with diabetes had a consistent twofold excess risk of CHD across all age groups. However, while there was a positive association between CHD and BMI in younger men (aged 45–54 years), the association became negative in those aged 75–93 years (*i.e.* a lower BMI was associated with excess risk) (Abbott *et al.* 2002). Due to a reduction in the frequency of smoking with increasing age (the result of smoking cessation as well as earlier losses to smoking-related diseases), the association between smoking and CHD weakened with age, whilst adverse effects of a sedentary lifestyle appeared to strengthen (Abbott *et al.* 2002). The relative importance of elevated blood levels of total cholesterol and blood pressure for CHD appeared to decline with advancing age, but the absolute importance of these risk factors is much greater in old age com-

pared with middle-aged individuals (Abbott *et al.* 2002) (Figure 10.11). Some of these age-related changes in risk factor effects may be due to difficulties in interpretation of results of epidemiological studies investigating the effects of risk factors in older groups because of the need to take into account the high prevalence of CVD in this age group, co-morbidity, the high mortality rate and natural selection. Furthermore, risk factors measured in advanced age may not reflect the lifetime level of exposure to them, thereby attenuating their observed impact on CVD.

As sub-clinical, severe coronary artery pathology afflicts one half of the elderly in affluent countries, the distinction between primary and secondary prevention is blurred. The Cardiovascular Health Study, for example, found a prevalence of sub-clinical vascular disease among participants aged 65 years and older with no evidence of clinical CVD of 54% (Kuller *et al.* 1995). Thus in this age group, factors that cause progression of established atherosclerosis or precipitated clinical events may be particularly important.

10.6.1 Dyslipidaemia and hypertension

There has been some uncertainty about the importance of elevated cholesterol levels for risk of CHD in the elderly. Many prospective studies have under-

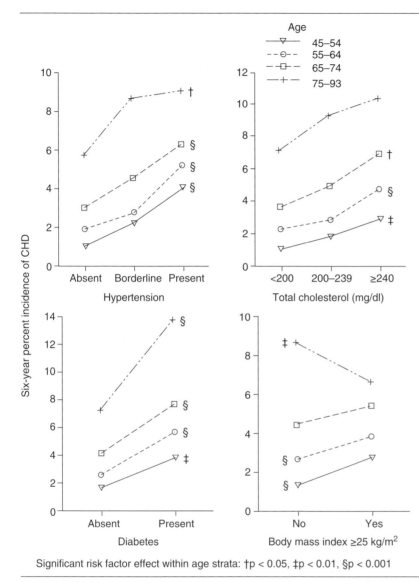

Figure 10.11: Effect of age on estimated relative risk of CHD associated with hypertension, high cholesterol levels, diabetes and being overweight in men from the Honolulu Heart Program.
Relative risk estimates have been adjusted for other risk factors.
Source: Abbott *et al.* (2002). Reproduced by permission of Elsevier.

estimated the strength of the association between total cholesterol and CHD by failing to take account of within-person variation or 'regression dilution' bias (Clarke *et al.* 1999). The magnitude of regression dilution bias is greater at longer intervals between measurements. Since much of the evidence on cholesterol and risk of CHD in older people has come from long-term follow-up of middle-aged cohorts, data from such studies have systematically under-estimated the importance of cholesterol in older people (Clarke *et al.* 2002). For example, in the Whitehall study 18,841 men aged 40–69 years had their cholesterol measured in middle age in 1967 to 1970 and 2,858 died from CHD over a 26-year period. The mean interval from baseline visit until CHD death was nine years for those dying at ages 40–64, 15 years for those dying at ages 65–74 and 21 years for those dying over the age of 75. After correction for regression dilution appropriate for the variable follow-up, a 1 mmol/L lower total

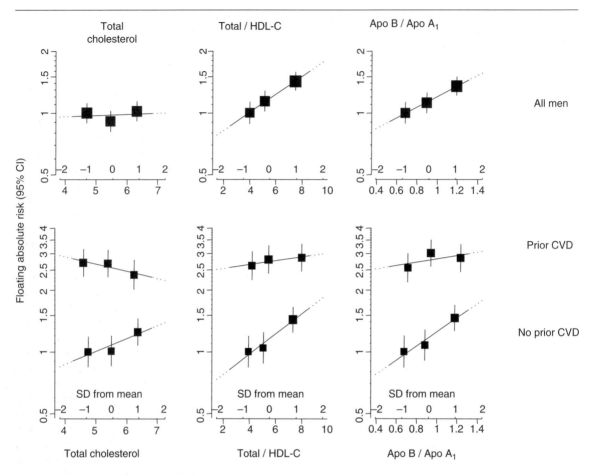

Figure 10.12: Blood lipids and CHD risk in old age according to the presence or absence of prior CVD. Seven-year follow-up of 5341 men in the Whitehall study (n = 447 CHD deaths). Apo: apolipoprotein; CI: confidence interval; CVD: cardiovascular disease; HDL-C: high-density lipoprotein cholesterol; SD: standard devidation. Source: Clarke *et al.* (2007). © American Medical Association 2007. All rights reserved.

cholesterol was associated with 27%, 26% and 21% fewer deaths at ages <65, 65–74 and >75 respectively (Clarke *et al.* 2002). A prospective cohort study of 5344 surviving participants in the Whitehall study (mean age 77 years) involving 447 CHD deaths (Clarke *et al.* 2008) demonstrated that there was no significant association of CHD mortality with total cholesterol levels when measured in old age in all men. But this apparent lack of an association masked a positive association of CHD risk with total cholesterol levels in men without prior diagnosed cardiovascular disease (CVD) and a non-significant inverse association in men with prior diagnosed

CVD (or statin use) (Figure 10.12). A similar pattern was observed for LDL-cholesterol and for Apo B, with strong positive associations in those without CVD and non-significant inverse associations among those with CVD. In contrast, CHD mortality was inversely associated with HDL and with Apo A_1 irrespective of the presence or absence of CVD. Differences in lipids that are achievable by statins were associated with about one-third lower risk of CHD, irrespective of age. Strategies to raise plasma Apo A_1 levels may be associated with even greater benefits than those achieved by solely lowering Apo B levels. Thus, while there is some attenuation in the proportional relationship of CHD with total cholesterol with increasing age, it remains a strongly positive risk factor for CHD at all ages, when studies take account of prior diagnosed CVD.

As with cholesterol, many studies assessing the relevance of blood pressure for CVD have underestimated its importance in older people because of failing to account for regression dilution bias. The Prospective Studies Collaboration meta-analysis of one million people involving 120,000 deaths had a mean age of death of 67 years. After appropriate correction for regression dilution bias, a 20 mmHg lower systolic blood pressure was associated with a 46%, 40% and 31% lower risk of CHD mortality among people aged 60–69 years, 70–79 years and 80–89 years respectively. The association between blood pressure and risk of stroke is even stronger, with 20 mmHg lower systolic blood pressure being associated with 43%, 38% and 38% lower risk of stroke deaths at ages 60–69 years, 70–79 years and 80–89 years respectively (see Chapter 8, Section 8.2.1).

The slight attenuation in relative risks associated with dyslipidaemia and hypertension should not be used as an argument not to intervene in the elderly. Primary and secondary prevention trials using lipid-lowering drugs (statins) have clearly demonstrated benefits of lowering cholesterol in older people (Miettinen *et al.* 1997; Downs *et al.* 1998; Hunt *et al.* 2001; Shepherd *et al.* 2002) with similar proportional effects to those observed in younger people. Similarly for antihypertensive treatment; large trials involving older patients, such as the Systolic Hypertension in the Elderly Program (SHEP Cooperative Research Group 1991) and the Systolic Hypertension in Europe trial (Staessen *et al.* 1997) have demonstrated a similar proportional benefit for prevention of CHD and stroke in older patients at least until the age of 80. Ongoing clinical trials, such as the Hypertension in the Very Elderly Trial, will clarify whether such treatments are effective in the very elderly (Bulpitt *et al.* 2003). Furthermore, although the relative risk of hypertension or hypercholesterolaemia for CVD incidence may be attenuated with advancing age, the absolute risk rises due to the higher event rates in older groups. The absolute risk reduction associated with preventive interventions to lower CVD risk factors (see Section 10.10) is, therefore, much greater in old age. Lifestyle modifications to alter these risk factors have

also been shown to be effective in reducing CVD risk in the elderly (Fair 2003).

10.6.2 Obesity and diabetes

Obesity has been widely recognised as a risk factor for CHD and stroke in older people. The most widely used marker for obesity in epidemiological studies is BMI (weight in kg divided by the square of height in metres). BMI measured in middle age is an important predictor of CVD risk in later life. However, when BMI is measured in older age groups, weaker or even inverse associations with CVD mortality have been reported (Price *et al.* 2006). This has led to suggestions that BMI may not be a good measure of body fat in older people. Unreliable assessment of height may also be a problem in older subjects (due to shrinkage and vertebral collapse). However, recent data from the Whitehall cohort of male civil servants demonstrated a doubling of risk of CVD mortality among those in the heaviest category in old age (BMI >26.1 kg/m^2) compared with the same reference group during the first two years of follow-up and also showed weight gain over a 30-year period to be a strong risk factor for cardiovascular disease mortality (Breeze *et al.* 2006). Further work is needed to clarify the usefulness of other indices, such as waist measurement or waist: hip ratio, as predictors of CVD risk in older age groups, as well as the cut-off points that should be used to identify those at risk.

Diabetes and impaired glucose tolerance are some of the most common diseases in older people and are considered to be an important risk factor until the age of 75, although their role in the oldest old remains unclear. Older patients with type 2 diabetes are at increased risk for both symptomatic and asymptomatic myocardial infarction, and appear to have worse outcomes than non-diabetics with these same conditions. Older people with diabetes also have a greater risk than those without diabetes of developing hypertension and stroke. Due to a lack of controlled trials investigating the effects of blood glucose control in the elderly, it is unknown whether treatment of hyperglycaemia in older patients will decrease the risk of cardiovascular and cerebrovascular disease, but it is proposed that treating diabetes along with other commonly associated risk factors for CVD may provide the best outlook for such patients.

10.6.3 The metabolic syndrome

Epidemiological studies have revealed an increasing prevalence of the metabolic syndrome in older populations (see Section 10.5). The presence of this syndrome increases the risk for the development of both CVD and type 2 diabetes in the general population and has been shown to be a significant predictor of cardiovascular events in older individuals (see Section 10.4.3). Scuteri and colleagues (2005) demonstrated a 38% increased risk of CVD among those with the syndrome (defined according to ATPIII criteria) (hazard ratio 1.38 (95% CI: 1.07–1.79), $P < 0.01$) and this predictive effect was independent of the individual components of the metabolic syndrome and of other traditional cardiovascular risk factors. Using a similar analytical approach, the syndrome was also shown to be an independent predictor of arterial stiffness and thickness in participants from the Baltimore Longitudinal Study of Aging (Scuteri *et al.* 2004). Identification and treatment of the metabolic syndrome may therefore represent an important approach to reducing the overall burden of CVD morbidity and mortality in the elderly.

10.6.4 Physical inactivity

The levels of activity recommended for health benefits in adults are also appropriate for older adults (*i.e.* at least 30 minutes of moderate intensity on five or more days of the week) (see Section 10.8) but a high proportion of older people in the UK are not meeting this target (Figure 10.9) (see Chapter 14, Section 14.6).

10.6.5 The relevance of novel risk factors in old age

Novel risk factors have the potential to offer further information about CVD risk in the elderly (see Section 10.4.2). Many of these emerging risk factors (*e.g.* homocysteine, inflammatory markers, endothelial dysfunction, oxidative stress) have been shown to increase with age (Herrmann *et al.* 1999; Wilkerson and Sane 2002) and to be associated with health-related behaviours such as physical inactivity, smoking and poor diet in older populations (*e.g.* Dankner *et al.* 2004). Whilst research into the effects of these risk factors has primarily focused on middle-

aged populations, data among older adults are emerging. For example, the Cardiovascular Health Study has identified a number of promising potential candidates in men and women aged 65 and over, including markers of haemostatic activation (fibrinogen, factor VIII coagulant activity), inflammation (C-reactive protein) (Cushman *et al.* 2005) and infection (exposure to herpes simplex virus-1 and possibly chlamydia which may be associated with increased CVD risk) (Siscovick *et al.* 2000). Elevated levels of more novel lipid-related factors, including Lp(a), have also been found to be associated with CHD risk in the elderly (Simons *et al.* 2001).

The strength of the association between these risk factors and CVD may alter with age. For example, the Framingham Study demonstrated a significant association with CVD risk across the whole age range but a weaker effect in the older (60–79 years) compared to younger age group (Kannel *et al.* 1987). In the Whitehall study of older men, Clarke *et al.* (2008) showed that CVD mortality was linearly related to increasing levels of CRP, fibrinogen and albumin in men with and without prior disease. A 2 standard deviation higher CRP or, equivalently, a 2 standard deviation lower albumin level, was associated with approximately a twofold higher risk of CVD.

There is some evidence that CRP levels increase with age (up to 70 years), however, some studies have shown its relationship with CVD to weaken beyond around 55 years (Kritchevsky *et al.* 2005), whilst others report similar findings to younger populations. For example, the Whitehall study demonstrated an association between CRP and cardiovascular mortality comparable in magnitude to that previously reported among middle-aged individuals, which was only partly attenuated by adjustment for a wide range of potential confounding factors measured in both middle and old age (Clarke *et al.* 2008). A causal association, however, remains to be established (see Section 10.4.2.6). Further research is, therefore, needed to clarify how effective these novel risk factors can be compared with traditional risk factors in estimating CVD mortality and morbidity in the elderly.

10.6.6 Periodontal disease and CVD

Periodontal disease is a chronic infection caused by predominantly Gram-negative bacteria that affects the supporting structures of the teeth. It has a high prevalence among adults, with reports of around 50% in the US (Albandar 2005). (For further information about factors influencing periodontal disease see Chapter 3.) Moderate and advanced periodontitis is more prevalent among the older age groups (Albandar 2005). Some prospective and retrospective cohort studies (using tooth loss and/or clinical signs of periodontal disease) have suggested periodontal infection to be associated with increased risk of CHD and stroke, although larger and better controlled studies are required to substantiate these findings (Khader *et al.* 2004). As dental infection and CVD have a multifactorial nature and share common risk factors, such as diabetes and smoking, and both increase with age, confirming a causal association is difficult. However, the presence of chronic oral inflammation has been shown to increase systemic pro-inflammatory mediators such as C-reactive protein, TNF-α and IL-6, which are thought to be initiating factors of CVD (Meurman *et al.* 2004; Taylor *et al.* 2006) (see Section 10.4.2.6). Short-term intervention studies have also demonstrated treatment of severe periodontal disease to reduce systemic inflammatory and thrombotic markers of cardiovascular risk and blood pressure (Montebugnoli *et al.* 2005; D'Aiuto *et al.* 2006; Taylor *et al.* 2006), as well as reverse endothelial dysfunction (Seinost *et al.* 2005). Whilst periodontal disease and infection may, therefore, be an additional modifiable risk factor for CVD in older people, further investigation of the link between oral health status, inflammatory and haemostatic markers and risk of CVD is needed to determine if treatment of poor dental health can play a significant role in CVD prevention.

10.7 The role of dietary and nutritional factors in CVD prevention

Adequate evidence is available from studies conducted within and across populations to link several nutrients, foods, food groups and dietary patterns with an increased or decreased risk of CVD. It is now universally recognised that a diet which is energy-dense, high in fat, salt and added sugars, and low in complex carbohydrates, fruit and vegetables, increases CVD risk (World Health Organization 2003a).

10.7.1 Energy density

The energy density of the diet is considered an important factor in terms of the likelihood of weight gain, over-consumption being more likely with energy-dense diets (Prentice and Jebb 2003). Appetite control appears to be undermined by passive over-consumption of energy-dense foods, particularly in sedentary individuals (Murgatroyd *et al.* 1999). The energy density of a meal is particularly influenced by its fat content (fat provides over twice the energy per gram as either protein or carbohydrate) and by its fibre and water content as foods rich in fibre or water are bulky yet the fibre itself contributes little to energy intake and the water contributes no energy. Consequently, diets rich in fruit and vegetables (which provide both water and fibre) and cereal foods and pulses (for fibre) have a lower energy density.

10.7.2 Dietary cholesterol

Reducing the amount of dietary cholesterol can lower blood LDL-cholesterol levels among those consuming a typical western diet, although there is considerable inter-individual variation in this response. A meta-analysis of metabolic ward studies of solid food diets in healthy volunteers reported lowering dietary cholesterol by 200 mg/day to be associated with reductions in total and LDL-cholesterol of 0.13 (SE 0.02) mmol/L and 0.10 (SE 0.02) mmol/L respectively (Clarke *et al.* 1997). For most individuals the influence of dietary cholesterol on plasma cholesterol level or CVD risk is small compared with the amount and type of fat in the diet (McNamara 2000). However, there is some evidence that people with diabetes may be more sensitive to dietary cholesterol because of heightened insulin resistance and dyslipidaemia in this group (Hu *et al.* 1999; Tanasescu *et al.* 2004).

10.7.3 Dietary fat intake

The association between dietary fat and CVD has been fundamental to health messages for several decades and the primary focus of national dietary recommendations for primary and secondary prevention (see Section 10.7.11). This was based on the understanding that consuming a low-fat diet reduces blood levels of total and LDL-cholesterol, whilst a

Table 10.2: Recommendations for CVD risk reduction in the UK, expressed as population averages

Nutrient	Recommendation	Mean daily UK intake (adults)
Fat	Decrease to 35% of food energy (33% total energy* including contribution from alcohol)	
Saturates	Decrease to 11% food energy (10% of total energy*)	Men 32.5 g (13.4% food energy); women 23.3 g (13.2% food energy)
Monounsaturates	No specific recommendations but, if the other guidance is followed, the level would be 13% of food energy (12% total energy*)	Men 29.1 g (12.1% food energy); women 20.2 g (11.5% food energy)
Polyunsaturates	No further increase in *n*-6 fatty acids (current level about 6.5% of food energy, 6% of total energy*). Concern expressed about intakes above 10% energy	Men 12.9 g (5.4% food energy); women 9.4 g (5.3% food energy)
	Long chain *n*-3 fatty acids: double average intake from 0.1 g/day to 0.2 g/day (1.5 g/week).	Men 2.3 g (1% food energy); women 1.7 g (1% food energy)
Trans fats	No more than 2% of energy intake	Current intake in men and women is 1.2% energy
Starch, intrinsic sugars, milk sugars	Increase to 39% of food energy (37% of total energy*)	
Non-milk extrinsic sugars	Restrict to 11% of food energy (10% of total energy*)	
Non-starch polysaccharides	Increase to 18 g per day in adults. Proportional, non-specified increase also recommended for children	
Sodium	Reduction in average intake from the current 150 mmol/day (equivalent to 9 g salt/day) to about 100 mmol/day (6 g salt per day). Specific targets for children have also been published (Scientific Advisory Committee on Nutrition 2003)	
Potassium	Increase in average intake in adults to 3.5 g/day (90 mmol/day). Proportional, non-specified increase also recommended for children.	

*Total energy includes contribution from alcohol.
DRV: dietary reference value.
Source: Department of Health (1991, 1994); Scientific Advisory Committee on Nutrition (2003). Material reproduced from these references is Crown copyright and is reproduced with the permission of the Controller of HMSO. From Stanner (2005).

high-fat diet is atherogenic. There has been considerable improvement in the average amount of fat consumed over the last 50 years, falling from 107 g/person/day in the UK in 1975 (Ministry of Agriculture 1997) to 76.2 g/day in 2000 (DEFRA 2001) (see Table 10.2). In fact, according to the NDNS (Henderson, Gregory, Irving and Swan 2003), the target for total fat intake has now been approximately reached in the adult population; although

some under-reporting of food intake often occurs in such surveys. However, while total fat intake, independent of fatty acid type, may contribute to obesity, it is not strongly associated with CHD. Accumulating evidence suggests that it is fat quality (*i.e.* the type of dietary fat), rather than the total amount of fat, that influences blood cholesterol levels and other risk factors and is therefore particularly important for CVD (Astrup *et al.* 2002). This is reflected in more recent national dietary guidelines (*e.g.* in the US and the Netherlands) which have shifted emphasis towards alteration of the fatty acid profile of the diet (Expert Panel on Detection, Evaluation and Treatment of High Blood Cholesterol in Adults 2001; Voedingsnormen 2001).

10.7.3.1 *Saturated fatty acids*

Associations between total fat intake and CHD are primarily mediated through the saturated fatty acid component. Intake of saturates is positively associated with higher levels of total and LDL-cholesterol and increased risk of CHD. Replacement of 5% of energy as saturated fatty acids (*e.g.* from 17% to 12%) by polyunsaturated fatty acids would be expected to lower total cholesterol by 0.39 mmol/L. Replacement of 5% of energy from saturated fatty acids (*e.g.* from 12% to 7%) by monounsaturates would be expected to lower total cholesterol by 0.24 mmol/L (Clarke *et al.* 1997). Different classes of saturates have different effects on plasma lipid and lipoprotein levels. Specifically, saturates with 12–16 carbon atoms tend to increase plasma total and LDL-cholesterol levels, whereas stearic acid (18:0) does not have a cholesterol-raising effect. Among the cholesterol-raising saturated fatty acids, myristic acid (14:0) appears to be more potent than lauric aicd (12:0) or palmitic acid (16:0) but the data are not entirely consistent (Hu *et al.* 2001). In addition, dietary saturates raise platelet activity and thus increase the tendency of blood to clot and may be associated with reduced insulin sensitivity, a key factor in the development of the metabolic syndrome (see Section 10.4.3).

10.7.3.2 **Trans** *fatty acids*

Trans fatty acids, produced during the partial hydrogenation of vegetable oils into semi-solid fats (see Table 10.3) appear to have a more potent effect on blood cholesterol than saturates and have been shown to adversely influence the ratio of total- to HDL-cholesterol when compared with *cis* unsaturated fatty acids (Mensink *et al.* 2003). Additionally, diets high in *trans* fatty acids have been shown in some studies to increase plasma levels of lipoprotein (a) and triglycerides and to reduce endothelial function by impairing flow-mediated dilatation (Buttriss

2005). There is also some evidence that they adversely affect essential fatty acid metabolism and prostaglandin balance, which may promote thrombogenesis (Buttriss 2005) and induce insulin resistance (Bray *et al.* 2002).

In a recent review of four prospective studies involving nearly 140,000 subjects, a 2% increase in energy intake from *trans* fatty acids was associated with a 23% increase in the incidence of CHD. The authors also reported that the adverse effects of *trans* fatty acids were observed even at very low intakes of 3% of total daily energy intake (2–7 g per day) (Mozaffarian *et al.* 2006).

Trans fatty acids are found in small amounts naturally, principally in animal-based foods (*e.g.* dairy and beef fat) as a result of bacterial transformation of unsaturated fatty acids in the rumen (first stomach) of ruminant animals. Despite inherent differences in chemical structure, industrially produced and ruminant *trans* fatty acids appear to have similar effects on serum lipoproteins, although direct evidence for an effect of ruminant fatty acids is limited (Scientific Advisory Committee on Nutrition 2007e). While ruminant *trans* fatty acids cannot be removed entirely from our diet, their intake is low enough in most populations not to constitute a significant health risk. However, intakes of *trans* fatty acids produced by the process of partial hydrogenation can be considerably higher in some populations and among individuals (often in low-income groups) who eat relatively large quantities of foods made with fats derived from partially hydrogenated oils (which are a source of *trans*), such as block margarines. Some experts have, therefore, advocated elimination of industrially produced *trans* fatty acids from the diet through voluntary agreement with industry or legislation (Mozaffarian *et al.* 2006). The food industry in some countries, including the UK, has responded to the scientific evidence by reformulating products (*e.g.* fat spreads) to reduce or in many cases eliminate their *trans* fatty acid content (see Chapter 14, Sections 14.3.8, 14.7 and 14.5.2). Current European diets are generally lower in these fatty acids than dietary recommendations advise, including in Britain, where mean adult intake has been estimated to be 1% of food energy (Scientific Advisory Committee on Nutrition 2007e) (dietary reference value is 2%). However, reductions in intake are less apparent in other countries, including North America.

Table 10.3: Sources of fatty acids in the UK diet (adults)

Type of fat	Sources in the UK diet (% of total intake) (descending order of importance)	Rich sources of individual fatty acids
Saturates	Milk and milk products (24%); meat and products (22%); cereal products (18%), *e.g.* cakes, biscuits, pastries; fat spreads (11%); potatoes and savoury snacks (7%)	Myristic acid (C14:0): particularly milk fat, coconut oil and products made from these Palmitic acid (C16:0): particularly animal fats, coconut oil, palm oil and products made from these Stearic acid (C18:0): particularly meat, cocoa butter (also present in dairy products)
Monounsaturates	Meat and products (27%); cereal products (17%); potatoes and savoury snacks (12%); fat and spreads (11%); milk and milk products (10%); egg and egg dishes (5%)	Oleic acid (C18:1): olive oil, rapeseed oil (moderate sources – meat, dairy products, peanut and palm oil)
Polyunsaturates – *n*-3 (omega 3) fatty acids	Meat and products (17%); cereal products (17%); potatoes and savoury snacks (17%); fish and fish dishes (oil-rich fish) (14%); vegetables (excluding potatoes) (11%); fat spreads (7%)	α-linolenic acid (C18:3): rapeseed, walnut, soya and blended vegetable oils, walnuts (moderate sources – meat from grass-fed ruminants, vegetables, meat and eggs from animals fed a diet enriched in C18:3) EPA (C20:5) and DHA (C22:6): oil-rich fish, fish oil (moderate sources: foods enriched or fortified with EPA/DHA)
– *n*-6 (omega 6) fatty acids	Cereal products (20%); meat and products (18%); fat spreads (14%); potatoes and savoury snacks (13%); vegetables (excluding potatoes) (9%)	Vegetable oils (*e.g.* sunflower, corn and soya bean) and spreads made from these (moderate sources: peanut and rapeseed oils)
Trans fatty acids	Cereal products (26%); meat and products (21%); fat spreads (18%); milk and milk products (16%); potatoes and savoury snacks (6%)	Partially hydrogenated oils and products made from these can potentially provide large amounts (see Section 10.7.3.2 and Chapter 14, Sections 14.3.8, 14.7 and 14.5.2)

DHA: docosahexaenoic acid; DRV: dietary reference value; EPA: eicosapentaenoic acid.
Source: Henderson, Gregory, Irving and Swan (2003). Material is Crown copyright and is reproduced with the permission of the Controller of HMSO. Table from Stanner (2005).

10.7.3.3 Low-fat vs. moderate-fat diets

The replacement of saturates with carbohydrates has traditionally been the standard advice for both weight loss and improvements in cardiovascular health. However, relatively recently this practice has been questioned and the issue of low-fat/high-carbohydrate vs. moderate-fat diets has become quite controversial (Katan *et al.* 1997; Astrup *et al.* 2002; Willett 2002; Sanders 2003). One of the principal areas of concern is the effect of low-fat/ high-carbohydrate diets on circulating lipids. Although LDL-cholesterol falls and beneficial effects can be expected in terms of bodyweight and haemostasis (decreases in factor VII coagulant activity and enhanced fibrinolysis), this may be accompanied by a concomitant reduction in HDL-cholesterol and/or an increase in serum triglycerides, and by an increased number of small dense LDL and remnant particles, all recognised as adverse factors for CVD risk (Katan *et al.* 1997; Katan 1998). There is evidence, however, that these effects may be transient. The Carmen study, a six-month intervention with a low-fat and high simple or complex carbohydrate diet, demonstrated no adverse effect on plasma lipids, but resulted in a modest but significant weight reduction (Saris *et al.* 2000). Nevertheless, isoenergetic replacement of saturates or *trans* fatty acids with either monounsaturates or polyunsaturates can lower total plasma and LDL-cholesterol (Poppitt *et al.* 2002) and reduce CHD risk. Thus, at least for those with a healthy bodyweight, moderate-fat diets rich in unsaturated fatty acids may offer an alternative to low-fat diets for CVD prevention. As such diets are often considered more palatable they are likely to promote better compliance.

10.7.3.4 n-6 polyunsaturated fatty acids

Few prospective studies have investigated the influence of *n*-6 polyunsaturates alone on CVD risk (most report on total polyunsaturated intake). Miettinen and colleagues (1982) reported an inverse association between the proportion of the polyunsaturated fatty acid, linoleic acid, in serum phospholipids at baseline and CHD incidence at five-year follow-up. The Kuopio Ischaemic Heart Study reported an inverse association between linoleic acid intake and serum levels and CVD mortality (Laaksonen *et al.* 2005) and higher intake of linoleic acid, as determined by the measurement of serum fatty acids, has been shown to be associated with a reduced risk of ischaemic stroke in Japanese men (Iso *et al.* 2002).

Numerous metabolic studies have shown cholesterol-lowering effects for vegetable oils rich in linoleic acid, when substituted for saturates. Some studies have demonstrated such a substitution to lead to a reduction in HDL-, as well as total and LDL-cholesterol levels and this, together with evidence of decreased protection from oxidation of polyunsaturated fatty acid-enriched LDL, have led many to recommend monounsaturates over polyunsaturates for CVD prevention (see Section 10.7.3.5) (Lunn and Theobald 2006). However, meta-analyses have shown energy substitution of polyunsaturates and monounsaturates for carbohydrate to result in an increase in HDL-cholesterol (*e.g.* Mensink *et al.* 2003), suggesting that it may be prudent to replace saturates with a mix of *n*-6 polyunsaturates and monounsaturates in order to ensure an appropriate balance of fatty acids is consumed (Lunn and Theobald 2006).

10.7.3.5 Monounsaturated fatty acids

The low incidence of CVD among Mediterranean populations has often been attributed to their relatively high intake of monounsaturated fatty acids as olive oil. Although the benefit of *n*-6 polyunsaturates on LDL-cholesterol is greater than the impact of monounsaturates, intakes of *n*-6 polyunsaturates greater than 10% energy (the recommended individual maximum level) may have adverse effects on HDL-cholesterol (Clarke *et al.* 1997). Whilst their effects on LDL-cholesterol may be more subtle, monounsaturates do not reduce protective HDL-cholesterol and may be more resistant than polyunsaturates to oxidation in the body. Intervention studies have also suggested other potential benefits of diets rich in monounsaturates in relation to haemostasis (Sirtori *et al.* 1986; Lopez-Segura *et al.* 1996), reduced inflammatory response (Yaqoob *et al.* 1998) and attenuated postprandial Factor VII responses to acute fat ingestion (Zampelas *et al.* 1994; Roche *et al.* 1998; Larsen *et al.* 1999; Kelly *et al.* 2001). While this may swing the balance in favour of monounsaturates as a replacement for saturates, further research is needed and advice at present is to replace saturates with unsaturated fatty acids (polyunsaturates and monounsaturates).

10.7.3.6 Long chain n-3 polyunsaturates

Oil-rich fish are the main dietary sources of the long chain *n*-3 (or omega 3) polyunsaturates, eicosapentaenoic acid (EPA) and docosahexaenoic acid (DHA). Randomised secondary prevention trials have demonstrated long chain *n*-3 fatty acids, taken as oil-rich fish (Burr *et al.* 1989) or as supplements (GISSI-Prevenzione Investigators 1999) to reduce cardiac events (*e.g.* death, non-fatal myocardial infarction and non-fatal stroke) in patients who had already had a heart attack, with an especially potent effect on sudden death. Some prospective studies (*e.g.* the Nurses' Health Study) have also shown an inverse association between fish consumption and *n*-3 fatty acids and CHD deaths (F. Hu *et al.* 2002), supporting a role in primary prevention. For example, the Physicians' Health Trial, a prospective study of over 20 years' duration, reported a strong inverse dose relationship between blood phospholipid long chain *n*-3 polyunsaturates content at baseline and subsequent mortality from CHD (Albert *et al.* 2002). As a result of the evidence in their favour, recommendations to increase intake of long-chain *n*-3 polyunsaturates have been made (Scientific Advisory Committee on Nutrition and COT 2004).

However, a recent meta-analysis of 89 randomised trials and cohort studies investigating the effect of *n*-3 polyunsaturates for at least six months was unable to show any clear evidence of a reduced risk of total mortality or cardiovascular events (Hooper *et al.* 2006). This finding was influenced by the inclusion of the Diet and Angina Randomised Trial (DART 2) of over 3000 men with stable angina, which reported an unexpected 26% increase in cardiac deaths in men increasing their intake of *n*-3 fatty acids; the effect was clearest in participants taking fish oil capsules rather than eating oil-rich fish (Burr *et al.* 2003). It is not clear why the results of this study conflict with findings of other trials, although possible explanations include the type of volunteers recruited (*i.e.* men with angina) and possible changes in other aspects of lifestyle as a result of the advice to increase *n*-3 intake.

Whilst the mechanism for their cardioprotective effect remains unclear, long chain *n*-3 polyunsaturates appear to decrease blood triglyceride concentrations (Lunn and Theobald 2006). In addition, they have been shown to decrease production of chemoattractants, growth factors, adhesion molecules, inflammatory eicosanoids and inflammatory cytokines, to lower blood pressure, to increase nitric oxide production, endothelial relaxation and vascular compliance, to decrease thrombosis and cardiac arrhythmias and to increase heart rate variability (Stanner 2005).

10.7.3.7 *α-linolenic acid*

An alternative dietary source of *n*-3 polyunsaturates is plant oils, such as linseed, rapeseed and nut oils, which are relatively rich in α-linolenic acid (ALNA) but do not contain the long chain *n*-3 fatty acids present in fish oil. Theoretically, ALNA can be elongated and desaturated to EPA and DHA, although in man the extent of this conversion appears limited (Lunn and Theobald 2006). In dietary studies, ALNA-rich oils do not appear to reproduce fish oil-like effects on CVD risk factors, including blood lipids, haemostatic factors, or immune, inflammatory and endothelial function or platelet function (Buttriss 2005). In adults, dietary ALNA seems to increase circulating levels of EPA, but not DHA (Burdge *et al.* 2003), which may explain the absence of the anticipated beneficial effects.

10.7.3.8 *Conjugated linoleic acid (CLA)*

Conjugated linoleic acid is a series of isomers of linoleic acid found predominantly in the meat and milk of ruminant animals. Some studies, primarily in animals, have suggested that CLA plays a role in modifying blood lipid profiles and influencing the lean/fat tissue ratio in favour of lean tissue. However, findings have been inconsistent, which might be attributed to the variability of the dose level and/or the mix of CLA isomers used in different studies, particularly as results from animal studies show that specific isomers of CLA may be responsible for specific biological effects (Buttriss 2005). Unfavourable effects of a high dose of one of the CLA isomers (*t*10*c*12 CLA, 3.4 g/day) have also been reported in relation to increased insulin resistance, oxidative stress and inflammatory biomarkers, and whilst such an intake is not consumed by diet alone, at present the effects of CLA on human health remain unclear (Tricon *et al.* 2005).

10.7.4 Protein

Some prospective studies have reported an inverse association between protein intake and CVD. For example, those in the highest quintile of protein intake (median 24% energy) in the Nurses' Health study had a relative risk of CHD of 0.74 (95% CI: 0.59–0.94) after controlling for age, smoking, total energy intake, percentage of energy from specific types of fat and other coronary risk factors compared to those in the lowest quintile (median 15% of energy). Iso *et al.* (2001) reported a similar inverse association between protein and stroke risk in the same cohort. The importance of the source of protein (*i.e.* animal- or plant-based) is currently not clear but different sources of protein appear to have different effects on CVD risk. Hu (2005) concluded that although optimal amounts and sources of protein cannot yet be determined, evidence suggests a potential benefit of partially replacing refined carbohydrates with protein sources low in saturates.

Large epidemiological studies (*e.g.* INTERSALT, MRFIT and the National Diet and Nutrition Survey of British Adults) have found an inverse association between dietary protein intake and blood pressure (Elliott 2003; Hu 2005). Clinical trials have also demonstrated blood pressure lowering from increased plant protein (soy) intake (*e.g.* Teede *et al.* 2001; Rivas *et al.* 2002), although findings have been inconsistent and a recent 12-month double-blind randomised trial in postmenopausal women (aged 60–75 years) demonstrating an increase in systolic blood pressure in the soy group compared to placebo (Kreijkamp-Kaspers *et al.* 2005) suggests that further research is needed before any recommendations can be made. Trials investigating the effects of animal protein are, as yet, limited but there is some evidence to suggest that replacement of refined carbohydrate-rich foods with protein in the form of lean red meat could have a blood pressure lowering effect (Hodgson *et al.* 2005). Emerging evidence from clinical trials also indicates that higher protein diets may increase short-term weight loss and improve blood lipids (Parker *et al.* 2002; Layman *et al.* 2003), although claims for the latter have generally been made with interventions that resulted in a concomitant reduction in weight.

10.7.5 Dietary fibre

Prospective studies have demonstrated high-fibre diets to reduce CHD risk. For example, a prospective study of 45,000 American male health professionals, followed for six years, demonstrated an age-adjusted relative risk of 0.59 among men in the highest quintile of dietary fibre (soluble and insoluble) intake compared with men in the lowest quintile (Rimm *et al.* 1996). The strongest association (a relative risk of 0.45) was for fatal coronary disease.

Soluble fibre (*e.g.* from oats) has been shown to lower plasma total and LDL-cholesterol, although the effect is small for those consuming moderate amounts (Truswell 2002). In a meta-analysis by Brown, Rosner *et al.* (1999) 2–10 g/day of soluble fibre was associated with a small, but significant, fall in total cholesterol (0.045 mmol/L per g fibre) and LDL-cholesterol (0.057 mmol/L per g fibre). Three apples or three 28 g servings of oatmeal, providing 3 g soluble fibre, decreased total and LDL-cholesterol by around 0.13 mmol/L. The effects on plasma lipids were not significantly influenced by source of the fibre (oats, psyllium or pectin) and were independent of background dietary fat intake. One of the components attracting interest is β-glucan, found in

oats (Amundsen *et al.* 2003), although not all studies show an effect (Lovegrove *et al.* 2000). The mechanism of this effect also remains undefined.

10.7.6 Micronutrients

10.7.6.1 Sodium (salt)

A number of micronutrients (*e.g.* potassium, calcium, magnesium) and other dietary factors (*e.g.* fruit and vegetable intake) have been reported to influence blood pressure. In particular, there has been considerable debate about the role of sodium (salt) on risk of hypertension and CVD (see Chapter 8, Section 8.2.2). Scientific Advisory Committee on Nutrition (2003) concluded that although studies that have prospectively collected 24-hour urine (a good marker of sodium intake) suggest that a high salt intake has adverse effects on CVD mortality, there are insufficient reliable data on morbidity and premature mortality outcomes to reach clear conclusions. However, SACN concluded that reducing the average salt intake in Britain would confer significant public health benefits by contributing to a reduction in CVD burden. Similar recommendations have been made elsewhere (American Heart Association 2006). SACN also concluded that the greatest reductions in blood pressure are observed when a diet rich in fruits, vegetables and low-fat dairy products, and reduced in saturates and total fat, is combined with a low salt intake. This was demonstrated by the DASH (Dietary Approaches to Stop Hypertension) study, which reported reductions in systolic blood pressure following salt modification (Sacks *et al.* 2001) but larger effects when sodium reduction was combined with other dietary interventions – a diet rich in fruit and vegetables (a source of potassium), low in fat, and incorporating low-fat dairy products (a source of calcium) (Appel *et al.* 1997).

10.7.6.2 Antioxidants

The cardioprotective effects of fruit and vegetables (see Section 10.7.7.1) has led to considerable interest in the role of dietary antioxidants (particularly vitamins C and E and β-carotene) in protecting against oxidative damage and thereby slowing the development of atherosclerosis. Although there are some exceptions, cross-sectional studies comparing different populations within one country or between different countries have found the incidence of CVD, particularly in Europe, to be inversely related to plasma levels of β-carotene, vitamin E (α-tocopherol) and, to a lesser extent, vitamin C (Gey *et al.* 1991; Su *et al.* 1998). Countries with a very high prevalence of CVD, such as Scotland, Northern Ireland and Finland, have significantly lower plasma levels of vitamin E and β-carotene, while the Mediterranean countries have relatively higher blood levels and a lower incidence of CVD. These findings have been supported by case-control studies, as patients with CVD commonly have lower levels of these nutrients. A number of large prospective studies have also provided stronger supportive evidence by demonstrating reduced CVD incidence and/or mortality with higher dietary intakes or plasma levels of these antioxidants (Bruckdorfer 2005). However, a number of large randomised primary and secondary intervention trials have failed to show any consistent benefit from the use of antioxidant supplements on CVD risk, with some trials even suggesting possible harm in certain subgroups (*e.g.* smokers) (Stanner *et al.* 2004; Bruckdorfer 2005). A causal link between lack of antioxidant vitamins and CVD or between antioxidant administration and CVD prevention therefore remains to be established.

Apart from the antioxidant vitamins, in plants there are many thousands of other substances with antioxidant properties, such as selenium (see Section 10.7.6.3) and flavonoids (British Nutrition Foundation 2003a). Flavonoids are found throughout the plant kingdom and are present in foods as diverse as wine, tea, fruit, onions and green vegetables. Flavonoid intake has been shown to be associated with a reduced risk of CHD (but not stroke) in most but not all studies (*e.g.* Hollman and Katan 1999; Yochum *et al.* 1999) but no long-term randomised controlled trials with hard end-points have yet been conducted.

10.7.6.3 Selenium

The role of selenium in the activity of specific antioxidant enzymes, particularly glutathione peroxidase, is well established (Holben and Smith 1999) and it is, therefore, considered to be an important antioxidant. Low levels of selenium have been associated with cardiomyopathy in China, but its importance in CVD remains controversial (Neve 1996). In case-control studies, patients with myocardial infarc-

tion have low plasma selenium concentrations, but this could be a consequence of the disease (British Nutrition Foundation 2001). Prospective studies investigating low selenium status and heart disease have produced mixed results (British Nutrition Foundation 2001). The two studies that found an association (Salonen *et al.* 1982; Virtamo *et al.* 1985) were conducted in Finland, where selenium intake was very low, one showing a 3.6-fold increase in coronary deaths and a 2.7-fold increase in heart attacks among men with low serum selenium levels (<45 μg/L) (Salonen *et al.* 1982; Virtamo *et al.* 1985). In populations with higher selenium intakes, no associations were found (Miettinen *et al.* 1983; Ringstad and Fonnebo 1987; Salvini *et al.* 1995), suggesting that cardiovascular risk may only be increased by very low selenium status (British Nutrition Foundation 2001).

10.7.6.4 Folate and B vitamins

Clinical trials have demonstrated that supplementation with folic acid lowers levels of homocysteine (see Section 10.4.2.2) and that inclusion of vitamins B_6 and B_{12} (which are also involved in homocysteine metabolism) amplify this effect (Clarke 2005a).

Several large randomised trials are being carried out to assess whether supplementation with folic acid and other B vitamins may impact on CVD risk. Few of these trials involve sufficient people or will last long enough to have a good chance on their own to reliably detect the epidemiologically predicted differences in risk of CVD (Clarke 2005b) but taken together they involve about 52,000 participants (32,000 with prior vascular disease in populations where the food supply is unfortified with folic acid, 14,000 with vascular disease and 6,000 with renal disease in fortified populations). A combined analysis of these trials should therefore have adequate power to detect whether lowering homocysteine by vitamin supplementation reduces the risk of CVD events within a few years (see Chapter 8, Section 8.2.4).

10.7.6.5 Milk peptides

Milk proteins, both caseins and whey proteins, are a rich source of angiotensin-1-converting enzyme

(ACE) inhibitory peptides (casokinins and lactokinins). Studies in spontaneously hypertensive rats have shown these milk protein-derived ACE inhibitors to significantly reduce blood pressure and a limited number of human studies have also associated milk protein-derived peptides with statistically significant hypotensive effects (see FitzGerald *et al.* 2004). Whilst functional foods (*e.g.* fermented milk drinks) containing these peptides are now being marketed, further evidence demonstrating the hypotensive effects of consuming specific milk protein-based ingredients and products is warranted.

10.7.7 Specific foods associated with CVD risk

10.7.7.1 Fruit and vegetables

Because many nutrients in fruit and vegetables, including antioxidant vitamins, folate and potassium, as well as flavonoids and dietary fibre (see Section 10.7.6), have been associated with reduced risk for CVD, it is widely believed that higher consumption of fruit and vegetables is cardioprotective. Populations and groups within populations consuming diets that contain a lot of fruit and vegetables (*e.g.* vegetarian diets, traditional Mediterranean diets) tend to have lower rates of heart disease and stroke. A number of prospective cohort studies have examined this relation and most have found protective effects for total fruit and vegetables for stroke, CHD and hypertension (Hu 2003). The largest study was performed by Joshipura *et al.* (1999), who conducted a pooled analysis of the Nurses' Health Study and the Health Professionals' Follow-up Study, including 2190 incident cases of CHD and 570 cases of ischaemic stroke. The multivariate relative risks comparing extreme quintiles of fruit and vegetable intake were 0.80 (95% CI: 0.69–0.92) for CHD and 0.69 (95% CI: 0.52–0.91) for ischaemic stroke. The inverse association between fruit and vegetables and CHD was graded in a dose–response fashion, with intake of at least eight servings/day associated with lowest risk. For stroke, the risk reduction reached a plateau at four or more servings/day. A similar risk reduction of around 30%, as well as a dose–response association, has also been demonstrated in other well-designed cohorts.

No clinical trials have been conducted to examine the effects of increased consumption of fruit and vegetables on CVD end-points. However, the Lyon Diet Heart Study showed that those who followed a Mediterranean-style diet, rich in fruit and vegetables and α-linolenic acid substantially reduced the recurrence of myocardial infarction and mortality over a four-year period compared with a regular low-fat diet (de Lorgeril *et al.* 1994). Among subjects with established CHD, a fat-modified diet enriched with fruit and vegetables, in conjunction with moderate physical activity for three years, was found to lead to a greater reduction in central obesity and a decline in cardiac events and total mortality compared to a control group (Singh *et al.* 1996). Experimental studies have also suggested beneficial effects of increased fruit and vegetables on blood pressure (Appel *et al.* 1997; John *et al.* 2002) and lipid levels (Jenkins *et al.* 1997).

The biological mechanisms whereby fruits and vegetables may exert their effects are not entirely clear and are likely to be multiple. Many nutrients and phytochemicals in fruits and vegetables, including fibre, potassium, folate, flavonoids and antioxidant vitamins, could be jointly responsible for the apparent reduction in CVD risk. Their low glycaemic load (see Chapter 13 for information about glycaemic index) and energy density may also play a significant role. The current advice to consume at least five portions of a variety of fruits and vegetables a day is, therefore, to be encouraged.

10.7.7.2 Whole-grains

Consumption of diets rich in whole-grain cereals (*e.g.* wholewheat cereals, wholemeal bread and brown rice) has been associated with a lower risk of CVD (Pietinen *et al.* 1996; Jacobs *et al.* 1999; Liu *et al.* 1999; Truswell 2002). In the Iowa Women's Health Study, after adjustment for CVD risk factors, the relative risks were 1.0, 0.96, 0.71, 0.64, and 0.70 in ascending quintiles of whole-grain intake (*p* for trend = 0.02) (Jacobs *et al.* 1998). The Nurses' Health Study observed a 25% reduction in risk of CHD among women who ate nearly three servings of whole-grains per day compared with those who ate less than a serving per week (Liu *et al.* 1999). In addition, higher consumption of whole-grains was associated with a 30% lower risk of ischaemic stroke (Liu *et al.* 2000), independent of known CVD risk factors (relative risk 0.69, 95% CI: 0.50–0.98 comparing the highest and lowest quintiles of intake). A recent study has also demonstrated benefits among older people (60–98 years), with regular whole-grain consumption associated with improved CVD risk factors (lower fasting glucose concentrations and BMI), lower prevalence of the metabolic syndrome and a lower incidence of CVD mortality (Sahyoun *et al.* 2006).

Vitamin E, dietary fibre (Richardson 2000), resistant starch and oligosaccharides (Cummings *et al.* 1992), as well as plant sterols (Jones *et al.* 1997), are some of the components of whole-grain cereals that may contribute to a reduced risk of heart disease. Eating a lot of whole-grain foods can also lower dietary glycaemic load (see Chapter 13, Section 13.4.2). Several ongoing studies may yield valuable information in this area. For example, the WHOLE-heart Study is a randomised controlled trial investigating the impact of whole-grain food consumption on lipid profiles, insulin sensitivity, endothelial function, inflammation and CVD risk, whilst RISCK is investigating the impact of types of carbohydrate consumed and the glycaemic load of the diet on CVD risk.

10.7.7.3 Soya

Legumes, particularly soya and its products, have been associated with decreased blood cholesterol levels. In a meta-analysis of 38 studies, an average of 47 g/day (range 17–124 g) of soya protein, led to an average reduction in total and LDL-cholesterol of 0.6 mmol/L and 0.56 mmol/L respectively (Anderson *et al.* 1995). The mechanism of action remains unclear (it may be partly linked to soya's soluble fibre content, see Section 10.7.5) and it is not known if this is a direct (causal) association or whether it results from the substitution of soya for other foods, or is influenced by other aspects of the diet or lifestyle of people who choose soy. In the UK, the Joint Health Claims Initiative (www.jhci. co.uk) has concluded that 'the inclusion of at least 25 g of soya protein per day, as part of a diet low in saturates, can help reduce blood cholesterol levels'. To carry the claim, a minimum of 5 g of soya protein (natural isoflavones intact) must be present per serving of a food. A similar health claim is also permitted in the US (www.cfsan.fda.gov). Achievement of an intake of 25 g soya protein is likely to require inclusion of soya-derived foods at each meal (see British Nutrition Foundation 2003b). There is also limited evidence to suggest that soya may exert effects other than cholesterol lowering. For example, there is some evidence that it can lower blood pressure, although findings from trials have been inconsistent (see Section 10.7.4) and further studies are needed before the true relation between soy protein or isoflavones and blood pressure is clear. The ISO-HEART study is currently investigating the effects of foods enhanced by soy-derived isoflavones on CVD risk among postmenopausal women (www. isoheart.kvl.dk).

10.7.7.4 Nuts

Nuts are high in fat, but most is in the form of monounsaturates and polyunsaturates. Numerous metabolic studies have found that a diet high in nuts (*e.g.* walnuts, almonds) significantly lowers LDL-cholesterol and decreases the ratio of total to HDL-cholesterol (Kris-Etherton *et al.* 2001). Besides this favourable effect on blood lipids, nuts contain a range of substances that may help to protect against CHD through other mechanisms, including magnesium, copper, folate, potassium, fibre and vitamin E. Cohort studies have generally shown eating nuts more than once per week to be associated with a decreased risk of CHD in both men and women (relative risks have ranged from 0.45 to 0.75) (Hu and Stampfer 1999; Kris-Etherton *et al.* 2001).

10.7.7.5 Plant phytosterol enriched foods

Spreads and other products that contain plant sterols or stanols have been shown to reduce LDL-cholesterol by approximately 10–15% (Law 2000) when consumed periodically during the day, over a period of time. Plant sterol and stanol esters seem to be equally effective at a daily dose of 2 g; larger doses do not increase efficacy (Wahle *et al.* 2005). Cholesterol uptake is inhibited by these phytosterols and its elimination facilitated (Trautwein *et al.* 2003).

10.7.7.6 Mycoprotein

There is some evidence that mycoprotein exerts a beneficial effect on total and LDL-cholesterol (Turnbull *et al.* 1990; 1992). A potential mechanism for this effect might concern the high fibre content of mycoprotein, which includes chitin and β-glucans.

10.7.7.7 Coffee

With the exception of boiled coffee, which has been shown to increase plasma cholesterol (Gross *et al.* 1997), there is little evidence that moderate coffee intake either increases or decreases cardiovascular risk (Woodward and Turnstall-Pedoe 1999). However, homocysteine levels are raised in heavy coffee drinkers (Grubben *et al.* 2000). Interestingly, a prospective study in the US of 6594 adults drinking caffeinated beverages on a regular basis demonstrated a significant protective effect against death from heart disease in people aged 65 years or older with normal blood pressure levels (Greenberg *et al.* 2007). The relative risk among those consuming more than four servings per day was 0.47 (95% CI: 0.32–0.69) compared with those consuming less than 0.5 servings/day over an 8.8-year follow-up. However, no effect was found in younger subjects. Thus some of the inconsistency in the findings of studies investigating the relationship between coffee and heart disease may be due to differences in the age of the subjects studied.

10.7.8 Alcohol

Regular light-to-moderate alcohol consumption (about two drinks per day) appears to provide some protection against heart disease and ischaemic stroke, particularly in postmenopausal women and middle-aged men (>40 years) (Foster and Marriott 2006). Data are emerging that alcohol, rather than some bioactive component in alcoholic drinks, is the predominant protective agent (British Nutrition Foundation 2003a). Likely mechanisms include an increase in HDL-cholesterol, improved endothelial function and beneficial changes in platelet function and fibrinolytic parameters (Redmond *et al.* 2000). Moderate consumption of alcohol is also associated with a modest decrease in homocysteine levels. However, excessive drinking, and in particular binge drinking, is associated with increased risk of cardiovascular disorders, including cardiomyopathy, hypertension, CHD and stroke (see Chapter 8, Section 8.2.2).

10.7.9 Dietary patterns and CVD risk

Prospective studies have shown composite diets (*e.g.* traditional Mediterranean diets, vegetarian diets, 'prudent' diets) to be associated with reduced risk of CVD and its risk factors. For example, in the Nurses' Health Study, a high dietary score for a 'prudent' diet with a high intake of fruit and vegetables, legumes, fish, poultry and whole-grains was associated with a significantly reduced risk of CHD after adjusting for other coronary risk factors (relative risk: 0.76, 95% CI: 0.60–0.98 comparing highest and lowest quintiles) (Fung *et al.* 2001). A similar association was demonstrated in the Health Professionals' Follow-up Study (relative risk: 0.70, 95% CI: 0.56–0.86 comparing lowest and highest quintiles) (Hu, Rimm *et al.* 2000). Metabolic studies have tested the effects of dietary patterns on CVD risk factors. Jenkins *et al.* (2002) found that a diet high in plant sterols, soy protein and viscous fibres significantly reduced LDL-cholesterol by 29% and the ratio of LDL to HDL by 26.5%. Several interventions have also supported benefits from a whole diet approach. The Dietary Approaches to Stop Hypertension Trial (DASH) dietary pattern (higher in fruit, vegetables, nuts, whole-grains and low-fat dairy products) was effective in lowering blood pressure (Appel *et al.* 1997) and serum homocysteine (Appel *et al.* 2000).

10.7.10 Diet–gene interactions

The study of interactions between nutritional and genetic factors is an emerging area of research and several polymorphisms have been identified that may influence an individual's response to specific dietary changes and impact on CVD risk. In particular, polymorphisms at various genetic loci that encode proteins involved in lipoprotein metabolism have shown gene–nutrient interactions in relation to the determination of plasma lipid profiles. For example, individuals with the E4 allelic variant of the apolipoprotein E (apoE) gene seem to exhibit greater LDL-cholesterol reductions on low-fat, low-cholesterol diets than subjects with other alleles (Ordovas 1999) and one study has suggested that they may respond to fish oil supplementation with an increase in LDL-cholesterol levels (Minihane *et al.* 2000). Another apolipoprotein structural variant, apo A-IV-2, appears to attenuate the response of LDL-cholesterol to dietary cholesterol (Dreon and Krauss 1997). Other studies have associated lipoprotein response to dietary modifications with DNA polymorphisms in the genes for apoB and the LDL receptor and in the promoter region of the apoA-I gene (Dreon and Krauss 1997).

Genetic influences on the impact of other dietary factors have also been demonstrated. For example, the cardioprotective effect of alcohol intake is greatest in individuals with a variant form of the alcohol dehydrogenase (ADH) enzyme (ADH3), who are slow metabolisers of alcohol (Hines *et al.* 2001). The 677 C→T polymorphism in the 5,10-methylenetetrahydrofolate reductase (MTHFR) gene interacts with folate status in determining elevated total plasma levels of homocysteine (Chiuve *et al.* 2005).

Research in this area is attracting considerable scientific interest and research funding. Lipgene, a programme funded by the European Commission, is investigating whether changing the fatty acid profile of the diet can improve insulin resistance in subjects with risk factors for the metabolic syndrome and studying the effect of common polymorphisms on response to dietary fat (www.lipgene.tcd.ie). The European Nutrigenomics Organisation (NuGO) is focusing on the links between genomics, nutrition and health research (www.nugo.org) and DiOGenes is investigating links between diet, obesity and genes (Saris 2005). Increased knowledge in this area and new techniques for measuring gene expression, gene polymorphisms (genomics), protein expression (proteomics) and metabolic profile (metabolomics) will eventually allow a more refined approach to reducing risk for CVD, with diet interventions targeted at individuals and sub-groups who are genetically susceptible and responsive to the effects of nutritional factors. However, the search for candidate genes has proved to be complex and their identification elusive (Williams 2003), largely because much of the variation in risk results from interactions between environmental exposures and the genome. As much of the data available currently on gene–nutrient interactions has been derived from retrospective genotyping, prospective studies are now required.

10.7.11 Current dietary recommendations in the UK

The recommended dietary changes to reduce rates of CVD in the UK population were detailed in the 1994 report by the Government's Committee on Medical Aspects of Food and Nutrition Policy

(COMA) (Department of Health 1994). These recommendations included reducing the average contribution of total fat to dietary energy (*i.e.* from food and alcohol) in the population to about 35% and reducing the average contribution of saturates to dietary energy to no more than 10% (Table 10.2). COMA recommended that average intakes of *trans* fatty acids should not increase, but made no specific recommendations for monounsaturates. The report recommended that average intakes of *n*-6 polyunsaturates need not increase above current levels and intakes of long chain *n*-3 polyunsaturates (EPA and DHA) should double from 0.1 g per day to 0.2 g per day. (Information about dietary sources of these fatty acids is presented in Table 10.3.) The population was also advised to increase the proportion of dietary energy derived from carbohydrate to approximately 50% and to reduce salt intake by at least one third from its current level of 9 g/day. In 2003, the Scientific Advisory Committee on Nutrition (SACN) repeated COMA's guidance on salt intake in adults and introduced additional guidance on reducing salt intake in children (Scientific Advisory Committee on Nutrition 2003). In 2005, these dietary objectives were repeated in 'Choosing a Better Diet, a Food and Health Action Plan', which further recommended a reduction in intake of added sugar (Department of Health 2004b). Dietary advice for those with established CVD is similar to that recommended for primary prevention (British Cardiac Society *et al.* 1998).

The practical food-based advice arising from the COMA recommendations for CVD prevention is, therefore, to maintain a healthy bodyweight, eat five or more portions of fruit and vegetables each day, reduce intake of fat (particularly saturates), reduce salt intake and eat at least two portions of fish, of which one should be oil-rich fish, each week (Table 10.4).

Given the wealth of published research investigating the role of diet in CVD risk, it appears timely to review the dietary recommendations in the UK for prevention of CHD and stroke, as has been done in the US (American Heart Association 2006) and the Netherlands (Fernandes 2002) (see Buttriss 2005). These have incorporated some of the newer insights into the role of different fatty acids in CVD risk. For example, they have included specific recommendations to increase the ratio of monounsaturates to other fatty acids (see Section 10.7.3.5).

Table 10.4: Summary of practical dietary advice to reduce risk of CVD

- Reduce consumption of all types of fat, for example by selecting lean cuts of meat and lower fat dairy products, by reducing use of oil and full-fat spreads (margarine, butter), by eating fewer fried foods and by moderating consumption of high-fat foods such as cakes, biscuits and savoury snacks.
- Opt for oils/spreads that are higher in monounsaturates or polyunsaturates and lower in saturates.
- Include oil-rich fish in the diet once a week (those with heart disease may benefit from higher intakes).*
- Include more fruit and vegetables in the diet, aiming for at least five portions of a variety of fruits and vegetables each day.
- Use less salt at the table and in cooking, and look for lower salt alternatives of manufactured foods. Reduce intake to <6 g/day (less for children).
- Include more starchy foods in the diet, *e.g.* bread, potatoes, yams, rice and pasta, so that at least 50% of energy intake comes from carbohydrate and increase consumption of whole-grain foods.
- Drink alcohol sensibly, *i.e.* no more than 2–3 units per day for women and no more than 3–4 units per day for men. Avoid binge drinking.

*The National Institute for Health and Clinical Excellence (2007) recommends that patients who have suffered a heart attack should consume 2–4 portions of oil-rich fish a week.
Source: Adapted from Department of Health (1994). Material is Crown copyright and is reproduced with the permission of the Controller of HMSO.

10.8 Physical activity and CVD

Physical inactivity and low fitness are major independent risk factors for CVD in both men and women (Department of Health 2004a; Buttriss and Hardman 2005). Epidemiological studies suggest that physically active individuals have a 30–50% lower risk of developing CHD than sedentary people and benefits are evident in both primary and secondary prevention (Wannamethee and Shaper 2002). Risk reductions have been observed with as little as 30 minutes of moderate-intensity activity a day. For example, the Nurses' Health Study showed a strong, graded inverse association between physical activity and risk of CHD, with regular brisk walking (three or more hours per week) and with vigorous exercise, both of which were associated with similar risk reductions in coronary events of around 30–40% (Manson *et al.* 1999). Protective mechanisms of physical activity include the regulation of body-weight, the reduction of insulin resistance, hypertension, dyslipidaemia and inflammation, and the enhancement of insulin sensitivity, glycaemic control and fibrinolytic and endothelial function.

The picture for stroke is less clear, perhaps because studies have generally not distinguished between ischaemic and haemorrhagic stoke, which have different pathophysiologies. However, the Nurses' Health Study showed moderate-intensity activity (*e.g.* brisk walking) to be associated with a substantial fall in risk of both total and ischaemic stroke, in a dose–response manner (Hu, Stampfer *et al.* 2000). This conclusion is supported by a review of population studies (Wannamethee and Shaper 2002).

No threshold for the minimal amount of exercise necessary to decrease CVD risk has been identified (Anderson *et al.* 1997; Mayer-Davis, D'Agostino *et al.* 1998) so any increase in daily energy expenditure is likely to be beneficial. However, as benefit increases in a dose-dependent fashion (Kohl 2001; Wannamethee and Shaper 2002), people who are already achieving moderate levels of activity can expect to derive additional benefit by increasing their activity. Although the available data are not totally consistent, it has been suggested that intermittent episodes of activity accumulated over the course of a day may have cardiorespiratory fitness benefits comparable to one longer continuous episode as long as total energy expended is equivalent (Buttriss and Hardman 2005). Accumulating activity in shorter bouts may help people to become more active in the longer term. A life-course approach to the promotion of physical activity is required as beneficial effects are evident from childhood through to older age, but most benefit appears to be lost if activity is not maintained (Department of Health 2004a).

The public health impact of physical activity may be especially important for older adults who are at high risk of CVD and often sedentary (see Section 10.6.4). There is good evidence that maintaining or taking up light or moderate physical activity can reduce mortality and heart attacks in older people with and without existing CVD (Donahue *et al.* 1988; Wannamethee *et al.* 1998; Manson *et al.* 1999; Manson *et al.* 2002). Activity can also prevent age-related weight gain and help with weight loss. Benefits are apparent even for men over the age of 60 who become physically active after years of a sedentary lifestyle (Blair *et al.* 1995). This supports public health recommendations for older sedentary people to increase physical activity and for active middle-aged people to continue their activity into old age.

Adults (including older adults) are recommended to take at least 30 minutes of at least moderate intensity activity on five or more days each week (although the optimal level of physical activity for CVD prevention remains unclear and this recommendation does not consider differences in age or ability). Moderate intensity activity should lead to an increase in breathing rate, an increase in heart rate and to a feeling of increased warmth, possibly accompanied by sweating. People who have been obese and who have lost weight may need to do 60–90 minutes of activity a day in order to maintain weight loss (Department of Health 2004a). Children and young people should achieve a total of at least 60 minutes of at least moderate intensity physical activity each day. At least twice a week this should include activities to improve bone health (activities that produce high physical stress on the bones), muscle strength and flexibility (Department of Health 2004a).

For those who are sedentary until old age, it can be harmful to engage in vigorous activity because of increased injury and heart attack risk, and physical activity with lower intensities, such as walking, cycling or gardening, are often preferable. Although older people should aim to meet the recommendation for physical activity for younger adults, even light activities conducted almost daily (≥ 5 times per week) may have substantial benefits for cardiovascular risk profile in this age group (Pols *et al.* 1997; Bijnen *et al.* 1998; Mensink *et al.* 1999). They may also result in improvements in many physical and psychological parameters (Department of Health 2004a).

10.9 The need for a life-course approach

As discussed in Section 10.6.1, several CVD risk factors, including blood pressure and cholesterol levels, are not as strongly or consistently predictive of CVD risk when measured after the age of 65 years. Whilst this is chiefly explained by methodological issues, such as possible confounding by drug treatment and co-morbidity (see Section 10.6.1), measurements in later life may not necessarily reflect lifetime exposure to these risk factors. The risk of CVD in old age is likely to be influenced by the combination, accumulation and/or interactions

of different environments and experiences across the life-course. This supports a whole-of-life approach to prevention and health promotion and highlights the need for heart disease prevention programmes to begin early in childhood and continue throughout adulthood to reduce the risk of atherosclerosis.

10.9.1 The fetal origins of adult disease (FOAD) hypothesis

Considerable evidence suggests that early life factors play an important role in the development of CVD. Studies have demonstrated consistent associations between low birthweight and low weight gain during infancy and increased adult blood pressure, type 2 diabetes, insulin resistance and incidence and mortality from CVD (Barker 1998; Fall 2005). This association appears to be independent of lifestyle risk factors such as smoking, adult weight, social class, alcohol and lack of exercise, although these are additive to the effect. Importantly, the association holds for the full range of birthweights, including those within the normal range (Figure 10.13), and is linked to restricted fetal growth rather than pre-term delivery (Osmond *et al.* 1993). There is also some evidence for associations between other markers of restricted growth (*e.g.* low ponderal index) and heart disease (Forsen *et al.* 1997; Eriksson *et al.* 1999). Other studies have suggested that faster postnatal catch-up growth may also be predictive of later risk of CVD (Eriksson *et al.* 1999; Bavdekar *et al.* 2000; Forsen *et al.* 2000; Law *et al.* 2002).

The fetal origins of adult disease (FOAD) hypothesis proposes that the association between low birthweight, childhood growth and subsequent CVD reflects permanent metabolic and structural changes resulting from under-nutrition during critical periods of early development (Barker 1998). This is well supported by animal studies, for example, demonstrating maternal protein restriction in pregnancy to be associated with higher blood pressure, impaired glucose tolerance, insulin resistance and altered hepatic architecture and function in the adult offspring (Fall 2005). However, at present the impact of maternal diet on fetal growth and adult disease in humans remains unclear. Despite some evidence that maternal protein and carbohydrate intake may influence blood pressure in the offspring (Campbell *et al.* 1996) and that intrauterine exposure to acute

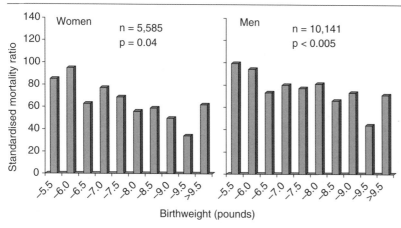

Figure 10.13: Deaths from CVD in men and women below the age of 65 years according to birthweight.
Source: Osmond *et al.* (1993).
Reproduced by permission of the BMJ Publishing Group.

1 pound (lb) = 2.5 kg.

famine may increase glucose intolerance in later life (Ravelli *et al.* 1998), studies in humans investigating the role of maternal and fetal nutrition are more limited. Some researchers have supported a genetic, rather than environmental, explanation, suggesting that genetic factors may lead to both low birthweight and subsequent risk of CVD. In support of this theory, genetic loci have been described which could link smallness at birth with adult disease (Dunger *et al.* 1998; Hattersley *et al.* 1998).

10.9.2 Intergenerational influences

Offspring birthweight is related to maternal height and birthweight (Drake and Walker 2004). In addition, lower maternal birthweight has been linked with CVD risk in the offspring. For example, babies of mothers who are small at birth are more likely to develop high blood pressure in later life and this association is largely independent of the relationship between maternal and offspring birthweight (Barker *et al.* 2000). There is also a substantial body of evidence from animal studies that programmed phenomena can be perpetuated in later generations. Animal models of prenatal programming by nutrition or exercise and postnatal programming by nutrition or handling have shown effects on birthweight, glucose tolerance and the hypothalamic–pituitary axis in subsequent generations (Drake and Walker 2004). Thus the effects of poor early growth may be self-perpetuating through several genera-

tions and policies aimed at improving maternal, fetal and infant health may have important benefits for succeeding generations.

10.10 Treating and preventing CVD in the elderly

The high proportion of older people with one or more CVD risk factors means that the distinction between primary and secondary prevention becomes blurred, but there are clear opportunities for intervention in later life. The major correctable risk factors remain relevant in older people for both primary and secondary CVD prevention and the response of these risk factors to treatment is as great in the elderly as in the middle-aged (see Section 10.6). Effective use of pharmacotherapy, including statins, antithrombotic agents, β-adrenoceptor antagonists and ACE inhibitors, therefore, play an important role in this age group and their widespread use has been supported in ageing populations. Wald and Law (2003) proposed that offering a combined intervention or 'poly-pill' containing a statin, three half-dose antihypertensives, aspirin and folic acid, to all those aged over 55 years could prevent heart disease and strokes by 80% or more in at-risk individuals (Wald and Law 2003). This concept met with a storm of controversy, with arguments raised regarding a lack of evidence for the magnitude of this effect, expected adherence problems, likely over-treatment of individuals and potential side-effects (Combination Pharmacotherapy and Public Health Research Working Group 2005). As well as quality of life benefits, there are clear economic advantages from avoiding the prolonged use of drugs, and lifestyle modifications offer a preferable strategy with more widespread benefits for protection against other conditions such as diabetes and cancer. Smoking cessation, regular physical activity, weight control and a healthy diet are, as in younger individuals, appropriate and effective measures for preventing cardiovascular events and prolonging survival in the elderly (Haveman-Nies *et al.* 2003). There is ample evidence from clinical trials that older people can make and sustain such lifestyle changes, perhaps even more so than younger adults (Applegate *et al.* 1992; Whelton *et al.* 1998). The high incidence of CVD events in older individuals means that relatively small improvements in risk factors, such as small reductions in blood pressure or LDL-cholesterol levels, through diet and lifestyle changes, can be of substantial benefit.

The most effective approach to promote dietary and lifestyle changes for CVD prevention in older people remains, however, unclear. A review for the Health Development Agency (Ebrahim and Davey Smith 1996) concluded that single lifestyle interventions for lowering risk factors such as blood cholesterol and blood pressure have had limited effect and their impact on disease outcome was uncertain, although weight reduction and low-fat diets appeared to have some value. Multiple interventions involving both lifestyle modifications and medication have had greater effects in terms of secondary prevention. Also, nutrition interventions, with or without exercise, after a heart attack have been highly effective in reducing mortality (Ebrahim and Davey Smith 1996). However, further research, particularly good quality evaluative studies, are needed to define the most effective interventions in older people (see Chapter 14, Section 14.7).

It is unlikely that all excess risk accumulated over many years can be erased by short-term prevention introduced in later life. Even the use of risk-reducing drugs, which can significantly lower risk when begun in later life, may not return an older individual to the low-risk status of a younger person. This reduction can only be accomplished by decreasing the magnitude of atherosclerosis by the long-term control of risk factors throughout the life-course. Appropriate interventions starting early in life and continuing into middle age have the potential to bring about greater reductions in long-term risk, and developing a healthy lifestyle and dietary habits in childhood is a pragmatic approach to preventing CVD.

10.11 Key points

- Cardiovascular disease (CVD), including coronary heart disease (CHD) and stroke, is the leading cause of morbidity and mortality in older men and women; those aged over 65 years represent an increasing proportion of the population treated for the condition.
- Ageing is clearly an important risk factor as the prevalence of CVD rises steeply with age and the outcome is more often fatal. This is thought to primarily reflect the length of time that people are exposed to the recognised risk factors.
- There is consensus on the importance of the main modifiable risk factors for the development of CVD. These include obesity, dyslipidaemia, hypertension, smoking, low levels of physical obesity and diabetes. Exposure to these risk factors in middle age predicts risk of premature death from CVD and risk in old age.
- The magnitude of the association between CVD and some of these factors (*e.g.* hypercholesterolaemia and hypertension) appears to decline when measured after the age of 65, although this may be due in part to difficulties of interpreting epidemiological studies in older populations (*e.g.* eliminating confounding factors such as co-morbidity). Nevertheless, the classic risk factors remain predictive of CVD in later life and large trials have demonstrated similar benefits from interventions such as antihypertensive and lipid-lowering drugs to those found in younger individuals. Due to the higher event rates, the absolute risk reduction yielded by preventive interventions is much greater in the older age segments of populations.

Continued

- The connection between CVD and more novel risk factors such as lipoprotein (a), homocysteine and oxidative stress in the elderly and the value of modifying them requires further investigation.
- As the risk factors that predict CVD in younger individuals remain relevant in older people for both primary and secondary prevention, dietary and lifestyle advice remains the same for the elderly as in middle age. Substantial evidence shows that diets incorporating non-hydrogenated unsaturated fatty acids as the predominant form of fat, whole-grains as the main form of carbohydrate, an abundance of fruits and vegetables, adequate *n*-3 fatty acids and not too much salt can offer significant protection against CVD. Such diets, together with regular physical activity, avoidance of smoking and maintenance of a healthy bodyweight, may prevent the majority of CVD in western populations.
- Whilst substantial evidence demonstrates physical activity to be effective in reducing CVD risk, the proportion of older people participating in regular activity is low. In the UK adults, including older people, are advised to accumulate at least 30 minutes of moderate-intensity activity (*e.g.* brisk walking) on at least five days a week. For many benefits to cardiovascular health, intensity can be traded for duration, provided that total energy expenditure remains high. Light- or moderate-intensity activities often popular with older people, such as walking or gardening, can therefore be of benefit.
- The study of the interactions between nutritional and genetic factors is an emerging and important area of research, and has the potential to permit a more individual approach to dietary advice for CVD prevention.
- Because older people carry the greatest burden of CVD, risk factor interventions initiated or continued in later life can have considerable benefit. As CVD risk factors have multiplicative effects, a multifactorial approach is the best strategy for prevention. However, the greatest achievements will be gained from a life-course approach that considers the interacting roles of prenatal, childhood and adult life experiences in the prevention of adult CVD.

10.12 Recommendations for future research

- The predictive role of CVD risk factors is less clear at extreme ages and clarification is required regarding the likely benefits of treatments such as antihypertensives in the very elderly (some clinical trials are underway, *e.g.* the Hypertension the Very Elderly Trial).
- There is a need to clarify desirable values of BMI in the elderly and to determine if other indices, such as waist:hip ratio, are better at identifying older people at risk.
- Research is needed to provide more information about the relationship between novel risk factors and CVD in the elderly and the potential value of modifying them in later life.
- Further investigation of the link between oral health status, inflammatory and haemostatic markers and risk of CVD is needed to determine if treatment of poor dental health can play a significant role in CVD prevention.
- Further studies are needed to provide greater insight into the effects of low-fat diets (coupled with different sources of carbohydrate) and of different fatty acids on weight management and CVD, and to identify the optimal amounts of monounsaturates and polyunsaturates and the optimal balance of *n*-3 and *n*-6 fatty acids in the diet.
- Further research is needed regarding the role of phytochemicals in CVD prevention.
- Further studies are required to clarify the relationship between dietary protein (animal and plant) and blood pressure.
- Studies of diet–gene interactions in large population groups, in which subjects are recruited prospectively according to genotype, are required to determine the impact of genetic influences on individual responses to dietary change.

Continued

- Well-designed and evaluated studies are needed to gain a better understanding of the effect of altering lifestyle in the elderly on CVD risk.
- Further research is needed to identify effective dietary interventions in later life.
- A better understanding of the intensity, frequency and duration of physical activity required to protect against CVD in elderly populations is needed. This will allow specific recommendations reflecting differences in age and functional ability to be made.
- There is a need to identify ways of promoting physical activity as part of everyday life for older people.

10.13 Key references

British Heart Foundation (2006) *Coronary Heart Disease Statistics*. London, British Heart Foundation.

Department of Health (1991) *Dietary Reference Values for Food Energy and Nutrients for the United Kingdom. Report of the Panel on Dietary Reference Intakes of the Committee on Medical Aspects of Food Policy*. London, HMSO.

Ebrahim S and Davey Smith G (1996) *Health Promotion in Older People for the Prevention of Coronary Heart Disease and Stroke*. London, Health Education Authority.

Kannel W (2002) Coronary heart disease risk factors in the elderly. *American Journal of Geriatric Cardiology*, **11**, 101–7.

Lunn J (2006) The health effects of dietary unsaturated fatty acids. A British Nutrition Foundation Briefing Paper. *Nutrition Bulletin* **31**: 178–224.

Stanner S (2005) *Cardiovascular Disease: Diet, Nutrition and Emerging Risk Factors. The Report of the British Nutrition Foundation Task Force*. Oxford, Blackwell.

11
Healthy Ageing: The Immune System

The immune system is a powerful example of both the disposable soma (Kirkwood 1977) and antagonistic pleiotropy (Williams 1957) theories of ageing. In terms of the disposable soma theory: fertility and fecundity are compromised in the face of high levels of inflammation, yet a robust inflammatory response is a prerequisite for repair of potentially lethal wounds and resistance to infection, maximising survival. For the antagonistic pleiotropy theory: again, robust immune and inflammatory responses are vital for survival, but chronic inflammation, a feature of advancing age, contributes to polarisation of cell-mediated immune responses and metabolic dysregulations in old age, driving insulin resistance and ultimately contributing to the constellation of the major degenerative diseases of ageing (diabetes, cardiovascular and neurodegenerative diseases).

Evolution has, of course, found a satisfactory compromise; though it is one which is better suited to our ancestrally shorter lifespans. Indeed, many of the 'biological problems' associated with our increased longevity over our hunter-gatherer forebears stem from the lack of selective pressure on late-acting biological processes. Nevertheless, we are not 'programmed' to die; evolution has programmed us for context-specific survival, not death. But, in the last few thousand years, we have changed the context more quickly than our genes/physiology can adapt; we simply outlive our ability to maintain adequate repair standards and, ultimately, homeostasis.

11.1 Overview of the immune system

The immune system consists of a network of lymphoid organs, cells and soluble mediators, all of which are coordinated for host defence. Immune cells originate in the bone marrow and are found circulating in the bloodstream, organised into lymphoid organs (thymus, spleen and lymph nodes) and dispersed in tissues throughout the body.

The immune system comprises two functional arms: the innate (ancestral/non-specific) and the acquired (specific/adaptive) system. A non-specific first line of defence is provided by the innate system capable of distinguishing between dangerous pathogens and harmless self-molecules. The cells involved here include 'professional immune cells', such as neutrophils, monocytes, macrophages and natural killer cells (NK). However, it is becoming increasingly apparent that many non-immune cells, including fibroblasts and endothelial cells, also produce mediators and express surface markers which allow them to play an important role in innate immunity. In contrast, the adaptive immune response mediates recognition of specific antigens (Ag) and the formation of memory cells capable of rapid activation and proliferation upon re-exposure to each Ag. Lymphocytes, of which there are two types – T-cells (which develop in the thymus) and B-cells (which develop in the bone marrow) – are the cellular component of the acquired immune system.

Communication within the immune system is brought about by direct cell-to-cell contact involving adhesion/signalling molecules and through the production of chemical messengers. Cytokines are the small, soluble chemical messengers modulating inflammation and immune responses produced by a wide variety of cells. They are involved in all aspects of the immune response and play a major role in determining the type of immunity generated in response to pathogenic agents. These mediators have been divided into several families including interleukins (IL-1 to IL-27), growth factors, chemokines, the tumour necrosis factor family (TNF) and interferons (IFN).

Cytokines mediate a metabolic response to infections, including induction of fever and loss of appetite. They increase vascular permeability and expression of adhesion molecules by endothelial cells, allowing infiltration of immune cells into sites of injury and infection. The liver is an important target for the action of cytokines, responding through the synthesis of acute-phase proteins such as C-reactive protein and fibrinogen, which are required for repair and recovery. Although inflammation (redness, swelling, heat and pain) is an integral part of the immune response, failure to resolve the response can be detrimental and has been implicated in the aetiology of inflammatory diseases, such as rheumatoid arthritis, psoriasis and atherosclerosis.

11.2 Immune changes during ageing

The elderly suffer impairments to their immune system, evidenced by increasing incidence and severity of infectious disease, cancer and autoimmunity. This immune dysfunction is of considerable importance in the morbidity and mortality of the aged (Pawelec *et al.* 1997; Pawelec and Solana 1997; Lesourd 1999). Low-level chronic inflammation, due to overexpression of many pro-inflammatory cytokines, also contributes to immune dysfunction in the elderly (Franceschi *et al.* 2000).

Immunosenescence is the term that has been given to the deterioration and dysregulation of immune function. Although most components of the immune system are modified with advancing age, much of the immunosenescence is associated with changes in the T-cell population. Several studies have reported an association between poor *in vitro* T-cell function and subsequent mortality (Ferguson *et al.* 1995, reviewed by Pawelec *et al.* 1995). It is generally believed that good health in the older population can be associated with immune functions approximating that of normal younger individuals. Much essential information has been revealed by studying exceptional populations of the 'successfully' aged (*e.g.* centenarians). Screening very old individuals for biomarkers of ageing and comparing these with younger elderly populations may help to exclude those factors which are age-associated but not relevant to the healthy ageing process.

There is considerable inter-individual variability in immunosenescence and it is widely believed that age-related immune changes are influenced by a number of factors, including genetics, environment, health and nutritional status.

Ageing is characterised by a pro-inflammatory phenotype resulting in chronic low-level inflammation. Controlling inflammatory status may, therefore, provide a route to successful ageing. In fact, recent reports support this theory, suggesting that individuals who are genetically predisposed to produce low levels of inflammatory cytokines or high levels of anti-inflammatory cytokines have an increased probability of achieving extreme longevity (Bonafe *et al.* 2001; Lio *et al.* 2002a, 2002b; Giacconi *et al.* 2004; Van Den Biggelaar *et al.* 2004).

11.2.1 Thymic involution

The thymus is the principal location of T-cell maturation. Thymic involution is known to occur soon after puberty and continues throughout life (Lesourd 1999; Pawelec *et al.* 2002). It has been estimated that complete atrophy should occur at around the age of 120 years (Hartwig and Steinmann 1994). Despite this, limited T-cell maturation does still occur in the elderly, possibly taking place in a remnant of the thymus or other extra-thymic tissue sites. Extra-thymic maturation may lead to the production of auto-reactive T-cell clones which would normally be deleted in the thymus (Hartwig 1995). Some data suggest that the small proportion of centenarians who are very healthy represent a group showing the best retention of thymic structure and function, thereby decreasing the incidence of auto-reactive T-cell clones (Pawelec *et al.* 1997).

How changes in thymic function actually influence T-cell homeostasis is still unclear. The general consensus is that changes in T-cell numbers with age are relatively small and are influenced greatly by underlying disease (Miller 1998; Remarque and Pawelec 1998). As the change in absolute cell number is not dramatic this cannot represent the only mechanism responsible for immunosenescence.

11.2.2 T-cell ageing

When compared with T-cells from younger individuals, older human T-cells show reduced levels of activation and proliferation in response to antigenic and mitogenic stimuli (Pawelec *et al.* 2002). A number of factors have been implicated in this decline of function; including decreased cell numbers, loss of cellular adhesion/activation molecule expression, signalling defects and alterations in cell membrane viscosity.

Whilst T-cell numbers do not change substantially with age, there is some evidence for age-related changes in the proportions of T-cell subsets, with reports of decreased numbers of CD4+ T-cells, increased CD8+ T-cells and decreases in CD4+/CD8+ cell ratios. These data refer only to circulating cells; the situation in lymphoid tissues still remains to be explored.

In adults the numbers of memory T-cells gradually increase in comparison with naïve T-cell numbers, resulting in a marked difference between the young and elderly in the ratio of naïve to memory T-cells. Consequently, the elderly immune system cannot respond well to insults by novel antigens. In addition, the memory cell pool in the elderly shows signs of severely depressed T-cell function (Ohkusu *et al.* 1997; Weyand *et al.* 1998).

One of the most important advances in cellular immunology has been the discovery of functionally distinct T-cell subsets (Mosmann *et al.* 1986). Thus, type 1 T-cells (T1) generate cytokines such as IL-2 and IFNγ leading to cell-mediated responses, whereas type 2 (T2) cells generate IL-4 and IL-5, leading to enhanced antibody responses (Mosmann and Sad 1996). Cytokines, such as IL-12, IL-15 and IL-18, produced by monocytes/macrophages drive a T1 response, whereas IL-10 production favours a T2 profile. A third population of T-cells, regulatory/suppresser T-cells, capable of secreting immunosuppressive cytokines such as IL-10 and TGF-β, has also been described (Fehervari and Sakaguchi 2004; Jiang and Chess 2004). This population of cells is thought to be important in the regulation of all immune responses, including suppression of innate and adaptive immune cell responses, maintenance of self-tolerance and resolution of inflammation. There is still considerable debate in the literature regarding these T-cells, and their mechanisms of suppression are not fully understood.

Data from murine studies suggest that a switch from a T1 to a T2 profile with age is one mechanism responsible for the immune dysfunction associated with ageing (Hung *et al.* 1975; Miller and Stutman 1981). The general age-related decline in T1 function

is believed to be the driving force behind the skew towards a T2 profile, rather than greatly increased production of IL-4, IL-5 and IL-10 and may be partly responsible for the increased incidence of many diseases associated with ageing. This model has been suggested in humans, but remains to be clearly established in this more complex system (Shearer 1997; Castle *et al.* 1999).

Data on cytokine secretion in older humans are inconsistent and under-investigated. The most studied cytokine is the T-cell growth factor IL-2. Since the first report on IL-2 production in the elderly (Gillis *et al.* 1981) many groups have published on the subject, and although some controversies exist, the consensus is that there is an age-related decline in IL-2 production and IL-2 receptor (IL-2R) expression following activation (Caruso *et al.* 1996; Beiqing *et al.* 1997; Gorczynski *et al.* 1997; Berstein and Murasko 1998; Chakravarti and Abraham 1999; Ginaldi *et al.* 1999; Lesourd and Mazari 1999; Pawelec *et al.* 2002). Other T1 cell-derived cytokines, such as IFNγ, have been investigated to a lesser degree but with similar conclusions drawn (Ouyang *et al.* 2000).

IL-4 is considered to be the prototypical type 2 cytokine and has, for this reason, been investigated along with IL-2 in the context of ageing. Results are still controversial, with groups suggesting increased or unchanged levels of IL-4 production in the elderly compared with the young (Berstein and Murasko 1998). One publication, one of the few to study IL-5, has shown increased production of IL-5 in elderly T-cell cultures (Lio *et al.* 1999). IL-4 and IL-5 impair macrophage killing and their dysregulation may therefore significantly contribute to the increased susceptibility of the elderly to infections and tumours. Only a few studies have looked at IL-10 production, and the limited data suggest there may be increased expression of this T2 cytokine in older humans (Cakman *et al.* 1996; Castle *et al.* 1997).

Several co-stimulatory molecules are present in markedly decreased levels on activated T-cells from older compared to young individuals and contribute to the dysfunctional activation and proliferation observed in older human T-cells (Caruso *et al.* 1996; Ginaldi *et al.* 2001; Dennett *et al.* 2002). To date the co-stimulatory molecule CD28 is perhaps the closest to a biomarker of ageing in T-cells, with several studies showing that the proportion of CD28+ T-cells declines with age (Pawelec *et al.* 1997; Boucher *et al.* 1998, reviewed by Pawelec *et al.* 2002).

11.2.3 NK cell ageing

There is a population of large granular lymphocytes involved in the recognition and lysis of both tumour cells and virally infected cells. The relative expression of the NK cell marker CD56 defines two functionally distinct sub-populations of NK cells. Mature NK cells make up 95% of the total NK cell population and are strongly cytotoxic. In contrast, the remaining 5% of the population comprise immature NK cells, which are poorly cytotoxic and proliferate strongly in response to IL-2.

Studies have demonstrated age-associated alterations in the number, phenotype and function of NK cells (Borrego *et al.* 1999; Solana *et al.* 1999; Solana and Mariani 2000). An increased number of NK cells has been observed (Di Lorenzo *et al.* 1999), the majority of which are phenotypically mature and have decreased activity and proliferation (Borrego *et al.* 1999; Solana *et al.* 1999). The percentage of T-cells expressing NK cell markers is also increased in the elderly (Solana and Mariani 2000) and in clinical conditions involving chronic inflammation (Tarazona *et al.* 2000). Taken together these findings suggest that a phenotypic and functional shift towards a less functional NK population occurs with age contributing to the increased incidence and severity of infections in the older population.

11.2.4 Macrophage ageing

Monocyte/macrophage populations do not appear to decline in number with age, although they show some defects in their ability to interact with other immune cells. Functionally intact antigen presenting cells (APCs) have impaired capacity to cross tissue barriers and, due to a decrease in major histocompatibility complex class II (MHC II) expression, also show a diminished ability to present Ag to T-cells (Saurwein-Teissl *et al.* 1998; Solana and Pawelec 1998).

A significant increase in the production of macrophage-derived pro-inflammatory mediators, such as IL-6 and TNFα, occurs in mitogen-activated cultures of older compared with young donors (Cossarizza *et al.* 1997). Presumably, as a result of this, levels of IL-6 are often high enough to be detectable in serum even in the absence of an inflammatory response (Ershler *et al.* 1993). This increase in pro-inflammatory mediator production may play a role in the development of several age-associated diseases, including atherosclerosis, rheumatoid arthritis, fibrosis and dementia. Activated macrophages also produce suppressive factors such as prostaglandin E_2 and oxidants such as hydrogen peroxide, many of which depress lymphocyte proliferation contributing to the age-related decline in T-cell function (Meydani *et al.* 1995).

The macrophage-derived type 1 cytokine IL-12 may also be decreased in the majority of older individuals as suggested by data showing that addition of recombinant IL-12 to peripheral blood cultures returned proliferation levels comparable with those of younger individuals (Castle *et al.* 1999).

11.2.5 Neutrophil ageing

Neutrophils from older individuals often show decreased functional activity (Di Lorenzo *et al.* 1999; Ginaldi *et al.* 1999), defined by diminished phagocytic capacity, decreased superoxide production (Biasi *et al.* 1996; Di Lorenzo *et al.* 1999), and decreased chemotaxis (Di Lorenzo *et al.* 1999). Spontaneous and Fas-induced neutrophil apoptosis is not altered with age (Di Lorenzo *et al.* 1999; Tortorella *et al.* 1999). However, the apoptosis induced by inflammation-derived reactive oxygen species (ROS) is slightly increased and responsiveness to rescue signals from pro-inflammatory mediators is decreased (Tortorella *et al.* 1999). Since neutrophils are one of the first lines of defence against infection, decreased activity and changes in apoptosis may account, at least in part, for the increased incidence of life-threatening infections observed in the elderly.

11.2.6 B-cell ageing

B-cell proliferation seems unaffected by the ageing process (Fernandez-Gutierrez *et al.* 1999). However, groups have reported alterations in B-cell function. An age-related increase in the levels of IgG and IgA but not IgM has been observed (Paganelli *et al.* 1992; Cossarizza *et al.* 1997). There is a decrease in the generation of specific, high-affinity, high-avidity antibodies and an increase in non-specific antibodies against autologous antigens (Thoman and Weigle

1989; Dunn-Walters *et al.* 2003), implying some kind of defect in the mechanism of antibody affinity maturation. These B-cell changes are thought to arise as a result of defects in T-cell function as the ability of B-cells to respond to T-cell-independent antigen remains unchanged (Heuser and Adler 1997). It is possible that down-regulation or loss of T-cell adhesion molecules, such as CD40L, may be involved in the provision of B-cell help and may be partly responsible for age-related changes in B-cell function (Weyand *et al.* 1998). However, T-cell-independent B-cell responses exist and this is an area that needs to be investigated in the context of ageing.

11.2.7 Cytokines and ageing

Cytokines are central to immune cell communications and, therefore, age-related changes in cytokine profiles will contribute to many of the functional alterations observed in the ageing immune system. Cytokine expression is controlled at multiple levels and is linked not only with age but also with health, nutritional and hormonal status. Hormones and immune mediators interact in a very complex manner and many groups have now demonstrated that there is a complex interrelationship between the immune and endocrine systems, where endocrinosenescence contributes significantly to immunosenescence, and vice versa (Straub *et al.* 2000).

Although IL-6 is the most studied cytokine in the context of ageing and has been termed 'a cytokine for gerontologists' (Ershler *et al.* 1993), there is still some controversy in the literature regarding this pro-inflammatory mediator. The main consensus is that IL-6 increases with age (Hager *et al.* 1994; Mysliwska *et al.* 1998; Straub *et al.* 1998; Young *et al.* 1999; Forsey *et al.* 2003; Ferrucci *et al.* 2005), but groups have also reported decreased (Peterson *et al.* 1994) or unchanged levels (Beharka *et al.* 2001) and changes in males but not females (Young *et al.* 1999). These differences most probably arise because these groups are looking at either very healthy individuals and/or those under the age of 70.

It has been suggested that these age-related increases in IL-6 account for many of the phenotypic changes seen with advanced age, including decreased lean body mass, osteopenia, low-grade anaemia, decreased serum albumin and cholesterol, and increased inflammatory proteins such as C-reactive protein (CRP) and serum amyloid A.

Furthermore, the increase of IL-6 may contribute, along with other pro-inflammatory factors, to the onset of many of the chronic age-related diseases (Ershler *et al.* 1993; Cohen *et al.* 1997; Ferrucci *et al.* 1999). Higher circulating levels of IL-6 predict onset of disability (Ferrucci *et al.* 1999), frailty and mortality (Harris *et al.* 1999) and have been implicated in the pathogenesis of pathophysiologically unrelated diseases that are common in old age, including Alzheimer's disease (see Chapter 8) and cardiovascular disease (CVD) (see Chapter 10) (Hull *et al.* 1999; Ershler and Keller 2000).

It has been reported that levels of another major pro-inflammatory cytokine, TNFα, are increased in the elderly and can predict mortality (Mooradian *et al.* 1991). However, the picture with TNF is not as clear as that of IL-6, as some groups report no change in TNFα levels with age and in older patients with pneumonia levels are lower than in younger patients (Gon *et al.* 1996).

Levels of the soluble form of intercellular adhesion molecules (sICAM-1) have been shown to increase with age (Miles *et al.* 2001) and are also significantly associated with several established CVD risk factors, including smoking, hypertension, diabetes and serum levels of triglycerides, fibrinogen and homocysteine (Rohde *et al.* 1999). Due to this correlation several groups have now suggested that sICAM-1 may be an early marker of atherosclerosis (Noguchi *et al.* 1998; Rohde *et al.* 1999; Ikata *et al.* 2000). Further studies are needed to evaluate whether the use of sICAM as a marker of pre-clinical atherosclerosis is reliable.

Several studies have, however, looked at the *ex vivo* capacity of macrophages from older donors to produce IL-10. Data from murine (Hobbs *et al.* 1996; Spencer *et al.* 1996), primate (Mascarucci *et al.* 2001) and human (Castle *et al.* 1999; Sadeghi *et al.* 1999; Pawelec *et al.* 2000) studies have shown increased capacity to produce IL-10 in older subjects when compared to younger controls. Sadeghi and colleagues have suggested that the increased IL-10 and IL-6 in older humans is produced by an expanded pool of activated monocytes (CD14(dim)/ CD16(bright)) (Sadeghi *et al.* 1999).

11.2.8 Cytokine antagonists and ageing

As well as altered levels of cytokines, older individuals may also have altered levels of cytokine antagonists and it is the combination of these two changes that will impact on the individual. Only a few groups have investigated levels of these soluble receptors in older populations and this is an area that needs to be further explored. For example, one group has shown no change in soluble IL-6R with age (Young *et al.* 1999) and another has shown that the levels are significantly increased in men but not women (Ferrucci *et al.* 2005). Increased levels of IL-1 receptor antagonist (IL-1ra) (Roubenoff *et al.* 1998; Ferrucci *et al.* 2005) and soluble TNF receptor (sTNF-R) (type I and II) have also been reported in the elderly (Roubenoff *et al.* 1998; Hasegawa *et al.* 2000). The increase in sTNF-R is even more pronounced in centenarians (Gerli *et al.* 2000).

Centenarians have increased levels of serum IL-18 when compared to younger controls. However, more importantly they also have significantly increased levels of IL-18 binding protein and hence lower levels of free IL-18 in their serum (Gangemi *et al.* 2003). Increased levels of IL-18 have been associated with atherosclerosis (Gangemi *et al.* 2003) and diabetes (Esposito *et al.* 2004) and may, therefore, be linked with poor health outcomes in old age.

Overall, the evidence suggests that successfully aged centenarians manage the age-related upward drift in inflammatory tone, at least in part, by compensating with parallel increases in a range of soluble cytokine antagonists.

11.2.9 Immune risk profile

It is well known that ageing is associated with increased vulnerability to diseases and it may be that immune status contributes in a direct way to this. The most frequent diseases observed in the very elderly are infections, with age-associated increases in cancers, cardiovascular diseases based on atherosclerosis (see Chapter 10) and neurodegenerative diseases (including Alzheimer's and Parkinson's) (see Chapter 8), mostly occurring or beginning earlier on, in late middle age. We hypothesise that alterations to T-cell functions with ageing contribute in a very important way to all these age-associated diseases. How does the alteration of the immune response contribute to the increased incidence of these age-related diseases? The 'immune risk profile' (IRP) is derived from longitudinal

studies of naturally ageing populations, the Swedish OCTO and NONA immune longitudinal studies (Wikby *et al.* 1998, 2002, 2005; Nilsson *et al.* 2003). These studies identified factors predicting mortality and identified values for a cluster of parameters including high CD8, low CD4 and poor T-cell proliferative responses predicting higher two-year mortality after the age of 80 years. Most interestingly, cytomegalovirus (CMV) seropositivity and large increases in the number of $CD8^+CD28^-CD57^+$ T-cells, known to be associated with CMV carrier status, were significantly associated with the IRP (Olsson *et al.* 2000), which was also independent of health status (Nilsson *et al.* 2003). The IRP thus identifies a home-dwelling old population at increased risk of mortality, independently of current disease, but, rather unexpectedly, strongly influenced by CMV status. Thus, analysis of immune data at baseline in the OCTO study identified an IRP predictive of subsequent two-year mortality, the prevalence of which was 16% at baseline, with another 16% of the subjects moving into the IRP group over the eight-year study (Wikby *et al.* 1998). Significantly higher frequencies of cells with receptors specific for a certain CMV peptide in HLA-A2+ provide support for a major impact of CMV in driving the CD8+CD28- T-cell clonal expansions, especially predominant in the IRP group (Ouyang *et al.* 2003). The IRP correlated with the number of CMV-pp65-receptor-bearing CD8 cells present (Ouyang *et al.* 2003). The following NONA immune longitudinal study confirmed findings from the OCTO study of an association between the IRP and CMV infection. The results also confirmed an elevated mortality risk in individuals with the IRP (Wikby *et al.* 2005). Data consistent with this result have also been obtained in a UK sample, showing that the inverted CD4/CD8 ratio, associated with the IRP, predicted survival in younger olderly people stratified by age, above and below 75 years (Huppert *et al.* 2003). These studies demonstrated that the IRP concept explored in selected very old people in the Swedish OCTO immune longitudinal study could be generalised to a sample of younger elderly in a different country and also the more broadly defined NONA population-based sample of individuals who were not specifically selected for good health at baseline. The NONA immune sample did not exclude individuals with compromised health and focused particularly on those with cognitive impairment, suspected of being another major predictor of mortality in the old (Wikby *et al.* 2005). Here, increases of IL-6 in the plasma and decreases of IL-2 secretion by stimulated T-cells were also associated with the IRP.

11.3 Genetics and immune ageing

Data are beginning to emerge suggesting that a common core of master genes, many of which are involved in inflammation and metabolic signalling pathways, are responsible for successful ageing (Franceschi *et al.* 2005). Unsurprisingly, polymorphisms in such genes that affect functional levels can impact on ageing trajectories. Healthy, well-functioning centenarians are good subjects for the examination of genetic traits associated with ageing outcomes. Comparison of the frequencies of specific polymorphisms in these populations with healthy young controls can reveal enrichments or depletions in influential genes. As mentioned previously, ageing is not a programmed process and so one would expect a diverse range of polymorphisms affecting a number of key homeostatic pathways to be represented.

In support of this theory, a number of reports have shown that a range of pro-inflammatory genotypes are associated with poor ageing trajectories, such as CVD, Alzheimer's and diabetes, for example high IL-1, IL-6, TNF, CD14 LPS receptor, Toll like receptor 4, Metallothionine 2A and apolipoprotein E4 (Emahazion *et al.* 1999; Helisalmi *et al.* 1999; Papassotiropoulos *et al.* 1999; Grimaldi *et al.* 2000; Nicoll *et al.* 2000; Marculescu *et al.* 2002; Kubaszek *et al.* 2003; Landi *et al.* 2003; Guo *et al.* 2004; Van Den Biggelaar *et al.* 2004; Ophir *et al.* 2005; Kornman 2006; Mocchegiani *et al.* 2006; Olivieri *et al.* 2006). Recently, polymorphisms of the selenoprotein S gene (involved in stress responses), resulting in lower expression levels, were shown to be associated with increases in TNF and IL-1 (Curran *et al.* 2005). Conversely, weaker anti-inflammatory genotypes are similarly associated with poor ageing outcome, for example low IL-10, TGFβ-1 and heat shock protein 70 (Carrieri *et al.* 2004; Lio *et al.* 2004; Van Den Biggelaar *et al.* 2004; Giacconi *et al.* 2005; Capri *et al.* 2006). This is a very active area of research with much to be verified and more to be discovered.

11.4 Inflammation and ageing

Ageing is characterised by a pro-inflammatory phenotype resulting from chronic low-level inflammation. Inflammation is both caused by a variety of ageing processes and contributes to them. Progressive loss of control of inflammation leads to persistent low-level chronic inflammatory processes, which initiate and/or accelerate disease progression (Franceschi *et al.* 2000). Further, in the absence of frank disease, inflammation contributes directly to frailty and compromised function (Cohen *et al.* 1997; Grossmann *et al.* 1999).

The overwhelming majority of those aged over 55 (in Europe and the US) have chronic low-grade inflammation, underlying the progression of many of the chronic degenerative diseases of ageing (*e.g.* CVD, insulin resistance, diabetes, cognitive decline and frailty). Besides a high mortality rate, a huge social burden is created as a result of the extremely high morbidity and low quality of life resulting from these chronic diseases. Controlling inflammatory status may therefore provide a route to successful ageing. In fact, recent reports support this theory, suggesting that those individuals who are genetically predisposed to produce low levels of inflammatory cytokines or high levels of anti-inflammatory cytokines have an increased probability of achieving extreme longevity (Bonafe *et al.* 2001; Lio *et al.* 2002a, 2002b; Giacconi *et al.* 2004; Van Den Biggelaar *et al.* 2004).

11.4.1 Ageing processes contribute to increased inflammation

Several underlying age-related changes in gross physiology and loss of control of a number of cellular processes lead directly to inflammation. Glucocorticoid (GC) levels rise with age (Seeman *et al.* 2001; Valenti 2002). This has both direct and indirect effects on increasing inflammatory tone. Central (brain) elevations in GCs directly increase corticotrophin-releasing hormone, which in turn induces IL-1 (Reul *et al.* 1998). The peripheral increases in GCs with age are believed to be the result of developing GC insensitivity, based on changes in GC receptor signalling (Kino *et al.* 2003). This insensitivity to GCs takes the 'brake' off inflammatory signalling, leading to increased inflammatory tone. Similarly, age-related falls in peroxisome proliferator-activated receptor (PPAR) activity, which down-regulates inflammation, occur at the transcriptional level (C.K. Lee *et al.* 1999, 2000; Daynes and Jones 2002). This also increases inflammation. This is compounded by falls in dehydroepiandrosterone (DHEA), a GC antagonist and an anti-inflammatory endogenous ligand for PPARα (Poynter and Daynes 1998; Roth *et al.* 2002; Mattison *et al.* 2003).

Failing antioxidant defences (declines in glutathione, catalase, superoxide dismutase, etc.) allow the redox of cells to drift lower than is optimal or to reach lower levels more quickly under challenge. This facilitates the pro-inflammatory transcription factor signalling cascades (particularly NFκB and AP-1), resulting in increased inflammatory mediator production (Nuttall *et al.* 1998; Grossmann *et al.* 1999; Bierhaus *et al.* 2001; Erden-Inal *et al.* 2002; Jones *et al.* 2002; Maggio *et al.* 2003; Rebrin *et al.* 2003; Townsend *et al.* 2003).

Peroxidation of macromolecules increases with age due to failing antioxidant defences. Some peroxidised lipids can react directly with specific receptors on monocytes (OxLdlR) and directly signal inflammatory mediator gene transcription (Janciauskiene *et al.* 2001). Similarly, glycation of macromolecules increases with age due to both the failing antioxidant defences and hyperglycaemia resulting from changes in glucose and energy metabolism as a result of insulin resistance. Again, some glycated proteins can react directly with specific receptors on monocyte family members and endothelia (RAGE) and directly signal inflammatory mediator gene transcription (Hori *et al.* 1996; Kilhovd *et al.* 1999; Bierhaus *et al.* 2001; Basta *et al.* 2002; Bucciarelli *et al.* 2002; Stern *et al.* 2002; Wendt *et al.* 2002).

The chaperonin/proteasome axis suffers age-related decrements in function (Njemini *et al.* 2002). This has two related effects. First, poor chaperone function results in more misfolded protein (amyloidosis), which accumulates with age (Dobson 2002; Friguet 2002). This is exacerbated by compromised proteasome function unable to dispose of these molecules (Ponnappan 1998). These protein aggregates are directly pro-inflammatory. Some of these result in the classic autoimmune diseases, such as thyroiditis. Second, the poor performance of the proteasome with age means that protein turnover rates are extended. This may result in many transcription factors being active longer than is optimal. In summary, progressive failure of a number of homeostatic systems occurs with age and leads directly to increased baseline levels of inflammation.

11.4.2 External factors contribute to increased inflammation

A number of extrinsic factors/practices also drive inflammation; these may become particularly important when imposed on an already age-dysregulated pro-inflammatory background. UV exposure leads to poor skin ageing phenotypes (see Chapter 7) and increased risk of age-related cancer progression. Inflammation is a primary mediator of UV-induced dermal remodelling/elastosis and contributor to the carcinogenic processes (Strickland and Kripke 1997; Clydesdale *et al.* 2001; Garssen and van Loveren 2001).

Diet-induced hyperglycaemia induces inflammatory responses (Marfella *et al.* 2000; Schiekofer *et al.* 2003). These induce transient inflammatory responses which are exacerbated by pre-existing insulin resistance or frank diabetes (Esposito *et al.* 2002) and hence age. Similarly, diet-induced hyperlipidaemia is associated with a pro-inflammatory phenotype (*e.g.* elevated CRP/IL-6) (Nappo *et al.* 2002; Tselepis and Chapman 2002; Lundman *et al.* 2003). This possibly occurs due to the increased levels and hence availability of lipids for peroxidation. A 900 kcal mixed meal induced increases in free radical production by peripheral blood mononuclear cells, followed by decreases in Ikappa kinase α and β subunits, with increased DNA binding of NFK β and rises in CRP (Aljada *et al.* 2004). Obesity itself is associated with an oxidative and inflammatory phenotype, linked with dysregulated function of the hypothalamic–pituitary–adrenal (HPA) axis (Yudkin *et al.* 2000; Keaney *et al.* 2003). However, the risk of metabolic syndrome has also been associated with inflammation independently of obesity (Lubree *et al.* 2002). Recently, the ability of fat depots, whether central, perivascular or ectopic, to make major local and/or systemic contributions to the inflammatory milieu has begun to be more fully appreciated (Yudkin 2003; Yudkin *et al.* 2005). For instance, perivascular fat, which increases with age, has been shown to regulate vascular tone via TNF secretion. Locally, this impairs insulin-stimulated nitric oxide synthesis resulting in arteriole constriction (Yudkin *et al.* 2005).

Chronic stress is associated with acceleration of the progression of age-related diseases such as neurodegeneration and CVD. Stress induction techniques have been shown to directly induce inflammatory responses in blood (Bierhaus *et al.* 2003; Kiecolt-Glaser *et al.* 2003). Such responses underlie disease progression. Sleep deprivation also drives poor ageing trajectories, leading to pronounced changes in neuroendocrine, hormonal and sleep rhythmicity, quantity and quality both reduced during ageing.

Low-level chronic inflammation induced by subclinical infections such as *Chlamydia* drive microvascular inflammation, increasing risk of CVD (Xu *et al.* 2000). Further, persistent chronic viral infections (Epstein-Barr virus, cytomegalovirus, herpes simplex virus) are associated with drifting inflammation during ageing (Olsson *et al.* 2000; Wikby *et al.* 2002), leading to the proposition that 'immunosenescence is contagious' (Pawelec *et al.* 2005).

In summary, any 'stressor' seems to be able to evoke new or exacerbate existing inflammation; this may become particularly important when imposed on an already age-dysregulated background.

11.4.3 Inflammation contributes directly to poor ageing

Increases in inflammation directly contribute to a variety of poor ageing outcomes (Figure 11.1). Thus pre-existing chronic inflammatory diseases are associated with poor ageing trajectories; for example, Crohn's and rheumatoid patients have increased risk of colon cancers and CVD respectively (Persson

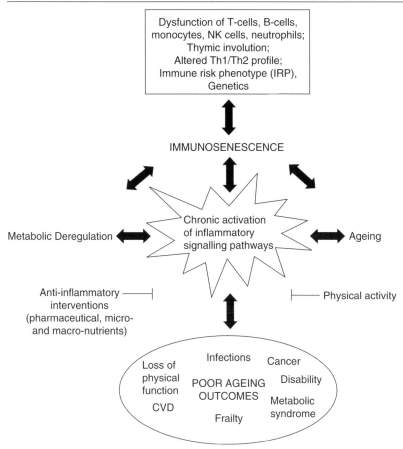

CVD: cardiovascular disease; Th1/Th2: helper T cells; NK cells: natural killer cells

Figure 11.1: Linkages between immune dysfunction, inflammation and poor ageing.

et al. 1996; Deon *et al.* 2001). Current inflammation is predictive of progression of diabetes (Spranger *et al.* 2003); both IL-1 and IL-6 levels being implicated. Chronic micro-inflammation drives age-associated reductions in muscle mass cachexia which compounds insulin resistance (Barbieri *et al.* 2003). Increases in inflammation are associated with obesity and dysregulation of the HPA axis, leading to increased risk of CVD (Yudkin *et al.* 2000). Inflammation is predictive of progression of CVD, independently of the traditional lipid metabolism-based measures (Chae *et al.* 2001; Walston *et al.* 2002; Murray and Freeman 2003; Vasan *et al.* 2003). CRP, IL-6, sICAM, fibrinogen and microalbuminuria have all been implicated.

Inflammation plays a major role in amyloid plaque progression, contributing to Alzheimer's disease. Remarque and colleagues (2001) have shown that individuals with a pro-inflammatory phenotype (high IL-1β/IL-10 ratio) have 13-fold higher odds of developing Alzheimer's disease. Inflammation is predictive of progression of Alzheimer's (Remarque *et al.* 2001; Weaver *et al.* 2002) and is associated with depression (Licinio and Wong 1999; Kop *et al.* 2002; Miller *et al.* 2002) and anhedonia (Dantzer *et al.* 1999; Dentino *et al.* 1999; Konsman *et al.* 2002).

Low-level inflammation is predictive of increasing mortality in older populations (Harris *et al.* 1999; Volpato *et al.* 2001; Cappola *et al.* 2003) and is predictive of increasing frailty/loss of function in older populations (Ferrucci *et al.* 1999, 2002; Reuben *et al.* 2002; Walston *et al.* 2002; Cappola *et al.* 2003), leading directly to losses of quality of life. Increases in inflammation, particularly as a result of oestrogen decline in post-menopausal women, underscore the age-associated loss of bone density associated with osteoporosis (di Minno and Mancini 1992; reviewed by Clowes *et al.* 2005 and Ginaldi *et al.* 2005) (see Chapter 4).

In summary, repeated episodes of low-level chronic inflammation exacerbate a wide range of age-associated morbidities.

11.5 Immune ageing and infections

The incidence and severity of infectious disease is increased in the elderly. This has been shown with many infections, including pneumonia, meningitis, sepsis, urinary tract infections, respiratory syncytial virus, human immunodeficiency virus and influenza (Barker and Mullooly 1980; Chattopadhyay and Al-Zahawi 1983; Gorse *et al.* 1984; La Croix *et al.* 1989; Sprenger *et al.* 1993; Ackermann and Munroe 1996, summarised in Falsey 2000). Additionally, the relative mortality rates of many infectious diseases in the elderly are more than twice those of the young. In the case of tuberculosis and urinary tract infection this rises to a factor of 10 (Yoshikawa 1997). The impact of age on severity of infection seems to be especially extreme for newly arisen pathogens, for example, SARS. In the young (<24 years), SARS caused 1% of mortality, whereas in the over 65s this figure was 50%.

11.6 Immune ageing and cancer

It has been suggested that all cancers are immunogenic because by virtue of malignant transformation, non-self, over-expressed or inappropriately expressed self proteins will provide antigens to the immune system. The reactivity of the immune system against such products of transformation and subsequent control of tumorigenesis is termed immunosurveillance, the existence of which is supported by a large body of data. Unsurprisingly, if the immune system functions suboptimally in the elderly, then so will immunosurveillance of cancer. But what is the evidence for this? The increased incidence of many cancers in the elderly is usually considered to be more a result of the time required for multi-hit carcinogenesis than to reflect decreased immune surveillance in the elderly. While in overtly immunosuppressed individuals, frequencies of certain cancers seem to be increased, in most older people there is little evidence for infection with opportunistic pathogens. Moreover, there is an increasingly clear correlation between chronic inflammatory states and carcinogenesis. For instance, there is a large literature associating inflammatory conditions of the gastrointestinal tract with increased incidence of cancers, from *H. pylori*–gastric cancer associations to inflammatory bowel disease associated colon cancers (Balkwill and Mantovani 2001). More recently, the mechanistic linkages between inflammation and cancer have begun to become better understood with clear involvement of the NFκB pathway; anti-inflammatory strategies have benefits in reducing the incidence of a range of cancers (Karin and Greten 2005).

As discussed above, many older people seem to suffer from low-grade chronic inflammation; perhaps it is this which contributes to increased cancer risk. It is, therefore, extremely difficult to identify clear associations between immunosenescence and cancer. Most still lie within the realm of speculation; for example, a commonly observed age-associated change in T-cells is increasing CD95 expression. Because some tumours are thought to express the ligand for this 'death receptor' it has been suggested that they can more easily neutralise tumour-specific T-cells by triggering their apoptosis following Fas/Fas-L interactions. This currently remains a hypothesis awaiting testing. So, can animal models tell us anything about this issue of cancer immunosurveillance and ageing? This is again, for different reasons, problematic, because the most common model, the mouse, may not be appropriate. Many age-associated changes are seen in murine immunity, and the most common cause of death in old laboratory mice is cancer, especially lymphoma. However, this may be more due to the common mouse strains used rather than evidence for weakening immunosurveillance. Experiments attempting to rejuvenate the immune system in mice have not resulted in extended longevity (Zhou *et al.* 1995).

In summary, the roles of declining immune surveillance and the contribution of increasing inflammation with age on cancer incidence and progression remain to be fully ascertained.

11.7 Diet and lifestyle routes to control inflammation

Current therapeutic intervention in chronic inflammatory diseases is relatively ineffective. New insights show that these diseases, although very different in nature, share common mechanisms. These conditions often start with an acute inflammatory response that later develops into a chronic phase, as the immune response switches from an adaptive to innate response.

A number of non-pharma, dietary and lifestyle interventions modulate inflammation. Moderate exercise is associated with many beneficial effects on degenerative diseases of ageing. It is associated with reduced all-cause mortality (Blair and Wei 2000), improved metabolic syndrome (Lakka *et al.* 2003) and cardiorespiratory fitness (Dunn *et al.* 1999; Gibbons *et al.* 2000). Human exercise intervention

studies show a causal reduction in CRP (Church *et al.* 2002; Ford and Norrie 2002). It is widely acknowledged that moderate exercise exerts many health benefits with no contraindications if prescription is tailored to an individual's health status.

The most consistent evidence of modulation of inflammation from dietary intervention studies involves antioxidants and polyunsaturated fatty acids. α-tocopherol supplemented at 1200 IU/day in type 2 diabetics with/without microvascular complications and matched controls leads to decreases in CRP and IL-6 (Devaraj and Jialal 2000). Vitamin C or vitamins C and E combinations have been shown to reduce exercise-induced inflammation (Thompson *et al.* 2001; Vassilakopoulos *et al.* 2003; Fischer *et al.* 2004). Vitamin E administered to older volunteers at 900 mg/d for four months potentiated insulin-mediated glucose disposal (Paolisso *et al.* 1994) and high doses of vitamins E and C supplementation immediately before a meal challenge attenuated the postprandial inflammatory responses (TNF, IL-6, ICAM, VCAM) (Esposito *et al.* 2003). Similarly, antioxidant administration blocks inflammation induced by a hyperglycaemic clamp procedure (Esposito *et al.* 2003). *n*-3 polyunsaturates may provide some protection against cardiovascular diseases in older men by lowering plasma triglycerides, decreasing lipoprotein peroxidation and the ratio of reduced to total glutathione, and decreasing soluble adhesion molecule 1 levels (a marker of vascular inflammation) (Yaqoob and Calder 2003; Cazzola *et al.* 2007).

Dietary fish oil suppresses the production of pro-inflammatory cytokines and expression of adhesion molecules. *n*-3 polyunsaturates can down-regulate NFκB activity. Clinical trials have shown oral fish oil to have beneficial effects in rheumatoid arthritis and asthma patients (Calder 2002). Nutritional supplementation of L-arginine, *n*-3 polyunsaturates and yeast RNA five days pre-operatively increased monocyte activation status (HLA-DR expression) and significantly lowered plasma IL-6. Further, delayed-type hypersensitivity (DTH) to recall antigens (T-cell memory responses) also improved (Tepaske *et al.* 2001). In patients with acute respiratory distress syndrome, reductions in bronchoalveolar lavage fluid levels of IL8, leukotriene B4 and neutrophil numbers followed enteric feeding of eicosapentaenoic acid (fish oil) and γ-linoleic acid (borage oil) with antioxidants. The findings suggest that this supplement may reduce pulmonary inflammation (Gadek *et al.* 1999; Pacht *et al.* 2003).

Caloric restriction (CR) is the 'gold standard' ageing intervention. It increases both mean and maximum lifespan in a very broad range of species from yeast to rodents; rhesus monkey (Mattison *et al.* 2003; Sell 2003) and human (Roth *et al.* 2002) data suggest that this is transferable to the higher primates. Contemporary reports are now beginning to unravel the mechanisms that underpin the beneficial affects of CR on ageing trajectories. Specifically, accumulating gene array data are showing that optimised energy metabolism profiles (low blood sugar, high insulin sensitivity), improved PPAR functionality and lower inflammation/stress responses are common features of the CR phenotype (C.K. Lee *et al.* 1999; 2000). Thus, CR, including weight loss, down-regulates inflammation (Gallistl *et al.* 2001; Heilbronn and Clifton 2002; Ziccardi *et al.* 2002) and at least partially rebalances endogenous antioxidant levels (Rebrin *et al.* 2003). CR in man has recently been shown to improve insulin sensitivity and lower core body temperature (Heilbronn *et al.* 2006), in common with the rodent and monkey data. Combinations of dietary restriction with exercise were particularly effective at improving insulin sensitivity, and increases of circulating adiponectin were seen with parallel decreases in monocyte chemotactic protein-1, CRP and IL-6. Macrophage activation markers were also decreased in terms of falls in mRNA for IL-6, IL-8 and TNF (Bruun *et al.* 2006).

11.8 Nutrition and immunity

Under-nutrition is common in the elderly and may be an important factor in influencing diminished elderly immune responses (Heuser and Adler 1997; Lesourd *et al.* 1998; Lesourd and Mazari 1999). Indeed, it has even been suggested that a deficit in the intake of antioxidant vitamins and trace elements may accelerate the ageing process (Richard and Roussel 1999). Further, infections (increasingly prevalent in the elderly), even when mild, can compromise nutritional status or lead to recompartmentalisation of trace elements as part of the acute adaptive response. This can lead to a spiral of impaired immunity and exacerbated infections. However, whilst nutrition, immune function and infection are clearly interrelated, it is no simple matter to quantify

these relationships. Most of what we know is related to nutrient deficiency states, acute infections and often hospitalised patient settings. Findings are confounded by changes in diet as a result of age (*e.g.* changes in dentition, cognitive function, mobility/independence), changes in physical activity (well known to modulate inflammatory processes) and unreliable dietary intake records (particularly those trying to assess earlier life-course consumption patterns) on which to base cause-and-effect relationships. Very few studies have been conducted on primary outcomes, such as infection/inflammation, disease severity/resistance or quality of life endpoints. Most studies have been carried out in populations already micronutrient-replete and usually over short periods. Few genuine attempts have been made to investigate micronutrient dose–response relationships and most work has been done on individual micronutrients, rather than the complex mixtures which our diets normally supply. Most studies have focused on secondary immune function outcomes such as antibody production, mitogenic responses, phagocyte functions or cytokine production. Whilst these are potentially highly relevant, the enormous redundancy and pleiotropy of the immune system makes it hard to predict what the consequences at the level of the fully integrated individual might be.

In an attempt to provide a framework for evaluation of immune responsiveness, an ILSI Task Force met to propose standards for measurements (Albers *et al.* 2005). This group, having surveyed the broad literature and practices, suggested that three categories with high, medium or low suitability for the evaluation of immune responsiveness be adopted. Vaccine-specific serum or salivary antibody responses, DTH or response to attenuated pathogens were considered highly suitable outcome measures. NK cytotoxicity, phagocyte oxidative burst, lymphocyte proliferative capacity and cytokine production patterns were considered of medium suitability. They further concluded that no single marker allowed conclusions to be drawn; the clinical outcome of an infection being the definitive measure. They recommended that combinations of markers with high and medium suitability be adopted and that in future clinical outcomes should be reported, as there remains little evidence linking markers of immune function with global health outcomes. This is a rather narrow view of the immune system as it is predominantly preoccupied with resistance to infectious disease. It fails to embrace the broader concept of immune surveillance and neglects the autonomous parts of the role of inflammation. Nevertheless, the problems of evaluating the current literature on interventions designed to improve immune function are thrown into stark relief by the ILSI conclusions.

11.8.1 Macronutrient deficiencies

At a gross macro-nutrition level, given the synthetic and proliferative needs of an orchestrated immune response, it is unsurprising that protein- and calorie-deficient diets lead to compromised immunity and increased risk and severity of infections (Weksler 1981; McMurray 1984). However, it would be naïve to imagine such situations are restricted to the developing world; institutionalisation, hospitalisation and social inequalities result in older populations being at risk for these reasons also. Even moderate to mild malnutrition has been shown to compromise immunity (McMurray *et al.* 1981; Dowd and Heatley 1984).

11.8.2 Micronutrient deficiencies

Deficiencies of specific micronutrients/trace elements may also compromise immune function. Deficiencies in vitamins C, A, E, D, B_6 and B_{12}, folate, biotin and zinc, copper, iron and selenium all result in poor T-cell differentiation and subsequent DTH responses (Beisel 1982; Meydani *et al.* 1995). Again, many older individuals are borderline or below the proposed US and UK recommended daily allowances (RDAs) and reference nutrient intakes (RNIs) for these micronutrients (Chernoff 1995).

Cross-sectional studies have attempted to identify relationships between the levels of various micronutrients and immune function. However, where these have employed healthy, affluent older subjects, little in the way of relationships was seen (Goodwin and Garry 1983, 1988). A more recent study (Kemp *et al.* 2002) did reveal reduced T-cell numbers and significant anergy (unresponsiveness) to a panel of seven skin recall antigens to be related to low serum copper in a population aged 58–86 years. In the same study, NK cell numbers were positively associated with dietary folate and vitamin B_6 and soluble IL-2R levels were positively correlated with body

mass index (BMI), serum vitamin B_6 and homocysteine, and negatively correlated with serum β-carotene and lycopene. Post-flu vaccination antibody titres in a group of 153 elderly (mean age 84.4 years) were positively associated with vitamin E status (Hara *et al.* 2005) and individuals with plasma vitamin E levels above 1670 μg/dl had fewer infections than those with less than 1200 μg/dl (Chavance *et al.* 1989).

In areas of low soil selenium content (mainly parts of South America and China) Coxsackie B3 virus causes cardiomyopathy (Keshan disease), linked to the reductions seen in the selenium-dependent glutathione peroxidase. Low selenium status drops cellular redox providing a free radical environment conducive to DNA damage and mutations; a change of 6–7 amino acids in the viral proteome is necessary for pathogenic transformation (Beck *et al.* 2003) and resultant cardiopathology. Selenium supplementation in this context is of great value (Ge *et al.* 1983).

11.8.3 Single micronutrient interventions

Several studies have been conducted employing β-carotene. UV-induced photo-suppression of DTH responses was reduced in an older group of men following supplementation (Herraiz *et al.* 1994, 1998) and in a very limited study of men and women with a mean age of 56 years, T helper and NK cell numbers increased in a dose-responsive manner after two months of supplementation (Watson *et al.* 1991). In a more robust study, 12 years of alternate day 50 mg β-carotene supplementation of men in the Physicians Health Study revealed improvements in NK cell activity, particularly in the older age groups (Santos *et al.* 1996). Overall the evidence suggests that β-carotene may improve T and NK cell functionality in older individuals, particularly in situations where a decrement has occurred or been induced. However, high-dose β-carotene supplementation has been associated with increased lung cancer development in smokers (Albanes *et al.* 1996; Omenn *et al.* 1996). Whilst the bases of these observations remain unclear, caution should be exercised when considering high-dose β-carotene supplementation of smokers.

There have also been many studies investigating the effect of vitamin E supplementation. When 50, 200 or 800 mg of vitamin E were given to older individuals for 4–5 months, antibody titres to hepatitis B vaccine and DTH responses improved, particularly in the 200 mg group (Meydani *et al.* 1997). In a separate study, 50 or 100 mg day supplementation of men (65–80 years) for six months also improved DTH responses. Interestingly, the benefits were greatest in those with the lowest baseline starting levels (Pallast *et al.* 1999). Recently, Meydani has reported in a large study that one year of supplementation with vitamin E at 200 IU day of 431 institutionalised (aged 65 years and over) individuals resulted in some protection against upper, though not lower, respiratory tract infections (Meydani *et al.* 2004). The effects were, however, quite modest. In contrast, a study of vitamin E supplementation in a Dutch older population failed to reveal any benefits on respiratory tract infections (Graat *et al.* 2002). Overall, vitamin E supplementation may have modest benefits in improving immunity in the elderly.

There are clear associations between low serum zinc levels and wide-ranging compromised immune function (Ibs and Rink 2004). Furthermore, zinc deficiency in the elderly is very prevalent. Data from 29,103 individuals from the Third National Health and Nutrition Examination Survey (1988–94) showed that only 51.1% of 51–71-year-olds and 42.5% of 71+-year-old adults in the US had adequate zinc levels (defined as ≥77% 1989 RDA) (Briefel *et al.* 2000), institutionalised elderly were at greater risk, showing lower zinc levels than free-living peers (Worwag *et al.* 1999). However, disappointingly, studies on zinc supplementation in the elderly have been discouraging, with either no benefit or even adverse affects (Bogden *et al.* 1988; Chandra *et al.* 1993). Dose seems to be absolutely key, with the best evidence suggesting that low- (Girodon *et al.* 1999), but not high-dose (Provinciali *et al.* 1998) zinc supplementation improves vaccine responses in the elderly. High doses, resulting in >30 µM plasma zinc levels, most likely inhibit a range of T-cell functionalities (Cakman *et al.* 1997; Wellinghausen *et al.* 1997, reviewed by Ibs and Rink 2004).

A small study, mostly of women aged 65–81 years, has shown vitamin B_6 supplementation at 50 mg/day to increase *in vitro* proliferative responses to mitogens (Talbott *et al.* 1987). Depletion/repletion experiments in older adults have shown that IL-2 production and lymphocyte proliferative responses are sensitive to vitamin B_6 (Meydani *et al.* 1991).

Increasing intakes of *n*-3 long chain polyunsaturates curtail inflammatory processes; this is generally construed as a favourable outcome (Calder 2002; Sijben and Calder 2007) particularly in the context of rising baseline chronic inflammation with age. However, it is also the case that reduced lymphocyte proliferative responses are often seen in the elderly (Thies *et al.* 2001) and decreased phagocytic activity associated with increased *n*-3 consumption may occur (Rees *et al.* 2006). Thus, there may be a trade-off between beneficial decreases in age-related inflammation and reduced immunity. Recent work has shown that older subjects (Rees *et al.* 2006) incorporate more *n*-3 into their plasma and mononuclear cell phospholipids than younger peers.

11.8.4 Micronutrient combination interventions

Interpretation of the results of micronutrient combination interventions is fraught with difficulties. As mentioned previously, few dose–response studies have been carried out with single micronutrients let alone with combinations. Interactions between supplemented micronutrients can and do occur. Most studies comprise small numbers of individuals, often already with reasonable starting background levels of micronutrients. Results can be confounded by improvements in function post-intervention from individuals who are deficient in particular micronutrients alongside no, or even deleterious, responses from those who were already replete prior to the intervention. Finally, interventions are short, even those of one year duration, while what is needed is trials demonstrating long-term readouts such as changes in immune function and disease resistance.

Administration of standard, over-the-counter multivitamin/mineral supplements for one year to older individuals improved DTH and mitogen responses (Bogden *et al.* 1990, 1994). Improvements were slow; little being seen at six months. Importantly, zinc, at 15 mg and especially at 100 mg, when given in addition to the supplements, reduced and delayed the positive effects (Bogden *et al.* 1990). A similar study deployed low-dose multivitamins vs. placebo in 60-year-olds for four months, but failed to see any effects on incidence of infections (Chavance *et al.* 1993). However, in this study no laboratory measures of immune function were taken, or data on duration of infections. A more recent study of 30 healthy elderly aged 70 or more given a nutritional (480 Kcals/31 g protein) supplement which included 120 mg vitamin E, 400 µg folic acid, 3.8 µg of vitamin B_{12} and a lactobacillus species probiotic/ 6 g oligosaccharides for one year showed increased NK cell numbers and activity, increased monocyte IL-2 production at four months and fewer infections at one year than the 30 non-supplemented controls (Bunout *et al.* 2004). Again, a recent small study involving a macro- and micronutrient-enriched drink administered to frail elderly (aged 65 years or more, 20 supplemented vs. 13 placebo over six months) showed maintained lymphocyte proliferative responses, whilst the placebo group declined (Wouters-Wesseling *et al.* 2005).

Twenty-eight days of vitamins A (800 IU), C (100 mg) and E (50 mg) supplementation of a group of older patients, who had been hospitalised for three months and who had evidence of some pre-existing vitamin A, C, and E deficiencies, again improved proliferative responses and numbers/% of CD4+ and CD8+ T-cells (Penn *et al.* 1991). In a similarly vulnerable group with poor micronutrient/ trace element status, trace element (20 mg zinc/ 100 µg selenium) and vitamin (6 mg β-carotene, 120 mg vitamin C, 15 mg vitamin E) supplementation of a large group (n = 725) of institutionalised over-65-year-old elderly improved influenza vaccine responses and marginally reduced incidence of infections in those groups given zinc and selenium (Girodon *et al.* 1999). DTH was unchanged in this study. Patients with degenerative aortic stenosis given either 400 mg vitamin E and 1000 mg vitamin C or vitamin C alone for six months revealed significantly reduced serum ICAM or P selectin respec-

tively (Tahir *et al.* 2005). Interestingly, ICAM levels returned to baseline six months after cessation of the intervention.

In contrast, a randomised, double-blind, placebo-controlled study of 652 over-60-year-old Dutch men and women of a multivitamin/mineral supplement (200 mg α-tocopherol) for around one year revealed no effect on incidence of infection by any of the treatments (Graat *et al.* 2002). However, in this essentially already micronutrient-replete group, a worsening of severity of symptoms was seen in the vitamin E-supplemented groups. Similarly, a study of 910 over-65-year-olds, not previously taking multivitamins/multiminerals and subsequently supplemented with them over one year, failed to reveal any benefits on primary outcomes of self-reported infection rates, primary physician contact times or quality of life and secondary outcomes such as hospitalisation or antibiotic prescription (Avenell, Campbell *et al.* 2005). A recent meta-analysis, in which eight studies met inclusion criteria, concluded that 'the evidence for routine use of multivitamin and multimineral supplements to reduce infections is weak and conflicting ... and confounded by outcome measure' (El-Kadiki and Sutton 2005). Dangour *et al.* (2004) conclude that the evidence does not support the use of supplements in well-nourished populations.

Overall, vulnerable groups with poor macro- and/ or micronutrient status, particularly the institutionalised or hospitalised elderly, benefit from micronutrient supplementation. The value of supplementation for those with adequate macro- and micronutrient status is much less compelling and may even be detrimental.

11.9 Key points

- Aggressive immune and inflammatory responses are highly adaptive and have been selected through evolution. However, there are trade-offs between inflammation and fertility/fecundity. Further, whilst such responses may be beneficial acutely and at young ages, they tend to be maladaptive when chronic and at late ages.
- The immune system ages (immunosenescence); innate immune responses tend to be exaggerated, while humoral immunity is compromised.

This leads to increased susceptibility to infectious diseases and cancers with age, and higher levels of inflammation.

- The immune system is not autonomous; it suffers from organismal ageing of its many compartments. But it also has to function in an ageing environment where the metabolic, trophic and regulatory contexts have changed and continue to change.
- 'Successful agers', such as high-functioning centenarians, have robust T-cell proliferative

Continued

responses, potent natural killer cell function and low levels of inflammation.

- The rise in levels of inflammatory mediators with age is due not solely to dysregulations of the 'professional immune cells' but also to increasing production from stromal cells, such as fibroblasts.
- The B-cell compartment and antibody production is less affected by age than the T-cell compartment. T-cell proliferative responses are compromised with age and probably skewed to a T1 (antibody production > cell-mediated immunity) profile.
- Natural killer cell functionality (kill of viral-infected targets) declines with age.
- Macrophages become more activated with age, but are poorer at antigen presentation. Neutrophil function probably declines with age, contributing to more or poorly resolved infections.
- An 'immune risk profile' consisting of high CD8, low CD4, poor T-cell proliferative responses and cytomegalovirus seropositivity predicts morbidity and mortality.
- Polymorphisms which drive higher levels of inflammatory mediator production are associated with poor ageing trajectories.
- Inflammation is caused by the ageing process and by external factors such as sleep loss, postprandial responses, obesity, environmental toxicants and pollutants.
- Inflammation contributes to poor ageing outcomes, particularly by exacerbating insulin resistance and vascular dysfunction, but probably also by leading directly to cancers.

- Controlling inflammation is beneficial in terms of a range of ageing outcomes. Improvements in insulin sensitivity and vascular function underpin many of the benefits.
- Diet and lifestyle interventions reduce acute and probably chronic inflammation. Fish oil, antioxidants and increasing physical activity (and weight loss) are all effective.
- Macro- or micronutrient deficiencies are detrimental to immune function and increase both the risk and severity of infections. Such deficiencies are common in the elderly due to poor diets associated with compromised dentition, hospitalisation and institutionalisation.
- There is no compelling evidence for the benefits of micronutrient supplementation on immune responses of those already replete. Indeed, there is evidence that it may be damaging. There is no evidence for the immune benefits of dietary interventions.
- There are no good randomised control trials in humans assessing the influence of dietary or lifestyle interventions on immunity as a function of age. The cost and duration of such studies is limiting and the ethics of performing such studies could be problematic.
- Redundancy and pleiotropy of the immune system makes it very challenging to design and perform nutritional interventions.
- With the exception of studies looking at macro- and micronutrient deficiency states and immune function, the results of animal model and particularly *in vitro* experiments on immune function are poorly transferable to human populations.

11.10 Recommendations for future research

- Controlling age-related increases in inflammatory tone is a more worthy and potentially more tractable target than improving disease resistance.
- The contribution and underlying mechanistic basis of the effects of inflammation on insulin resistance merit more attention.
- The mechanisms by which the gradual accrual of genomic damage (see Chapter 2) are sensed and subsequently lead to age-related increases in inflammatory tone should be determined.

This may lead to the identification of new intervention strategies.

- The contribution of low-level, sustained viral infections to poor ageing trajectories should be investigated.
- Short-term human models for modulation of both inflammation and broader immune functions need to be developed. These could be based on sleep deprivation, postprandial excursion or exercise as a starting point.

Continued

- The potentially detrimental effects of micronutrient supplementation of the 'replete' individual require further investigation; particularly given the very high penetration of these practices. Simple, rapid, low-cost, accurate diagnostics for a range of micronutrients should be developed.

- More thought needs to be given to the perennial problem of how to target appropriate interventions to those most in need; the elderly, vulnerable, isolated and members of low socio-economic groups in our societies.

11.11 Key references

Bjelakovic G, Nikolova D, Gluud LL, Simonetti RG and Gluud C (2007) Mortality in randomized trials of antioxidant supplements for primary and secondary prevention: systematic review and meta-analysis. *Journal of the American Medical Association*, **297**, 842–57.

Calder, PC (2006) n-3 polyunsaturated fatty acids, inflammation, and inflammatory diseases. *American Journal of Clinical Nutrition*, **83(6 Suppl)**, 1505S–19S.

Franceschi C, Capri M, Monti D, *et al.* (2007) Inflammaging and anti-inflammaging: a systemic perspective on aging and longevity emerged from studies in humans. *Mechanisms of Ageing & Development*, **128**, 92–105.

Pawelec G, Akbar A, Caruso C *et al.* (2005) Human immunosenescence: is it infectious? *Immunological Reviews*, **205**, 257–68.

Poynter ME and Daynes RA (1998) Peroxisome proliferator-activated receptor alpha activation modulates cellular redox status, represses nuclear factor-kappaB signaling, and reduces inflammatory cytokine production in aging. *Journal of Biological Chemistry*, **273**, 32833–41.

12
Healthy Ageing:
The Gastrointestinal Tract

12.1 Introduction

Many sections of the gastrointestinal (GI) tract exhibit physiological and histological changes during ageing, with implications for functional alterations in terms of digestion and absorption and in some cases pathological damage to the mucosa. With the increase in the ageing population in Europe and many other developed nations, GI disorders in older people have become priority areas for clinicians and researchers. Recent studies suggest that, in older subjects (over 65 years), disorders of the GI tract are the third most prevalent cause of visits to family doctors (Destro *et al.* 2003).

12.2 The oesophagus

12.2.1 Gastro-oesophageal reflux disease, Barrett's oesophagus, achalasia

Pilotto (2004), in a review of age-related changes in the upper GI tract, has listed a number of patho-physiological changes in oesophageal functions. Changes seen in older people include a shorter intra-abdominal segment of the lower oesophageal sphincter, a reduction of secondary peristalsis and an increase in the prevalence of tertiary contractions. One important consequence of such changes is gastro-oesophageal reflux disease (GERD), the prevalence of which increases with age, although there are notable differences in clinical expression between young and older patients. GERD can lead to oesophagitis and in some instances to Barrett's oesophagus (an acquired condition secondary to longstanding gastro-oesophageal reflux disease

involving development of columnar metaplasia in the lower oesophagus), the incidence of which is rising dramatically (van Soest *et al.* 2005). The pathogenesis of Barrett's oesophagus is poorly understood. As some individuals have severe erosive oesophagitis and never develop Barrett's oesophagus, host factors must be important (Shaheen 2005). As discussed below, GERD, oesophagitis and Barrett's oesophagus are important since they are risk factors for adenocarcinoma (Lagergren 2005).

There is no reported dietary association with GERD, although a recent meta-analysis found a significant association between body mass index (BMI) and GERD symptoms in six out of nine epidemiological studies with pooled adjusted odds ratios (ORs) of 1.43 and 1.94 for BMIs of 25–30 and >30 kg/m^2 respectively (Hampel *et al.* 2005). Furthermore, six of seven studies found a significant association of BMI with erosive oesophagitis.

A recent case-control study has reported that patients with Barrett's oesophagus had significantly lower plasma concentrations of selenium, vitamin C, β-cryptoxanthine and xanthophyll compared with controls (Clements *et al.* 2005).

The incidence and prevalence of achalasia has been reported from a limited number of centres in the US, UK, Israel, Zimbabwe, Singapore and New Zealand (Mayberry 2001). The disease is relatively rare, with an incidence of about 0.3–1.1/100,000/year, although there are marked variations between and within countries, suggesting that environmental factors may be involved in the cause of the disease. Genetic predisposition seems minimal (Podas *et al.* 1998). The disease occurs with equal frequency in men and women and is more common with ageing, with those over 70 years being most at risk, although absolute numbers are still small. Diagnosis of achalasia is based on classic manometric criteria – hypertensive lower oesophageal sphincter with incomplete relaxation on swallowing, elevated oesophageal baseline pressure and complete absence of oesophageal peristalsis (Podas *et al.* 1998; Brucher *et al.* 2001). The rarity of the disease has hampered attempts to investigate aetiological factors and early reports of links between achalasia and infections (parasitic and viral) and B vitamin deficiency have not been substantiated in subsequent studies (Podas *et al.* 1998).

12.2.2 Oesophageal cancer

Cancer of the oesophagus is the eighth most common cancer worldwide, with 462,000 cases/year, accounting for approximately 4.6% of new cancer cases, and has a particularly high incidence in China and Central Asia (Ferlay *et al.* 2004). In the UK more than 7600 people are diagnosed with the disease each year and there are about 7400 deaths (Cancer Research UK 2007). It is more commonly diagnosed in men and 80% of cases are diagnosed in people over 60 years. It has a very poor prognosis with five-year survival rates of 10% (World Cancer Research Fund/American Institute for Cancer Research 2007).

The majority of oesophageal cancers are squamous cell carcinomas. However, in western societies the incidence of adenocarcinoma of the oesophagus has increased dramatically over the last 40 years, at a rate faster than any other type of cancer, and adenocarcinoma is now the predominant form of oesophageal cancer in the US (Levi *et al.* 2001; American Cancer Society 2004; Shaheen 2005). The highest incidence is in the UK, although incidences in the US, Australia and the Netherlands are also relatively high. Low incidence areas include Scandinavia and Eastern Europe (Lagergren 2005). The cause of the increase is unknown but possible explanations include an increase in the prevalence of risk factors such as GERD and obesity, and a decrease in the prevalence of *Helicobacter pylori* (*H. pylori*) infection, although the sex distribution of these factors does not match well with the trends in cancer incidence (Lagergren 2005). Changes in diagnostic methods do not appear to be responsible (Hampel *et al.* 2005).

The risk factors for the two cancers are quite distinct. In developed countries, over 80% of the risk of squamous cell carcinoma of the oesophagus can be attributed to consumption of alcohol and tobacco (Schottenfeld 1984; Castelletto *et al.* 1992), which appear to act independently (Tuyns 1983). There is ample evidence from both cohort and case-control studies of an increased risk of oesophageal cancer with increasing consumption of alcoholic drinks (World Cancer Research Fund/American Institute for Cancer Research 2007). The type of alcoholic beverage associated with the greatest risk of oesophageal cancer in the majority of the American studies was spirits (Pottern *et al.* 1981; Brown *et al.* 1988; Yu *et al.* 1988).

Epidemiological studies, mostly with South American and Asian populations, indicate increased risk associated with consumption of very hot beverages, especially maté, the risk rising with duration of use. Increased risk associated with hot foods or drinks consumption has also been seen in case-control studies in these populations, although it appears that it is the high temperature of consumption rather than the beverages *per se* that is responsible, probably via thermal damage to the mucosa resulting in inflammation (World Cancer Research Fund/American Institute for Cancer Research 2007). Measures of BMI appear to be inversely related to risk of squamous cell carcinoma (D'Avanzo *et al.* 1996; Chow *et al.* 1998).

For adenocarcinoma of the oesophagus, the majority of cases arise from Barrett's oesophagus, which is associated with a 30–60-fold increase in risk (Lagergren 2005). It should be noted, however, that Barrett's patients progress to cancer at the rate of approximately 0.5% per year, so the majority die from unrelated causes (Oberg *et al.* 2005). GERD is also associated with increased risk: the more frequent, persistent and severe symptoms of reflux, the greater the risk with ORs of 8–40 (Lagergren 2005). The association with smoking is weak and alcohol consumption shows no consistent relationship. There appears to be an inverse relationship with *H. pylori* infection and some evidence of a protective effect of non-steroidal anti-inflammatory drugs (NSAIDs) (Lagergren 2005).

In contrast to the situation for squamous cell carcinoma, several, though not all, case-control studies have found a high BMI to be a risk factor for adenocarcinoma of the oesophagus (Lagergren 2005).

Three recent, large studies with a population-based design indicated a strong, dose-dependent association between increasing BMI and risk of oesophageal adenocarcinoma (Chow *et al.* 1998; Lagergren *et al.* 1999; Wu *et al.* 2001). In a meta-analysis, Hampel *et al.* (2005) calculated pooled adjusted ORs for adenocarcinoma of 1.52 and 2.78 for BMIs of 25–30 and >30 kg/m^2, respectively. The mechanism behind this association remains to be identified.

A German study of 124 patients with long-standing achalasia found that the risk for developing oesophageal cancer was increased about 140-fold over that of the general population although the prognosis was not worse than that of patients with squamous cell oesophageal cancer but no achalasia (Brucher *et al.* 2001).

12.2.2.1 Nutritional approaches

Case-control studies conducted in the western and developing worlds indicate a protective association with fruit and vegetable consumption, even after correction for smoking and alcohol consumption, with odds ratios for most studies around 0.3–0.8 (Chainani-Wu 2002; World Cancer Research Fund/ American Institute for Cancer Research 2007). Two recent, large, case-control studies, one conducted in the US (Mayne *et al.* 2001) and the other in Sweden (Terry *et al.* 2000; Terry, Lagergren, Hansen *et al.*

2001; Terry, Lagergren, Ye *et al.* 2001), have explored the associations between a wide range of food and nutrient intakes with both forms of oesophageal cancer. The results of the two studies are remarkably consistent and indicate similar dietary risk factors for squamous cell carcinoma and adenocarcinoma. Generally, higher intake of nutrients of animal origin was associated with increased risk, *e.g.* animal protein (OR for 75th vs. 25th percentile 1.79–2.14), cholesterol (OR 1.63–1.74) and vitamin B_{12} (OR 1.39–1.51). Dietary fat intake was associated with increased risk of adenocarcinoma (OR 2.18), but not squamous cell carcinoma (OR 0.98) (Mayne *et al.* 2001) (Table 12.1). In contrast, increased intake of plant-based foods and nutrients was associated with decreased risk (Table 12.1). Comparing individuals in the highest and lowest quartile of fruit and vegetable consumption (4.8 vs. 1.5 servings/d), Terry, Lagergren, Hansen *et al.* (2001) reported a 40–50% lower risk of the two forms of cancer. Negative associations with both cancer types were seen in the US and Swedish studies for fibre, β-carotene, vitamins C and E, with ORs between 0.28 and 0.73. Mayne *et al.* (2001) also found negative associations with dietary folate and vitamin B_6, but not with any type of vitamin supplement use, multiple or single.

It should be noted that the odds ratios associated with diet are considerably smaller than those found

Table 12.1: Nutrient intake and risk of oesophageal adenocarcinoma and squamous cell carcinoma

Nutrient	Adjusted ORs (95% CI) 75 vs. 25 percentile of intake	
	Adenocarcinoma	Squamous cell carcinoma
Energy	1.12 (0.91–1.38)	0.77 (0.59–1.01)
Total fat	2.18 (1.27–3.76)*	0.98 (0.52–1.86)
Total fibre	0.28 (0.19–0.40)*	0.24 (0.14–0.38)*
Insoluble	0.28 (0.19–0.41)*	0.24 (0.15–0.38)*
Soluble	0.30 (0.21–0.443)*	0.27 (0.16–0.43)*
Total protein	1.49 (1.02–2.18)*	1.75 (1.07–2.88)*
Animal protein	1.79 (1.33–2.41)*	2.14 (1.47–3.12)*
Vegetable protein	0.39 (0.27–0.58)*	0.34 (0.21–0.56)*
Cholesterol	1.74 (1.36–2.23)*	1.63 (1.22–2.18)*
Calcium	1.00 (0.77–1.30)	1.26 (0.91–1.75)
β-carotene	0.43 (0.32–0.59)*	0.43 (0.29–0.63)*
Vitamin E	0.73 (0.54–1.00)	1.00 (0.74–1.36)
Folate	0.48 (0.36–0.73)*	0.58 (0.39–0.86)*
Vitamin C	0.45 (0.33–0.61)*	0.53 (0.36–0.79)*
Vitamin B_{12}	1.39 (1.10–1.76)*	1.51 (1.15–2.00)*

*Statistically significant ($P < 0.05$).
CI: confidence interval; OR: odds ratio.
Source: Mayne *et al.* (2001).

for smoking and alcohol and in translating their percentage risk reductions into absolute decreases in risks, Terry, Lagergren, Hansen *et al.* (2001) commented that a moderate increase in plant food consumption by a large number of subjects (>25,000) would prevent only one case of oesophageal cancer per year. For squamous cell carcinoma at least, reduction in smoking and in excessive alcohol intake would be more effective.

Hsing *et al.* (1993) found some evidence of increased oesophageal cancer incidence among patients with pernicious anaemia and this has been confirmed by Ye and Nyren (2003), who showed a significantly increased risk for oesophageal squamous cell carcinoma, but not for adenocarcinoma, in a population of mean age 71 years. In the light of the Mayne *et al.* (2001) study showing that vitamin B_{12} intake was significantly positively associated with risk for squamous cell carcinoma and adenocarcinoma, it is likely that the association with pernicious anaemia may be due to chronic achlorhydria seen in the patients (see Section 12.3.1). Pernicious anaemia is the end-stage of type A atrophic gastritis and achlorhydria may exist many years before a clinical diagnosis of gastritis, resulting in an intragastric environment favouring bacterial overgrowth and consequent formation of N-nitrosamines, which are thought to be a risk factor for oesophageal squamous cell carcinoma.

12.3 The stomach

12.3.1 Gastric pH

The pH of the stomach contents of the fasting normal human is usually less than 3, which is sufficient to kill most commensal bacteria (Draser 1988). However, during a meal, the gastric acid is buffered, allowing bacteria ingested with food to survive at least until the pH falls and thus permitting a transient gastric flora. In situations where gastric acid secretion is impaired, bacteria can survive longer and may even proliferate in the elevated pH conditions. Reduced gastric acid secretion (hypochlorhydria) is common after gastric surgery (Hill 1995). Hypochlorhydria is also seen in patients with atrophic gastritis associated with chronic *H. pylori* infection. Certain diseases, such as pernicious anaemia and hypogammaglobulinaemia, are associated with achlorhydria, which results in the gastric pH rising

to 7 and above (Hill 1995). Such reductions in gastric acidity allow a diverse flora with up to 10^9 organisms per gram to establish in the stomach, consisting usually of species of salivary bacteria of the genera *Streptococcus*, *Neisseria*, *Staphylococcus* and *Veillonella*, although *Bacteroides*, *Lactobacillus* (*Lact.*) and *Escherichia* species are also found (Hill 1995).

The presence of a gastric microflora in hypochlorhydric and achlorhydric individuals has potential toxicological sequelae since it increases the probability of xenobiotic metabolism by the bacteria and may exacerbate vitamin B_{12} deficiency. It has been suggested that the increased gastric cancer risk of achlorhydric patients is linked to increased formation of N-nitroso compounds by their gastric bacterial flora (Hill 1988).

A number of early studies reviewed by Hill (1995) suggested that gastric acid secretion decreases naturally with ageing, with an associated increase in a range of bacterial types colonising the stomach. A study by Husebye *et al.* (2001) of 15 healthy older subjects (range 80–91 years) found 12 (80%) to be hypochlorhydric (mean pH 6.6 +/– 0.3) with an elevated bacterial count of 10^5–10^{10} colony forming units (CFU) per ml in fasting gastric aspirate. Normochlorhydric subjects had low counts (<10^1 CFU/ml). The microbial flora was dominated by streptococci, staphylococci and *Haemophilus* spp., but few if any Gram-negative organisms or strict anaerobes. They concluded that advanced age is accompanied by fasting hypochlorhydria and colonisation with mainly Gram-positive bacteria in the upper gut.

However, most recent studies have not confirmed a decrease in acid secretion with age. A study by Feldman *et al.* (1996) reported that gastric acid and pepsin output were similar in young (18–34 years) and middle-aged (35–64 years) groups, but that stimulated acid output was reduced by approximately 30% in older people (65–98 years). However, after adjustment for atrophic gastritis, *H. pylori* infection and other variables, age had no independent effect on acid output. The decline in acid secretion in older people was primarily related to a higher prevalence of chronic atrophic gastritis and a lower prevalence of smoking. Notably, however, pepsin output was decreased by about 40% in older people independently of atrophic gastritis, *H. pylori* infection and smoking (Feldman *et al.* 1996).

Similarly, Katelaris *et al.* (1993) found that in healthy men without atrophy, gastric acid secretion was unaffected by ageing. Gastritis with atrophy, which is closely related to *H. pylori* infection, was the only factor that had an independent negative effect on acid secretion. Increased basal serum gastrin was related to both atrophy and *H. pylori* infection but not to ageing *per se*. More recently, two large-scale studies have confirmed these observations. Hurwitz *et al.* (1997) conducted a cross-sectional study of basal gastric acidity and atrophic gastritis in 248 volunteers aged 65 years or older living independently. Basal unstimulated gastric content was acidic (pH < 3.5) in 84% of the subjects. Of those who were consistent hyposecretors of acid, most had serum markers indicative of atrophic gastritis. In a retrospective study of 753 subjects (aged under 35 to over 70 years), Shih *et al.* (2003) assessed a variety of ambulatory gastric pH measurements (baseline acidity, and nocturnal, daytime and postprandial acidities) and found no relationship with age.

12.3.2 Gastric motility

Data on the effect of ageing on GI motility are few and somewhat inconsistent, which may reflect the methodology used to assess the end-points. A number of studies have reported that older people frequently have symptoms of fullness and loss of appetite, which can be attributed to impaired gastric motor activity and which can lead to malnutrition and other complications. For example, changes in interdigestive gastric motor activity and related serum motilin (steadily high without the normal cyclic fluctuations) have been noted in older subjects in comparison with younger adults (Bortolotti *et al.* 1987). The effects of age seem to be independent of gastric acidity and chronic atrophic gastritis, suggesting that other factors, such as alterations in the neurohormonal control system of gut motility, should be considered in the genesis of these age-related disorders. Similarly, Shimamoto *et al.* (2002) found various measures of gastric motor activity (postprandial peristalsis and gastric contractile force) were reduced and gastric emptying delayed in a small group of older subjects compared with younger volunteers, and the reduction was greater in an inactive older cohort.

In contrast to the above reports, a recent study of 16 healthy older (74–85 years) and young (20–30 years) volunteers, which measured gastric emptying, small intestinal and colonic transit rates, and postprandial frequency of antral contractions by gamma camera technique, found no effect of age on any of the end-points. Older individuals, however, had a slower colonic transit than young individuals (Madsen and Graff 2004).

One of the suggested consequences of gastric motor impairment is functional dyspepsia (FD), a poorly characterised GI disorder of unknown aetiology that is frequently difficult to manage. Patients with FD often report symptoms after meal ingestion, including fullness, bloating, epigastric pain, nausea and vomiting (Feinle-Bisset *et al.* 2004). Frequent reports by patients that their FD symptoms are often related to food ingestion suggest a relationship to food or dietary habits, although such an association has not been formally evaluated. The fact that dietary assessments have often implicated fatty foods in symptom induction suggests that dietary modification might ameliorate symptoms, but further studies are needed to establish whether dietary therapies have any place in the management of FD (Feinle-Bisset *et al.* 2004).

12.3.3 Gastric and duodenal ulcer

The incidence of gastric and duodenal ulcers and their bleeding complications is increasing in old-aged populations worldwide, the main risk factors being NSAID use and *H. pylori* infection (Pilotto 2004). Epidemiological studies have demonstrated that risk of NSAID-associated gastric and duodenal injuries tends to increase linearly with age. Many clinical studies have reported that 53–73% of older peptic ulcer patients are *H. pylori*-positive (Pilotto *et al.* 2000) and it has been reported from short-term studies that treatment of *H. pylori* infection healed ulcers and improved symptoms in the majority of patients (Pilotto 2004). Furthermore, a one-year follow-up study in older patients with peptic ulcer disease found that eradication of *H. pylori* infection improved clinical outcome, reducing ulcer recurrences and symptoms (Pilotto *et al.* 1998). It should be noted, however, that treatment with antibiotics to eradicate *H. pylori* can result in intestinal overgrowth of potentially pathogenic bacteria. There are several case reports (some in older people) suggesting increased risk of pseudomembranous colitis associated with *Clostridium difficile* (*C. difficile*) in patients receiving *H. pylori* therapies (Braegger and Nadal 1994; Archimandritis *et al.* 1998; Nawaz *et al.* 1998). In a study by Buhling *et al.* (2001), the faecal microflora of 51 *H. pylori* infected patients was shown to be different from that of 27 healthy controls, with higher counts of lactobacilli in the patients. Treatment of the patients with the most widely used drug therapy for *H. pylori* infection, namely a proton pump inhibitor (omeprazole 20 mg bd) and two antibiotics, clarithromycin (250 mg bd) and metronidazole (400 mg bd), resulted in increased colonisation by yeasts and a decrease in anaerobes including lactobacilli. *C. difficile* was cultured from three cases, but there was no toxin production and no clinical manifestation of pseudomembranous colitis occurred. Furthermore, after four weeks of therapy, the microflora became similar to that of the untreated healthy control group.

12.3.4 Chronic atrophic gastritis and gastric cancer

Chronic atrophic gastritis usually begins at the gastric antrum and extends proximally towards the cardia, resulting in a reduction in gastric secretory function. It is considered an early step in the sequence of mucosal changes in the stomach leading to cancer, namely gastritis, chronic atrophic gastritis, metaplasia, dysplasia and finally carcinoma (Correa 1992). This hypothesis is supported by a considerable number of epidemiological and clinical studies in countries with a high incidence of gastric cancer.

The prevalence of atrophic change of the gastric mucosa generally increases with age, as does intestinal metaplasia and gastric carcinoma. For example, in a study of a Japanese population (the Japanese have a high incidence of both atrophic gastritis and cancer), the incidences of atrophic gastritis and metaplasia were 49% and 38%, respectively, in the 30- to 39-year-old group compared with 89% and 82% respectively in those 60 years and older (Asaka *et al.* 1996). However, the major risk factor in atrophic gastritis and indeed the development of gastric cancer appears to be infection with *H. pylori* (Kuipers *et al.* 1995; Watanabe *et al.* 1997). In a

recent Japanese longitudinal cohort study of 4655 healthy asymptomatic subjects followed for a mean period of 7.7 years (Ohata *et al.* 2004), both *H. pylori* and chronic atrophic gastritis (CAG) were significantly associated with gastric cancer. No cancer developed in the *H. pylori*(-)/CAG(-) group during the study period. This supports the theory that it is quite rare for any type of gastric cancer to develop in an *H. pylori*-free healthy stomach. In the Asaka *et al.* (1996) study, the frequency of atrophic gastritis and intestinal metaplasia was extremely low in the *H. pylori* seronegative group regardless of age.

The *H. pylori* bacterium colonises the stomach mucosa and triggers a series of inflammatory reactions resulting in significant epithelial cell damage and epithelial proliferation, as well as an increased level of apoptosis. In addition, *H. pylori* infection has been associated with changes in oncogene and tumour suppressor gene expression as shown by increased ras p21 expression and p53 mutation in *H. pylori* positive cases of gastric cancer (J. Wang *et al.* 2002). It has also been shown that chronic *H. pylori* infection is associated with decreased expression of the cyclin-dependent kinase inhibitor (CDI) p27kip1.

It should be noted that bacterial colonisation is necessary, although not in itself sufficient, for the development of the cancer. Rather, it would appear that chronic inflammation caused by the bacterial colonisation is more important than *H. pylori* infection *per se*. The observed incidence rate of gastric cancer in subjects with *H. pylori* infection is comparatively low, suggesting that other environmental or genetic co-factors are involved in the progression to cancer (Ohata *et al.* 2004). The observed geographic variability in gastric cancer appears to be explained by a synergistic interaction between *H. pylori* infection and other environmental factors. For example, a cross-sectional study in Japan has shown consumption of highly salted foods increases the risk of *H. pylori* infection, possibly by causing mucosal damage (Tsugane 2005). It should be noted that the median urinary salt excretion in this study was 7–13 g/day. Additionally, a synergistic enhancing effect of *H. pylori* infection and salted food intake has been reported in a case-control study in Korea (Lee *et al.* 2003).

In older people, atrophic gastritis is an important cause of poor vitamin B_{12} (cobalamin) status

(Wolters *et al.* 2004). It is thought that atrophic gastritis results in declining gastric acid and pepsinogen secretion which results in decreased intestinal absorption of the cobalamin protein complexes from food. In addition, some drugs used in the treatment of gastritis, such as proton pump inhibitors or H2 receptor antagonists, inhibit the intestinal absorption of vitamin B_{12}.

The prevalence of vitamin B_{12} deficiency (serum cobalamin of <150 pmol/L) in older people has been estimated to be 10–15%, which can rise to over 34% for marginal deficiency (serum cobalamin of <220 pmol/L) (Wolters *et al.* 2004; Green *et al.* 2005; Paulionis *et al.* 2005). It should be noted that atrophic gastritis is not the only cause of vitamin B_{12} deficiency in older people. A small study of a French cohort estimated that about 40% of the vitamin-deficient patients had gastritis (Andres *et al.* 2002). A recent study in a New Zealand population (n = 466) concluded that while atrophic gastritis accounted for around 33% of cases of vitamin B_{12} deficiency, it increased the relative risk of deficiency by 21-fold (Green *et al.* 2005).

12.3.4.1 Nutritional approaches

The crucial role of *H. pylori* in the development of chronic atrophic gastritis and gastric cancer means that antibiotic treatment is a prime means of prevention and therapy in infected subjects. Equally, however, the strong association in many epidemiological studies of gastric cancer risk with dietary factors, such as salt, nitrates and low intake of fresh fruits and vegetables and vitamin C, suggests that dietary modification could modulate risk of the disease (Correa 1991; Kaaks *et al.* 1998; Terry *et al.* 1998).

Salt and salted foods: Evidence from ecological, case-control and cohort studies indicates an increased risk of gastric cancer with high intake of salt and salt-preserved foods, particularly those consumed in Japan and Korea (Tsugane 2005; World Cancer Research Fund/American Institute for Cancer Research 2007). Such data are supported by experimental studies in rodents which have shown that salt causes gastritis and other gastric damage, including mucosal erosion and degeneration, and enhances the carcinogenic effects of chemical carcinogens.

Fruits and vegetables: In a review of the epidemiological data, Correa *et al.* (1998) reported a consistent association between gastric cancer risk and low intakes of fruit and vegetables, which has been attributed to intake of antioxidant micronutrients, particularly vitamin C. The effect of vitamin C may be related to its ability to scavenge reactive oxygen species and inhibit N-nitroso compound formation, although high doses of the vitamin have been shown to inhibit *H. pylori* growth and colonisation (Zhang *et al.* 1997).

In vitro and animal experiments have shown that sulforaphane, a glucosinolate found in broccoli, inhibits *H. pylori* infection and blocks gastric tumour formation, however an epidemiological investigation of broccoli consumption and chronic atrophic gastritis among Japanese males did not find the expected negative correlation (Sato *et al.* 2004). In fact, the prevalence of chronic atrophic gastritis among men who ate broccoli once or more weekly was twice as high as that among men who consumed a negligible amount ($P < 0.05$).

The second World Cancer Research Fund report considered the evidence that fruit and non-starchy vegetables protect against stomach cancer was 'probable'. There were ample studies and evidence of benefit from a number of different fruits and vegetables (World Cancer Research Fund/American Institute for Cancer Research 2007).

Antioxidants: Marotta *et al.* (2004) reported an intervention study with antioxidant supplements in 60 older patients with *H. pylori*-negative atrophic gastritis and intestinal metaplasia. The patients were randomly allocated into three matched groups and supplemented for six months with vitamin E (300 mg/day), a multivitamin supplement or a proprietary fermented papaya preparation. Biopsy samples from the antrum at 0, 3 and 6 months were analysed for enzymatic abnormalities and free radical-modified DNA adducts associated with premalignant changes in the gastric mucosa: α-tocopherol, malonyl dialdehyde, xanthine oxidase, ornithine decarboxylase and 8-hydroxydeoxyguanidine. Ten dyspeptic patients served as controls. All supplements significantly decreased ornithine decarboxylase and the papaya extract significantly decreased 8-hydroxydeoxyguanidine levels in the mucosa. These preliminary data suggest that antioxidant supplementation might be a potential chemopreventive approach in *H. pylori*-eradicated chronic atrophic gastritis patients and especially in older populations.

Probiotics: Some well-designed human intervention studies and experiments in animal models have demonstrated that secreted products of *Lact. acidophilus* sp. can suppress the growth of *H. pylori* both *in vitro* and *in vivo* (Felley and Michetti 2003). For example, when *H. pylori* was incubated in the presence of serial dilutions of *Lact. salivarius* or *Lact. johnsonii* culture supernatants, growth of *H. pylori* was inhibited, whether or not it was bound to epithelial cells. Inhibitory effects of *Lact. salivarius* on *H. pylori* were also demonstrated in a gnotobiotic murine model (Aiba *et al.* 1998). This effect appeared to be due to the production of a large amount of lactic acid. In addition, the effect of *Lact. johnsonii* La1 supernatant on *H. pylori* colonisation was assessed in 20 human subjects in a double-blind, controlled study (Michetti *et al.* 1999). La1 showed inhibitory effects on *H. pylori* in infected subjects as assessed by the ^{14}C urea breath test. Furthermore, in a randomised trial of 53 subjects with *H. pylori* infections, those patients receiving *Lact. johnsonii* La1 (180 ml twice a day for three weeks), in addition to antibiotic therapy, showed significant, though modest, decreases (in comparison with placebo) in level of *H. pylori*, inflammation of the antrum and activity of the inflammation in both antrum and corpus (Felley and Michetti 2003). Similar results were obtained by Sakamoto *et al.* (2001), who investigated the effect of *Lact. gasseri* LG21 in 31 patients with *H. pylori* infections. LG21 suppressed *H. pylori* colonisation of the gastric mucosa and reduced mucosal inflammation. The studies provide some preliminary evidence that certain *Lact.* strains can both suppress *H. pylori* and reduce gastric mucosal inflammation. Further studies are needed to evaluate whether this effect is maintained with long-term ingestion of these probiotics (see Section 12.5.1.1 for definition).

Vitamin B$_{12}$: In terms of vitamin B$_{12}$ deficiency associated with atrophic gastritis in older people, Green *et al.* (2005) found that an intake of vitamin B$_{12}$ from food that exceeded the reference nutrient intake (1.5 µg/day) did not protect against deficient or marginal vitamin status. However, vitamin B$_{12}$ supplement users had a reduced risk of having deficient and marginal vitamin B$_{12}$ status. It has been recommended that general supplementation with vitamin B$_{12}$ of >50 µg/day should be considered for older people (Wolters *et al.* 2004).

12.4 The small intestine

The major roles of the gut include digestion and absorption, defence, excretion of exogenous and endogenous material, and communication. All of these roles are dependent on the correct functioning of the intestinal mucosa. This mucosa separates the external world (*i.e.* gut contents) from the body proper and consists of a single layer of columnar epithelial cells.

12.4.1 Biology of the intestinal epithelium

The small intestinal epithelial cells arise from pluripotent stem cells located approximately four cells up from the base of the intestinal crypt. Asymmetric division of the stem cell results in the production of a new stem cell and of a transit cell, which is capable of a number of further cell divisions. Mitosis is terminated with the onset of differentiation (Figure 12.1). Differentiation occurs as the cells leave the crypt and is completed during transit along the associated villus. Cells are shed continuously from the villus tip and, in health, the number of cells born in the crypt matches exactly those lost from the villus

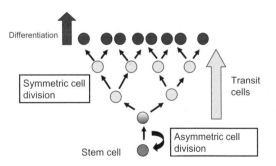

Figure 12.1: Model of cell proliferation in the small intestine.

tip and those dying by apoptosis. An imbalance in the numbers of cells born and those being shed or which die by apoptosis has significant implications for the health of the mucosa and is associated with disease (Mathers 2003). For example, excess cell proliferation may predispose to tumorigenesis, whilst an excess of cell death is associated with the blunting of the villi in coeliac disease, and with mucosal erosion in inflammatory bowel disease. Ciccocioppo *et al.* (2002) reported that both cell proliferation and apoptosis were increased in the duodenum of older (mean age 78 years) compared with younger (mean age 38 years) healthy human volunteers. This apparently hyper-proliferative mucosa, balanced by an exaggerated apoptotic state, maintains the integrity of the mucosal architecture during ageing but at the possible cost of reduced cellular maturity (since rapid proliferation reduces the time for cellular differentiation), which may impair absorptive function in stress conditions. There is also evidence of higher rates of cell proliferation in the jejunum of older (27 months) vs. young adult (4 months) rats (Mathers *et al.* 1993). Changes in the density and physical dimensions of ileal crypts accompanied by reduced ability to regenerate after damage (irradiation) have been reported for older (28–30 months) compared with young (6–7 months) mice (Martin *et al.* 1998).

Studies in rats have indicated an age-related loss of villous height, but most studies in humans have not shown any age-related morphological changes in the small intestine in terms of surface structure, crypt depth, villous height, brush border and Brunner glands (Hoffmann and Zeitz 2002).

Small intestinal stem cells give rise to four functionally different cell lineages, viz. the non-secretory enterocytes and three secretory cell lineages, namely goblet cells, Paneth cells and enteroendocrine cells. Differentiation into the secretory lineages appears to be dependent on expression of *MATH1* whilst expression of *NGN3* restricts differentiation to the endocrine cell lineages (Schonhoff *et al.* 2004).

12.4.1.1 Enterocytes

Enterocytes, which are by far the most numerous of the epithelial cells, are responsible for hydrolysis of food macromolecules via hydrolases expressed on the apical (brush border) membrane and for the transport (absorption) of digested end-products.

For some nutrients (*e.g.* peptides and fatty acids), there is further processing within the enterocyte before the molecules are exported into the portal blood stream or lymphatic system. There is considerable controversy around the influence of ageing on enterocyte function. Although there are some data from animal experiments that nutrient absorption declines with age (Woudstra and Thomson 2002), unequivocal evidence for loss of digestive or absorptive capacity with ageing in humans, in the absence of disease, is scanty (Harper 1998). Lactase, which hydrolyses lactose, is the mucosal disaccharidase showing the greatest age-related changes. Lactase expression in the fetal gut is detectable from week 8 of gestation and virtually all infants express lactase adequately. Weaning is followed by the loss of lactase expression in the majority of humans – a phenomenon that is probably genetically determined and associated with an SNP (T/C at position −13910) 14 kb upstream of the gene for lactase-phlorizin hydrolase (*LPH*) (Enattah *et al.* 2002). Interestingly, postmenopausal women who carried the CC genotype of *LPH* were lactose intolerant (could not digest lactose efficiently), had significantly greater aversion to milk, reduced bone mineral density and greater bone fracture incidence (Obermayer-Pietsch *et al.* 2004). Almost 100% of adults in Southeast Asia are lactose maldigesters compared with only 2% of the British population (Buttriss and Korpela 2002). Transient loss of lactase activity can be caused by episodes of diarrhoea, drug treatment or other factors that damage the small bowel mucosa.

In a study of duodenal biopsies from 38 individuals aged 55–91 years in the north-east of England, there was no detectable effect of age on the activities of six brush border hydrolases (including lactase and other disaccharidases), alkaline phosphatase and a peptidase (Wallis *et al.* 1993). In contrast, maldigestion of lactose (assessed by breath hydrogen response to a lactose challenge) increased with age in two separate studies of apparently healthy Italian volunteers (Carroccio *et al.* 1998; di Stefano *et al.* 2001). The larger of the two studies (Carroccio *et al.* 1998) enrolled 323 subjects aged 5–85 years, which was a random sample of 25% of the population of Ventimiglia di Sicilia. Figure 12.2 shows the increase in lactose maldigestion with age. It should be noted, however, that the breath hydrogen test used to diagnose lactose maldigestion is somewhat unphysiological (being based on a 50 g dose of lactose) and

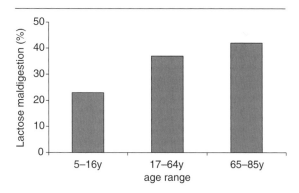

Figure 12.2: Lactose intolerance and maldigestion in a Sicilian town.
Source: Carroccio *et al.* (1998). Reproduced by permission of the American College of Nutrition, from the *Journal of the American College of Nutrition.* Permission conveyed through the Copyright Clearance Centre, Inc.

several controlled dietary intervention trials have shown that such lactose maldigesters tolerate cheese and yogurt and even milk when consumed with meals (Buttriss and Korpela 2002).

A study of calcium absorption (using a radio-labelled isotope) in healthy postmenopausal women aged 40–87 years reported a 28% decrease in calcium absorption in women over 75 years (Nordin *et al.* 2004). Because there was no concomitant decline in serum $1,25(OH)_2D$, the authors concluded that there was a decline in the responsiveness of the small intestine to serum calcitriol, analogous to the corresponding event at menopause.

12.4.1.2 Goblet cells

The primary function of goblet cells is to secrete mucus that consists of hydrated mucin (large glycopeptides) molecules. Mucus has virtually unparalleled lubricating properties and has roles in movement of digesta through the gut lumen and in protection of the epithelial surface. The expression of mucins, which are encoded by *MUC* genes, can be detected from as early as 12 weeks in the fetal small intestine with patterns of expression similar to those in the adult, in whom MUC2, MUC3 and MUC4 predominate (Buisine *et al.* 2000). There appears to be no information about changes in mucin expression or secretion during ageing.

12.4.1.3 Paneth cells

Unlike the other epithelial cell lineages in the small bowel, Paneth cells reside at the bottom of the crypt where they live for more than 20 days. They secrete lysozyme, secretory phospholipase A_2 and alpha-defensins, all of which contribute to the antimicrobial role of the Paneth cell. Forming a key element of intestinal innate immunity, alpha-defensins are small cysteine-rich peptides with broad spectrum antimicrobial activity against bacteria, fungi, protozoa and enveloped viruses (Ayabe *et al.* 2004). It has been hypothesised that increased numbers of Paneth cells might be produced in response to inflammation (Ayabe *et al.* 2004), but there is no information on changes in Paneth cell number or function with age. However, Paneth cells appear to become depleted of secretory granules (which store alpha-defensins) in response to infective and nutritional stress and P. Kelly *et al.* (2004) have postulated that this is one mechanism by which reduced zinc status can increase susceptibility to intestinal infection. Given the significant numbers of older people with zinc intakes below the lower reference nutrient intake (LRNI) (13% and 4% of older men and women living in institutions respectively), it will be important to ascertain whether this compromises their ability to defend against intestinal infections.

12.4.1.4 Enteroendocrine cells

Endocrine cells comprise approximately 1% of the cells in the gut epithelium and represent the largest population of hormone-producing cells in the human body (Schonhoff *et al.* 2004). These enteroendocrine cells produce an array of peptide hormones that regulate a wide range of GI processes including gastric emptying, pancreatic secretion, gall bladder contraction and the motor functions controlling intestinal transit of digesta. In addition, GI peptides act on distant organs, especially the brain, with profound implications for appetite and energy balance (see Chapter 13, Section 13.2.3). For example, cholecystokinin (CCK), which is released from endocrine cells in the proximal duodenum in response to the presence of fats and amino acids in the gut lumen, stimulates exocrine pancreatic enzyme secretion and gall bladder contraction and inhibits food intake. Older people appear to be more sensitive to the satiating effects of raised circulating concentrations of CCK (Parker and Chapman 2004). Glucagon-like peptide-1 (GLP-1) is a 30-amino acid residue peptide synthesised within the L-cells of the distal small intestine and colon, with about equal contributions by the two parts of the intestine to GLP-1 in the circulation (Robertson *et al.* 1999). GLP-1 stimulates glucose-dependent insulin secretion and inhibits gastric emptying, gastric acid secretion and food intake (Drucker 2003). Plasma GLP-1 concentrations are similar in younger and older persons with similar responses to nutrient challenges, but the influence of ageing on the satiating effects of GLP-1 is unknown (Parker and Chapman 2004).

12.4.2 Exocrine pancreas

Acinar cells within the pancreas are responsible for the synthesis, storage and, in response to GI peptide stimulation, the release into the proximal duodenum of a consortium of hydrolases, including lipases, amylases, proteases, DNAases and RNAases, thus having a major role in digestion. With the exception of the amylases, these hydrolytic enzymes are released as zymogens, which are activated within the gut lumen by partial hydrolysis by enterokinase (in the case of trypsinogen conversion to trypsin) and by trypsin for the other pro-enzymes. Pancreatic exocrine secretion in response to intravenous injection of secretin and CCK is lower in older people (Laugier *et al.* 1991; Vellas *et al.* 1998). Although this does not seem to have been studied systematically in humans, pancreatic enzymes are normally secreted in considerable excess, so it is unlikely that lack of pancreatic enzyme secretion plays a major role in malnutrition in older people. Small but significant reductions in the digestion of food within the small bowel of older compared with young adult rats has been observed (Mathers *et al.* 1993), but it is not known whether this is due to changes in pancreatic enzyme secretion or to other factors.

12.4.3 Coeliac disease

Coeliac disease is generally considered to be a disease of children and young adults, Recently, however, it is increasingly being diagnosed in older adults in the UK, Europe and the US (Freeman *et al.* 2002), as a direct result of relatively simple blood

tests now available for screening purposes (instead of the traditional and invasive intestinal biopsy). The symptoms in these patients include weight loss, diarrhoea and anaemia. Often the typical symptoms of malabsorption have been less apparent (Freeman *et al.* 2002). Development of malignancy, usually small intestinal lymphoma, is a serious concern, especially when diagnosis of coeliac disease is delayed into later adult life. Furthermore, decreased bone mineral density is frequently associated with coeliac disease, most likely because of reduced calcium absorption, and patients have a higher prevalence of fractures in the peripheral skeleton (Vazquez *et al.* 2000). As with younger patients, treatment of coeliac disease is by adoption of a gluten-free diet, which as well as alleviating symptoms has a protective effect on occurrence of malignancies and on fractures (Freeman *et al.* 2002). Older patients can have difficulties in adhering to a strict gluten-free diet and additional clinical and household support may be needed to ensure compliance. Nutritional assessment may indicate a need for supplementation with iron, folic acid and vitamin B_{12}, and a multivitamin preparation is recommended (Freeman *et al.* 2002).

12.4.4 Diarrhoea

Diarrhoea is a significant worldwide problem and is of particular concern for older people; about 85% of mortality associated with diarrhoea in the developed world involves the elderly (Gangarosa *et al.* 1992). Diarrhoea can be acute (<14 days' duration, usually caused by infection), persistent (>14 days) or chronic (>30 days). It is usually classified into inflammatory, secretory and osmotic (Hoffmann and Zeitz 2002). Secretory diarrhoea is a consequence of disturbed intestinal electrolyte (sodium, potassium, chloride, bicarbonate) transport. The most common causes in the elderly are infectious diarrhoea, diabetic diarrhoea, excessive use of laxatives/diuretics, food-borne toxins and alcohol-induced diarrhoea. Food allergies also fall into this group but are a much rarer cause. Osmotic diarrhoea is due to the presence in the gut of non-absorbable solutes either because of deficiencies in digestive processes (*e.g.* pancreatic insufficiency, coeliac disease, lactose intolerance) or ingested substances such as antacids, foods containing osmotically active substances such as the sugar substitute sorbitol, and certain osmotically active laxatives like lactulose. Diarrhoea associated with inflammation (as with Crohn's disease and ulcerative colitis) is less common.

In patients with acute diarrhoea lasting more than a day, the primary treatment is rehydration with oral rehydration solution or if necessary intravenous fluids. No evidence-based guidelines for treatment of persistent or chronic diarrhoea are available and treatment will depend on the cause established (Hoffmann and Zeitz 2002).

Diarrhoea is a familiar complication of antibiotic treatment. Although infrequent in non-hospitalised patients, antibiotic-associated diarrhoea (AAD) is common in hospitals, nursing homes and other types of chronic care facilities, where the frequency can range from 3% to 60% (McFarland 1993, 1998). AAD usually occurs 2–8 weeks after treatment with antibiotics, especially broad spectrum type antibiotics, probably due to disruption of the intestinal microflora. This results in breakdown of its colonisation resistance to opportunistic enteric pathogens, in particular *C. difficile* which has been implicated in about 10–26% of AAD patients and is now one of the most common causes of infectious diarrhoea in hospitals and nursing homes (Oldfield 2004).

Older patients are particularly susceptible to diarrhoea induced by *C. difficile*, which in addition to severe diarrhoea can result in pseudomembranous colitis and 2–3-fold increases in mortality (Spencer 1998). Recurrence of symptoms following treatment of the infection is a particular problem, with up to 66% of patients suffering from recurrences.

There have been four meta-analyses of the impact of probiotics on AAD of which the largest and most comprehensive is that of McFarland (2006). Of the 25 trials that met the inclusion criteria, 13 (52%) reported a significant reduction of AAD in the probiotic-treated group vs. placebo. The other 12 reported non-significant effects. In the meta-analysis, probiotics had a significant effect (overall RR = 0.43, 95% CI: 0.31–0.58, $p < 0.001$). The diversity of study populations (children/adults), range of probiotic types, doses 10^7–10^{11} organisms per day and treatment duration probably contributed to the contradictory results. It was noted that use of daily doses of $>10^{10}$ per day was associated with significant efficacy.

Amongst the probiotic preparations used, three were associated with overall significant reductions in

risk of AAD, namely *Saccharomyces boulardii* (six studies, combined RR: 0.37, 95% CI: 0.26–0.52, $p < 0.0001$), *Lact. rhamnosus* GG (six studies, combined RR: 0.31, 95% CI: 0.13–0.72, $p < 0.006$), and various mixtures of probiotics (seven studies, RR: 0.51, 95% CI: 0.38–0.68, $p < 0.0001$). Studies with other individual probiotics overall just failed to reach statistical significance ($p = 0.06$).

Six of the randomised, placebo-controlled trials in the meta-analysis investigated *C. difficile*-associated diarrhoea and two of these, both using *S. boulardii*, reported significant reduction in risk of recurrence vs. placebo (McFarland 2006). The combined RR for all six studies (which involved, in addition to *S. boulardii*, *Lact. rhamnosus* GG, *Lact. plantarum* 299v and a *Lact. Bifidobacterium* mixture) was 0.59, (95% CI: 041–0.85 $p < 0.005$). Furthermore, a recent randomised placebo-controlled trial, not included in the meta-analysis, reported the effect of a probiotic yogurt drink containing *Lact. casei* DN114001 together with *Lact. delbrueckii subsp. bulgaricus* and *Streptococcus thermophilus* in older (>50 years; mean age 74 years) hospitalised patients receiving a new course of antibiotics (Hickson *et al.* 2007). The probiotic drink was given during antibiotic treatment plus one week after and fewer patients in this group developed diarrhoea (odds ratio 0.25, 95% CI: 0.07–0.85). The probiotic also prevented *C. difficile* infection (0% vs. 17% in the placebo group).

Thus overall, probiotics show considerable promise as therapies for AAD and there is some evidence for efficacy of *S. boulardii* for *C. difficile*-associated diarrhoea, although more extensive trials, particularly in older people, are needed in the latter area.

In the light of the positive effects of probiotics, it seems reasonable that prebiotics might exert similar beneficial effects on AAD by elevating the concentration of bifidobacteria in the gut and increasing colonisation resistance. This hypothesis has been tested in two large-scale interventions, with differing results. In the first of these placebo-controlled, randomised, double-blind trials (Lewis *et al.* 2005b), 435 hospital inpatients over 65 years who had been prescribed a broad-spectrum antibiotic in the preceding 24 hours were allocated to either fructooligosaccharides (FOS) or sucrose (12 g/day), which were consumed for the duration of the antibiotic treatment and for one week afterwards. Subjects were then followed up for a further week since *C. difficile*-

associated diarrhoea occurs within 14 days of anti-biotic treatment. Of the 435 subjects, 116 developed diarrhoea, of which 49 were positive for *C. difficile* toxin. However, there were no significant differences between FOS and placebo, despite a significant increase in faecal bifidobacteria counts in the FOS group indicating good compliance with the treatment. Thus in this study FOS did not protect older patients treated with broad spectrum antibiotics from AAD, whether or not associated with *C. difficile*.

In a second study (Lewis *et al.* 2005a), the same authors investigated the effect of FOS on relapse of *C. difficile* diarrhoea after antibiotic treatment, which occurs in about 10–20% of patients (Kelly *et al.* 1994). The study was a randomised double-blind, placebo-controlled design in which 142 adult patients with *C. difficile*-associated diarrhoea (treated with metronidazole and vancomycin) were allocated to FOS or sucrose (12 g/day). The treatments were taken as soon as possible after diagnosis until 30 days after cessation of diarrhoea, with a further 30-day follow-up. Relapse occurred in 30 patients after about 18 days and was more common in subjects on placebo (34.3%) than those taking FOS (8.3% $p <$ 0.001). The length of stay in hospital was also reduced in those on FOS.

Orrhage *et al.* (2000) compared the effect of pre-biotic (see Section 12.5.1. for definition) and synbi-otic (pro- and prebiotic) treatments on faecal microflora and *C. difficile* carriage in a placebo-controlled, parallel design intervention. Three groups of 10 healthy subjects (21–50 years) were given oral cefpodoxime proxetil for seven days. One group was given a placebo milk, a second group was given the same milk with 15 g FOS/day and the third group consumed a synbiotic comprising 15 g/day FOS and a fermented milk providing *B. longum* BB536 (2–10 $\times 10^{10}$ cfu/d) + *L. acidophilus* NCFB 1748 (10–15 $\times$ 10^{10} cfu/d). The milks were consumed for 21 days along with the antibiotic treatment. In the placebo and prebiotic-treated volunteers, six out of 10 subjects in each group were colonised by *C. difficile* and half were cytotoxin-positive. In contrast, in the synbiotic group, only one subject harboured detectable numbers of *C. difficile* and only at one sampling occasion. Thus a combination of pro- and prebiotics, although not prebiotics alone, decreased *C. difficile* carriage after antibiotic treatment.

12.5 The large intestine

12.5.1 The microflora of the large intestine

The microflora of the human GI tract, and in particular the large intestine, comprises a large and diverse range of microorganisms, with over 10^{12} bacteria per gram of contents (Cummings and Macfarlane 1991). It is, therefore, not surprising that the activities of this microbial population can have a significant impact on the health of the host. The microflora interacts with its host at both the local (intestinal mucosa) and systemic levels, resulting in a broad range of immunological, physiological and metabolic effects. From the standpoint of the host, these effects have both beneficial and detrimental outcomes for nutrition, infections, xenobiotic metabolism, ingested chemicals and cancer (Rowland and Gangolli 1999).

The faecal microflora undergoes dramatic changes during early life particularly during weaning. However, modification of the flora during later life has until recently received little attention. The first study was by Mitsuoka (1992), who reported that older adults had fewer of bifidobacteria and elevated clostridia and lactobacilli in faeces than younger adults. However, this study was conducted with classic microbiological methods (culturing of viable bacteria on selective and non-selective media) and there is now evidence that these methods grossly underestimate microbial diversity within the human gut. Currently a number of studies are being conducted on the faecal flora during ageing using more sophisticated and accurate molecular methods of analysis, in particular those exploiting 16S ribosomal RNA sequences and PCR (Blaut *et al.* 2002). These indicate that <25% of the molecular species found in adults correspond to known organisms (Suau *et al.* 1999). Sequence analysis of over 280 clones from a single older person's faecal sample (only one subject was studied) showed that the flora was even more diverse than that of an adult (Table 12.2). Furthermore, the proportion of unknown molecular species was much higher among the clones derived from the older subject and 22% of the flora comprised species outside the major groups found in younger adults, *i.e. Bacteroides/Prevotella*, *Clostridium coccoides*, *Clostridium leptum* groups (Blaut *et al.* 2002).

Table 12.2: Increase in microbial diversity with age

Subjects (number)	Number of clones	Number of species	% described species
Infants (2)	164	15	70
Adults (5)	619	160	19
Elderly (1)	280	168	8

Source: Blaut *et al.* (2002).

A somewhat more extensive study of the faecal flora of humans in different age groups was conducted by Hopkins *et al.* (2001), who compared, using both conventional microbiological and molecular methods, children (16 months–7 years), adults (21–34 years) and healthy older subjects (67–88 years). Although total bacterial counts were similar in all age groups, bacterial composition varied considerably. Most notably, bifidobacterial numbers were significantly lower in older people: in two of the four subjects numbers of bifidobacteria were undetectable and in one the count was very low. However, in the final older subject, very high numbers (approximately 10^{10}/g faeces) were detected. Data from 16S rRNA analyses confirmed the results obtained by conventional bacteriology.

The same research group recently reported a further study in which the faecal microfloras of healthy young adults (19–35 years), healthy elderly (67–75 years) and hospitalised antibiotic-treated elderly (73–101 years) were compared using conventional microbiological methods (Woodmansey *et al.* 2004). The results showed that total anaerobe numbers remained relatively constant with age, although, as before, individual bacterial genera changed markedly. Reductions in both numbers and species diversity of bacteroides and bifidobacteria in both older groups were seen. In particular, bifidobacterial populations showed marked variations in the dominant species, with *Bifidobacterium angulatum* and *Bifidobacterium adolescentis* being isolated from older people and *Bifidobacterium longum*, *Bifidobacterium catenulatum*, *Bifidobacterium boum*, and *Bifidobacterium infantis* being detected only in the healthy young volunteers. Other differences in the intestinal ecosystem in older subjects were observed, with alterations in the dominant clostridial species in combination with greater numbers of facultative anaerobes. It is not clear why this study

showed decreased species diversity in the faecal flora of older subjects, although it may be related to the methodology used (conventional microbiology rather than molecular methods) or to the study being conducted in a different location from the Hopkins *et al.* (2001) investigation.

12.5.1.1 Nutritional approaches: modification of gut microflora by probiotics and prebiotics

There is evidence that bifidobacteria exert inhibitory effects on potential pathogens such as *C. difficile* and may be involved in colonisation resistance and immune function (Yamazaki *et al.* 1985; Gibson and Wang 1994). Other studies demonstrate reduced precancerous lesions and tumours in the colon of laboratory animals given strains of bifidobacteria (Reddy and Rivenson 1993; Rowland *et al.* 1998). On the basis of such evidence it has been suggested that the decline in faecal bifidobacteria numbers with age plays a role in the increased risk of infections and some chronic degenerative diseases in older people.

One implication of this is that it should be possible to restore to some extent the original balance of the microflora by supplementing the diet with probiotic bifidobacteria or bifidogenic products, *i.e.* prebiotics such as non-digestible oligosaccharides (NDOs) which selectively stimulate the growth of bifidobacteria in the gut. Probiotics have been defined as live microorganisms which when administered in adequate amounts confer a health benefit on the host (FAO/WHO 2002) whereas a prebiotic is described as a non-digestible food ingredient that beneficially affects the host by selectively stimulating the growth and/or activity of one or a limited number of bacteria (*e.g.* bifidobacteria and lactobacilli) in the colon that have the potential to improve host health (Gibson and Roberfroid 1995).

There is extensive evidence that NDOs modulate the composition of the gut microflora in adults. This has been observed in a large number of dietary intervention trials (Roberfroid 1993). There is evidence from some studies that the stimulatory effects of prebiotics on bifidobacteria numbers in the gut are more apparent when the initial levels are low (Tuohy *et al.* 2001), suggesting that prebiotics would be particularly effective in older people. To date, however, there have been few reported studies in this area.

Kleessen *et al.* (1997) conducted a study in which groups of 15 and 10 patients received lactose or inulin, respectively, for a period of 19 days. The dose, 20 g/day from days 1 to 8, was gradually increased to 40 g/day from days 9 to 11 and was kept at this level from days 12 to 19. Despite considerable inter-individual variations, inulin was found to increase bifidobacteria significantly from 7.9 to 9.2 log^{10}/g dry faeces, and to decrease enterococci in number and enterobacteria in frequency. Further studies on the effects of pro- and prebiotics in older people are underway in a major EU project (www. crownalife.be).

12.5.2 Constipation

Bowel dysfunction is a major problem for older people, with constipation being one of their commonest complaints. Although constipation is often defined clinically as fewer than three bowel movements a week (Whitehead *et al.* 1989), in practice it covers a wide range of reported symptoms, including straining, hard stools, pain and incomplete evacuation, even though bowel movements may be within the physiological norm (Potter 2003).

Estimates of the prevalence of constipation vary between 2 and 34%, in part because of inconsistencies in the use of criteria to define the condition (Garrigues *et al.* 2004; Higgins and Johanson 2004). Some, but not all, studies indicate a relationship between age and prevalence. A recent systematic review of American studies revealed that four out of six found an increase in constipation with age (Higgins and Johanson 2004), although a cross-sectional survey in Spain found no relationship (Garrigues *et al.* 2004). Constipation is not only distressing for the patient, it has a negative impact on quality of life, places great strain on carers and generates significant health care costs (Higgins and Johanson 2004). Side-effects include hernias, loss of appetite, GI obstruction and inflammation (Alessi 1988; Dahl *et al.* 2003).

The pathophysiology underlying constipation in older people is complex and is thought to include alteration in neural innervation, smooth muscle activity and neuroendrocrine function, resulting in changes in colonic transit time, difficulty in defaecation and changes in rectal sensation (Potter 2003). Constipation has also been reported as an adverse side-effect in the use of a number of drugs, in par-

ticular, opioids (population attributable risk (PAR) = 2.6%), diuretics (PAR = 5.6%), antidepressants (PAR = 8.2%), antihistamines (PAR = 9.2%), antispasmodics (PAR = 11.6%), anticonvulsants (PAR = 2.5%) and aluminium antacids (PAR = 3.0%) (Talley *et al.* 2003). In this context, it is noteworthy that the National Diet and Nutrition Survey reported that in free-living, older age groups 75% of men and 79% of women were taking medications. These figures rise to 97% and 92% respectively when those living in institutions are considered (Finch *et al.* 1998).

12.5.2.1 Nutritional approaches

The complex and varied aetiology of constipation in older people suggests that nutritional solutions may be too simplistic an approach. Epidemiological studies are few and conflicting. In a community-based study in New Zealand of 778 older adults (>70 years), 34 were considered to have constipation. Analysis of this sub-group showed that constipation was more common in women than men, increased with age and was associated with the use of constipating drugs. This group was frailer and less physically active. Low intakes of dietary fibre, fruit, vegetables, bread and cereals or fluid were not associated with an increased occurrence of constipation (Campbell *et al.* 1993). In a random sample of 2807 residents, aged 60 years or more in Singapore, surveyed by questionnaire, the overall age- and gender-adjusted prevalence rate of constipation was 11.6 per 100 persons. There were no gender or ethnic differences in constipation rates, but rates of constipation were significantly associated with advancing age and with lower intake of rice, fruits and vegetables, but no dose–response gradient was seen (Wong *et al.* 1999).

Dietary remedies represent a less invasive strategy than enemas and laxatives, with minimal side-effects, and there is some evidence that dietary fibre, non-digestible oligosaccharides and probiotics may be effective.

Fruit and vegetables: Anecdotal reports suggest that the use of fruit as a laxative is effective, although there are few controlled trials in this area. A recent study investigated the effect of consumption of kiwi fruit on laxation in older people (Rush *et al.* 2002). Thirty-eight free-living, healthy adults (>60 years old) consumed their normal diet, with or without one kiwi fruit per 30 kg body weight daily for three weeks, followed by a three-week crossover period. Kiwi fruit significantly enhanced all tested measures of laxation (stool frequency, volume, consistency and ease of defaecation) in these adults. It is likely that a number of factors in the whole fruit are involved, but the nature of the stools suggests fibre is important.

Dietary fibre: A number of studies have evaluated the effect of adding dietary fibre to the diets of older people, usually those in nursing homes or similar institutions. The results are variable due in part to palatability and acceptability problems associated with some fibre sources (Hankey *et al.* 1993; Lengyel *et al.* 2003). However, some studies reported considerable success. For example, a 12-month study in institutionalised older patients (average age 83.5 years) showed that constipation was eliminated effectively and safely by the use of dietary fibre (daily intake of 25 g) and a controlled fluid intake (Hope and Down 1986). Similarly a randomised placebo-controlled trial in older hospitalised patients given a 150 ml portion of yogurt containing lactitol, guar gum and wheat bran twice daily reported a significant increase in faecal output compared with a control yogurt without fibre (Rajala *et al.* 1988). Dahl *et al.* (2003) demonstrated that the addition of modest amounts of finely processed pea fibre (4 g fibre/day) to various foods for older subjects in long-term residential care significantly increased the frequency of bowel movements and reduced laxative use (Figure 12.3). A community intervention trial in small retirement communities (age >55 years) in Australia involving media, community activities and social marketing principles resulted in an increase in sales of wholemeal bread and decreased sales of laxatives (Egger *et al.* 1991).

It is clear that the type of non-digestible carbohydrate selected can have a major impact on the extent of laxation. In studies of the effects of carbohydrates on faecal bulking in healthy subjects, it has been shown that wheat bran (insoluble fibre) increases stool weight by 5 g per g carbohydrate consumed (Cummings *et al.* 1992), whereas soluble fibre in the form of pectin and guar gum has relatively minor effects (1–2 g increase in faecal weight per g carbohydrate) (Cummings *et al.* 1976). Resistant starch and non-digestible oligosaccharides induce increases

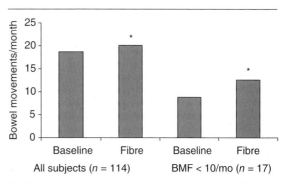

BMF: Bowel frequency.

Figure 12.3: Effect of fibre intake on constipation in older subjects.
Effect of fibre (finely processed pea hull fibre 4 g/day) on bowel movement frequency among elderly institutionalised residents. Data were collected for the same elderly residents before and during a six-week intervention. Results are shown for all subjects and for those with <10 bowel movements per month.
*Statistically different from corresponding baseline value, $p < 0.05$.
Source: Dahl *et al.* (2003).

in stool weight of 1.5–2.2 g per g carbohydrate (Cummings *et al.* 1992; Gibson and Roberfroid 1995; Heijnen *et al.* 1998).

Probiotics and prebiotics: It is not clear whether the changes in microflora apparent in older people are causally related to constipation, but it is known that changes in intestinal flora can alter intestinal motility (Husebye *et al.* 2001), and the short chain fatty acids produced by bacteria in the gut can influence transit time (Scheppach 1994). A potential approach to relieving constipation is, therefore, to increase the numbers of bifidobacteria and/or lactobacilli using pro- or prebiotics. A number of clinical trials have been conducted with conventional and probiotic-enriched yogurts and fermented milks in older subjects with constipation. These have been reviewed in detail by Pathmakanthan *et al.* (2000). Of seven studies, five showed significant laxative effects and one showed a significant improvement in transit time. In general, similar studies in younger subjects supported these results. For example, Alm *et al.* (1983) conducted a crossover study with acidophilus milk and buttermilk in 42 hospitalised geriatric patients and found a reduced need for laxatives during the acidophilus period. The largest study

(350 healthy older subjects) tested the effect in a double-blind parallel study of yogurt containing *Bifidobacterium animalis* DN-173-010 on oro–anal transit time. There was a significant, dose-related reduction in transit time with the effect lasting 2–6 weeks after the two-week period of consumption ceased (Meance *et al.* 1999). Ouwehand *et al.* (2002) reported that a commercially available mixture of *Lact. rhamnosus* LC705 and *Propionibacter freund-reichii* JS brought about a 24% increase in defaecation frequency in a group of older subjects.

The widely used laxative lactulose has prebiotic effects, as it is not digested by mammalian disac-charidases and stimulates numbers of bifidobacteria in the colonic flora that catabolise it to short chain fatty acids, creating an osmotic effect (Kot and Pettit-Young 1992). There are reports that other prebiotics such as fructooligosaccharides, galactool-igosaccharides and inulin may also exert mild laxa-tive effects, although in most studies the effects do not reach statistical significance. For example, Kleessen *et al.* (1997) found some subject-to-subject variation in their study comparing lactose and inulin given to older subjects in dosages of 20 g increasing to 40 g/day, but inulin had the more effective laxa-tive action; while Teuri and Korpela (1998) found that galactooligosaccharides (9 g/day) relieved con-stipation in some, but not all, older subjects.

Physical activity: Studies on the influence of physi-cal activity on gut transit and constipation have yielded inconsistent results. In a prospective study in 62,000 women aged 36–61 years, those who reported daily physical activity had a significantly lower prevalence of constipation (prevalence ratio 0.56) (Dukas *et al.* 2003). However, intervention studies in healthy subjects do not provide supportive evidence. For example, Coenen *et al.* (1992) found moderate physical activity (jogging) had no effect on oro–anal transit time (measured by radio-opaque markers) or stool frequency of 20 healthy young men in whom diet remained constant, although stool weight was increased.

In a similar study, Robertson *et al.* (1993) inves-tigated the effect of one week of moderate aerobic (treadmill) exercise on total GI and segmental colon transit in 16 men with a sedentary lifestyle. Total transit time was not significantly changed by the exercise (24.5 h before and 20.9 h after exercise). Meshkinpour *et al.* (1998) used longer periods of

moderate exercise (one hour a day, five days a week for four weeks) in eight subjects aged 27–72 years with chronic idiopathic constipation. The subjects were asked to maintain their routine dietary intake throughout the study. Again, there was no effect of exercise on constipation, assessed using an index that took into consideration three parameters of bowel function.

In a controlled, clinical intervention trial of regular daily exercise over a period of 32 weeks with 89 nursing home residents, bowel movement fre-quency, measured at baseline and 32 weeks, showed no significant change in the control or intervention group (Simmons and Schnelle 2004). Food and fluid consumption during meals was measured at baseline and 32 weeks and showed no change over time in either group. In contrast, a randomised, controlled study in middle-aged (>45 years) subjects with chronic idiopathic constipation found that a 12-week physical activity programme (30 min of brisk walking and a daily 11-min period of home-based exercise) significantly reduced three out of four of the Rome I criteria for constipation (De Schryver *et al.* 2005). Fibre and fluid intake was unchanged. Furthermore, the rectosigmoid and total colonic transit time decreased (from 17.5 to 9.6 h and 79.2 to 58.4 h, respectively; $p < 0.05$).

Overall, therefore, well-designed studies of sub-stantial duration have not shown a consistent effect of regular exercise, especially in older subjects and in those with chronic constipation.

12.5.3 Irritable bowel syndrome

Irritable bowel syndrome (IBS) is a highly prevalent disorder associated with a wide range of symptoms, including abdominal pain or discomfort, loose or hard stools, flatulence and bloating. It does not appear to be a disorder related to ageing and epide-miological evidence indicates that prevalence declines with age, although it remains common in older people (Bennett and Talley 2002). Generally, treatment of IBS in older people is focused on drugs rather than nutritional approaches. Increased fibre intake with adequate fluids may help patients with constipation, although symptoms of bloating may be aggravated (Bennett and Talley 2002). The ability of various probiotics, including *Lact. plantarum* v299, *Bif. infantis* 35624, *Lact. reuteri* and *Lact. aci-dophilus*, to ameliorate the symptoms of IBS has been studied in randomised placebo-controlled trials, over 1–6 months. The results of the nine trials are variable. Three trials, on *Lact. acidophilus* (Halpern *et al.* 1996), *Lact. plantarum* v299 (Niedzielin *et al.* 2001) and *Bifidobacterium infantis* 35624 (Whorwell *et al.* 2006), showed significant improvements in a wide range of symptoms, whereas others reported improvements in only one symptom. For example, *Lact. plantarum* DSM 9843 improved flatulence (Nobaek *et al.* 2000) and VSL#3 (probiotic mixture) improved bloating in one study (Kim *et al.* 2003) and flatulence in another (Kim *et al.* 2005). One study (on *Lact. reuteri*) showed no effect (Niv *et al.* 2005).

12.5.4 Diverticular disease

Diverticular disease is uncommon before the age of 40 years and the incidence increases with age. Many patients are asymptomatic or exhibit mild symptoms such as irregular defaecation. However, in others it presents with a wide range of symptoms, from abdominal pain, bloating, flatulence, diarrhoea, rectal bleeding and intestinal obstruction (diverticulosis) to inflammation, abscesses and perforation (diverticulitis, occurring in 10–25% of patients with diverticulosis) (Place and Simmang 2002). The majority of diverticula occurs in the sigmoid colon in western societies and consists of herniations of the mucosa and submucosa through the muscular wall of the colon. This is considered to be a consequence of the low bulk of the western diet causing intracolonic hypertension (Painter 1985). Epidemiological studies show an inverse relationship between dietary fibre intake and colonic diverticula and the principal treatment for diverticular disease is increased fibre intake. Consumption of 20–30 g per day of wheat bran is recommended (Place and Simmang 2002) and coarse bran appears to be more effective than finely ground bran (Smith *et al.* 1981). There is also epidemiological evidence that increased physical activity is protective (Aldoori *et al.* 1995).

12.5.5 Colorectal cancer

Ageing is the major risk factor for development of colorectal cancer: the incidence increases dramatically with age, from 10 per 100,000 at 40 years to 345 and 235 per 100,000 at 75 years for men and women respectively (Figure 12.4). Colorectal cancer

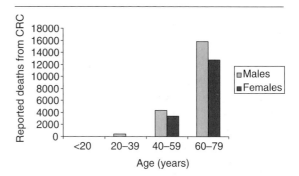

Figure 12.4: Reported deaths from colorectal cancer (CRC) in US, 1997.
Source: Greenlee *et al.* (2000).

is the fourth most common cause of cancer-related mortality in the world, accounting for 9.2% of all new cancer cases (Globocan 2002). In Europe, North America, Australia and New Zealand, it is the most common cancer after lung and breast (Boyle and Langman 2000).

Colorectal cancer is considered to develop via a sequence of changes to normal mucosa involving hyper-proliferation, adenoma formation and growth, and finally carcinoma. Extensive studies have identified specific genetic changes in various proto-oncogenes, tumour suppressor genes and DNA mismatch repair genes, as well as alterations in DNA methylation status and inherited genetic defects. In this adenoma–carcinoma sequence, at least 5–7 major molecular alterations need to occur for a normal epithelial cell to proceed to carcinoma (Fearon and Vogelstein 1990).

12.5.5.1 Nutritional strategies

Epidemiological evidence suggests that diet plays a significant role in the aetiology of colorectal cancer. However, identifying conclusively which constituents exert an effect on risk has been more problematic owing to inconsistent data (Heavey *et al.* 2004). Recent, prospective studies, including the European Prospective Investigation into Cancer and Nutrition (EPIC), a large (500,000 subjects) observational study in 10 European countries, have weakened the negative association previously found with fruit and vegetables, and overall the data for protective effects appear less convincing (World Cancer Research Fund/American Institute for Cancer Research 2007).

Dietary fibre intake has been identified in a large body of epidemiological and experimental studies to be associated with reduced risk (Department of Health 1998b; World Cancer Research Fund/American Institute for Cancer Research 2007). Furthermore, intervention trials with fibre supplements had no effect on recurrence of colorectal polyps (Alberts *et al.* 2000; Bonithon-Kopp *et al.* 2000). However, the EPIC study reported an adjusted relative risk of 0.58 for the highest (33 g/day) vs. lowest (12.6 g/day) quintiles of fibre intake, with a significant trend across the quintiles and a prediction of an 8% reduction in risk for each quintile intake of fibre (Bingham *et al.* 2003). No particular source of fibre was significantly more protective than another.

Red and processed meats appear to be associated with an elevated risk in nearly all studies (Department of Health 1998b; World Cancer Research Fund/American Institute for Cancer Research 2007). The latest results from the EPIC European Cancer study have reported hazard ratios (HR) for colorectal cancer of 1.42 for intakes of processed meat of >80 g/day vs. <10 g/day ($P_{trend} = 0.02$). For red meat the corresponding value was 1.17 and was not statistically significant ($P_{trend} = 0.08$) (Norat *et al.* 2005). It was not possible to determine if any particular type of processed or red meat was more strongly associated with colorectal cancer risk than others. It is noteworthy that the increase in colorectal cancer risk associated with red and processed meats combined was more apparent in groups with low (<17 g/day) and medium (17–26 g/day) fibre intake in comparison to those with high fibre intake (>26 g/day) with HR of 1.50, 1.20 and 1.09 respectively. The risk reduction associated with high fibre intake was of similar magnitude in all categories of intake of red and processed meat, indicating that a high fibre intake attenuates any risk associated with meat. There was no significant association with poultry, which is consistent with other cohort studies. Interestingly the EPIC study detected a significant inverse association with fish intake (>80 g/day vs. <10 g/day; hazard ratio 0.69; $P_{trend} = 0.001$) (Norat *et al.* 2005). However, such an association has not been found in most other prospective studies of fish and cancer risk.

In terms of specific nutrients and other dietary components, a high intake of saturated/animal fat is possibly related to increased risk (Potter 1999; Zock 2001). Additionally, several micronutrients, including carotenoids, ascorbate and folate, have been examined epidemiologically to seek an explanation of the protective effect associated with vegetables, but the results have frequently been discordant and, coupled with the paucity of data, no strong associations have been observed (Giovannucci *et al.* 1993, 1995, 1998; Glynn *et al.* 1996; Slattery *et al.* 1997; Kato *et al.* 1999; Su and Arab 2001).

Results of both cohort and case studies for calcium are inconsistent, although most evidence suggests a reduced risk of colorectal cancer or no association (Potter *et al.* 1993). However, a randomised, double-blind trial of 930 patients with a recent history of colorectal adenomas given calcium carbonate (3 g daily; 1200 mg elemental calcium) or placebo for four years found a lower risk of recurrent adenomas in subjects assigned calcium (Baron *et al.* 1999). The adjusted risk ratio of one or more adenomas was 0.81 (95% CI: 0.67–0.99); the adjusted ratio of the average number of adenomas was 0.76 (95% CI: 0.60–0.96). The effect of calcium seemed independent of initial dietary fat and calcium intake. These findings indicate that calcium supplementation had a modest protective effect against colorectal adenomas.

Studies in animal models provide evidence that pro- and prebiotics can beneficially influence various stages in the initiation and development of colon cancer. There is, however, limited evidence from epidemiological studies for protective effects of products containing pro- and prebiotics in humans, but recent dietary intervention studies in healthy subjects and in polyp and cancer patients have yielded promising results on the basis of biomarkers of cancer risk (decreased cell proliferation and reduction in DNA damage in rectal biopsies), and in terms of grade of colorectal tumours (Ishikawa *et al.* 2005; Rafter *et al.* 2007).

Alcohol has long been suspected as a risk factor for colorectal neoplasms, although results are inconsistent (Potter *et al.* 1993). The World Cancer Research Fund Report concluded that elevated alcohol consumption increases the risk of cancers of the colon and rectum, was convincing for men and probable for women (*i.e.* the evidence is stronger for men than women due to fewer data for women), and that this association is related to total ethanol intake rather than the type of alcoholic drink. Elevated risk is apparent at an intake of 30 g or more per day for both sexes (World Cancer Research Fund/American

Institute for Cancer Research 2007). In addition, in some cohort studies low folate intake in the presence of alcohol has been associated with a higher risk of colon cancer (Giovannucci *et al.* 1995; Glynn *et al.* 1996; Su and Arab 2001; Fuchs *et al.* 2002).

It should be mentioned that the majority of case-control and cohort studies have reported a significant protective effect of physical activity on colorectal cancer risk (Berglund 2002; World Cancer Research Fund/American Institute for Cancer Research 2007). Evidence is emerging of an increased risk of colorectal cancer among people who are obese (Frezza *et al.* 2006). Three prospective studies, the American Cancer Society's Cancer Prevention Study II (Murphy *et al.* 2000), the Framingham cohort (L.L. Moore *et al.* 2004) and EPIC (Pischon *et al.* 2006), have reported increased risk of colon cancer with increasing BMI and/or body weight. The effects were stronger in men than in women in all the studies. For example, the EPIC study found both bodyweight and BMI were significantly associated with increased risk of colon cancer in men (RR: 1.55, 95% CI: 1.12–2.15) but not women, and the Cancer Prevention Study II reported an RR of 1.90 (95% CI: 1.46–2.47) for men with a BMI > 32 kg/m^2 compared with an RR of 1.23 (95% CI: 0.96–1.59)

for women of the same BMI. In contrast, anthropometric measures of abdominal obesity (waist circumference and waist:hip ratio) showed significant increased risk for colon cancer in both men and women (Moore *et al.* 2004; Pischon *et al.* 2006). The second World Cancer Research Fund report concluded that the evidence for body fatness and abdominal fatness and colorectal cancer was convincing (World Cancer Research Fund/American Institute for Cancer Research 2007).

It may be concluded that consumption of diets high in vegetables and fibre and low–moderate amounts of processed and red meat, together with increased physical activity, could represent an effective strategy for reducing risk of colorectal cancer. Indeed, the conclusions of the UK COMA committee, which considered nutritional aspects of cancer risk (Department of Health 1998b), recommended an increase in fruit and vegetable consumption to at least five portions a day, with the emphasis on variety rather than any specific types and an increase in fibre intake from 12 to 18 g/day, again from a variety of food sources. The committee also suggested that high consumers of red meat (>140 g/day; 12–14 portions a week) should reduce their consumption to the current average of about 90 g/day.

12.6 Key points

- Recent studies suggest that, in older subjects (>65 years), disorders of the GI tract are the third most prevalent cause of visits to the GP.
- Gastro-oesophageal reflux disease (GERD) prevalence increases with age. GERD can lead to oesophagitis and in some instances to Barrett's oesophagus, which are risk factors for oesophageal adenocarcinoma. GERD is positively associated with BMI.
- Incidence of oesophageal cancer (squamous cell carcinoma and adenocarcinoma) increases with age. It is not a very common malignancy but it has a poor prognosis. Adenocarcinoma of the oesophagus has increased dramatically over the last 40 years and is now the predominant form of oesophageal cancer in the US and UK. Smoking and high alcohol consumption are risk factors for squamous cell carcinoma. There is epidemiological evidence that high consump-

tion of fruit and vegetables is protective for both types of cancer.
- The incidence of gastric and duodenal ulcers is increasing in older populations worldwide, the main risk factors being use of non-steroidal anti-inflammatory drugs and *H. pylori* infection.
- The prevalence of atrophic change of the gastric mucosa generally increases with age, as does intestinal metaplasia and gastric carcinoma.
- In older people, atrophic gastritis is an important cause of poor vitamin B$_{12}$ status.
- The crucial role of *H. pylori* in the development of chronic atrophic gastritis and gastric cancer means antibiotic treatment is a primary means of prevention and therapy in infected subjects.
- A consistent association exists between gastric cancer risk and low intakes of fruit and vegetables, which has been attributed to intake of

Continued

antioxidant micronutrients and vitamin C in particular.

- Studies in humans have not shown any age-related morphological changes in the small intestine in terms of surface structure, crypt depth, villous height, brush border and Brunner glands. Evidence for age-related changes in small intestinal hydrolases is limited and inconsistent.
- Diarrhoea is a significant worldwide problem; about 85% of deaths associated with diarrhoea in the developed world involve older people.
- There is evidence that the gut microflora of the colon alters with age, with an increase in species diversity and fewer bifidobacteria. The implications for health have not been established. Prebiotics have been shown to increase the numbers of bifidobacteria, but there are few studies in older people.
- Probiotics show considerable promise as therapies for antibiotic-associated diarrhoea and there is some evidence for efficacy of *S. boulardii* for *C. difficile* associated diarrhoea, although more extensive trials, particularly in older people, are needed in the latter area. Further studies are also required to investigate the role of prebiotics on antibiotic-associated diarrhoea.
- Bowel dysfunction is a major problem for older people, especially constipation. The effect of adding dietary fibre to the diets of older people is variable, but some studies report success, especially when fibre is combined with increased fluid intake. Insoluble fibre, such as wheat bran, appears to be more effective in increasing stool bulk than soluble fibre, resistant starch or prebiotics. A number of intervention trials have

shown that probiotics relieve constipation in older subjects. In general, studies do not indicate that increased physical activity alleviates constipation.

- Diverticular disease is uncommon before the age of 40 years and increases with age. There is an inverse relationship between dietary fibre intake and colonic diverticula and the principal treatment for diverticular disease is increased fibre intake. Consumption of 20–30 g of wheat bran per day is recommended for people with diverticular disease.
- Colorectal cancer incidence increases dramatically with age. In Europe, North America, Australia and New Zealand it is the second most common cancer after lung cancer in men and breast cancer in women. Epidemiological evidence suggests that diet plays a significant role in the aetiology of colorectal cancer. Processed meats, and to a lesser extent red meat, appear to be associated with a slightly elevated risk. Case-control studies indicate that increased vegetable intake is associated with reduced risk, but a beneficial effect of fruit is less clear. Case-control and recent prospective studies indicate that high dietary fibre intakes are protective. Case-control and cohort studies have reported a significant protective effect of physical activity on colorectal cancer risk, with high levels of activity at work and leisure time throughout life appearing to carry the lowest risk (approximately 50% reduction). Recent prospective studies have indicated a significant effect of high body mass index or waist circumference on colon cancer risk, with the effects being more apparent in men than women.

12.7 Recommendations for future research

- In general, further research is needed to identify effective dietary interventions throughout life to help prevent a wide range of gastrointestinal disorders in later life.
- Impaired gastric motility with age appears to have consequences for malnutrition and other complications. There is a need to investigate the aetiology of the disorder and to elucidate the nutritional factors involved.

- Further investigations are recommended to extend promising data suggesting that probiotics may suppress *H. pylori* and reduce inflammation in the gastric mucosa.
- Further investigations are needed into the health implications for older people of the changes in gut microflora composition with age and the potential for modifying such changes by dietary means, *e.g.* with pre- and probiotics.

Continued

- Research is needed to develop more effective dietary and lifestyle strategies for alleviating and preventing constipation in older people.
- Research is needed to validate potential biomarkers of cancer risk and to assess the potential for modifying them by diet and physical activity.
- Randomised controlled trials are required to provide greater insight into the role of specific dietary components in the aetiology and prevention of cancers of the GI tract. Such trials will however need to employ validated biomarkers of disease, of which few are currently available.

- Further research is needed regarding the role of phytochemicals in reducing risk of GI cancer. Primary prevention trials with validated biomarkers of risk are needed.
- Studies of diet–gene interactions in large population groups, in which subjects are recruited prospectively according to genotype, are required to determine the impact of genetic influences on individual responses to dietary change in GI cancers.
- A better understanding of the intensity, frequency and duration of physical activity required to reduce cancer risk in older populations is needed.

12.8 Key references

Cancer Research UK (2007) UK oesophageal cancer statistics. info.cancerresearchuk.org/cancerstats/types/oesophagus.

Destro C, Maggi S and Crepaldi G (2003) Epidemiology of gastrointestinal disorders in the elderly. In *Aging and the Gastrointestinal Tract*. Ed. A Pilotto, P Malfertheiner and P Holt. Basel, Karger Press: 1–11.

Hoffmann JC and Zeitz M (2002) Small bowel disease in the elderly: diarrhoea and malabsorption. *Best Practice & Research: Clinical Gastroenterology*, **16**, 17–36.

Pathmakanthan S, Meance S and Edwards CA (2000) Probiotics: A review of human studies to date and methodological approaches. *Microbial Ecology in Health & Disease*, **12 (Suppl 12)**: 10–30.

World Cancer Research Fund (2007) *Food, Nutrition, Physical Activity and the Prevention of Cancer: A Global Perspective*. Washington, DC, American Institute for Cancer Research.

13
Healthy Ageing: The Endocrine System

13.1 Introduction

This chapter considers the impact of ageing on the endocrine system and highlights interactions with disease, focusing on conditions known to be important in older people and those that may be influenced by diet or physical activity.

The endocrine system is one of two major communication systems within the body (the nervous system being the other) and is involved in all the body's functions. Hormones are produced in one organ or cell and travel in the blood to a target organ or cell where they regulate function. Hormonal regulation of some physiological processes involves a hierarchy of responses, using a series of chemical signals coordinated by the hypothalamus, which acts on input from the central nervous system. A key group of hormones within the hierarchy are the tropic hormones, which stimulate hormone production from other endocrine glands, such as thyroid stimulating hormone (TSH) which increases output of thyroid hormones, and follicle stimulating hormone (FSH), which influences output of female sex hormones.

There are a large number of endocrine glands, such as the thyroid, pituitary, adrenal and parathyroid glands, the ovaries, testes and pancreatic islets. Also, organs such as the heart, liver and gastrointestinal (GI) tract have an endocrine role, along with other functions. Some individual glands produce a number of different hormones (*e.g.* the pituitary gland), and some hormones are produced by more than one type of endocrine gland, for example, somatostatin is produced by the pancreas (where it inhibits the release of another hormone, somatotropin) and the GI tract (where it inhibits gastric secretion and motility). Different tissue types may respond differently to the same hormonal signal and a particular hormone; for example, insulin can trigger a number of different systemic physiological effects. Most hormones initiate a cellular response by combining with a specific intracellular or membrane-associated receptor protein; there may be several different receptors that recognise the same hormone and activate different signal transduction pathways. Consequently, hormonal signalling is very complex.

There are three classes of hormones, all of which regulate the function of their target cells, *i.e.* cells that express a receptor for the hormone:

- amine hormones are nitrogen-containing derivatives of the amino acids tyrosine and tryptophan (*e.g.* thyroxine and catecholamines);
- peptide hormones are the most abundant (*e.g.* insulin, growth hormone, thyroid stimulating hormone [TSH]);
- lipid-derived hormones (*e.g.* steroid hormones such as testosterone and cortisol, and sterol-derived hormones such as vitamin D [1,25-dihydroxy D3]).

A large number of other hormone-like substances, known as cytokines, are also produced; these act more locally as cell-to-cell signalling proteins. Cytokines are involved in a diverse number of immunological and inflammatory responses and infectious diseases (see Chapter 11, Sections 11.1 and 11.2.7) but also in developmental processes during embryogenesis. For example, in the face of infection, cytokines signal immune cells to travel to the site of infection and in addition activate cells, stimulating them to produce more cytokines. Adipokines are cytokine signalling molecules originating specifically from, or expressed in, adipose tissue. Examples of adipokines include tumour necrosis factor-alpha (TNF-α), interleukin-6 (IL-6), leptin, adiponectin (see Chapter 11, Section 11.2.7). As with hormones, cytokines bind to receptors and whereas there seems to be some degree of duplication (or redundancy) in the functions of specific cytokines, the receptors themselves appear remarkably function-specific and many authorities are now of the opinion that classification of cytokine receptors on the basis of their three-dimensional structure may be clinically useful, not least because a deficiency of cytokine receptors has been linked to debilitating immunodeficiency.

13.2 The endocrine system and the effects of ageing

Hormonal changes are associated with ageing, perhaps because endocrine organs have decreased functional reserves causing hormone secretion to fall, because hormone receptors become less responsive or sensitive to hormones or because the 'normal' range changes with age (Morley 2001). This section highlights some of the changes observed.

Over the past 15 years it has become evident that lifespan can be prolonged by mutations in genes that regulate endocrine signalling pathways. A review by Russell and Kahn (2007) describes how alterations in endocrine signalling in a group of cells or a single tissue can influence lifespan, which they suggest indicates that cross-talk between tissues coordinates the ageing of the organism. They propose that these endocrine pathways may serve as targets for the manipulation of the ageing process and prevention of age-related diseases.

An association between endocrine signalling and lifespan has been recognised for many years, stemming from work with lower species such as flies. Findings in several model organisms suggest that the relationship between decreased insulin levels and longevity might not be an epiphenomenon, particularly as a lower insulin level coupled with normal blood glucose is a consistent characteristic of food-restricted animals, and food restriction without malnutrition prolongs the lifespan of animal species, from single-cell organisms to mammals (Russell and Kahn 2007) (see Chapter 2, Section 2.5). To date, the insulin-like growth factor-1 (IGF-1) signalling pathways of worms and flies are the best studied models, but similar pathways exist in mammals and

have been studied in IGF-1 receptor-mutant mice, for example. In mammals, owing to the key role of insulin in the regulation of carbohydrate and lipid metabolism, dramatic reductions in insulin signalling lead to metabolic disarray and shortened lifespan. In non-obese, otherwise healthy humans, insulin resistance is a predictor of age-related disease.

As well as involvement of peptide hormone receptor signalling, which is now well established (see Section 13.2.1), a role for lipophilic hormones, including steroid hormones, has been identified in model systems (Russell and Kahn 2007). Based on work in mice and lower species, a role for steroid hormones (*e.g.* pregnenolone, oestrogen) has been proposed, involving the class O forkhead box transcription factor, FOXO1, but supportive evidence in mammals is still very limited.

Hofman and Swaab (2006) have proposed the existence in older people of progressive disruption to what they call the circadian pacemaker. The suprachiasmatic nucleus (SCN) located in the hypothalamus is considered to be a critical component in the timing of a wide variety of biological processes. The circadian cycles established by this biological clock occur throughout nature and have a period of approximately 24 hours. With advancing age, however, these daily fluctuations deteriorate, leading to disrupted cycles with reduced amplitude.

In humans, alterations in the regulation of circadian rhythms are thought to lead to an imbalance of the hormonal system and contribute to the symptoms of a number of conditions for which the risk is increased in old age (*e.g.* sleep disturbances, dementia and depression). This may exacerbate the impact of characteristics of the ageing process. It appears that the disruption of circadian rhythms and the increased incidence of disturbed sleep during ageing are paralleled by age-related alterations in the neural and temporal organization of the SCN and a decreased photic input to the clock, *i.e.* the biological clock is synchronised to the environmental light–dark cycle by photic information from the retina to the SCN in the hypothalamus. The many lines of evidence of age-related decrements in circadian timekeeping and the observed neuronal degeneration of the SCN in senescence strongly suggest that the circadian pacemaker in the human brain becomes progressively disturbed during ageing. If light is important, disturbance in processing of light information in older people and in some neurode-generative diseases may have a profound effect on the timing of a variety of physiological and behavioural activities, including sleep.

13.2.1 The growth hormone/insulin-like growth factor-1 axis

Growth hormone (GH) release and IGF-1 synthesis decrease with increasing age. The regulation of the GH/IGF-1 system is dependent on the integrity of the hypothalamus, pituitary and liver. During ageing there are several changes that contribute to the decline in GH/IGF-1, including changes in the signal to the somatotrophes from the growth hormone-releasing hormone somatostatin. Other relevant factors include body composition, exercise, diet and sleep. All of these factors are discussed in detail in Sherlock and Toogood (2007). The phenotypic similarities between ageing and adult growth hormone deficiency syndrome, combined with this decrease in GH/IGF-1 with ageing, have prompted the question whether ageing is a GH-deficient state and therefore whether GH may have a role as an 'anti-ageing' drug. The advent of recombinant growth hormone has led to a number of studies treating older patients with GH alone or in combination with sex steroids or exercise. However, Sherlock and Toogood conclude that the results do not support the use of GH in older patients with normal pituitary function as they did not show efficacy and reported high rates of serious adverse events (*e.g.* peripheral oedema, impaired glucose tolerance/diabetes mellitus, carpal tunnel syndrome), which were dose-dependent and resolved with dose reduction or drug discontinuation. There is also some evidence associating GH/IGF-1 with increased cancer risk.

13.2.2 Insulin and related hormones

Age-related changes in insulin secretion and/or function may, at least in part, be responsible for the increased number of older adults with type 2 diabetes (see Section 13.3.1 and Chapter 10, Section 10.5). Although the mechanisms are not understood, it is generally acknowledged that ageing is associated with a decline in beta-cell function, the pancreatic cells that produce insulin (Thearle and Brillantes 2005). There appears to be a decrease in the normal

pattern of insulin secretion among older adults; decreased frequency and amplitude of normal periodic pulses of insulin secretion during the fasting state and during glucose infusion have been observed (Scheen *et al.* 1996; Meneilly *et al.* 1997, 1999). However, there is a great deal of variability in beta-cell function. For example, it can be affected by weight loss, and in a study of obese patients with type 2 diabetes, weight loss led to an increase in beta-cell activity (Ferrannini *et al.* 2004). It is also worth noting that normal fasting insulin levels in older adults may reflect a deterioration in insulin secretion as insulin clearance from the blood may be decreased (Thearle and Brillantes 2005).

There are a number of glucose-stimulated gut hormones (incretin hormones) that affect the release of insulin (see Chapter 12, Section 12.4.1.4). Examples include glucose-dependent insulinotrophic polypeptide (GIP, also known as glucose-dependent insulinotrophic polypeptide) and glucagon-like peptide-1 (GLP-1). GIP's main action is stimulation of glucose-dependent insulin secretion, while GLP-1 does this as well as stimulating insulin biosynthesis and inhibiting glucagon secretion and gastric emptying, and food intake. Basal levels of the incretin hormone GIP do not seem to be affected by ageing; however, there is a suggestion that beta-cell sensitivity to GIP may be impaired in older people, which may contribute to a decrease in glucose-induced insulin release in normal ageing (Meneilly *et al.* 1998). Similarly, it is thought that decreased beta-cell sensitivity to the incretin hormones GLP-1 and GIP may account for the increased levels of these hormones seen following a glucose challenge in older subjects, *i.e.* a greater amount of these hormones is produced in an attempt to compensate for their decreased effect on the beta-cells (Thearle and Brillantes 2005).

13.2.3 Hormones relating to feeding

In addition to changes in taste, flavour perception and dentition that occur with ageing (see Chapter 3), a number of hormones influence feeding. It has been suggested that changes in endocrine factors with age may contribute to the decrease in appetite and food intake seen in some older adults. In older individuals there appears to be a decrease in feeding drive and an increase in satiety signalling, thus diminishing appetite and causing the so-called 'anorexia of ageing'. This is reflected in appetite scales, which confirm that older people are less hungry and have a higher degree of satiety during fasting than their younger counterparts (Sturm *et al.* 2003).

Cholecystokinin (CCK) regulates gastric motility and secretion, gall bladder contraction and pancreatic enzyme secretion, as well as having a possible role in satiety. Current evidence suggests that increased activity of CCK and decreased levels of androgens (especially in men) with ageing may contribute to the anorexia of ageing. CCK elicits a dose-dependent reduction in food intake in young healthy individuals (Kissileff *et al.* 1981). It is present in greater concentrations in older people and there is a suggestion that, in undernourished older people, CCK concentrations are greater still (Berthelemy *et al.* 1992). Another satiety hormone, leptin, does not appear to differ between young and older individuals (Isidori *et al.* 2000; MacIntosh *et al.* 2001). However, its production is cyclical, dependent on adipose tissue mass and stimulated by inflammatory cytokines. Thus measuring blood concentrations on a single occasion may not truly reflect hormone activity. Furthermore, changes in the expression of the leptin receptor (b-Rb) are significantly correlated with age as well as adiposity, implying that leptin sensitivity declines with age, contributing to age-associated adiposity and metabolic syndrome (Wang *et al.* 2005).

Elevated leptin levels would be expected in individuals with low-grade chronic inflammation and reduced lean body mass, as seen in sarcopenia (see Chapter 6, Section 6.3). Other hormones that suppress hunger include α-melanocyte-stimulating hormone, cocaine and amphetamine regulating transcript, and corticotrophin-releasing hormone, although none have been specifically studied in relation to ageing.

Secretion of the appetite stimulant ghrelin may be affected by ageing (Chapman 2004). Ghrelin is produced mainly by the gastric mucosa and acts on the hypothalamus to induce feeding. However, reduced concentrations have been found in older rats compared with their younger counterparts (Liu *et al.* 2002) and there is some evidence that this is also true for humans (Rigamonti *et al.* 2002), especially undernourished older people (Sturm *et al.* 2003),

suggesting an additional mechanism of appetite suppression. Neuropeptide Y, orexin A and B, and melanin-concentrating hormone (MCH) also trigger appetite through the hypothalamic feeding centre, but again the effects of ageing on these hormone have not been studied.

13.2.4 Sex hormones

Hormones play an important role in sexual health. In men testosterone is essential for the production of sperm as well as having a role in maintaining sex drive. Androgens also have a role in maintenance of sexual drive in women, while other hormones control ovarian function. It has been suggested that age-related changes in the hypothalamus may be an important contributing factor in reproductive ageing (Brann and Mahesh 2005). As women age, their ovaries stop responding to follicle stimulating hormone and luteinising hormone, and the production of oestrogen and progesterone progressively slows down and eventually stops (menopause). For about 75% of women, the menopause is associated with vasomotor symptoms such as hot flushes and night sweats, which may be associated with sleep and mood disturbances (Utian 2005). There has been interest in the role of diet in controlling or alleviating such symptoms (see Section 13.4.4) and some studies have suggested that the increase in blood pressure in women after menopause is associated with the reduction in oestrogen synthesis or an imbalance between androgens and female sex hormones, but this needs to be substantiated (Pechere-Bertschi and Burnier 2004).

A decrease in sex steroids affects hormone-controlled skin functions, such as the function of keratinocytes, Langerhans' cells, melanocytes and sebaceous glands and the synthesis of hyaluronic acid (Sator *et al.* 2004). Hence oestrogen deprivation in women is associated with skin dryness, atrophy, fine wrinkling, poor healing and hot flushes. Epidermal thinning, declining dermal collagen content, diminished skin moisture, decreased laxity and impaired wound healing have been reported in post-menopausal women (Hall and Phillips 2005) (see Chapter 7, Section 7.6.5). Systemic hormone replacement treatment (HRT) has a beneficial effect on skin ageing and topical application of oestrogens may also have a positive effect.

Long-term supplementation with dehydroepiandrosterone (DHEA, an adrenal steroid) has also been suggested to benefit skin (*e.g.* improved hydration, epidermal thickness, sebum production and pigmentation) in healthy older people compared to those in a placebo group (Baulieu *et al.* 2000), but there is little consensus on the benefits of DHEA replacement therapy.

The sex hormones play a critical role in bone health (see Section 13.3.5). The sex steroids also influence the development and function of cells in the immune system (see Chapter 11). This leads to a gender difference in immune function, with premenopausal women having higher immunoglobulin levels and mounting stronger immune responses following immunisation or infection than men. Studies show that DHEA promotes the production of type I cytokines (IL-2 and IFNγ) and the development of cell-mediated immunity, while oestrogen fosters B-cell activation (Verthelyi 2001).

Many women experience weight gain around the time of the menopause and both cross-sectional and longitudinal studies suggest the reduction in oestrogen at menopause is an independent factor increasing intra-abdominal fat in women; interventions with oestrogen replacement therapy have been able to reduce the degree of central obesity (Tchernof *et al.* 1998). Changes in testosterone production may also play a role in intra-abdominal fat accumulation in both men and women (Beaufrere and Morio 2000) and testosterone replacement therapy in older men has been shown to attenuate central fat accumulation (Mayes and Watson 2004).

A long-term decline in testosterone, DHEA and cortisol with ageing has also been reported (Gray *et al.* 1991; Feldman *et al.* 2002). This decrease in testosterone has been associated with a decline in sexual function, a decrease in bone density and an atherogenic lipid profile, as well as fatigue, depression, a decrease in lean body mass and an increase in visceral fat and obesity (Wespes and Schulman 2002). The Baltimore Longitudinal Study of Aging also suggested a detrimental effect of lower circulating free testosterone concentrations on cognitive performance in older men (Moffat *et al.* 2002).

13.2.5 Hormones related to bone health

Bone, acting as a calcium reservoir, has an important role in calcium homeostasis. If plasma calcium levels drop, secretion of parathyroid hormone (PTH) increases. This leads to an increased release of calcium from bone via an increase in bone resorption. PTH also stimulates the production of 1,25 hydroxyvitamin D (1,25 $(OH)_2 D_3$), the active form of vitamin D, produced from precursors in the diet and/or from exposure of skin to sunlight (see Chapter 4, Section 4.2.3), causing an increase in intestinal absorption of calcium. Problems with PTH status may affect bone health. For example, hypoparathyroidism is associated with low bone turnover and high bone mass if it occurs once the skeleton is fully formed, while an excess of PTH (hyperparathyroidism) can lead to bone loss and may play a role in the development of osteoporosis.

It has also been suggested that there may be a slight increase in PTH with age. However, this increase could be in response to low vitamin D status (which was found in 6% and 10% respectively of free-living British men and women, and 38% and 37% respectively of institutionalised men and women), leading to less calcium being absorbed from the gut (Sawin 2001), and hence the fall in PTH with age may not be inevitable.

Oestrogen has a direct effect on cartilage and bone cells, with bone turnover being decreased by low levels of oestrogen possibly through inhibition of resorption. It has been suggested that oestrogen deficiency is the single most important factor in the development of osteoporosis in men and women (Raisz 2004a) (see Section 13.3.5). The role of testosterone in bone metabolism is less clear as it can be converted to oestrogen in many tissues, perhaps including bone tissue. However, studies suggest it may also have a role in stimulating bone formation and inhibiting resorption.

The major growth-regulating hormones, such as the GH-IGF axis (see Section 13.2.1) (Raisz 2004a), thyroid hormones (Vestergaard and Mosekilde 2002) and adrenal glucocorticoids (Canalis and Delany 2002) also influence skeletal growth and remodelling. While IGF-1 concentration seems to be positively associated with cancer risk in adults (see Section 13.3.4), IGF-1 is very important in prepubertal growth, with higher IGF-1 levels associated with an increase in bone mineral density. For example, the Avon Longitudinal Study of Parents and Children showed a positive association between protein intake, leg length and IGF-1, especially in boys (Rogers *et al.* 2006) (see Chapter 4 on bone).

13.2.6 Hormones related to muscle mass

Several hormones are known to be important in the regulation of muscle protein turnover, including testosterone, GH, IGF-1 and DHEA (Greenlund and Nair 2003) (see Chapter 6, Section 6.7).

13.2.7 The thyroid gland

A range of disorders can affect the thyroid gland. In addition to clinical hyperthyroidism (over-production of the thyroid hormones thyroxine and tri-iodothyronine) and hypothyroidism (under-production of the thyroid hormones), there is also sub-clinical hyper- and hypothyroidism. These conditions are characterised by normal serum levels of free thyroxine and tri-iodothyronine but mildly decreased serum levels of thyroid-stimulating hormone (thyrotropin) in sub-clinical hyperthyroidism and mildly increased serum levels of thyrotropin in sub-clinical hypothyroidism.

Thyroid abnormalities affect a considerable proportion of all populations, but seem to be more common in older populations (Laurberg *et al.* 1998). While hypothyroidism can occur at any age, the incidence increases from middle age onwards. For example, in a coastal area in the north-west of Ireland the prevalence of one form of hypothyroidism was 8.6% in women aged 50 years or more but only 0.9% in women aged 18–50 years (Bonar *et al.* 2000). Women appear to be more affected than men; *e.g.* in the US Framingham Study, 5.9% of women but only 2.3% of men aged 60 or over were found have a thyroid deficiency (Sawin *et al.* 1985).

Fewer studies have compared the prevalence of hyperthyroidism in older and younger populations. Wilson and colleagues (2006) found a prevalence of undiagnosed hyperthyroidism of 0.3% in a large group aged over 65 years in the UK, with an additional prevalence of previously diagnosed overt hyperthyroidism of 0.3%. However, the prevalence of sub-clinical hyperthyroidism is much higher than that of overt disease. Low serum thyroid stimulating hormone (TSH) levels have been reported in about 5% of older subjects (Parle *et al.* 1991), a value significantly higher than in younger age groups, and estimates of sub-clinical hyperthyroidism in older groups range from 0.8% (Pirich *et al.* 2000) to 5.8% (Parle *et al.* 1991).

Virtually every tissue in the body is affected by the thyroid hormones. They have a role in regulation of metabolic rate, brain development and function, and growth (Vander *et al.* 1990). Low levels of thyroxine can, in some cases, lead to an increase in blood cholesterol and therefore an increased risk of CVD (British Heart Foundation 2005b).

13.2.8 Hormones related to stress

Stress can be defined as internal or external events (stressors) which threaten or challenge an organism's existence and well-being, and the responses made to reduce the impact of such events (Faraday 2006). During periods of stress, corticotrophin-releasing hormone (CRH) is released from the hypothalamus, inducing the release of the adrenocortico-trophic hormone (ACTH) from the pituitary, which in turn activates the production and release of glucocorticoids from the adrenal gland (Pedersen *et al.* 2001). The adrenal medulla (the central part of the adrenal gland) releases norepinephrine (noradrenaline) and epinephrine (adrenaline) directly into blood, while the adrenal cortex (the outer covering of the gland) releases cortisol, a glucocorticoid, and a small amount of aldosterone (Foy *et al.* 2006). This pathway, known as the hypothalamic–pituitary–adrenal (HPA) axis, is the major regulator of stress responses.

The main consequence of activation of the HPA axis is a change in glucose metabolism. Glucocorticoids promote mobilisation of glucose from glycogen stores (they can regulate expression and/or activity of the membrane glucose transporter protein). This ensures that the glucose supply is maintained to essential tissues but uptake and metabolism in non-essential peripheral tissues is inhibited.

Ageing is correlated with increased glucocorticoid levels and may also be associated with an altered function of the HPA axis. Several studies involving patients with Alzheimer's disease have found disturbances in HPA axis function (Pedersen *et al.* 2001).

13.3 Effect of age-related changes in hormonal status on risk of disease

The diversity and complexity of the endocrine system means that it has the potential to influence health

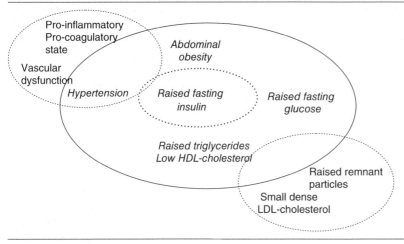

Figure 13.1: Cluster of disorders linked with resistance to normal insulin action. HDL: high-density lipoprotein; LDL: low-density lipoprotein. Source: Shaw *et al.* (2005). Reproduced by permission of Cambridge University Press.

and disease in a number of ways. Some examples pertinent to the topic are given below.

13.3.1 Diabetes

Diabetes mellitus is one of the most common chronic disorders and there are two distinct forms:

- Type 1 diabetes is characterised by partial or total failure of insulin production by the beta-cells of the pancreas. This type of diabetes usually appears before the age of 40. It is treated by insulin injections and diet, and regular exercise is recommended.
- Type 2 diabetes occurs when insufficient amounts of insulin are produced or the body's cells are less responsive to insulin (insulin resistance). Insulin resistance, a feature of the metabolic syndrome (see Figure 13.1 and Chapter 10, Section 10.4.3), is a risk marker for diabetes. Typically, insulin resistance is coupled with higher blood insulin levels, as individuals with insulin resistance need to produce more insulin to maintain their blood glucose levels (Bonora *et al.* 1998). Bodyweight and physical activity levels can directly affect insulin sensitivity; sedentary behaviours can lead to increased insulin requirements and are associated with a decreased ability to secrete insulin (National Institutes of Health, Lung and Blood Institute 1998; Turner and Clapham 1998). Around 90% of people with diabetes have this form of diabetes (see British Nutrition Foundation 2005).

Changes in glucose metabolism have been observed with age and increasing age is positively associated with risk of type 2 diabetes (Nugent 2004) (see Section 13.2.2 and Chapter 10, Section 10.5). The American National Health and Nutrition Examination Survey (NHANES) III found the prevalence of type 2 diabetes in those aged 60–74 years to be more than 20%, with an additional 20% meeting the criteria for impaired glucose tolerance. Similar levels were found in the previous NHANES study (Chang and Halter 2003). The Health Survey for England 2003 also showed that the prevalence of total diabetes increased with age; less than 1% of men and women aged 16–34 years reported having diabetes, while diabetes was reported by 2.8% of men and 1.5% in women aged 35–44 years and 10% and 8.9% respectively in those aged 75 and over. While these figures reflect both type 1 and type 2 diabetes, type 2 diabetes dominated, with <1% of all men and women having type 1 diabetes (Sproston and Primatesta 2004). There are ethnic differences with respect to risk of developing diabetes, *e.g.* in the UK, South Asians are more susceptible (see Chapter 14, Section 14.2.5).

13.3.2 Cardiovascular disease (CVD)

A protective role for the female sex hormones in CVD has been suggested from human observational studies and animal experimental studies. However, several large studies, including the Women's Health

Initiative Study (a primary prevention study) and two secondary prevention studies, the Heart and Estrogen/Progestin Replacement Study and the Women's Estrogen for Stroke Trial, did not find that hormone replacement therapy (HRT) gave protection from CVD; it actually increased risk (Brass 2004; Dubey *et al.* 2004).

13.3.3 Obesity

Excess body fat induces a wide range of metabolic changes, including insulin resistance, glucose intolerance, dyslipidaemia (see Chapter 10, Section 10.6.1), elevated blood pressure, impaired removal of blood clots from the circulation (fibrinolysis) and endothelial function, collectively referred to as the metabolic syndrome (Hauner 2002) (Figure 13.1) (see Chapter 10, Section 10.4.3 for more on the metabolic syndrome). It is now known that adipose tissue is metabolically active, producing more than 100 different factors. For example, it produces leptin, a protein with a cytokine-like structure that has a central role in fat metabolism (Hauner 2005). Circulating levels of most of the hormones produced by adipose tissue are positively related to body adiposity (Havel 2004). Human adipose tissue may also express the components of the renin-angiotensin system, and may be involved in the regulation of adipocyte formation and lipid metabolism (as angiotensin II produced in adipocytes may trigger conversion of pre-adipocytes to adipocytes, and increase lipid synthesis and storage in adipocytes), as well as involvement in the development of secondary diseases such as hypertension (Karlsson *et al.* 1998). The British Nutrition Foundation Task Force report (2005) on cardiovascular disease includes a chapter on these adipose tissue-derived factors.

Polycystic ovary syndrome (PCOS) is one of the most common endocrine disorders in women of fertile age (San Millan *et al.* 2004), with an estimated prevalence of 5–10% among pre-menopausal women (Hassan and Gordon 2007). A substantial proportion of women with PCOS are overweight and many are obese, but obesity *per se* is not considered to be the initiating event of the syndrome (Ehrmann 2005). PCOS is characterised by over-production of androgens (sex hormones) and irregular or no ovulation. It is often associated with peripheral insulin resistance (where the body's cells are less responsive to the action of insulin) and chronic hyperinsulinae-

mia, both of which are features of the metabolic syndrome (Pasquali and Gambineri 2006). Although its association with obesity is unclear, in older women obesity (particularly abdominal obesity) and PCOS increases susceptibility to impaired glucose tolerance and type 2 diabetes (Pasquali and Gambineri 2006). The American Diabetes Association recognises PCOS as a risk factor that justifies screening for type 2 diabetes (Ehrmann 2005).

13.3.4 Cancer

Hormonal factors have been identified as risk factors for some cancers, especially those of the breast and prostate. Of particular note are IGF-1 and its main binding protein (IGF-binding protein 3, IGFBP-3), which have been associated with increased risk of breast and prostate cancers, and exposure to oestrogen across the life-course, which increases the risk of breast, ovarian and endometrial cancers. The duration of exposure to oestrogen is increased by early menarche, late menopause, not bearing children and late (age >30) first pregnancy (World Cancer Research Fund/American Institute for Cancer Research 2007).

13.3.4.1 Breast cancer

Plasma levels of endogenous sex hormones (androgens and oestrogens) are major determinants of the subsequent occurrence of breast cancer after the menopause. Before the menopause, breast cancer risk is associated with high androgen levels and low progesterone levels in the luteal phase of the cycle. One of the most established risk factors in postmenopausal women is being overweight, which is associated with higher plasma levels of oestrogens (Franco 2006).

Pooled data from nine studies found that high levels of free oestradiol (the active form of oestrogen) more than doubled the risk of postmenopausal breast cancer; women with high levels of testosterone had a similarly increased risk of breast cancer (Key *et al.* 2002). Similar conclusions were reached in a review by Hankinson and Eliassen (2007).

The findings of studies considering synthetic hormones are inconsistent. On the one hand, no benefit on breast cancer risk was found in a large UK cohort study of oral contraceptive use (Hannaford *et al.*

2007). But Nelson and colleagues (2002) have reported that five or more years' use of HRT increases the risk of breast cancer and The Million Women Study also demonstrated an increased risk of breast cancer mortality with use of HRT (Beral and Million Women Study Collaborators 2003).

Serum levels of C-peptide and IGF-1 are also associated with the subsequent occurrence of breast cancer in prospective studies. These factors cooperate in stimulating breast epithelial cell proliferation and preventing apoptosis. Insulin resistance may also be important as insulin may increase the availability of both sex hormones (Franco 2006). A systematic review of case-control and nested case-control studies of IGF-1 and IGFBP-3 and cancer (Renehan *et al.* 2004) found a significantly increased risk for IGF-1 (OR: 2.08 (1.37, 3.15)) and a non-significantly increased risk for IGFBP-3 for premenopausal breast cancer. For postmenopausal breast cancer, there was a non-significant decrease in risk for IGF-1 and IGFBP-3. Findings from EPIC also showed an increased risk for postmenopausal but not premenopausal breast cancer for IGF-1 and IGFBP-3 (Rinaldi *et al.* 2006).

13.3.4.2 Prostate cancer

A systematic review of case-control and nested case-control studies of IGF-1 and IGFBP-3 and cancer found a significantly increased risk with high circulating levels of IGF-1 and a non-significantly decreased risk with elevated levels of IGFBP-3 (Renehan *et al.* 2004). The prospective Prostate, Lung, Colorectal and Ovarian Cancer Screening Trial examined associations between IGF-1 and IGFBP-3 and risk of prostate cancer; the IGF-1: IGFBP-3 molar ratio was associated with a doubling of risk in obese men. Risk was specifically increased for aggressive disease in obese men (OR 2.80, 95% CI: 1.11–7.08) (Weiss *et al.* 2007).

13.3.4.3 Other cancers

Most of the known risk factors for ovarian and endometrial cancers are related to hormonal and reproductive events (Lukanova and Kaaks 2005), although the results of studies are not consistent. Use of oral contraceptives significantly decreased risk of ovarian cancer and uterine body cancer in a

large UK cohort (Hannaford *et al.* 2007). The risk of invasive cervical cancer was non-significantly increased. With HRT, Nelson and colleagues (2002) concluded that unopposed oestrogen increases the risk of endometrial cancer, but mixed regimens (oestrogen and progesterone) do not.

For colorectal cancer, Nelson and colleagues (2002) reported a 20% reduction in risk with HRT use and Renehan and colleagues (2004) reported a significantly increased risk with raised IGF-1 and a non-significantly decreased risk with IGFBP-3. The EPIC study reported that hyperinsulinaemia, as determined by C-peptide levels, is associated with increased risk of colorectal cancer after adjustment for body mass index (BMI) and physical activity, but there was no clear association for IGF binding proteins 1 and 2 (Jenab *et al.* 2007).

13.3.5 Bone health

A number of hormones, including activated vitamin D, influence the risk of osteoporosis and fracture with ageing (see Chapter 4). Oestrogen deficiency has been recognised as a major cause of bone loss in the first decade after the menopause and a number of studies have found a strong relationship between endogenous oestrogen level and bone mass in both older men and women (see Raisz 2004a; see also Chapter 4).

Changes in the GH–IGF-1 axis (Section 13.2.1) may also contribute to age-related bone loss (Figure 13.2). It is estimated that GH secretion decreases by 14% per decade (Wolk 2004), accounting for the low serum IGF-1 concentrations seen in older men and women (along with reduced nutrient intake). Ageing can also affect circulating IGF binding proteins (IGFBPs), for example, increased serum IGFBP-4 levels have been observed in both men and women as they age, while IGFBP-3 and IGFBP-5 are lower in older adults compared with younger adults (Rosen 1999).

Studies have shown that small amounts of PTH given daily by injection can lead to increases in bone formation. A multinational study on postmenopausal women with prior vertebral fractures demonstrated that use of a synthetic fragment of PTH reduced risk of further vertebral fracture by 70% over 18 months of treatment. Non-vertebral fracture risk was reduced by 50% (Neer *et al.* 2001).

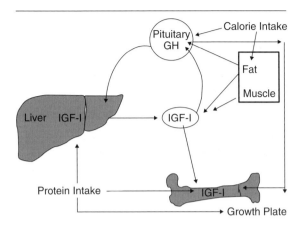

Figure 13.2: Nutrient regulation of systemic and skeletal IGF-1. Skeletal IGF-1 regulates trabecular bone, while systemic IGF-1 regulates cortical bone. GH: growth hormone; IGF-1: insulin-like growth factor 1.
Source: Rosen (2004). Reproduced with kind permission of Springer Science and Business Media.

13.3.6 Sarcopenia

The Amsterdam Longitudinal Aging Study found that higher PTH levels (≥4 pmol/L) were associated with an increased risk of sarcopenia compared with low PTH (<3.0 pmol/L) as measured by grip strength and muscle mass (Visser, Deeg *et al.* 2003).

Some, but not all, studies have found that men treated with testosterone have increased measures of muscle mass or strength (Brodsky *et al.* 1996; Katznelson *et al.* 1996; Bhasin *et al.* 1997; Synder *et al.* 2000) (see Chapter 6, Section 6.3.3). However, testosterone therapy may be associated with some adverse effects (P. Liu *et al.* 2004). GH deficiency results in loss of muscle mass and increased adipose mass. GH replacement can reverse this in both children and adults but its use in older adults remains controversial (Greenlund and Nair 2003) (see Section 13.2.1).

13.3.7 Stress

Repeated stress can inhibit neurogenesis (formation of new neurons) and dendritic remodelling. It has been suggested that chronic exposure to glucocorticoids can result in dendritic atrophy in hippocampal neurons in the brain, therefore impairing learning and memory processing (Pedersen *et al.* 2001).

13.4 The influence of diet and physical activity on the endocrine system

This section highlights certain dietary patterns, specific dietary components and lifestyle factors that may directly influence the endocrine system.

13.4.1 Appropriate weight and physical activity

While chronic energy (caloric) restriction has been shown to slow ageing in a variety of species, it is believed that this is unlikely to be the case for humans (see Chapter 2, Section 2.5). However, achieving an appropriate weight and being physically active are important for all age groups and have a number of benefits. Bodyweight and physical activity have been shown to influence the endocrine system. For example, physical activity has been shown to be beneficial in the treatment of sarcopenia, with combinations of aerobic and resistance exercise, and stretching programmes having well-established beneficial effects (Greenlund and Nair 2003) (see Chapter 6, Section 6.10). Physical activity has also been shown to decrease levels of testosterone (free and bound) in postmenopausal women, which may decrease breast cancer risk (McTiernan *et al.* 2004). Insulin sensitivity can be improved through regular physical activity and is therefore an important component in the prevention and treatment of diabetes (see Section 13.4.1.2).

13.4.1.1 Obesity

Weight reduction by dietary means can restore normal adipokine secretions. It is likely that improvements are proportionate to weight loss (Hauner 2005). Body size may also influence binding globulins, the carriers of hormones in the blood. For example, among the men in the Massachusetts Male Aging Study, sex hormone binding globulin (SHBG) was negatively associated with body size (both BMI and waist:hip ratio) as well as intakes of protein and animal fat, and was positively associated with intakes of fibre (Longcope *et al.* 2000). These observations may help explain some of the associations found between bodyweight (and testosterone) and prostate cancer. Similarly, work in postmenopausal women found that those who were obese had low levels of SHBG, which may increase breast cancer risk (Key *et al.* 2002).

13.4.1.2 *Diabetes*

Modification of weight and activity levels is an important aspect of prevention and treatment of type 2 diabetes (see Section 13.3.1 and Chapter 14, Section 14.2.5). Physical inactivity is associated with increased insulin resistance (IR), while an increase in activity level can increase sensitivity to insulin. The US Diabetes Prevention Program enrolled older adults with impaired glucose tolerance. Both metformin treatment and lifestyle changes (which aimed for 150 minutes of physical activity per week and 7% weight loss) significantly reduced incidence of diabetes by 31% and 58% respectively (compared with placebo). The lifestyle intervention was particularly effective in older people, with a 71% reduction in diabetes incidence (compared with an 11% reduction in incidence among those taking metformin in this age group) (Knowler *et al.* 2002). Similar findings have been reported in other studies (see Chapter 14, Section 14.2.5).

13.4.2 Carbohydrates and fibre

The quantity and quality of carbohydrate in the diet are major determinants of postprandial blood glucose concentrations and the resulting fluctuations in circulating insulin. There has, therefore, been much interest in carbohydrates with respect to diabetes and insulin resistance. The role of carbohydrate and fibre in the diet for management of diabetes is well established, with increased intakes of fruit and vegetables being advocated as well as regular meals based on starchy carbohydrates. A high-fibre diet is particularly recommended because studies have shown benefits in glycaemic control among people with type 2 diabetes (British Nutrition Foundation 2005; Lunn and Buttriss 2007). There is also a subsidiary role for low glycaemic index (GI) foods in the management of diabetes, with medium-term studies showing improvements in glycaemic control when high GI foods are replaced with low GI foods (Frost *et al.* 1994; Willett *et al.* 2002; World Health Organization 2003a; S. Kelly *et al.* 2004).

Research has also investigated the role of GI and glycaemic load (GL) in the prevention of diabetes. In the Nurses' Health Study, risk of developing diabetes was increased by 37% in the highest GI vs. lowest GI quintile and GL was also positively associated with diabetes (relative risk, RR: 1.47) (Salmeron *et al.* 1997a). Similarly, in the Health Professionals' Follow-Up Study, men with a high GI diet had an increased risk of diabetes (comparing the highest with the lowest quintile, RR: 1.37). Those men with a high GL diet and a low cereal fibre intake (<2.5 g/day) had a further increase in risk (RR: 2.50 when compared to men with a low GL diet and high cereal fibre intake) (Salmeron *et al.* 1997a). In contrast, The Iowa Women's Health Study found no significant association of either GI or GL with diabetes incidence (Meyer *et al.* 2000). This study used an older cohort, which may have introduced selection bias (Augustin *et al.* 2002). A strong inverse association was found, however, between diabetes incidence over six years and total grain, whole-grain, total dietary fibre and cereal fibre intake, after adjustment for non-dietary confounding variables. The multivariate adjusted relative risks for diabetes across quintiles of whole-grain intake were 1.0, 0.99, 0.98, 0.92 and 0.79 (for trend $p = 0.005$) (<3 servings/week in lowest quintile vs. >17.5 servings/week in highest quintile); across quintiles of total dietary fibre intake the relative risks were 1.0, 1.09, 1.00, 0.94 and 0.78 (for trend $p = 0.005$) (intake in lowest quintile of <15.3 g/day vs. >23.6 g/day in highest quintile) (Meyer *et al.* 2000).

The long-term effects of lower vs. higher postprandial blood glucose concentrations within the normal range need to be studied, as does the impact (if any) of an elevated insulin concentration (Lineback 2005). Longer-term studies are needed to confirm the impact of a lower GL/GI diet and whether any changes observed in short-term studies persist in the long term.

With respect to insulin sensitivity, it is known that a diet rich in carbohydrate can increase insulin output, which may exacerbate insulin resistance. However, the type of carbohydrate appears to be important and there are some studies suggesting that a diet based on low GI foods may improve insulin sensitivity (Frost *et al.* 1998; Brynes *et al.* 2003).

It has been suggested that dietary patterns that promote elevated plasma insulin (transiently by diet or by underlying insulin resistance) might increase the risk of breast cancer through an effect on IGF-1 activity (see Section 13.3.4). A large prospective study of women (n = 63,307) investigated the association between breast cancer risk and diets with a high GL. At five-year follow-up, there was no evidence of increased risk for breast cancer with high GL (RR: 0.90; 95% confidence interval, CI: 0.76–1.08; highest vs. lowest quintile) or GI (RR: 1.03; 95% CI: 0.87–1.22; highest vs. lowest quintile) (Jonas *et al.* 2003).

There is also interest in the effect of resistant starch (the portions of starch and starch products that resist digestion as they pass through the gastro-intestinal tract) on glycaemic and insulinaemic responses. At least 15 studies have found an improvement in these measures after a resistant starch-rich test meal, while 10 have found no effect or no physiologically relevant effect (for a recent review see Nugent 2005).

13.4.3 Plant-based diets

There is now considerable evidence that diets rich in plant foods are generally associated with a reduced risk of a range of chronic diseases. It has been suggested that plant-based diets could modulate disease risk through effects on steroid hormones (Lampe 1999). While not all studies have found hormonal differences between people following a vegetarian diet and those following an omnivorous diet (Bennett and Ingram 1990; Remer *et al.* 1998), some studies have. For example, a cross-sectional study found vegan women (eating no animal products) had a mean serum IGF-1 concentration that was 13% lower than that of both meat-eaters and vegetarians (those avoiding meat and fish but eating eggs and dairy products) ($p = 0.0006$). The mean concentrations of both serum IGF-binding protein-1 (IGFBP-1) and IGFBP-2 were 20–30% higher in vegan women compared with meat-eaters and vegetarians (Allen *et al.* 2002). Another small study found mean concentrations of prolactin were significantly higher in non-vegetarians and lacto-ovo-vegetarians than in vegans. On average, vegans (in comparison with non-vegetarians and lacto-ovo-vegetarians) had 48% higher concentrations of faecal oestrone and 35% higher levels of faecal oestrone plus oestradiol-17 β ($p < 0.01$). No differences were found between the three groups with regard to plasma oestrone, oestradiol-17β and testosterone (Pusateri *et al.* 1990).

13.4.3.1 Menopause onset and symptoms

Few studies have investigated the association between age at menopause and diet. A relatively small prospective study in Japan following 1,130 women over a six-year period found green and yellow vegetable intake was significantly inversely associated with menopause. Women in the highest tertile group for intake of these vegetables were 30% less likely to have entered menopause compared to those in the lowest group during the six-year period, after adjustment for a range of factors, including age, body mass index, smoking status and age at which regular menstruation began (Nagata *et al.* 2000).

It has been suggested that plant-based diets and in particular phytoestrogens (see Section 13.4.4) may affect the risk of ovarian cancer through their effect on endogenous hormones. Lower levels of oestradiol and its metabolite oestrone have been reported for women consuming vegetarian diets vs. omnivore diets and, while this link has not been conclusively proven, there is some evidence of a protective effect against ovarian cancer with components of a plant-based diet. Pooled analysis from 12 cohort studies showed a non-significantly reduced risk when comparing high- against lowintake groups (0.90, 95% CI: 0.78–1.04) (Koushik *et al.* 2005). The World Cancer Research Fund (WCRF) second expert report on 'Food, Nutrition, Physical Activity and Prevention of Cancer' reviewed evidence on non-starchy vegetables and green vegetables (World Cancer Research Fund/American Institute for Cancer Research 2007). Meta-analysis of four of the five cohort studies reporting on non-starchy vegetables showed a decreased risk (RR: 0.64 (0.33, 0.97)) for an increase of one serving a day. There was also evidence of a reduced risk for green vegetables. Together with the evidence from the pooling project, the Panel considered the evidence to be only 'limited-suggestive' of a protective effect of vegetables on ovarian cancer.

13.4.4 Phytoestrogen-containing foods

Phytoestrogens (isoflavones, lignans and stilbenes) occur in a range of plant foods, with soya beans and soya products being the major source of isoflavones in the diet. Linseed is a source of lignans, and stilbenes are widely distributed in plants including peanuts which contain resveratrol (Cassidy 2003). Phytoestrogens have structures similar to oestradiol and can bind weakly to oestrogen receptors (see Chapter 4, Section 4.2.8 for the role in bone health; Chapter 7, Section 7.12.4 for the role in skin ageing; Chapter 10, Section 10.7.7.3 for heart health and Chapter 14, Section 14.2.6 for cancer risk). It has been suggested that phytoestrogens may be beneficial in a number of hormone-related conditions, such as relief from menopausal symptoms and breast cancer, although evidence to support this has not always been forthcoming.

While a cross-sectional survey of Japanese women found an association between consumption of soy products and timing of the menopause, with women consuming higher amounts of soy products entering the menopause later, a prospective study by the same group failed to observe an association (Nagata *et al.* 1998, 2000). A recent systematic review concluded that the available evidence did not suggest phytoestrogens alleviated hot flushes or other menopausal symptoms (Krebs *et al.* 2004).

A network on the health aspects of phytoestrogens has been built around three EU-funded projects (PHYTOS, PHYTOPREVENT and ISO-HEART). This network, the PHYTOHEALTH Thematic Network, aims to establish a pan-European network of institutions dealing with safety and health effects of phytoestrogens, and identification of optimal sources and processing technologies. A critical review of the health effects of soy phytoestrogens in postmenopausal women by this network concluded that there was limited evidence that soy protein isolates, soy foods or red clover extract were effective in reducing hot flushes; soy isoflavone extracts may also be effective. The group found there were too few randomised controlled trials to draw any conclusions on the effects of isoflavones on breast or colon cancer or diabetes (Cassidy *et al.* 2006). The data with regard to bone health are unclear (see Chapter 4, Section 4.2.8) (British Nutrition Foundation 2003b).

There is some suggestion that diet–gene interactions may play a role. Low and colleagues (2005) found that urinary and serum levels of phytoestrogens were negatively correlated with plasma oestradiol among a small group of postmenopausal women, and a particularly strong association was found among those women with a specific polymorphism (CC genotype for ESR PvuII polymorphism).

13.4.5 Fat

There is evidence from studies in rodents that a very high fat intake (compared to a low fat intake) can cause insulin resistance, impair glucose tolerance and elevate glucose levels (Winzell *et al.* 2004), and it has been suggested that changes in cell membrane properties and changes in insulin receptor binding or activation may be involved (British Nutrition Foundation 2005).

Observational and prospective studies in humans have generally supported the hypothesis that unsaturated fatty acids have a protective role with regard to insulin resistance and saturated fatty acids a potentially harmful role. For example, in a study of healthy men and women there was no effect on insulin secretion but insulin sensitivity increased by 12% when saturates were replaced with monounsaturates (but only when the total intake from fat was below 37% of energy intake) (Vessby *et al.* 2001). It is unclear whether polyunsaturates have a similar effect to monounsaturates, although one crossover study of short duration found insulin sensitivity to be increased after a polyunsaturates-rich diet (Summers *et al.* 2002).

There has also been interest in the effects of long chain *n*-3 polyunsaturates on insulin sensitivity because of the protective effect of fish consumption in type 2 diabetes seen in epidemiological studies. A review by another British Nutrition Foundation Task Force concluded that while there was moderately strong evidence for an effect of long chain *n*-3 fatty acids on insulin sensitivity among people with type 2 diabetes, this benefit has not been seen in 'healthy' people without diabetes (British Nutrition Foundation 2005).

Work in animals (Winzell *et al.* 2004) suggests that there may be a role for adiponectin in modifying insulin secretion during insulin resistance, possibly by helping the pancreatic islets to compensate for the reduced insulin action.

13.4.6 Protein

Severe protein under-nutrition can impair GH secretion and leads to even lower levels of IGF-1 in older adults (Rosen 2004). The Health Professionals' Follow-Up Study found that among 753 generally well-nourished men (middle-aged or older), plasma IGF-1 and the ratio of IGF-1 to IGF-binding protein tended to increase with higher intakes of protein (and minerals, including potassium, zinc, calcium and phosphorus). The major sources of protein (including vegetable protein, milk, fish and poultry but not red meat) were associated with an increase in IGF-1 levels. Energy intake was positively associated with plasma IGF-1 level, but only in men with BMI <25 kg/m^2. The authors suggest that the age-related decline in IGF-1 may be exacerbated by low protein and mineral intakes (Giovannucci *et al.* 2003).

In a small ($n = 82$), randomised, double-blind placebo-controlled trial, serum levels of IGF-1 increased in older adults with recent hip fracture who received a protein supplement (20 g/day) for six months; proximal femur bone loss was also attenuated, resulting in shorter hospital stays (Schurch *et al.* 1998).

13.4.7 Iodine

Diets that are deficient in iodine, as well as those which contain an excess, have been associated with thyroid tumour formation in humans and experimental animals. Low levels of dietary iodine cause a decrease in the level of thyroid hormones, therefore increasing the release of thyroid stimulating hormone (TSH) from the pituitary gland. High levels of TSH can lead to increased production of thyroid follicular cells as well as an increase in cell size, leading to an enlargement of the gland (goitre). On the other hand, elevated TSH levels can occur with long-term excessive intakes of iodine by blocking the uptake of iodine by the thyroid gland. Iodine intakes of older UK adults have generally been found to be adequate; average intakes for free-living men and women being 134% and 106% of the reference nutrient intake (RNI) respectively. For those men and women living in institutions, intakes of the RNI were 138% and 125% respectively (Finch *et al.* 1998). However, elsewhere in the world (*e.g.* the Middle East) iodine deficiency is common, whilst in parts of Europe (*e.g.* Switzerland), it is prevented by use of iodised salt.

While some plant foods contain compounds referred to as goitrogens that can impair iodine metabolism leading to an increase in TSH secretion, there is no evidence from human studies that goitrogens increase the risk of cancer.

13.4.8 Zinc

Zinc deficiency is associated with reduced IGF-1 levels, which can be normalised by zinc supplementation (Allen *et al.* 2005). However, the exact role of zinc with respect to IGF-1 levels is unclear. While one study in postmenopausal women found zinc intake to be strongly correlated to IGF-1 levels (Devine *et al.* 1998), two other studies, including one in older adults, did not find a correlation between these two factors (Allen *et al.* 2002).

13.4.9 Other dietary components

It has been suggested that lycopene (a carotenoid present in tomatoes and tomato-based products) may be able to modulate hormones important in prostate cancer (see Section 13.3.4.2). For example, in a prostate cancer model, lycopene (200 ppm) and vitamin E (540 ppm) supplementation interfered with local testosterone activation by down-regulating 5-alpha-reductase and consequently reduced steroid target genes expression (Siler *et al.* 2004). A very small trial of men with metastatic hormone refractory cancer ($n = 20$) suggested that lycopene may have a role in treatment, but larger, controlled studies would be needed to substantiate this (Ansari and Gupta 2004). However, the European Prospective Investigation into Cancer and Nutrition (EPIC) found no significant associations between fruit and vegetable consumption and prostate cancer risk (Key *et al.* 2004a). The WCRF second expert report on 'Food, Nutrition, Physical Activity and Prevention of Cancer' reviewed evidence on the effect of foods containing lycopene on prostate cancer. The Panel considered there was a substantial amount of consistent evidence that tomato products probably protect against prostate cancer. Meta-analysis of cohort studies on serum or plasma lycopene, which are likely to be more precise and accurate than dietary assessments, showed a 4% decreased risk per 10 µg lycopene/L. Studies of cumulative lycopene intake or of tomato sauce products (from which lycopene is highly bioavailable) showed a statistically significantly decreased risk (World Cancer Research Fund/American Institute for Cancer Research 2007).

Although it is referred to as a vitamin, the active form of vitamin D (1,25 dihydroxyvitamin D) is an important factor in bone health (see Chapter 4,

Section 4.2.3) and is now thought to have a role in a variety of other aspects of health (see Chapter 14).

There has been some interest in coffee and its association with type 2 diabetes. A recent systematic review supported the hypothesis that habitual coffee consumption is associated with a substantially lower risk of type 2 diabetes (relative risk of type 2 diabetes was 0.65 (95%, CI: 0.54–0.78) for the highest (six or more cups per day) and 0.72 (95% CI: 0.62–0.83) for the second highest (4–6 cups per day) category of

coffee consumption vs. the lowest consumption category (≤2 cups per day) (van Dam and Hu 2005). A possible mechanism for this association has been suggested following a small, three-way, randomised crossover study, which found that caffeinated coffee significantly altered the secretion of GIP and GLP-1 (see Section 13.2.2) compared with the control (Johnston *et al.* 2003). However, longer-term intervention studies are needed on coffee consumption and glucose metabolism to explore the possible underlying mechanisms.

13.5 Key points

- The endocrine system is one of the major communication systems in the human body. Hormones are produced in one organ or cell and travel in the blood to a target organ or cell, where they elicit a response.
- The endocrine system plays an important role in health and is involved in all of the body's functions. Hormonal imbalances and dysfunctions are associated with a number of diseases, including chronic conditions such as diabetes, cardiovascular disease, obesity and some cancers.
- Older age appears to be associated with a number of changes to the endocrine system. These include a decrease in hormone secretion, a decrease in the sensitivity of the body's tissues to these hormones, and a change in hormone binding capacity/efficiency. Relatively little is known about hormones and ageing, especially with respect to different ethnic groups. However, there is now particular interest in some aspects of the endocrine system, *e.g.* the growth hormone/insulin-like growth factor-1 axis.
- Dietary treatment of type 2 diabetes has focused on modification of bodyweight and activity levels. A high-fibre diet, rich in fruits and vegetables, is advocated. More recently glycaemic index (GI) and glycaemic load (GL) have been

included in some treatment plans, although the role of GI and GL in prevention of type 2 diabetes remains to be proven.

- The role of diet and physical activity in modulating hormonal changes is a relatively new area of research. Diets rich in plant foods are generally associated with a reduced risk of a range of chronic diseases. It has been suggested that plant-based diets might modulate disease risk through effects on steroid hormones, but this remains to be shown.
- It has been suggested that because of their structural similarity to oestrogen, phytoestrogens may be beneficial in a number of hormonal-related conditions. However, evidence of their ability to reduce hot flushes in menopausal women remains conflicting and there is, as yet, insufficient evidence to draw conclusions about the effects of phytoestrogens in diabetes, colon cancer or breast cancer or bone health.
- There is growing evidence that the quality and quantity of dietary fat can affect hormones that may impact on a number of health outcomes, including insulin resistance, and perhaps even some cancers.
- It appears that protein and perhaps zinc may affect a number of hormones, including growth hormone and insulin-like growth factor-1.

13.6 Recommendations for future research

The role of diet and physical activity in modulating hormonal changes is a relatively new area of research. Further work is needed to explore the effects of diet (including dietary patterns and specific components) and physical activity on the ageing endocrine system and the impact of dietary and lifestyle changes in relation to risk of disease and ill health in later life. For example:

- The long-term effects on health of higher post-prandial blood glucose concentrations within the normal range need to be investigated further.

- Well-designed studies are required to investigate the ability of phytoestrogens to reduce menopausal symptoms, especially given the consumer interest in alternative treatments and concerns about hormone replacement therapy.
- Further research is needed to investigate the effect of various nutrients on a number of hormones, including growth hormone and insulin-like growth factor-1, given the important role these hormones have in bone health and other body systems.

13.7 Key references

Hannaford PC, Selvaraj S, Elliott AM, *et al.* (2007) Cancer risk among users of oral contraceptives: cohort data from the Royal College of General Practitioners' oral contraception study. *British Medical Journal*, **335**, 651.

Morley JE (2001) Hormones, aging and endocrine disease in the elderly. *Endocrinology and Metabolism* 4th edition. Ed. P Felig and LA Frohman. New York, McGraw-Hill: 1455–82.

Russell SJ and Kahn CR (2007) Endocrine regulation of ageing. *Nature Reviews Molecular Cell Biology*, **8**, 681–91.

14
Taking the Science Forward:
Public Health Implications

14.1 Introduction

Ageing begins at birth and increases in rate at puberty (House of Lords 2005). Once adulthood is reached, the annual risk of dying approximately doubles with every eight additional years that pass (Figure 14.1). The traditional view that the ageing process is controlled by self-destruct programming has largely been abandoned in favour of the concept that ageing is the result of a gradual build-up of subtle defects in the cells and organs that constitute the human body, which eventually disrupt cell function, with genes (and possibly nutrient supply) influencing repair to this molecular damage (see Figure 14.2) (Chapter 2, Section 2.2).

This change in thinking indicates that the ageing process is more malleable than generally assumed and that the mechanisms governing health in old age are functioning throughout life. It also opens up the prospect of healthy ageing. Nutrition, lifestyle and environment all have the potential to influence the rate at which damage to cells is accumulated, by modifying exposure to intrinsic and extrinsic triggers of damage or by acting via the body's repair and maintenance processes (Figure 14.2). These factors may in turn be modified by socio-economic circumstances (Kirkwood 2006).

Research is gradually unravelling how and why we age and what opportunities might exist for intervention, but there is considerable variability in individual health trajectories through life and also difficulties associated with applying objective measures of health and quality of life across different age groups. A House of Lords report (2005) suggests that freedom from disability provides a more easily ascertainable objective measure of the quality of life. However, regardless of which measure is adopted,

there is a period (about eight years for men and 11 years for women) during which older people regard themselves as not being in generally good health, or as having a limiting long-standing illness or disability. The evidence suggests that this period of perceived ill health is not decreasing and may well be increasing (House of Lords 2005) (Figure 14.3).

This Task Force Report has discussed the effect of ageing on various organ systems and the purpose of this chapter is to integrate current evidence on how a life-course nutrition and physical activity approach may minimise or even negate the effects of ageing. A life-course approach is recognised as important because the risk of chronic disease is not only influenced by adult life experiences; risk factors often begin to take effect in early life onwards.

Over the past century there have been considerable improvements in life expectancy, which has almost doubled in some parts of the world (see Chapter 1, Section 1.1.1). As a result of this and also the concomitant fall in birth rate in recent years in many parts of the world, the proportion of older people in the population is rising, a trend that is set to continue. Growth of 223% is estimated for the period 1970–2025, so that by 2025 there will be around 1.2 billion people over the age of 60 years (see Chapter 1, Section 1.1.1). Across Europe, the proportion of the population over the age of 60 years has been increasing. In 2002, it had reached 20–25% in countries such as Italy, Spain, France and the UK, and it is expected to reach 30–35% in these countries by 2025 (World Health Organization 2002a). In Britain, women tend to live longer than men, although the gap is narrowing. In 1951 there were 77 men aged 50 years and over for every 100 women of the same age. By 2003, the proportions were 85 men per 100 women and by 2031 there are

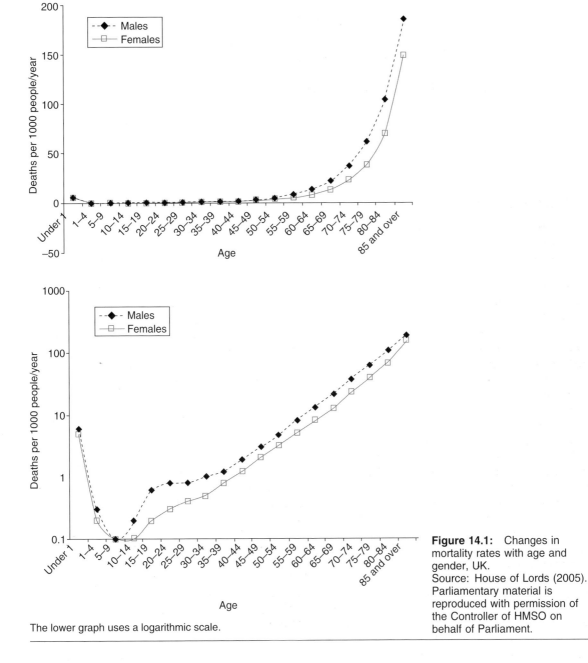

Figure 14.1: Changes in mortality rates with age and gender, UK.
Source: House of Lords (2005). Parliamentary material is reproduced with permission of the Controller of HMSO on behalf of Parliament.

The lower graph uses a logarithmic scale.

expected to be 90 men per 100 women aged 50 years and over (www.statistics.gov.uk). Among people aged over 85 years, the ratio in 2003 was 40 men per 100 women and this is expected to rise to 65 per 100 by 2031. These trends carry considerable public health implications, especially as experience of long-standing illness (see Chapter 1, Section 1.2) and associated medical spending (see Chapter 1, Section 1.4) increases with age.

In this chapter, the term health embraces quality of life issues (*i.e.* self-esteem, independence and socio-economic security) as well as absence of

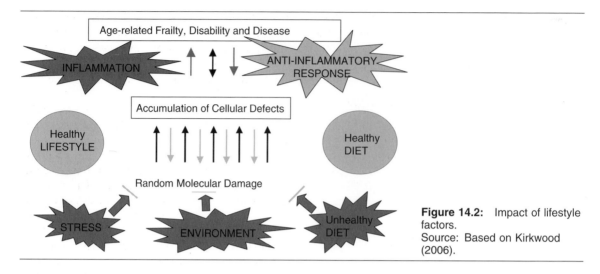

Figure 14.2: Impact of lifestyle factors.
Source: Based on Kirkwood (2006).

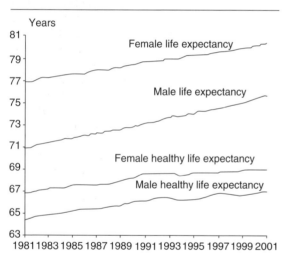

Figure 14.3: Life expectancy and healthy life expectancy.
Source: House of Lords (2005). Parliamentary material is reproduced with the permission of the Controller of HMSO on behalf of Parliament.

disease, as defined by the World Health Organization (2001). The House of Lords' report lists having a social role and function as influences on healthy ageing, alongside good nutrition, physical activity, not smoking and not drinking to excess, and good mental health and wellbeing. Long-term population-based studies show that social and productive activities are as important as physical activity in reducing the likelihood of illness and institutionalisation, although the mechanisms of these effects are unclear.

Ethnic differences in risk are also important (see Chapter 1, Section 1.3), as are related differences in nutrient intake, physical activity level and experience of various lifestyle factors. The Policy Research Institute on Ageing and Ethnicity (PRIAE) (2004) has published information from a survey of older people from ethnic minority groups across 10 EU countries (UK, Finland, France, Netherlands, Spain, Germany, Hungary Bosnia-Herzegovina, Croatia and Switzerland), which was conducted to inform and help plan the nature and direction of provision of future health and social care services. The research encompassed more than 20 ethnic groups. The survey revealed that in every country there were significant numbers of older people from minority ethnic groups living on incomes which were substantially less than the average for older people in the country concerned. In many of the countries one or two groups stood out as being in a worse socio-economic situation than other groups (*e.g.* Turks in Germany and the Netherlands, and Chinese/Vietnamese in the UK). There were also striking differences in the incidence of serious diseases such as diabetes and cardiovascular disease (CVD) (see Chapter 1, Section 1.3). In those from the UK, diabetes was most prevalent among African-Caribbeans and South Asians; heart disease and lung/breathing conditions were highest among the South Asians; and osteoporosis was highest among the Chinese/Vietnamese (Policy

Research Institute on Ageing and Ethnicity 2004). Men had a higher incidence of diabetes compared to women; and women had a much higher incidence of musculoskeletal disorders (*e.g.* osteoporosis).

14.2 Current trends in morbidity and quality of life

In this section the prevalence of chronic disease and other major causes of morbidity that affect older people is summarised, including diseases and conditions not covered elsewhere in the report, such as cancer and obesity.

14.2.1 Common causes of morbidity during adulthood

Data on morbidity (illness) is relatively difficult to collect compared to mortality. The General Household Survey (2004) provides information on the most common conditions resulting in chronic illness (see Figure 14.4) (General Household Survey 2004). Figure 14.5 provides information on specific illnesses in three of the most common categories. From this it is evident that the burden of these conditions generally increases with age and some affect one sex more than the other, *e.g.* arthritis and rheumatism are particularly prominent among women (see Chapter 5). Osteoarthritis is estimated to affect

about five million people in the UK (House of Lords 2005). Conditions that often result in death (*e.g.* stroke and cancer) (see Sections 14.2.2 and 14.2.6) are less prominent causes of long-term ill health, but nevertheless are major contributors to deterioration in quality of life.

These statistics emphasise that a substantial number of people, even in middle age, have their quality of life affected adversely by potentially preventable chronic illness and there is good reason to adopt a life-course approach to promote better health and quality of life in old age. This warrants that greater attention is paid to nutrition, physical activity and obesity prevention throughout the life-course (World Health Organization 2003a, 2004b). In this context, particular attention has focused to date on prevention of coronary heart disease (CHD), and more recently on obesity and diabetes. A lifestyle approach to cancer prevention has also been adopted in recent decades (see Section 14.2.6), initially focusing on smoking and more recently on aspects of diet.

However, any condition that affects a person's ability to live independently or to be active will also have a major impact on quality of life, for instance, sarcopenia (see Chapter 6) and skeletal problems such as osteoporosis (see Chapter 4) reduce mobility. CVD (see Chapter 10), resulting in shortness of breath on exertion, will similarly impact on the

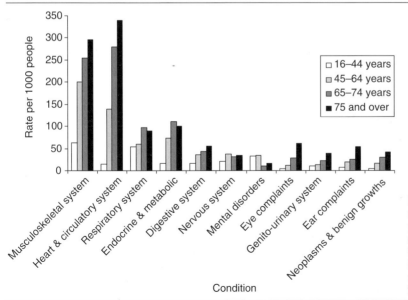

Figure 14.4: Chronic illness, rate per 1000 people reporting particular longstanding conditions, by age, Great Britain. Source: General Household Survey 2004 (www.statistics.gov.uk). Reproduced under the terms of the Click-Use Licence.

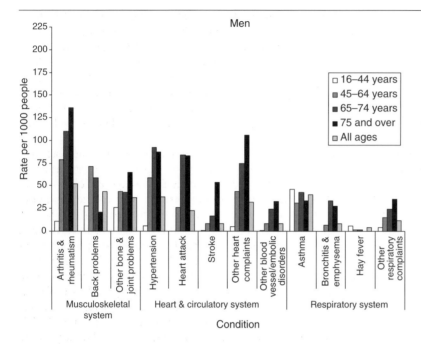

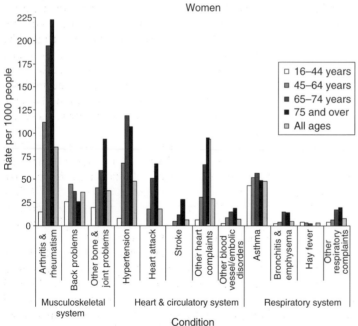

Figure 14.5: Chronic illness affecting the musculoskeletal, circulatory and respiratory systems, rate per 1000 people reporting particular longstanding condition, by age and sex, Great Britain.
Source: General Household Survey 2004 (www.statistics.gov.uk). Reproduced under the terms of the Click-Use Licence.

ability to live a full and active life, as will peripheral vascular disease, stroke, dementia (see Chapter 8) and diseases of the eye (see Chapter 9).

14.2.2 Cardiovascular disease (CVD)

Death rates from CHD have been falling in the UK since the late 1970s; rates have fallen by 44% over the last 10 years among those under 65 years (British Heart Foundation 2006). For stroke, death rates have also fallen; in people under 65 they fell by 25% between 1993 and 2003 (British Heart Foundation 2006). Recent trends indicate that the *Our Healthier Nation* target to reduce the death rate from CHD, stroke and related diseases in people under 75 years by at least two-fifths by 2010 will be met. Nevertheless, CVD remains a major cause of death in the UK and rates are falling faster in some other countries: in the UK the death rate for men aged 35–74 years fell by 42% between 1990 and 2000, compared with 48% in Australia and 54% in Norway.

Over 70% of all cardiovascular deaths now occur after the age of 75 (British Heart Foundation 2006). Men are around four times more likely to die from heart disease than women up to the age of 65, but the gap between the sexes narrows with advancing age. Women's risk escalates rapidly from around 55 years and by the age of 65–70 is the same as men's (British Heart Foundation 2006).

Regional, socio-economic and ethnic differences also exist. Death rates are highest in Scotland and the North of England, lowest in the South of England, and intermediate in Wales and Northern Ireland. Although at the end of the 1980s rates for premature deaths from CHD had been falling in the UK, rates had fallen faster in non-manual classes than in manual workers, hence the gap had widened over time. From data for 1991–93 it was estimated that each year 5000 lives and 47,000 working years are lost in men aged 20–64 years due to social inequalities in CHD death rates (British Heart Foundation 2006). Since 1994 the socio-economic inequality has been decreasing (from 37.2% in 1994 to 27.6% in 2003). If current trends continue, the target to reduce the inequalities gap in premature death from CVD (between the fifth of areas with the worst health and deprivation indicators and the population as a whole) to 22% by 2010 will be met.

South Asians (Indians, Bangladeshis, Pakistanis and Sri Lankans) living in the UK have a higher premature death rate from CHD and from stroke than the UK average. On the other hand, West Africans and African-Caribbeans have a lower rate for premature CHD death, although their death rate for stroke is considerably higher (Sproston and Mindell 2006) (see Sections 14.3.8 and Chapter 10, Section 10.4.1).

The strong association between increased age and raised CVD risk is thought to reflect primarily the length of time that people are exposed to the modifiable risk factors. Scientific consensus exists about the importance of the main modifiable risk factors for the development of CVD. These include obesity, dyslipidaemia, hypertension, smoking, physical inactivity and diabetes. Exposure to these risk factors in middle age predicts risk of premature death from CVD and risk in old age. The prevalence of most modifiable risk factors for CVD increases with age but as discussed in Chapter 10, Section 10.6.1, several CVD risk factors, including blood pressure and cholesterol levels, are not as strongly or consistently predictive of CVD risk when measured after the age of 65 years. This may be partly explained by difficulties with interpreting epidemiological studies in older populations (such as possible confounding by drug treatment and co-morbidity) and methodological issues, and measurements in later life may not necessarily reflect lifetime exposure to these risk factors.

Blood lipid measurements, in particular HDL-cholesterol and triglyceride concentrations, are able to predict risk of CVD well into old age; for example in subjects over the age of 85 years, low HDL-cholesterol concentrations carry a 2–3-fold increased mortality risk from coronary heart disease and stroke (see Chapter 10, Section 10.6.1).

As discussed in Chapter 10, Section 10.6.1, the age-related reduction in relative risk associated with dyslipidaemia and hypertension should not be used as an argument not to intervene as both drug and lifestyle modifications to these risk factors have been demonstrated to be effective, irrespective of age, up until the age of 80. Furthermore, because of the increased incidence of heart attacks and stroke with age, the absolute risk reduction yielded by risk factor reduction is substantial in older age groups. Nevertheless as some of the traditional risk factors (*e.g.*

LDL-cholesterol) lose some of their importance as predictors of CVD with age, novel risk factors may have particular value in predicting risk in older age groups. Promising candidates include markers of haemostatic activation and of inflammation, and possibly homocysteine (see Chapter 10, Section 10.6.5).

The incidence of stroke, a major cause of disability, increases exponentially with age and, with increasing life expectancy, is a common condition among the older population (see Chapter 8). It is the third most common cause of death in older people and rates are higher in women than men. Stroke and dementia (see Section 14.2.3) are the two most common reasons for admission to long-term institutional care.

About 82% of strokes are ischaemic (due to a blood vessel blockage), 15% are haemorrhagic and 3% arise from a subarachnoid haemorrhage. In the UK, 97% of strokes occur in people over the age of 55 and 81% occur in people over the age of 75. The severity and risk of dying also increase with age. Age-specific incidence of stroke is falling in many developed countries due to control of blood pressure and reduction in smoking, but the absolute number of cases continues to rise as people live longer, about 60% of whom die or become dependent as a result of the stroke.

14.2.3 Dementia and depression

The incidence of dementia, Parkinson's disease and depression increase exponentially with age and, with increasing life expectancy, have become common among the older population (see Chapter 8). Dementia affects 1 in 20 people over the age of 65 and again more women than men are affected. The age-specific incidence of dementia in the UK increases from 7/1000/year at age 65 to 85/1000/year at age 85 (see Chapter 8, Section 8.3). In addition, many more people suffer from mild cognitive impairment that does not progress to dementia. Dementia and stroke are the two most common reasons for admission to long-term institutional care. Many of the established risk factors for stroke are also thought to be relevant to dementia, Parkinson's disease (which affects 3% of the population aged 65 years and above) and depression. Depression in older people is closely associated with poor physical health; recent research has focused on the role of vascular factors and nutri-

tion in determining risk in this age group (see Chapter 8, Section 8.4).

14.2.4 Obesity

Although often not considered as a chronic illness, obesity can influence quality of life to a significant degree. The prevalence of overweight and obesity is increasing around the world, but prevalence rates in the UK are among the highest in Europe (World Health Organization 2005). In 2004 in England, 44% of men and 34% of women were overweight (BMI 25–30 kg/m^2) and a further 23% of men and 23% of women were obese (BMI >30) (Health & Social Care Information Centre 2005) (see Table 14.1). Central obesity, recognised as being associated with the metabolic syndrome (see Chapter 10, Section 10.4.3) and CHD (see Chapter 10, Section 10.4.1) is also common, affecting 33% of men and 30% of women (Department of Health 2004c).

Overweight and obesity increase with age, peaking in those aged 55–64 (see Table 14.1). About 31% of men and 38% of women aged 16–24 have a BMI >25 but this increases to 78% and 70%, respectively, in those aged 55–64 years. Prevalence of central obesity also increases with age, especially in men – 57% of men compared with 45% of women at 65–74 years.

There are marked social class differences in obesity prevalence in women but not in men. In men in manual occupations the prevalence of obesity is 23% compared with 21% in those in non-manual jobs (the values for overweight are 42% and 44% respectively) (Zaninotto *et al.* 2006). In contrast in women the prevalence of obesity in those in manual households is 28% compared with 19% in non-manual households (the respective percentages for overweight are 33% and 32%).

With the exception of Black Caribbean and Irish men in the UK, men from ethnic minority groups have markedly lower obesity prevalence rates than the general population: Bangladeshi and Chinese men have the lowest rates, 5.8% and 6% respectively. Among women, prevalence is highest in Black Caribbean (32.1%), Black African (38.5%) and Pakistani (28.1%) groups, and lowest (7.6%) in the Chinese group (Sproston and Mindell 2006).

Obesity prevention is a public health goal, therefore, given that prevalence has been rising in recent decades around the world (see Figure 14.6). Obesity has increased by over 50% in adults aged 16–64

Table 14.1: Body mass index (BMI)* by sex and age, England, 2004. Data expressed as percentage of age category

BMI (kg/m²)	All ages	16–24	25–34	35–44	45–54	55–64	65–74	75 and over
Men								
20 or under	4.7	20.2	4.1	2.1	0.5	0.7	1.6	2.5
Over 20–25	28.8	48.8	37.0	22.4	21.7	21.7	22.2	24.1
Over 25–30	43.9	23.1	41.0	50.3	48.2	47.5	48.4	54.4
Over 30	22.7	7.9	17.9	25.2	29.6	27.8	27.8	19.0
Women								
20 or under	6.3	16.4	8.7	5.5	3.8	1.7	3.5	3.8
Over 20–25	36.7	47.4	43.2	40.1	33.0	29.3	27.9	29.7
Over 25–30	33.9	24.1	31.2	30.4	35.9	37.0	39.9	45.9
Over 30	23.2	12.1	16.9	24.0	27.3	32.0	28.7	20.6

*Weighted for non-response.
BMI: 25–30 = overweight; BMI: >30 = obese.
Source: Health & Social Care Information Centre (2005). © 2007, reproduced by permission of the Information Centre. All rights reserved.

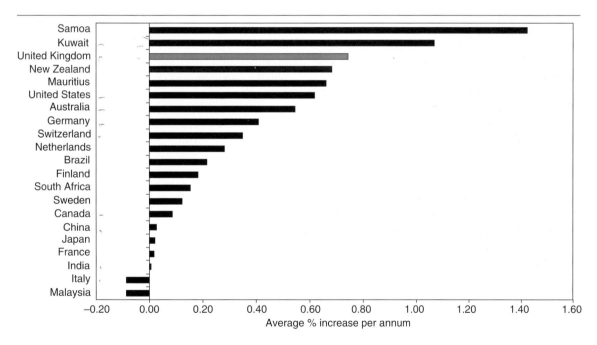

Figure 14.6: Annual increase in prevalence of obesity, 1980–98, all available countries worldwide.
Source: British Heart Foundation (2006).

years in England in the last decade (Zaninotto *et al.* 2006) and the rise is particularly marked in men in whom rates have tripled since the mid-1980s. Recent projections are that, by 2010, 33% of men and 30% of women will be obese and a further 42% of men and 30% of women will be overweight (Zaninotto *et al.* 2006) (see Table 14.1 for the percentages in 2004; the most recent data available in autumn 2006). Estimates by Foresight (Government Office for Science 2007) suggest that by 2050 60% of men and 50% of women will be defined as obese (McPherson *et al.* 2007).

There has also been a steady increase in prevalence among children (Health & Social Care Information Centre 2006). Overall, the prevalence of obesity in 2–15-year-olds in England in 2004 was 19% among boys and 18% among girls (in 1995 it was 11% and 12% respectively). An additional 14% of boys and 16% of girls can be classed as overweight (above the 85th percentile) resulting in a total of 33% of boys and 34% of girls being heavier than they should be for their age (in 1995 overweight/obesity affected 24% of boys and 25% girls). Of particular concern is the recognition that the rate of increase seems to be rising, and this suggests that the prevalence in adulthood is set to increase further unless action is taken. By 2010, it is estimated that 19% of boys and 22% of girls aged 2–15 years will be obese (and a further 14% of boys and 14% of girls overweight) (Zaninotto *et al.* 2006).

Statistics summarised by the British Heart Foundation suggest that although Italy, Greece and Portugal have the highest prevalence of overweight among children aged 4–11 years, England is not far behind and is well ahead of many other EU countries (British Heart Foundation 2005a).

In the 2004 Health Survey for England, overweight/obesity was higher (compared with the general population) among Black Caribbean, Black African and Pakistani boys, and Black Caribbean and Black African girls (Sproston and Mindell 2006).

In 2004, the UK Department of Health introduced an obesity target: to halt the year-on-year rise in obesity among children under 11 by 2010, in the context of a broader strategy to tackle obesity in the population as a whole. The Department of Health has developed an Obesity Prevention social marketing programme to help achieve this target, focusing on families with young children. However, there is almost no evidence that policies have changed the

trajectory of obesity growth and the scale of the challenge is influenced by the many competing priorities that parents face. In a study among disadvantaged families in Scotland with young teenagers, parents attached a low priority to monitoring their children's diets, especially outside the home (Backett-Milburn *et al.* 2006). Therefore, the challenge for public health is to acknowledge and work with the wider social, media and community influences on teenage behaviour, as well as engaging with parents.

14.2.5 Type 2 diabetes

In parallel with increases in bodyweight are changes in insulin resistance and hence risk of the metabolic syndrome (see Chapter 10, Section 10.4.3 and Chapter 13, Section 13.3.1) and diabetes. Type 2 diabetes substantially increases the risk of developing CHD: men with type 2 diabetes have a 2–4-fold greater annual risk and women an even greater risk (3–5-fold) (British Heart Foundation 2006). It also magnifies the impact of risk factors for CHD (*i.e.* obesity, smoking and raised blood pressure and blood cholesterol). Diabetes is now one of the most common non-communicable diseases globally, currently affecting an estimated 194 million people aged 20–79 years and projected to affect 333 million by 2025 (British Heart Foundation 2006). The UK prevalence is average for developed countries.

Data for the UK show that the prevalence of diagnosed type 2 diabetes rises with age (see Figure 14.7). There is an estimated 1.9 million (total of 4% of men and 3% of women) diagnosed with type 2 diabetes in the UK (British Heart Foundation 2006) and it is suggested that a further 3% of men and 0.7% of women have undiagnosed type 2 diabetes, amounting to 2.5 million people overall. However, changes in diet and physical activity can have a major impact on development of type 2 diabetes in people with impaired glucose tolerance. Studies in Finland (Tuomilehto *et al.* 2001) and the US (Knowler *et al.* 2002) have shown that intensive lifestyle modification slows progression to diabetes by 58% over 3–4 years compared with usual lifestyle recommendations. Furthermore, extended follow-up of the Finnish subjects indicates that despite cessation of active counselling, the group that received this continued to have a lower incidence of diabetes over a further median three years of follow-up com-

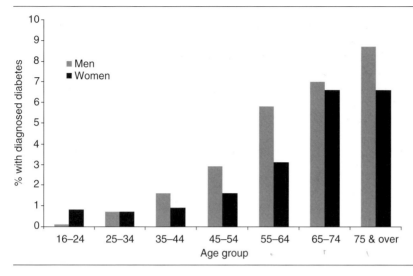

Figure 14.7: Prevalence of diagnosed diabetes by sex and age, 1998, England.
Source: British Heart Foundation (2006).

pared with the control group (36% lower during this period) (Lindstrom *et al.* 2006). Overall, the reduction during the total seven years of follow-up was 43%, similar to the 46% reduction reported in the Da Qing study which had a six-year follow-up (Pan *et al.* 1997).

Preservation of beta cell function seems to be particularly important because deterioration in insulin secretion capacity appears to limit the effectiveness of both lifestyle and drug interventions. Projections indicate that intensive lifestyle change is cost-effective in the long term, so a crucial question is how intensive the lifestyle intervention has to be to be effective (Goldberg 2006).

As with obesity, the prevalence of type 2 diabetes is increasing, having more than doubled in men and increased by 80% in women since 1991. Furthermore, it is estimated that by 2010 the prevalence will be about 7% for men and 5% for women (*i.e.* about three million people). Also, as with obesity, there are socio-economic differences, as shown in the Health Survey for England of 2003, with men in the highest income quintile having a prevalence of 2.3% compared with 6.1% in the lowest income quintile. The comparative figures in women were 1.7% and 4% (Sproston and Primatesta 2004). There are also variations in prevalence among ethnic groups, with the highest prevalence of type 2 diabetes being seen in men and women from India, Bangladesh and Pakistan (British Heart Foundation 2006) (Figure 14.8).

It is particularly alarming that type 2 diabetes is now being diagnosed in obese adolescents, having previously been considered a disease of adults (Drake *et al.* 2002).

14.2.6 Cancer

Cancer has not been covered in depth in the preceding chapters and so this section provides additional detail. It is recognised that diet and lifestyle factors can influence risk of developing cancer, with associations with lifestyle characteristics being stronger for some forms of cancer than others (World Cancer Research Fund 1997; Department of Health 1998b; Key *et al.* 2004b; World Cancer Research Fund/ American Institute for Cancer Research 2007). It has been estimated that approximately 30% of cancers could be prevented by dietary means in western countries (World Cancer Research Fund 1997).

Avoiding overweight/obesity, increasing physical activity level, limiting alcohol intake and not smoking decrease cancer risk (Key *et al.* 2004b). Overweight/ obesity increases risk for cancers of the oesophagus (adenocarcinoma), colorectum, breast (postmenopausal women), endometrium and kidney. Observational data suggest that increased physical activity reduces the risk of colon cancer and probably breast cancer. A review of studies suggests that 30–60 minutes/day of moderate to vigorous activity reduces colon cancer risk by 30–40% in a dose-dependent manner and breast cancer risk by 20–30%, compared

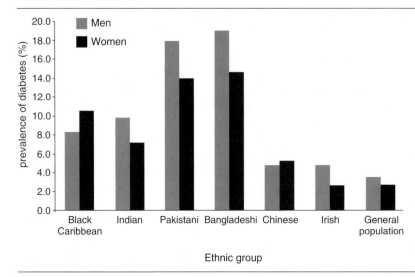

Figure 14.8: Prevalence of diagnosed diabetes by sex and ethnic group, 1999, England. Source: British Heart Foundation (2006).

to those who are inactive (Lee 2003; see Miles 2007a for a review). Various mechanisms for the apparently protective effect of greater physical activity have been suggested, but weight control is the most favoured because of the association between obesity and cancer risk at several sites (Key *et al.* 2004b; Miles 2007a). Consumption of alcoholic beverages causes cancers of the oral cavity, pharynx, oesophagus (with the effect being exacerbated by smoking) and the liver, and current UK recommendations are to limit consumption to a total of 3–4 units (24–32 g) a day for men and 2–3 units (16–24 g) a day for women (see Foster and Marriott 2006). An association between alcohol intake and colon cancer has also been suggested. A pooling study of eight cohorts in five countries revealed a clear increase in risk with intakes of over 30 g alcohol per day compared with non-drinkers (Cho, Smith-Warner *et al.* 2004a). WCRF (World Cancer Research Fund/American Institute for Cancer Research 2007) recommends no more than two drinks a day for men and one a day for women.

Few dietary effects on cancer risk have been established as convincing. The review by WCRF found that vegetables probably protect against cancers of the oral cavity, oesophagus and stomach (allium vegetables including garlic are specifically associated with the latter and garlic also probably protects against colon cancer). Fruits probably protect against cancers of the lung, oral cavity, oesophagus and stomach and there is limited evidence that non-starchy vegetables protect against

cancers of the lung, colorectum, ovary and endometrium and that fruits protect against cancers of the pancreas, liver and colorectum. Probable protection at specific sites was identified by WCRF for particular constituents of these foods, in particular fibre, vitamin C and carotenoids.

The WCRF Panel found that, since the mid-1990s, support for a broad and strong protective effect of fruit and vegetables has weakened, although modest benefits probably do exist. Key and colleagues (2004b) discuss the heterogeneity of the composition of fruits and vegetables as a category, and the possibility that specific types are associated with risk reduction of specific cancers (*e.g.* brassica vegetables, citrus fruits). High intakes of preserved and red meats have been linked with increased risk of colorectal cancer, and recently attention has focused on preserved meats in particular (World Cancer Research Fund/American Institute for Cancer Research 2007). However, the association with high meat intake seems to be offset by high fibre intake. In the European Prospective Investigation into Cancer and Nutrition (EPIC), among high meat consumers, the hazard ratio fell from 1.50 (95% CI: 1.06–1.80) at a low fibre intake (<17 g/d) to a statistically non-significant 1.09 (95% CI: 0.83–1.42) with a high fibre intake (>26 g/d in women and 28 g/d in men) (Norat *et al.* 2005). Salt-preserved foods and high salt intakes probably increase the risk of stomach cancer (World Cancer Research Fund/American Institute for Cancer Research 2007).

A number of meta-analyses of cohort studies have been published by the Harvard-based pooling project (www.hsph.harvard.edu/poolingproject/publications.html). For example, a meta-analysis focusing on lung cancer (Smith-Warner *et al.* 2003) found a modest reduction in risk associated with elevated fruit and vegetable intake, which was mostly attributable to fruit. Another meta-analysis (Mannisto *et al.* 2004) has shown an apparent benefit of certain carotenoids in relation to lung cancer risk, especially β-cryptoxanthin (RR 0.76; 95% CI: 0.67–0.85, highest vs. lowest quintile), which is found in citrus fruit in particular. However, the primary factor linked with lung cancer risk is smoking, and residual confounding associated with smoking leads to difficulties in investigation of associations between diet and lung cancer risk. It should be noted, however, that β-carotene supplementation in high-risk individuals increased the incidence of lung cancer (Alpha-Tocopherol Beta-Carotene Cancer Prevention Study Group 1994).

Colorectal cancer offers the strongest evidence of a dietary involvement in cancer (Cummings and Bingham 1998). Fibre is believed to be one of the most important, yet controversial, dietary factors linked to reduction in colorectal cancer risk and there are well-studied mechanisms that support this hypothesis. Fibre is thought to reduce the risk of colorectal cancer in a number of ways. It increases faecal bulk and reduces transit time through the large bowel, which has the effect of diluting genotoxins in the stool and reducing the amount of time that the contents of the faecal stream are in contact with the colonic mucosa. This limits the potential amount of DNA damage (Y. Hu *et al.* 2002). Most dietary fibre subtypes are also fermented by the anaerobic bacteria in the gut to short chain fatty acids including butyrate (Nordgaard *et al.* 1995; Lunn and Buttriss 2007). Butyrate is an antiproliferative agent and has been shown to induce apoptosis in colon cancer cell lines so is therefore important for maintaining a healthy, functional epithelium (Blottiere *et al.* 2003).

A major source of recent data, derived from a large number of subjects across Europe, is the EPIC study (summarised in Table 14.2). The EPIC data suggest a protective effect of fibre in colon cancer. There was a 40% reduction in risk between the lowest (15 g/day) and the highest (35 g/day) quintiles of intake (Bingham *et al.* 2003) but this has proved to be controversial (Bingham 2006) as a protective

effect of a high-fibre diet has not been seen in cohorts in the US, Finland and Sweden (Fuchs *et al.* 1999; Pietinen *et al.* 1999; Terry, Giovannucci *et al.* 2001); indeed, some studies (*e.g.* Potter and McMichael 1986) have reported an increased risk of high-fibre diets. Also, although a pooled analysis of prospective studies conducted by Park *et al.* (2005) found that dietary fibre was associated inversely with age-adjusted colorectal cancer risk, this association was eliminated when other dietary risk factors were taken into account. However, there was some support for a specific, weak effect of fibre from cereals and from whole-grain foods. Confounding by folate intake has been suggested to explain the discrepancy with the EPIC data but re-analysis of the EPIC cohort data found that even after adjusting for folate intake, an inverse association between dietary fibre intake and colorectal cancer risk remained (Bingham *et al.* 2005). The recent report by the World Cancer Research Fund (WCRF)/American Institute for Cancer Research (2007) has supported a probably decreased risk between fibre and colorectal cancer.

The subject is further complicated when trials looking at intermediate-stage biomarkers are considered. Large intervention trials have shown that supplements of soluble fibre, bran or vegetables have not reduced recurrence rates in patients with adenomatous polyps, which are precursors to cancerous lesions (Alberts *et al.* 2000; Bonithon-Kopp *et al.* 2000; Schatzkin *et al.* 2000), and this has been confirmed by a Cochrane Review (Asano and McLeod 2002).

A beneficial effect on colon cancer risk of higher calcium (and milk) intake has also been proposed (Cho, Smith-Warner *et al.* 2004b). In a pooled analysis of 10 cohort studies, the relative risk for the highest vs. the lowest quintile was 0.78 for total calcium intake (95% CI: 0.69–0.88; *P* (trend) <0.001). WCRF concluded that milk and calcium probably protect against colon cancer.

Interest is also growing in the hypothesis that low folate status may contribute to carcinogenesis by alteration of gene expression and increased DNA damage (Choi and Mason 2000) and the finding that a common polymorphism in the methyltetrahydrofolate reductase gene, involved in folate metabolism, may also be associated with colorectal cancer is supportive (Key *et al.* 2004b). Associations between folate intake and cancer risk have been reviewed in the context of the case for folic acid fortification (Scientific Advisory Committee on Nutrition 2006). The review found that although

Table 14.2: Findings from EPIC, by main cancer site

Topic	Publications	Main results
Breast cancer		
Fruits and vegetables	van Gils *et al.* (2005)	No statistically significant decreased risks for fruits and vegetables
Body size	Lahmann *et al.* (2004)	Statistically significant increased risk for postmenopausal but not for premenopausal breast cancer. In postmenopausal breast cancer cases the effect is limited to women not using HRT
Adult weight gain	Lahmann *et al.* (2005)	Findings suggest that large adult weight gain was a significant predictor of breast cancer in postmenopausal women not taking exogenous hormones
Phytoestrogens	Grace *et al.* (2004) Keinan-Boker *et al.* (2004)	One study found positive association with isoflavones in the EPIC-Norfolk cohort. But no association was found with these phytoestrogens in the EPIC-Utrecht cohort. Further analyses with pooled data are ongoing
Fish	Engeset *et al.* (2006)	No significant associations between total fish intake and breast cancer
Physical activity	Lahmann *et al.* (2007)	Total physical activity level was associated with a reduction in breast cancer among postmenopausal women. Household activity was significantly associated with reduced risk in both pre- and postmenopausal women. Occupational and recreational activity was not significantly associated with breast cancer
Colon cancer		
Fibre	Bingham *et al.* (2003)	Inverse relation of dietary fibre with colorectal cancer incidence with the greatest protective effect in the left colon, and least in the rectum. No food source of fibre is significantly more protective than others
	Bingham *et al.* (2005)	Confirmation of the above findings after adjustment for folate and with a longer follow-up
Nuts	Jenab *et al.* (2004)	Higher nut and seed intake not significantly associated to the risk of colorectal, colon and rectal cancers in men but did show an inverse association with colon cancer in women
Meat, fish, poultry	Norat *et al.* (2005)	High consumption of processed and red meat associated with an increase in colorectal cancer risk; the association with high intakes of meat was more apparent in people with low/medium compared to high intakes of fibre (see earlier text). The effect was strongest for processed meat. Fish consumption is significantly inversely associated with risk and there is no association with poultry
Obesity	Pischon *et al.* (2006)	Higher bodyweight and BMI significantly associated with colon cancer in men, but not women. Anthropometric measures of abdominal obesity showed a significant increased risk for colon cancer in men and women
Physical activity	Friedenreich *et al.* (2006)	Most active compared with inactive had a non-significant decreased risk of colon cancer. The effect was stronger for right-sided colon cancers and for lean participants compared with obese. No association was shown for rectal cancer

Table 14.2: *Continued*

Topic	Publications	Main results
Gastric cancer		
Meat, nitrosamines and nitrites	Gonzalez *et al.* (2006a)	Gastric non-cardia cancer risk was statistically significantly associated with intakes of total meat, red meat and processed meat, especially in subjects with *H. pylori* infection. Intakes of total, red or processed meat were not associated with the risk of gastric cardia cancer.
Fruit and vegetables intake	Gonzalez *et al.* (2006b)	No association with total vegetable intake or specific groups of vegetables, except for the intestinal type, where a negative association is possible regarding total vegetable intake and onion and garlic intake. No evidence of association with fresh fruit intake. An inverse but non-significant association was found between citrus fruit intake and the cardia site but no association was observed with the non-cardia site
Retinol, tocopherol and carotenoids	Jenab *et al.* (2006a)	Significant decreased risk was observed for plasma levels of β-cryptoxanthin, zeaxanthin, retinol and lipid-unadjusted α-tocopherol
Vitamin C	Jenab *et al.* (2006b)	No association with dietary vitamin C, whereas a significant protective effect was seen for plasma vitamin C. This protective effect was more pronounced in subjects consuming higher levels of red and processed meats, which may increase endogenous *N*-nitroso compound production

EPIC: European Prospective Investigation into Cancer; HRT: hormone replacement therapy.
Source: www.iarc.fr/epic.

there is some evidence of an inverse association between low intake and/or status and risk of cancer (most of the evidence is for colon cancer), folate may have a dual modulatory role, at high intakes promoting progression of existing cancerous lesions.

Despite the large amount of case-control and prospective evidence concerning diet and cancer, there have been relatively few intervention studies, and some notable large studies have not been supportive. For example, the US Women's Heath Initiative, which randomly assigned almost 50,000 postmenopausal women to either a control group or an intensive behaviour modification programme designed to reduce fat intake and increase fruit, vegetable and grain intake, found no statistically significant association with colorectal cancer risk (Beresford *et al.* 2006) or breast cancer risk (Prentice *et al.* 2006).

14.2.7 Osteoporosis

Osteoporosis affects an estimated 1 in 3 women and 1 in 12 men over the age of 55 years in the UK; about 200,000 osteoporotic fractures occurred in 2000 (see Chapter 4, Section 4.1.2), costing the NHS in excess of £1.7 billion per annum. Worldwide, the annual rate of osteoporotic fractures is expected to rise to 6.26 million by 2050, from 1.66 million in 1990. Considerable skeletal changes occur with age and the two principal determinants of adult bone health are the peak bone mass attained during growth and early adulthood, and the rate at which bone is lost with advancing age, with the menopause years of women resulting in particularly rapid loss. Both of these determinants are influenced by a combination of genetic, endocrine, mechanical and nutritional factors (see Chapter 14, Section 14.3.2).

The overall lifetime risk of fragility fractures in the UK at the age of 50 years is 53.2% in women and 20.7% in men. The risk of hip fracture increases 10-fold every 20 years as we age, associated with changed bone architecture and also increased risk of falling (see Chapter 14, Section 14.3.2).

14.2.8 Arthritis and joint pain

Many adults report musculoskeletal pain and impairment; the prevalence of self-reported chronic pain increases with age. The more common forms of arthritis fall into two categories: those that involve inflammation of joints, such as rheumatoid arthritis and gout, and age-related degenerative conditions, such as osteoarthritis. The inflammatory forms together affect about 1 in 100 people, whereas osteoarthritis is far more common, affecting 10 out of 100 people aged over 65 years (see Chapter 5, Section 5.1.1 and Section 14.3.3).

14.2.9 Oral health

Dental care used to be dominated by tooth extraction but is now more focused on restoration of teeth. There is also a greater social awareness of the benefits of retaining some natural teeth for both aesthetic and functional reasons. Indeed, the National Diet and Nutrition Survey (NDNS) of adults aged 65 years and over clearly showed that overall nutrient intake and nutritional status were greater in those who had retained some natural teeth (Steele *et al.* 1998) (see Chapter 3).

Root caries is a feature of the dentition of older people, associated with progressive erosion of the gum margin over time, which is often the result of long-term periodontal disease (the single most common chronic inflammatory disease in humans) and sometimes over-aggressive brushing of teeth. There is now compelling evidence from the US and Ireland that water fluoridation can reduce both the prevalence and severity of root caries in older people (see Chapter 3, Section 3.2.1.2). Currently, as little as 10% of the UK domestic water supply provides either natural or added fluoride at the optimal level of 1 mg/L.

Deterioration in oral health has a major impact on quality of life, both directly and indirectly. Not only can it affect how people chew, taste and enjoy food, it can also exert profound physical and psychological effects on enjoyment of life. For example, how people look, talk and socialise, as well as their self-esteem, self-image and sense of social wellbeing can be affected. Yet much can be done to prevent poor oral health (see Chapter 3 and Section 14.3.1).

In the UK, 58% of adults aged 75 and over are edentulous and rely on dentures; this influences their ability to consume certain foods, including fresh fruit and raw vegetables. Although modern dentures make chewing easier, many wearers seem reluctant to change their habits. However, tailored dietary intervention at the time when dentures are replaced can positively change dietary behaviour, with fruit and vegetable intake increasing by 210 g/day (>2.5 servings) (Bradbury *et al.* 2006).

In 2005, the Department of Health published *Choosing Better Oral Health*, which recognises the importance of good oral health among older people.

14.2.10 Other conditions

Although they have a lesser overall impact, eye and ear complaints affect over 50% of the population over the age of 75 years (see Chapter 1, Section 1.2). One in eight people over 75 in the UK suffers from severe vision impairment (see Chapter 9, Section 9.1) and 1 in 50 over the age of 75 is blind. The prevalence of vision impairment increases with age, affecting 20% of those over 80 years compared to 6% of those aged 75–79. Women are affected disproportionately (House of Lords 2005). The major causes of vision impairment are refractive errors (presbyopia, inability to focus on close objects which is corrected with spectacles), cataract (opacity of the lens) and age-related macular degeneration (AMD), which affects the central field of vision. Loss of vision due to cataract can easily be treated by replacement of the affected lens by an artificial lens, whereas AMD is the main cause of blindness among older people in developed countries. Currently, for those with AMD, there are no effective therapies to restore vision, although progression of some forms of AMD can be delayed (see Chapter 9, Section 9.1.3). Other causes of vision impairment or loss are diabetic retinopathy (associated with poorly controlled diabetes) and glaucoma (caused by optic nerve damage, which can be associated with untreated raised pressure within the eye), both of which are progressively more common with ageing (see Chapter 9, Section 9.1.5 and 9.1.4 respectively).

Despite the prevalence of severe vision impairment, some degree of hearing loss is the commonest sensory impairment in old age, affecting approximately nine million people in the UK in total and half of people over the age of 60 years (House of Lords 2005). Virtually nothing is known about the cause of hearing impairment in old age, but there seems to be a heritability of about 50%.

14.3 Summary of the Task Force's findings for different organ systems

The purpose of this section is to begin to tease out the common strands that could be part of a health promotion package targeted at healthy ageing.

14.3.1 Teeth and the oral cavity

Dental caries arises through the interaction between bacteria in dental plaque on the tooth surface and fermentable sugars derived from food and drink, resulting in acid production and demineralisation of tooth enamel (see Chapter 3). The frequency of consumption of sugar-releasing foods and drinks is considered more important than the total amount consumed in predicting caries severity. The protective effect of fluoride is important in this respect (see below). With a relatively low frequency, natural defences (saliva production) and repair mechanisms (remineralisation) can function efficiently. But with a high frequency of intake, demineralisation dominates. To prevent ordinary enamel caries in younger people, dentists normally recommend no more than four episodes of sugar-containing foods or drinks a day to allow normal remineralisation following any demineralisation resulting from acid challenge. For prevention of root caries (common in older people), there is no evidence about the specific frequency of sugars intake that might be regarded as safe but, in the NDNS of older people (Steele *et al.* 1998), the mean number of episodes was 5.1 in those living in their own homes, rising to 7.9 in those in residential homes and other types of institution. A specific problem that arises among ill older people relates to the use of energy supplements and sugar-containing medicines (see Chapter 3, Sections 3.2.2.2 and 3.2.2.3).

A problem that is gaining prominence among children and young adults is dental erosion, caused by consumption of acidic foods and drinks (and also by stomach acid regurgitation). Dental erosion is currently not a problem among older people but may become a feature in future generations of older people, as loss of significant quantities of enamel through erosion is irreversible (see Chapter 3, Section 3.2.3).

Some minerals, including calcium, zinc, magnesium, strontium and fluoride, can strengthen the crystalline structure of tooth tissue, and regular use of fluoride toothpaste can help teeth resist decay. Fluoride also enhances the remineralisation process of demineralised enamel.

Iron, vitamin B_{12} and folate are among the nutrients critical for maintenance of oral mucosa integrity, and oral health is reduced in subjects with relatively high alcohol intake and in smokers. Smoking not only influences the development and flora of bacterial plaque, it also exerts direct effects on the gingival and periodontal tissues by modifying the rate of blood flow through these tissues. Tobacco use and a high alcohol intake are both risk factors for oral cancer (see Chapter 3, Section 3.2.6).

Taste perception changes with age and these effects are amplified in people who take multiple medications and in those who are chronically ill, which may be a consequence of changes in saliva flow and composition. Related to taste, sense of smell also changes with age; nearly two-thirds of adults over the age of 80 years show some level of disturbance with men particularly affected. Ability to process food in the mouth also diminishes with age, in parallel with changes in dentition and oral status in general. This impacts on the length of time it takes to chew foods and also the types of food chosen (see Chapter 3, Section 3.3.1).

In summary:

- Children and younger adults are advised to look after their teeth because having natural teeth in old age is positively associated with nutritional status. Steps to avoid dental caries and dental erosion are important.
- Dentists normally recommend that sugar-containing foods and drinks should be limited to a maximum of four episodes per day, and fluoridated toothpaste should be used regularly.
- Use of fluoride toothpaste and limiting the frequency of sugars intake remains important into old age.
- Adequate intakes of various minerals (*e.g.* calcium, zinc) are needed for remineralisation of teeth, and iron and various B vitamins (folate and B_{12} in particular) are needed for gum health.
- Use of sugars in medicines consumed regularly by older people should be avoided where possible.
- Alcohol consumption should be restricted and tobacco use avoided.
- Avoidance of periodontal disease should continue as a high priority in dental practice.
- When advising older people on healthy eating, the effects of changes in taste, smell and food handling efficiency in the mouth need to be taken into account.

14.3.2 Bones

Weight-bearing physical activity (*e.g.* brisk walking, jogging, running, step aerobics) is crucial for maintaining a healthy skeleton into old age, and may have a synergistic effect with nutrition. In general, physical activity promotes muscle strength, mobility and balance, hence reducing the likelihood of falls among older people. Physical activity may also have a significant direct effect on bone, with data indicating both improvements in bone mass and a reduction in bone resorption with weight-bearing physical activity. Both calcium and vitamin D are key nutrients in optimisation of bone health, and vitamin K is thought to be important (possibly by reducing postmenopausal bone loss). An adequate calcium intake is essential throughout life and, for women five or more years postmenopause, calcium supplementation can reduce bone loss, particularly if habitual calcium intake is low. Among children and young adults, there is concern that soft drinks are displacing milk (a major dietary source of calcium) from the diet.

Combined supplementation with vitamin D and calcium has significantly reduced fractures in institutionalised elderly, and supportive evidence exists from studies among community-based older people, although not all studies have reported benefit (see Chapter 4, Section 4.2.2.4). A recent review suggests that a vitamin D intake of 17.5–20 µg/day (700–800 IU/day) combined with calcium supplementation is associated with fewer hip and non-vertebral fractures in frail older people in institutions (Avenell, Gillespie *et al.* 2005). The current dietary recommendation for this age group is 10 µg/day (Department of Health 1991). The benefit of vitamin D supplementation in the absence of calcium remains unclear. However, trials using higher supplementation levels have found a lower fracture incidence, with and without supplemental calcium (Bischoff-Ferrari *et al.* 2005), and it has been reported that a mean serum 25 hydroxyvitamin D (25 OHD) level of at least 75 nmol/L is required to reduce fracture incidence, *i.e.* a level considerably higher than the value of 25 nmol/L considered to be sufficient to prevent rickets and osteomalacia (Bischoff-Ferrari *et al.* 2006) (see Chapter 4, Section 4.2.3).

Season, geography, skin colour and sunlight exposure are the main predictors of vitamin D status. Oil-rich fish is the richest dietary source, margarine is fortified by law in the UK and some vitamin D is added voluntarily to other foods, including fat spreads. Evidence of widespread vitamin D insufficiency has been recognised for some time (see Table

Table 14.3: Prevalence (%) of low vitamin D status in the UK (25 OHD <25 nmol/L)

Age (years)	Males (%)	Females (%)
4–6	3	2
7–10	4	7
11–14	11	11
15–18	16	10
19–24	24	28
25–34	16	13
35–49	12	15
50–64	9	11
65–74 (living in the community)	5	6
75–84 (living in the community)	5	15
85+ (living in the community)	13	25
65–84 (in institutions)	36	38
85+ (in institutions)	42	37

Source: Finch *et al.* (1998); Bates *et al.* (2000); Ruston *et al.* (2004).

Table 14.4: Prevalence of serum levels of the active form of vitamin D, 25 OHD, below several thresholds in British adults aged 47 years

25 OHD threshold	Winter/Spring	Summer/Autumn
<25 nmol/L	15.5%	3.2%
<40 nmol/L	46.6%	15.4%
<75 nmol/L	87.1%	60.9%

Source: Hypponen and Power (2007).

14.3), particularly among housebound older people and those in institutions (up to 47% are affected) (Finch *et al.* 1998). This requires urgent action in the light of recent findings from the UK 1958 birth cohort (Hypponen and Power 2007) (see Table 14.4) demonstrating evidence of widespread low status of the active form of vitamin D (25 OHD) in middle-aged adults, particularly in the winter months. These data are consistent with the NDNS of adults; the mean serum 25 OHD concentration in those aged 35–49 years was 48 nmol/L (Ruston *et al.* 2004). There is also evidence of poor vitamin D status in older children and younger adults (24% of men and 28% of women aged 19–24 years have serum levels below 25 nmol/L; Table 14.3), and this may result in problems in the future. Indeed, if Bischoff-Ferrari and colleagues are correct, a substantial proportion of the UK population would seem to have a vitamin D status that is increasing their risk of fracture. In the NDNS of adults over 65, the highest 25 OHD threshold examined was 60 nmol/L; 62% of the free-living subjects had serum levels below this threshold and this rose to 92% in those living in institutions (Finch *et al.* 1998). In the more recent survey of adults under 65 years (Ruston *et al.* 2004), higher thresholds were examined; 84% of men and 80% of women were below the 70 nmol/L threshold.

Vitamin D receptors are found in various cell types (*e.g.* lymphocytes and monocytes) and in different tissues (*e.g.* brain, heart, pancreas, intestine and placenta) and vitamin D is involved in regulation of gene transcription, suggesting that it has wide-ranging health effects. Indeed, although it has yet to be demonstrated in clinical trials, it is suggested that higher status may reduce risk of colon and other cancers (Vieth *et al.* 2007), and in the 1958 birth cohort, lower 25 OHD is associated with poorer long-term blood glucose control (Hypponen and Power 2007). Low vitamin D status has also been implicated in tuberculosis, multiple sclerosis and type 1 diabetes, although evidence remains inconclusive (Scientific Advisory Committee on Nutrition 2007c). Furthermore, a recent meta-analysis (Pittas *et al.* 2007) discusses the possibility that vitamin D in combination with calcium may have a role in the prevention of type 2 diabetes, perhaps influencing pancreatic beta-cell function, insulin resistance or systemic inflammation. So, risks from low vitamin D status may be greater than previously thought.

Vegetables are a major source of vitamin K and this may in part explain the positive association between fruit and vegetables and bone health. Diets rich in fruit and vegetables are typically alkaline in nature, which is also suggested to be beneficial (see Chapter 4, Section 4.2.6), and are rich in potassium which is able to conserve calcium. The evidence for beneficial effects of phytoestrogens is now looking weaker than originally anticipated (see Chapter 4, Section 4.2.8) and the evidence that high sodium intake leads to an increased rate of bone resorption is limited, although there is good evidence for an increase in urinary calcium excretion, which in the long term may be detrimental to health if not countered by increased absorption (see Chapter 4, Section 4.2.11). Recent evidence suggests that high vitamin A intakes by postmenopausal women may lead to low bone mineral density and increased risk of osteoporosis (see Chapter 4, Section 4.2.9); current

UK government advice is that intakes above 1500 mg of retinol equivalents should be avoided, which in practice means avoiding high-dose supplements (including cod-liver oil) and not eating liver or liver products (*e.g.* pâté, more than once a week).

The precise role of other nutrients (vitamins C and B complex, copper, zinc and magnesium) is yet to be fully elucidated. Low protein intake in older people is associated with low bone mass and increased risk of fracture, and is an important additional risk factor for falling through an effect on muscle mass (see Chapter 6, Section 6.7). However, overall, the data concerning the role of protein are conflicting (see Chapter 4, Section 4.2.4) and evidence discussed in Chapter 6 suggests that, in general, protein intakes in older adults are not a cause for concern. It has been suggested that *n*-3 fatty acid intake (especially docosahexaenoic acid, DHA) is positively associated with bone mineral accrual, although the evidence is sparse (Hogstrom *et al.* 2007; Vanek and Connor 2007) (see Chapter 4, Section 4.2.13). High alcohol intake is a risk factor for osteoporosis and osteoporotic fracture, but the effect of moderate drinking is unclear (see Chapter 4, Section 4.2.12.1). Other risk factors include low bodyweight and smoking.

In summary:

- By 2030, an estimated one in four of the population will be 'elderly' and it is very important that attention is paid to nutritional status and physical activity levels across the population to help optimise skeletal health later in life.
- Weight-bearing exercise is crucial for maintaining a healthy skeleton into old age.
- Calcium and vitamin D are key nutrients for bone health; vitamin K is also important.
- Calcium supplementation can reduce bone loss in postmenopausal women with habitually low calcium intakes, and a combination of calcium and vitamin D can significantly reduce fractures in frail institutionalised older people.
- There is widespread evidence of low vitamin D status and an urgent need to review current recommendations on vitamin D.
- A positive association between fruit and vegetable consumption and bone health has been reported, although the mechanism is not clear.
- High intakes of vitamin A by postmenopausal women may be detrimental to bone health.

14.3.3 Joints

Very little is known about whether diet has a role in the prevention of arthritis (see Chapter 5). There is weak evidence linking a diet low in fish/fish oil with an increased risk of acquiring the disease, but the data are inconsistent and lacking in strength. Avoidance of joint injury and regular physical activity are regarded as important in the prevention of osteoarthritis.

With regard to treatment of existing disease, the most promising evidence in the treatment of symptoms of existing rheumatoid arthritis concerns the use of fatty acid supplements, such as fish oils, at levels of 2.7–4 g/day eicosapentaenoic acid (EPA) and DHA (similar to those levels linked with heart health benefit) (see Chapter 5, Section 5.2.2; Chapter 10, Section 10.7.3.6). Osteoarthritis is often associated with overweight, and weight loss has been shown to have a dose–response effect in reducing pain and disability in osteoarthritis of the knee (see Chapter 5, Section 5.3.8.3).

Gout is an inflammatory arthritis caused by crystals of uric acid, affecting the base of the big toe in particular (see Chapter 5, Section 5.2.4). Obesity and high alcohol intakes are both risk factors for gout, and reduction of these, along with following a diet low in purines, constitutes nutritional management.

A wide range of supplements are available and in common use (see Chapter 5, Section 5.3.8.3). A recent survey of patients with knee osteoarthritis found that 15.9% were taking glucosamine and 5.4% were taking chondroitin (see Chapter 5, Table 5.3). By comparison, 38.2% were taking cod-liver oil and 45.5% and 42.5% respectively were taking anti-inflammatory drugs and paracetamol. Other popular products are referred to in Chapter 5. Meta-analysis of the available data from large trials suggests that small positive effects exist for glucosamine and, in particular, chondroitin. In contrast to rheumatoid arthritis, there is almost no evidence to support the use of cod-liver oil in osteoarthritis (see Chapter 5, Section 5.3.8.3). Limited evidence exists for some of the other popular remedies (see Chapter 5, Section 5.3.8.3).

In summary:

- Little is known about the role of diet in prevention of arthritis but regular physical activity and avoidance of joint injury are important.

- High-dose supplements providing EPA and DHA (2.7–4 g/day) are the most promising dietary approach for existing rheumatoid arthritis.
- Weight loss can improve pain and disability associated with osteoarthritis, and glucosamine and chondroitin have been shown to have small positive effects. There is almost no rationale to support the use of fish oils in osteoarthritis.
- Weight loss, dietary restrictions and reduction in alcohol consumption are used to manage gout.

14.3.4 Muscle

The principal functions of muscle are to enable the body to move and to maintain posture (see Chapter 6). Muscle also has important metabolic functions. These functions all depend on an adequate tissue mass and appropriate composition of muscle, and a properly functioning motor control system. Sarcopenia (age-related loss of skeletal muscle) affects up to a quarter of those over 65 years, more than half of those aged over 80 years, and is associated with considerable economic costs to society through its impact on morbidity and mortality. Established risk factors are advanced age, low bodyweight, physical inactivity, low birthweight and impaired lower limb function. Other possible risk factors include smoking, excess alcohol, stress (corticosteroid secretion) and chronic low-grade inflammation. Another cause of sarcopenia in older subjects is thought to be vitamin D deficiency (see Chapter 6, Section 6.7.1) through vitamin D's role in activation of insulin-like growth factor (IGF-1) (see Section 14.3.2 for more information on vitamin D).

Loss of skeletal muscle adversely affects glucose handling and this is exacerbated as we age because muscle progressively becomes more insulin-resistant. However, strenuous activity can help reverse this resistance to insulin (see Chapter 6, Section 6.6).

To preserve muscle mass and function through to the ninth and tenth decades of life, muscle must be used frequently and supplied with essential nutrients. The UK Department of Health (2004a) recommends that all adults, including older adults, should take a minimum of 30 minutes of moderate activity at least five times a week, although benefit is also achieved by taking multiple shorter bouts throughout the day, including brisk walking. For many older people, structured, supervised exercise programmes are essential. Physical activity (combinations of aerobic, resistance and stretching) is effective in treating sarcopenia. When planning resources for such a programme, provision must be made for the house-bound, whether this is due to infirmity or lack of confidence, as this older group stands to benefit the most.

Motivation and support of younger age groups through education programmes encouraging physical activity and avoidance of smoking and excessive alcohol consumption facilitate prevention of sarcopenia by increasing muscle bulk in younger life, and thus minimise the impact of ageing. Screening for mineral and vitamin deficiencies and providing meals soon after physical activity should be considered, particularly in at-risk populations such as older people in hospitals and nursing homes.

Contrary to predictions that older subjects would benefit from increased protein intake, the information presented in Chapter 6, Section 6.8 demonstrates that, if anything, requirements fall. However, the timing of protein intake after exercise is thought to be important in older subjects. With both aerobic exercise and resistance training, intake of protein-containing foods soon after exercise results in a bigger anabolic response in muscle, hence improving the impact on skeletal muscle of the meal.

In summary:

- Sarcopenia affects up to 25% of those over 65 years and more than half of those over 85 years.
- Frequent use through regular physical activity (throughout life) and appropriate supply of essential nutrients through a varied diet can help build and later preserve muscle mass and function.
- Avoidance of smoking and excess alcohol intake may be important.
- A combination of aerobic, resistance and stretching exercise is an effective treatment for sarcopenia.
- Eating protein-containing foods soon after exercise increases the anabolic response in muscle in older people. This should be considered for those older people in hospitals or nursing homes.
- Low vitamin D status, which is particularly prevalent among house-bound older people, should be prevented.

14.3.5 Skin

Skin contributes at least 3 kg to the weight of the average adult, covering an area of 1.8 m². Over a lifetime, over 40 kg of skin cells are shed, the equivalent of 3–5 million cells a day. The epidermis provides a highly water impermeable barrier, which is dependent on a supply of essential fatty acids (see Chapter 7, Section 7.2) and the dermis provides skin with almost all of its structural resilience. Two of the most noticeable changes as skin ages are alterations in pigment production (resulting in age spots, for example) and wrinkles. Altered melanocyte (pigment-generating cell) function and reorganisation of collagen cross-linking in the dermis directly drive these changes, but the primary cause is excessive lifetime exposure to sunlight, which can also increase the risk of skin cancer.

Relatively little exposure to sunlight is needed to produce sufficient vitamin D (Chapter 7, Section 7.5) and synthesis still occurs after application of sunscreen. Exposure for 15–30 minutes each day has been recommended for older people during the summer months (Ley *et al.* 1999). Solar UV radiation varies with latitude, time of year and time of day. Complete cloud cover reduces the energy of the radiation arriving from the sun by 50%, and about 40% of available UV radiation can be detected in shade. There is no UV radiation of appropriate wavelength in Britain between the end of October and the end of March (see Section 14.3.2 for more information on vitamin D).

The high dependency of skin health on adequate nutrition and hydration is evident from the development of serious skin lesions in response to a variety of nutritional deficiencies, particularly in developing countries. Of particular note are vitamin A (which influences cell differentiation and proliferation); vitamin C (maintenance of connective tissue); B vitamins including riboflavin (energy conversion from substrates and also maintenance of skin and mucous membranes), niacin (energy production, DNA synthesis and skin maintenance) and pyridoxine (energy production, essential co-factor for cell renewal); and vitamin E (cellular protection against free radical damage) (see Chapter 7, Section 7.8). Adequate intakes of these nutrients can be acquired from a healthy and varied diet.

Some vitamins (E and C), carotenoids (*e.g.* β-carotene and lycopene), minerals, *n*-3 PUFA and some plant polyphenols (evidence almost exclusively from animal or *in vitro* studies) have been suggested to provide some degree of protection against UV-induced reddening of the skin (erythema) when taken as high-dose supplements for a period of time (see Chapter 7, Section 7.9.1), although this is not comparable to the use of sunscreen and it remains untested as to whether these effects will translate into measurable effects on skin ageing or skin health.

Protein, specific amino acids (*e.g.* proline and arginine), energy sources (fat and carbohydrate) and specific micronutrients (vitamins A, C, E and zinc) all play a crucial role in wound healing (see Chapter 7, Section 7.10).

All the cell types in skin are subject to hormonal influences and so there are marked changes in skin in women after the menopause, including loss of elasticity and strength, and increased dryness (see Section 7.12.4). Despite claims about the potential value of plant phytoestrogens (isoflavones) in the prevention and treatment of skin ageing, there is a lack of supporting clinical data.

In summary:

- Excessive exposure to sunlight results in photo-ageing of skin and increases skin cancer risk.
- Smoking and other lifestyle factors, such as stress and excessive alcohol intake, can contribute to skin ageing, as can hormonal status in women.
- Relatively little exposure to sunlight during the summer months is needed to produce sufficient vitamin D (although a substantial proportion of the UK population has low vitamin D status).
- Skin health is dependent on adequate nutrition and hydration.
- There is some evidence that high-dose supplements of some nutrients and plant polyphenols may offer some degree of protection against UV-induced skin reddening, but the impact on skin ageing and skin health has yet to be ascertained.
- Protein, especially the amino acids proline and arginine, energy sources and some micronutrients are crucial in wound healing.

14.3.6 Brain

Stroke and dementia are the two most common reasons for admission to long-term institutional care (see Chapter 8 and Chapter 14, Sections 14.2.2 and 14.2.3). The most important risk factor for stroke is high blood pressure. Others include tobacco use, unhealthy diet and lack of physical activity. Weight reduction and increased physical activity result in blood pressure reduction. Many of the established

risk factors for stroke are also thought to be relevant to dementia, Parkinson's disease (which affects 3% of the population aged 65 years and above) and depression. Depression in older people is closely associated with poor physical health; recent research has focused on the role of vascular factors and nutrition in determining risk in this age group, for example there have been many reports of links between low folate status and depression and also of possible associations with vitamin B_{12} status, *n*-3 fatty acid status and selenium intake, although data are inconsistent (see Chapter 8, Section 8.4).

The most important dietary determinants of blood pressure are intakes of sodium, fatty acids, energy and alcohol (see Chapter 8, Section 8.2.2). The most reliable evidence for an effect of sodium comes from the Dietary Approaches to Stop Hypertension (DASH) trial and the DASH-sodium trial. The DASH trial randomised subjects to receive either the standard US diet or a diet low in total fat and saturates (utilising low-fat dairy products), and high in fruit and vegetables; the latter diet was associated with a reduction in systolic/diastolic blood pressure of 5.5/3.0 mmHg (Appel *et al.* 1997). The follow-on trial investigated combining the DASH diet with reduced sodium intake and this reduced blood pressure by a further 2.5/1.2 mmHg (Sacks *et al.* 2001). It is well recognised that many individuals are not able to follow dietary advice sufficiently closely to achieve risk factor reduction and hence a population approach to sodium reduction has been adopted in the UK, through which manufacturers have been encouraged by the Food Standards Agency to reduce the sodium content of their products (see www.food. gov.uk) (see Section 14.5.2).

An inverse association between fish intake and risk of stroke (particularly thrombotic stroke) has been reported in several, but not all, prospective studies (see Chapter 8, Section 8.2.7). Large trials are currently assessing the effects of supplementation with long chain *n*-3 fatty acids on risk of heart disease and stroke (see Chapter 8, Section 8.2.7; Chapter 10, Section 10.7.3.6). With regard to dementia, a recent review reported that data are insufficient to draw any strong conclusions about the effect of oil-rich fish on cognitive function in normal ageing or on the incidence or treatment of dementia (Issa *et al.* 2006). However, one recent study suggests a significant delay in rate of cognitive decline in those with mild compared with more advanced cognitive decline (see

Chapter 8, Section 8.3.4). Whilst unsaturated fatty acids may reduce risk of Alzheimer's disease, saturates and in particular *trans* fatty acids appear to be associated with increased risk (a four-fold difference in risk between high and low intakes of *trans* fatty acids) (see Chapter 8, Section 8.3.4).

Alcohol intake is an independent risk factor for hypertension (and some cancers), but there is some evidence that the benefits of moderate drinking (up to 3–4 units per day for men and 2–3 units per day for women) may extend beyond heart disease (see Chapter 10, Section 10.7.8) to ischaemic stroke, Alzheimer's disease and vascular dementia (see Chapter 8, Sections 8.3.7 and 8.5.1).

An elevated plasma concentration of homocysteine (which may be influenced by diet) has been suggested as a modifiable risk factor for stroke. After adjustment for the effects of smoking, cholesterol and blood pressure, a meta-analysis of 30 prospective studies suggests that a 25% lower plasma homocysteine level is associated with a 19% lower risk of stroke (Homocysteine Studies Collaboration 2002) (see Chapter 8, Section 8.2.3). A similar effect (18% reduction in risk of stroke) has been reported in a recent meta-analysis of randomised controlled trials using folic acid (Wang *et al.* 2007). Associations have also been reported with age-related cognitive decline, vascular dementia and Alzheimer's disease (see Chapter 8, Section 8.3.1) but there is substantial uncertainty about whether these associations are causal. Dietary intake of folate/folic acid is a major determinant of plasma homocysteine level in the general population but, in the older population, low vitamin B_{12} status is a more important cause of elevated levels. A high proportion of older people have biochemical evidence of low vitamin B_{12} status and this increases with age from 5% at age 65 to 20% at age 80 (Clarke, Refsum *et al.* 2003). Although it is evident that homocysteine levels can be lowered by B vitamin supplementation, it is not yet clear whether this reduction is causally related to a reduction in risk of stroke (or CHD) (see Chapter 8, Section 8.2.4) or other conditions referred to here. Trials are underway to assess this (see Chapter 8, Section 8.2.4).

Poor vitamin B_{12} status is considered likely to be a more important cause of cognitive impairment in older people than poor folate status (see Chapter 8, Section 8.3.2). Given the ability of folic acid fortification to mask B_{12} deficiency, there are concerns that B_{12} deficiency may go unnoticed in countries with mandatory folic acid fortification and thus adversely influence deterioration in neurological function. According to a recent study, only a small proportion of older people with biochemical evidence of B_{12} deficiency have anaemia, neuropathy or cognitive impairment (Hin *et al.* 2006). However, the need for a management strategy to identify and treat low B_{12} status in older people (which is often not dietary in origin) has been recognised by the Scientific Advisory Committee on Nutrition (2006) in the UK (see Chapter 8, Section 8.6). Various vitamin B_{12} supplementation trials are underway (see Chapter 8, Section 8.3.2).

Prevalence of dementia is predicted to rise considerably over the coming decades (Ferri *et al.* 2005). The OPAL study (Dangour *et al.* 2006) is currently examining the influence of long chain *n*-3 fatty acids relative to olive oil on cognition (and retinal function) of 70–79-year-olds. A recent study investigated prediction of risk of late-life dementia in people of middle age on the basis of their risk profiles. Occurrence of dementia in the 20 years of follow-up was 4% and was significantly predicted by age, low education (<10 years), hypertension, hypercholesterolaemia and obesity (Kivipelto *et al.* 2006). Blood pressure in mid-life has also been reported as predictive.

Despite promising information from observational studies regarding fruits and vegetables, large-scale trials using antioxidant supplements have failed to demonstrate a reduction in risk of stroke, any other vascular events (see Chapter 8, Section 8.2.6) or Alzheimer's disease (see Chapter 8, Section 8.3.3). Composite dietary patterns such as the Mediterranean diet (see Section 14.5.5) have been linked with lower risk of Alzheimer's disease (Scarmeas *et al.* 2006), but such studies are difficult to interpret and extrapolate because of clustering of various relevant dietary and lifestyle factors.

Low doses of caffeine have been suggested to enhance cognitive function (see Chapter 8, Section 8.3.7), but high doses should be avoided as they can cause side-effects in vulnerable people. Vitamin D deficiency is common in older adults (see Section 14.3.2 and Chapter 4, Section 4.2.3) and has been implicated in low mood and impaired cognitive performance (Wilkins *et al.* 2006).

Recent cohort studies suggest an association between regular physical activity and reduced cognitive decline (see Section 14.6, and Chapter 8, Section 8.3.8), but evidence from randomised controlled trials is still awaited.

Low vitamin B_{12} and folate status may be associated with depression, but there is no clear evidence from randomised trials that *n*-3 supplements or selenium status protect against depression (see Chapter 8, Section 8.4).

With regard to Parkinson's disease, a number of foods and nutrients have been implicated in risk but a systematic review has concluded that significant associations are lacking (Ishihara and Brayne 2005) (see Chapter 8, Section 8.5.1). The strongest evidence concerns caffeine and alcohol, but findings are not entirely consistent.

In summary:

- The most important risk factor for stroke is high blood pressure, the dietary determinants of which are high intakes of sodium, alcohol and energy (hence emphasising the relevance of bodyweight and activity levels). Smoking is another important risk factor for stroke.
- On the other hand, light to moderate alcohol consumption may be linked to reduced cognitive decline.
- The DASH dietary pattern is an effective means of reducing blood pressure, as are weight reduction and increased physical activity.
- A possible protective role of long chain *n*-3 fatty acids (or oil-rich fish) is being investigated.
- There is also interest in a potential role of folate and/or vitamin B_{12} in stroke prevention; trials are underway.
- Many of the established risk factors for stroke (high blood pressure, obesity, inactivity) may also be important for dementia, and there is growing interest in the potential of specific dietary interventions, *e.g.* a link with low status of *n*-3 fatty acids and vitamin D.

14.3.7 Eyes

Laboratory and animal studies have demonstrated the important role of antioxidants in the lens and retina. Epidemiological studies have also suggested that dietary antioxidants, *e.g.* vitamins C and E, carotenoids and, more recently, lutein and zeaxanthin, may provide protection against cataract and AMD (see Chapter 9, Sections 9.5.2 and 9.5.4). This evidence supports general dietary recommendations

concerning the importance of fruits and vegetables, especially citrus fruit and other rich sources of vitamin C, and vegetables rich in lutein and zeaxanthin, such as spinach, broccoli, kale, and red and orange peppers. Although the evidence is less robust, it is likely that consuming at least one serving of oil-rich fish per week will help reduce the risk of AMD. In contrast, there is no evidence that the use of vitamin supplements is of proven benefit in the prevention of age-related eye disease. However, multivitamin supplements with zinc have been shown to be of benefit in patients with intermediate AMD in one or both eyes.

As with other diseases, such as CVD, there is evidence of an association between overall dietary quality and reduced risk of eye disease. For example, in the Nurses' Health Study, adherence to recommended dietary guidelines for five food groups (grains, vegetables, fruit and fruit juice, milk and milk products, meat/alternatives including fish, nuts and beans) reduced risk by 50%, which was increased to 70% when those taking vitamin C supplements were excluded (Moeller *et al.* 2004) (see Chapter 9, Section 9.5.2).

Claims have been made for a wide variety of other foods and supplements, such as blue/purple fruits and gingko biloba; although plausible mechanisms have been proposed there is minimal evidence to date to demonstrate benefit in humans (see Chapter 9, Section 9.7).

Smoking is a major risk factor for both cataract and AMD, and smokers with AMD are at a high risk of progression of damage to their vision. There is moderately strong evidence that high exposure to sunlight is associated with increased risk of cataract and AMD, and this can be avoided by use of sunglasses and wide-brimmed hats when outdoors during the middle of the day. Another risk factor is obesity, especially high abdominal adiposity or high waist:hip ratio, independently of the increased risk associated with type 2 diabetes.

In summary:

- Smoking is a major risk factor for both cataract and AMD and there is moderate evidence of a detrimental effect of high exposure to sunlight.
- Good nutrition in general appears to be protective.
- In particular, intake of fruits and vegetables is likely to be protective, especially citrus fruit and

other rich sources of vitamin C, and vegetables rich in lutein and zeaxanthin, such as spinach, broccoli, kale, and red and orange peppers.

- Consuming at least one serving of oil-rich fish per week may help reduce the risk of AMD.
- In contrast, there is no evidence that the use of vitamin supplements is of proven benefit in the prevention of age-related eye disease.
- Another risk factor is obesity, especially abdominal obesity.

14.3.8 Cardiovascular system

The risk of CVD in old age is likely to be influenced by the combination, accumulation, and/or interactions of different environments and experiences across the life-course. This supports a life-course approach to prevention and health promotion, and highlights the need for CVD prevention programmes to begin early in childhood (perhaps even earlier, given the relationship between birthweight and CVD risk) and continue throughout adulthood to reduce the risk of atherosclerosis. Nevertheless, risk factors such as high blood pressure and high blood cholesterol are still predictive of CVD among older people and changing habits in later life can still impact on risk. Dietary and lifestyle advice therefore remains the same for older people as in middle age. Furthermore, there is evidence of effective dietary interventions in older populations (see Chapter 10, Section 10.10).

The connection between most of the more novel risk factors (lipoprotein (a), homocysteine, oxidative stress) in older people and the value of modifying these requires further investigation. A report from the UK Scientific Advisory Committee on Nutrition (SACN) (2006) on folate confirmed that whilst an inverse relationship exists between folate status and homocysteine, it is still too early to predict whether folic acid supplementation can reduce risk of CVD (see Chapter 10, Sections 10.4.2.2 and 10.7.6.4). To date the results of trials have been mixed, with several showing no effect on CVD (see Chapter 8).

The clustering of several vascular risk factors, including obesity (particularly abdominal obesity), dyslipidaemia, impaired glucose metabolism and hypertension, is called the metabolic syndrome (also known as insulin resistance syndrome or Syndrome X). This often precedes the onset of type 2 diabetes

and substantially increases risk of CVD mortality and morbidity (Coppack *et al.* 2005) (see Section 14.2.5 and Chapter 10, Section 10.4.3).

Substantial evidence shows that diets incorporating non-hydrogenated unsaturated (*cis*) fatty acids as the predominant form of fat, starchy foods especially whole-grains as the main form of carbohydrate, an abundance of fruits and vegetables, a modest salt intake (<6 g/day for adults) and adequate n-3 fatty acids (specifically those derived from oil-rich fish) can offer significant protection against CVD (Table 14.5). The shorter chain length n-3 fatty acid, alpha-linolenic acid (ALNA), has not been shown to have the same effect as those characteristic of oil-rich fish, although it may be important as a displacer of other dietary fatty acids (*i.e.* saturates of chain length C12–C16) (see Lunn and Theobald 2006). Cholesterol-lowering effects have been

Table 14.5: Summary of practical dietary advice to reduce risk of CVD

- Reduce consumption of all types of fat, for example by selecting lean cuts of meat and lower fat dairy products, by reducing use of oil and full-fat spreads (margarine, butter), by eating less fried foods and by moderating consumption of high-fat foods, such as cakes, biscuits and savoury snacks.
- Opt for oils/spreads that are higher in monounsaturates or polyunsaturates and lower in saturates.
- Include oil-rich fish in the diet at least once a week (those with heart disease may benefit from higher intakes).*
- Include more fruit and vegetables in the diet, aiming for at least five portions of a variety of fruits and vegetables each day.
- Use less salt at the table and in cooking, and look for lower salt alternatives of manufactured foods. Reduce intake to <6 g/day (less for children).
- Include more starchy foods in the diet, *e.g.* bread, potatoes, yams, rice and pasta, so that at least 50% of energy intake comes from carbohydrate. Increase consumption of whole-grain foods.
- Drink alcohol sensibly, *i.e.* no more than 2–3 units per day for women and no more than 3–4 units per day for men (see Section 14.5.4). Avoid binge drinking.

*The National Institute for Health and Clinical Excellence (2007) recommends that patients who have suffered a heart attack should consume 2–4 portions of oil-rich fish a week.
Source: Based on Department of Health (1994).
Material is Crown copyright and is reproduced with the permission of the Controller of HMSO.

demonstrated for phytosterols/-stanols (British Nutrition Foundation 2008) and, to a lesser extent, for legumes, nuts and some whole-grain cereals. Such diets, together with regular physical activity, avoidance of smoking and maintenance of a healthy bodyweight, may prevent the greater part of CVD in western populations. The study of the interactions between nutritional and genetic factors is an emerging and important area of research, and has the potential to permit a more individual approach to dietary advice for CVD prevention.

Recently, consideration has been given as to whether legislation should be put in place to further reduce *trans* fatty acid intake in the UK. It has been concluded that no action is needed. Although there is evidence that dietary *trans* fatty acids have a moderate impact on risk of CHD, average intakes in the UK have now fallen to 1%, well below the maximum of 2% of energy (see Section 14.5.2) (Scientific Advisory Committee on Nutrition 2007e).

As described in Chapter 10, Section 10.7.6.2, randomised controlled trials have not revealed a beneficial effect on heart disease risk of supplementation with antioxidant vitamins. Indeed, supplements of β-carotene may increase disease risk in high-risk groups such as smokers.

The importance of avoiding tobacco is now widely recognised but less attention has been paid to discouraging physical inactivity (Fox and Hillsdon 2007). Having a sedentary lifestyle increases cardiovascular risk and also influences other risk factors and co-morbidities such as high blood pressure, obesity and diabetes (Buttriss and Hardman 2005; Miles 2007b) (see Chapter 10, Section 10.8).

The public health impact of physical activity may be especially important for older adults who are at high risk of CVD and are often sedentary (see Chapter 10, Section 10.6.4). There is good evidence that maintaining or taking up light or moderate physical activity can reduce mortality and heart attacks in older people with and without existing CVD. Activity can also prevent age-related weight gain and help with weight loss. Benefits are apparent even for men over the age of 60 who become physically active after years of a sedentary lifestyle (Blair *et al.* 1995). This supports public health recommendations for older sedentary people to increase physical activity and for active middle-aged people to continue their activity into old age (see Section 14.6 and Chapter 10, Section 10.8).

For those who are sedentary until old age, it can be harmful to engage in vigorous activity because of increased injury and heart attack risk. Initially at least, types of physical activity with lower intensities, such as walking, cycling or gardening, are often preferable. Although older people should aim to meet the recommendation for physical activity for younger adults, even light activities conducted almost daily (≥5 times per week) may have substantial benefits for cardiovascular risk profile in this age group. They may also result in improvements in many physical and psychological parameters (Department of Health 2004a).

In summary:

- Current dietary advice to reduce CVD risk is summarised in Table 14.5.
- A cholesterol-lowering effect has also been demonstrated for phytosterol/phytostanol-enriched foods and modest cholesterol-lowering effects for legumes (*e.g.* soya) and nuts.
- It is still unclear whether folate-rich foods or folic acid supplementation specifically benefit heart health.
- The importance of physical activity urgently needs greater emphasis.
- Maintenance of a healthy bodyweight is important.
- No convincing evidence exists for antioxidant supplementation (and it may increase risk in smokers).
- The impact of birthweight on cardiovascular risk highlights the importance of a life-course approach.

14.3.9 Immune system

Impairments to the immune system occur with ageing, with low-level chronic inflammation, due to over-expression of inflammatory cytokines, being common and a contributing factor (see Chapter 11, Section 11.2). The increase in pro-inflammatory mediator production may play a role in the development of several age-related conditions, including atherosclerosis (see Chapter 10), rheumatoid arthritis (see Chapter 5), fibrosis, sarcopenia (Chapter 6) and dementia (Chapter 8).

Much of the age-related immune system dysfunction (*i.e.* exaggeration of innate responses) is associated with changes to the T lymphocyte (T cell) population (see Chapter 11, Section 11.2.2), although all components of the immune system are modified to some extent and inter-individual variability in response to ageing is thought to be due to differences in genetics, environment, health and nutritional status. Control of the pro-inflammatory response to ageing has been suggested to provide a route to healthy ageing (see Chapter 11, Section 11.2). Improvements in insulin sensitivity and vascular function underpin many of the benefits.

Diet and lifestyle interventions have been shown to reduce acute and probably chronic inflammation: long chain *n*-3 PUFA supplementation (*e.g.* fish oil), antioxidants, weight loss and increased physical activity level are all effective (see Chapter 11, Section 11.7).

Protein- and energy-deficient diets and various micronutrient deficiencies are detrimental to immune function (see Chapter 11, Section 11.8), and increase both the risk and severity of infections. Micronutrient deficiencies are common in the elderly, resulting from poor diets associated with compromised dentition, hospitalisation and institutionalisation (see Section 14.5). Rectification of deficiencies in nutritionally compromised individuals improves markers of immune function but there is currently no evidence to support the routine use of micronutrient supplementation to improve immune responses among those already well nourished. Indeed, there is evidence that it may be damaging (see Chapter 11, Section 11.8.4).

In summary:

- Immune system impairment occurs with ageing and is associated with low-level chronic inflammation which is thought to have a role in development of chronic disease.
- Protein- and energy-deficient diets and some micronutrient deficiencies (which can be common in some older people) are detrimental to immune function and increase both the risk and severity of infections.
- Diet and lifestyle interventions such as long chain *n*-3 fatty acid supplementation, sufficient supply of antioxidants and increased physical activity (and weight loss) reduce acute (and probably chronic) inflammation.
- There is currently no evidence to support the routine use of micronutrient supplementation to improve immune responses in well-nourished subjects.

14.3.10 Digestive system

Table 14.6 describes the changes that occur to the gastrointestinal tract with ageing, the factors involved and opportunities for diet or lifestyle intervention (see Chapter 12).

Disorders of the GI tract are the third most common cause of GP consultations in the UK. Gastro-oesophageal reflux, which is positively associated with BMI, increases with age and can lead to oesophagitis, a risk factor for oesophageal adenocarcinoma (the commonest form of oesophageal cancer in the UK and US). Smoking and high alcohol intake are risk factors for squamous cell carcinomas of the oesophagus, and have adverse effects on other parts of the gut. High fruit and vegetable consumption is protective for both forms of cancer (see Section 14.2.6). Consumption of very hot drinks is said to increase the risk of oesophageal cancer.

The prevalence of atrophic change to the gastric mucosa generally increases with age, as does gastric metaplasia and gastric carcinoma. *H. pylori* plays a direct role in the development of chronic atrophic gastritis and gastric cancer, and antibiotic treatment can eradicate the infection. In older people, atrophic gastritis is an important cause of malabsorption of vitamin B_{12} and hence poor vitamin B_{12} status (see Section 14.2.6). The association between gastric cancer risk and fruit and vegetable intake has been attributed to vitamin C in particular (see Section 14.2.6).

There is evidence that the colonic microflora changes with age, with an increase in species diversity and lower numbers of bifidobacteria, although the implications of these changes for health have yet to be established (see Chapter 12, Section 12.5.1). Prebiotics have been shown to increase the numbers of bifidobacteria, but there are few studies in older people. Bowel dysfunction, especially constipation, is a major problem for older people; some studies have shown that increasing fibre intake, especially when fluid intake is also increased, provides relief. Insoluble fibre (*e.g.* wheat bran) appears more effective than soluble fibre, resistant starch or prebiotics. A number of intervention studies have shown that prebiotics relieve constipation in older subjects (see Chapter 12, Section 12.5.2.1).

Antibiotic-associated diarrhoea (AAD) is common in hospitals, nursing homes and other chronic care facilities (see Chapter 12, Section 12.4.4) and results

Table 14.6: Changes in the gastrointestinal tract with age, and dietary and lifestyle factors that may influence risk of ill health

Major changes in the gastrointestinal tract as a consequence of ageing	Factors involved	Dietary and lifestyle approaches that may be of benefit
Reflux of stomach juice into the oesophagus (gullet) leading to inflammation of the oesophagus (oesophagitis) and changes in the cells of the lining (Barrett's oesophagus). May develop into cancer.	Changes in sphincter and peristalsis. High BMI associated with reflux and Barrett's oesophagus.	Maintenance of healthy bodyweight. Increased consumption of fruit and vegetables.
Oesophageal cancer.	Gastric reflux, Barrett's oesophagus. Smoking, excessive alcohol (convincing evidence). Being overweight (convincing evidence). Low intake of fruits and non-starchy vegetables (probably increase risk).	Giving up smoking. Avoidance of excess alcohol consumption and excess body fat. Increased fruit and non-starchy vegetable consumption, especially those providing β-carotene and/or vitamin C.
Gastric and duodenal ulcers, bleeding complications.	Infection with *H. pylori*. Use of NSAIDs.	Antibiotic therapy.
Stomach (gastric) cancer.	Infection with *H. pylori*. High intake of highly salted food (probably increase risk). Low fruit and non-starchy vegetable (especially allium vegetables) consumption (probably increase risk).	Antibiotic therapy to eliminate *H. pylori*. Increased fruit and non-starchy vegetable (especially allium vegetable) consumption.
Diarrhoea: this is a significant worldwide problem and is of particular concern for older people. About 85% of mortality associated with diarrhoea in the developed world affects older people.	Infections, diabetes, excessive use of laxatives/diuretics, food-borne toxins, and alcohol. Food allergies/intolerances (rarer). Poor digestion (*e.g.* pancreatic insufficiency, coeliac disease, lactose intolerance) or ingested substances such as antacids, foods containing substances such as sorbitol. Diarrhoea associated with inflammation (such as with Crohn's disease and ulcerative colitis) is less common.	Probiotics, alone or in combination with prebiotics, may be useful in treatment of antibiotic-associated diarrhoea.
Constipation.	Changes in muscle activity in gut, drugs (analgesic, opioids, diuretics, antidepressants). Low fibre intake.	Increased intake of dietary fibre, especially insoluble fibre, increased fluid intake. Consumption of prebiotics.
Changes in gut bacteria in colon (lower numbers of bifidobacteria).	Not known.	Consumption of prebiotics, *e.g.* oligosaccharides.
Diverticular disease (rare in people <40 years).	Low fibre intake.	Increased intake of dietary fibre (20–30 g wheat bran/day).

Table 14.6: *Continued*

Major changes in the gastrointestinal tract as a consequence of ageing	Factors involved	Dietary and lifestyle approaches that may be of benefit
Colorectal cancer (third most common cancer worldwide).	Hereditary factors are a minor component. Low physical activity (convincing evidence). Obesity, especially abdominal obesity (convincing evidence). High alcohol intake (convincing evidence in men, probably increases risk in women). Processed meat and to a lesser extent red meat associated with a slightly elevated risk, which is attenuated by a high fibre intake.	Increased physical activity, avoidance of obesity especially abdominal obesity. Moderate alcohol intake (see Section 14.2.6). Increased intake of dietary fibre. Moderated intake of processed and red meats. In the UK, government advice is that intakes should not rise above the current average of 90 g/day and those with intakes above 140 g/day (cooked weight, 12–14 portions per week) should consider a reduction (Department of Health 1998). WCRF advice to minimise cancer risk focuses particularly on processed meat: maximum of 500 g/week red and processed meat (cooked weight; equivalent to 700–750 g raw weight), very little of which to be processed meat. Milk and calcium probably protect against colon cancer and there is limited evidence suggesting protection via non-starchy vegetables, fruit, folate-rich foods, fish and vitamin D.

BMI: body mass index; *H. pylori: Helicobacter pylori*; NSAIDs: non-steroidal anti-inflammatory drugs; WCRF: World Cancer Research Fund.

from disruption of the intestinal microflora enabling opportunistic colonisation by enteric pathogens, in particular *C. difficile*. Older patients are particularly susceptible to AAD and it can increase mortality risk by 2–3-fold. Probiotics (at doses of 10^{10} organisms per day) show considerable promise as therapies for AAD and a combination of pro- and prebiotics (but not prebiotics alone) have been reported to decrease *C. difficile* colonisation after antibiotic treatment.

The incidence of diverticular disease increases with age, but is uncommon in those under the age of 40. There is an inverse relationship between dietary fibre intake and colonic diverticular disease. The incidence of colorectal cancer increases dramatically with age. In Europe, the US, Australia and New Zealand it is the second most common cancer. Epidemiological evidence (Miles 2007a) suggests that physical activity patterns in particular and diet play a significant role in the aetiology (see Chapter 12, Section 12.5.5.1). High intakes of vegetables (World Cancer Research Fund 1997) and fibre (Bingham *et al.* 2003) are protective. Processed meats and, to a lesser extent, red meat appear to be associated with a slightly elevated risk (World Cancer Research Fund/American Institute for Cancer Research 2007). In EPIC, a high-fibre intake attenuated any risk associated with meat (Norat *et al.* 2005) (see Chapter 12, Section 12.5.5.1). Associations have also been reported with overweight and obesity. Higher bodyweight and BMI significantly increase colorectal cancer risk in men but not women. Abdominal obesity was significantly associated in both men and women (Pischon *et al.* 2006). Calcium supplementation has been shown to have a modest protective effect against colorectal adenomas. High alcohol consumption increases risk of colorectal cancer, and may also exacerbate the impact on risk of low folate status (see Section 14.2.6 and Chapter 12, Section 12.5.5.1).

In summary:

- Smoking and high alcohol intake increase the risk of cancer at a number of sites.
- High intakes of vegetables and fruit are probably protective against cancer in the gut.
- High fibre intake also seems to be protective and can offset the modest adverse effect of high meat intake. The effect of meat appears strongest for processed meat. Calcium supplementation is moderately important (providing protection against colon cancer). An effect is also reported for milk.
- Physical activity exerts a significant protective effect on colon cancer risk and there is now convincing evidence that obesity, especially abdominal obesity, is a risk factor.
- Gastric and duodenal ulcers are increasing among older people worldwide, linked to *H. pylori* infection (eradicated by antibiotics) and use of non-steroidal anti-inflammatory drugs (NSAIDs). Treatment of *H. pylori* infection is important.
- The gut flora in the colon changes with age, with a reduction in bifidobacteria; prebiotics may help reverse this but there are few studies in older people.
- Probiotics, alone or in combination with prebiotics, show considerable promise as therapy for antibiotic-associated diarrhoea.
- There is an inverse relationship between fibre intake and risk of diverticular disease. Fibre, combined with adequate fluid intake, helps protect against constipation (physical activity may also be important).

14.3.11 Endocrine system

Hormonal regulation is central to many physiological processes, *e.g.* maintenance of blood pressure, bone density and blood sugar levels (see Chapter 13). Dysfunction in these regulatory processes leads to increased risk of disease, either directly (as in the case of diabetes and osteoporosis) or indirectly (via action through a risk factor for disease, *e.g.* raised blood pressure as a risk factor for CVD). Weight reduction can help normalise adipokine production and can also have beneficial effects on blood hormone levels. In several diabetes studies, a combination of diet and physical activity has been shown to be particularly effective. For example, in the US Diabetes Prevention Program, lifestyle changes, 150 minutes of physical activity per week plus a 7% weight loss, reduced diabetes incidence by 58% compared to a control group, whereas metformin treatment resulted in only a 31% reduction (Knowler *et al.* 2002). The intervention was particularly successful in the older age group, who experienced a 71% reduction compared to the control group.

Changes in endocrine factors with age have been suggested to be responsible for the diminished appetite associated with ageing (see Chapter 13, Section 13.2.3). Conversely, lifestyle factors, dietary patterns and specific dietary components may directly influence the endocrine system (see Chapter 13, Section 13.4), although there is little information available about interactions between the endocrine system, ageing and these factors *per se*. For example, the nature and quantity of dietary carbohydrates and fibre are major determinants of postprandial blood glucose level and subsequent fluctuations in circulating insulin (see Chapter 13, Section 13.4.2). There is also a subsidiary role for glycaemic index and interest is growing in the ability of resistant starch to beneficially influence glycaemic and insulinaemic responses (Nugent 2005). Fat quality has also been shown to influence hormonal responses. For example, replacing dietary saturates with monounsaturates in a study of healthy men and women resulted in a 12% increase in insulin sensitivity in those with a total fat intake below 37% of energy (Vessby *et al.* 2001) and there may also be a beneficial effect of long chain *n*-3 fatty acids in people with diabetes (see Buttriss 2005).

Dietary patterns characterised as being rich in plant-derived foods have been reported to have beneficial effects on the endocrine system in some studies, although findings are inconsistent (see Chapter 13, Section 13.4.3). Specific plant components have been highlighted, such as phytoestrogens (isoflavones, lignans and stilbenes), which have structures similar to oestradiol and can bind weakly to oestrogen receptors (see Chapter 13, Section 13.4.4). A recent review found that although there was some, albeit conflicting, evidence to support a role for phytoestrogens in reducing hot flushes in menopausal women, there was insufficient evidence to draw conclusions about the effects of phytoestrogens in diabetes, colon cancer or breast cancer (Cassidy *et al.* 2006).

In summary:

- Lifestyle factors (physical activity), dietary patterns (*e.g.* diet rich in plant-derived foods) and specific dietary components (type of fat or carbohydrate) may directly influence the endocrine system, but there is little information available about interactions between such factors, the endocrine system and ageing.
- Diet and physical activity in combination have been shown to reduce significantly the incidence of diabetes in high-risk subjects, particularly in older age groups.

14.4 Common themes

Some common themes are evident. For example, regular physical activity and maintenance of a healthy bodyweight benefit most organ systems (bones, muscles, cardiovascular system, immune function, gastrointestinal system) and help minimise disease risk, *e.g.* colon cancer (see Section 14.2.6), obesity (see Section 14.2.4), type 2 diabetes (see Section 14.2.5), coronary heart disease (see Section 14.3.8 and Chapter 10), osteoporosis (see Section 14.3.2 and Chapter 4), osteoarthritis (see Section 14.3.3 and Chapter 5), stroke risk and cognitive decline (see Sections 14.2.2, 14.2.3 and Chapter 8). To date, the need to tackle inactivity has not received the attention it deserves and avoidance of smoking and excessive alcohol consumption are key characteristics of reduced health risk. Excess alcohol intake can result in interactions with drugs and hence poor control of blood pressure and other risk factors. However, modest intake seems to carry some benefits (Table 14.7).

Among dietary factors, common themes are fat quality; the importance of long chain *n*-3 fatty acid in particular, and certain micronutrients (*e.g.* folate, vitamin B_{12} and vitamin D), and the importance of fruit and vegetables and other fibre-containing foods, including pulses and whole-grain cereals (see Table 14.7).These themes are discussed in Sections 14.5 and 14.6 in the context of the need for action in terms of future health.

Nothing in the review suggests that current diet and lifestyle recommendations need to change radi-

cally, but there is need for changes in emphasis. This is discussed further in Section 14.7.

14.5 Current trends in diet and the way forward

Current trends in nutrient intakes, dietary patterns, nutrient status and physical activity patterns among older people are discussed in Chapter 1, Sections 1.5 and 1.6. Two surveys by SACN (2007a, 2007b) have summarised respectively available evidence about the nutritional health of the UK population and the dietary patterns associated with poor micronutrient intake and status.

14.5.1 Fruit and vegetables

These analyses have identified a number of areas for concern. Consumption of fruit and vegetables is below the recommendation of at least five servings a day in all age groups, and is particularly low for young adults and people in lower socio-economic groups (Scientific Advisory Committee on Nutrition 2007a). Figure 14.9 shows consumption in different age groups of adults in 2000/1. In women aged 19–64, average intake was 282 g/d, and in men 273 g/d. In older free-living people (65+ years), intakes were lower at 244 g/day and 230 g/day in men and women, respectively. They were lower still among those older people in institutions: 171 g/day and 163 g/day, respectively. In children aged 4–18 years, average intakes in age sub-groups ranged between 167 and 216 g/day; 20% did not consume any fruit (excluding

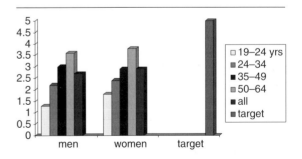

Figure 14.9: Consumption of fruit and vegetables in British adults aged 19–64 (using five-a-day criterion), portions per day.
Source: Scientific Advisory Committee on Nutrition (2007a).

Table 14.7: Diet and lifestyle messages emerging from the Task Force, and associated benefits

Diet and lifestyle messages	Associated benefits
Fat quality: ↓ SFA and *trans* fatty acids, ↑ *cis* MUFA and PUFA	↓ risk of CHD and stroke; improved insulin sensitivity.
↑ EPA and DHA, fish oils (increase; see oil-rich fish below)	↓ risk of CHD and possibly stroke; reduced symptoms of rheumatoid arthritis; may have an effect on eye health and help prevent cognitive decline; improved immune function; very limited data suggesting improved bone mineral accrual (DHA).
Starchy carbohydrates (increase intake)	See dietary fibres and whole-grain sections below. Slow release carbohydrates have a role in diabetic control.
Dietary fibres (increase intake)	Improved gut health (↓ constipation, ↓ diverticular disease risk, ↓ colon cancer risk); cardiovascular health (soluble fibre ↓ plasma cholesterol); satiety effects with some fibre types, *e.g.* viscous fibres such as guar gum, pectin, psyllium, β-glucan.
Sugars (moderation)	Dental health benefits associated with moderation of frequency of sugars consumption but regular use of fluoridated toothpaste is the most important message.
Alcohol (in moderation)	↓ risk of CHD but high intake increases risk of stroke, osteoporosis, sarcopenia and some cancers and carries effects associated with dehydration. Light to moderate intake may help prevent cognitive decline.
Protein (adequate dietary supply)	Preserves skeletal muscle mass, ↓ risk of falls (hence ↓ fracture risk).
Folate	↓ neural tube defects in fetus (maternal intake of 400 μg/d); effect on CVD and dementia still unclear (possible adverse effect of fortification on cancer progression is currently under review); low status may be predictive of depression.
Vitamin B_{12} (ensure adequate supply)	↓ risk of neurological problems, *e.g.* peripheral neuropathy and possibly dementia; low status may be predictive of depression.
Vitamin K (ensure adequate supply)	↑ bone mineral density; ↓ osteoporotic fractures.
Salt/sodium (moderation)	Positively associated with blood pressure (raised blood pressure is a major risk factor for stroke and heart disease).
Calcium (ensure adequate supply)	Improves bone health (↑ bone mineral density; ↓ postmenopausal bone loss); some evidence for ↓ colon cancer risk (milk and supplemental calcium).
Vitamin D status (ensure adequate status)	Essential for bone mineralisation; ↓ sarcopenia risk; limited evidence that it may ↓ (colon) cancer risk, delay cognitive decline, improve low mood.
Vitamin A (avoid excess)	Excess (>1500 μg retinol equivalents/day) associated with low bone mineral density in postmenopausal women.
Antioxidant vitamins	Dietary supply (via food and drink) essential for good health, *e.g.* immune function. Evidence not supportive of a role for supplements in heart health, cancer or eye health (may be adverse effects).
Plant bioactives	Only limited evidence exists. For example, eye health (*e.g.* fruits and vegetables rich in lutein, zeaxanthin); heart health (phytosterol/-stanol enriched foods).

Table 14.7:   *Continued*

Diet and lifestyle messages	Associated benefits
Pre- and probiotics	Some evidence for a benefit with digestive health through effect on colonic flora.
Fruit and vegetables (increased intake)	High intake associated with ↓ risk of CHD, and of stroke (especially fruit). Probably protects against some cancers; limited evidence for a benefit for dementia and bone health.
Nuts (in moderation)	Positive association with heart health.
Whole-grain cereals (increased intake)	Positive association with heart health and gut health (via fibre content).
Soya	Positive association with heart health (via LDL-cholesterol).
Fish (especially oil-rich fish)	Positive association with heart health and cancer risk. Possible beneficial effect with dementia (studies underway).
Meat	Modest ↑ risk of colon cancer with processed meat in particular; also some evidence of an increase with red meat particularly in association with low fibre intake (*i.e.* effect attenuated by high fibre intake).
Low-fat dairy products (in moderation)	Calcium content important for bone health; ↓ blood pressure (as part of the DASH diet); possible ↓ risk of colon cancer.
Fluid intake	Important for general health and wellbeing; associated with ↓ risk of constipation; possibly associated with better skin health.
Tobacco (avoidance)	Strong evidence of causal link between smoking and heart disease and cancer. Tobacco use also associated with ↑ risk of eye damage; osteoporosis, premature skin ageing; poor periodontal (gum) health and possible ↑ risk of sarcopenia.
Healthy bodyweight	↓ risk of CHD and stroke; ↓ colon, oesophageal, breast (postmenopause), endometrial and kidney cancer risk; ↓ risk of osteoarthritis, improved immune function and gastrointestinal health; low bodyweight is a risk factor for low bone mass.
Physical activity (be more active more often)	↓ risk of CHD, stroke and type 2 diabetes; ↓ colon and breast cancer risk; ↓ risk of osteoarthritis; ↑ bone mass; improvements in cognitive function and wellbeing, and ↓ in sarcopenia. Benefits to gastrointestinal health.
Sunlight (avoid excess)	Sunlight important for vitamin D synthesis (low status widespread) but too much associated with photo-ageing and risk of skin cancer.

CHD: coronary heart disease; CVD: cardiovascular disease; DASH: Dietary Approaches to Stop Hypertension; DHA: docosahexaenoic acid; EPA: eicosapentaenoic acid, MUFA: monounsaturated fatty acids; PUFA: polyunsaturated fatty acids; SFA: saturated fatty acids.

juice) during the survey week and 4% ate no vegetables.

The Health Survey for England of 2004 shows that, among the general population, a significantly higher proportion of women than men met the five-a-day recommendation (27% vs. 23%) (Health & Social Care Information Centre 2005). A comparison of the NDNS surveys of adults in the 1980s and 2000/1 reveals that mean daily consumption has risen by 0.4 portions (to a total of 2.8 servings), but

in 2000/1, 86% still consumed less than the recommended five or more portions a day (Scientific Advisory Committee on Nutrition 2007a). The greatest increase was in the 50–64 age group, but the picture was particularly poor among those aged 19–24, almost all of whom (98%) consumed less than five servings a day.

In a comparison of ethnic minority groups, the proportion of Chinese and Indian women achieving the target was 42% and 36%, respectively; in men, the percentages were 36% and 37% respectively (and 33% in Pakistani men) (Sproston and Mindell 2006). Mean daily intake of fruit and vegetables was also higher in most ethnic groups compared with the general population, in whom it was 3.3/day in men and 3.6/day in women. For example, mean intakes in Chinese men and women were 4.4 and 4.9 servings/day, respectively, and in Indian men and women, 4.2 and 4.4 servings/day, respectively.

Data are available for English children aged 5–15 years: 11% of boys and 12% of girls ate five or more servings of fruit and vegetables a day. Children in most of the minority ethnic groups had higher consumption levels: they were highest in Indian and Bangladeshi boys (each 22%) and Chinese girls (24%). The average number of portions a day was also higher, reaching 3.4/day in Indian boys and 3.6/day in Chinese girls, compared to 2.5 and 2.6 in boys and girls, respectively, in the general population (Sproston and Mindell 2006).

14.5.2 Sugars, fibre, fat and salt

The proportion of energy intake derived from non-milk extrinsic sugars (NMES) exceeds the recommendation of 11% of food energy in most age groups, particularly children and young adults. In adults (19–64 years) intakes were 13.6% of food energy in men and 11.9% in women. But in those aged 19–24 years, intakes were 17.4% and 14.2% of food energy, respectively, in men and women, and intakes were 16–17% of food energy in older children (Scientific Advisory Committee on Nutrition 2007a). Among the highest consuming group of adults, intake reached 30% of food energy. The main sources of NMES were table sugar, soft drinks and biscuits, buns, cakes and pastries; soft drinks were the single largest contributor in the diets of children and younger adults. In adults aged over 65, whose diets were studied in the mid-1990s, NMES intake was 13% of food energy in men and just exceeded the dietary reference value (DRV) (11%) in women. However, in those living in institutions, average NMES intake reached 17.9% of food energy in men and 18.5% in women. In this group, table sugar was the greatest contributor, and together sugars, preserves and confectionery provided about half of the intake (Scientific Advisory Committee on Nutrition 2007a).

In 2000/1, intakes of non-starch polysaccharides (NSP) were 15.2 g/day in men and 12.6 g/day in women (DRV 18 g/d). A third of men and half of women had intakes <12 g/day (the minimum for individuals) (Scientific Advisory Committee on Nutrition 2007a). Cereals and cereal products were the main source, providing over 40%, followed by vegetables/vegetable dishes, which provided 20%.

On a positive note, intakes of total dietary fat and saturated fatty acids have both been falling over the past 20 years, in line with recommendations. In adults, in 1986/7, over 40% of food energy was provided as fat; by 2000/1, this had fallen to 35.8% in men and 34.9% in women (DRV 35%). Similarly, during this period saturates intake has fallen from about 17% of food energy to about 13%, but remains above the DRV of 11%. Also during this period, *trans* fatty acids intake has fallen. In 2000/1 intake was already below the DRV (2% of food energy) at 1.2% of food energy among adults, and has continued to fall as a direct result of the food industry's removal of *trans* fatty acids from many product ranges, including snack foods, baked goods and spreads. A review by the UK government's Scientific Advisory Committee on Nutrition (SACN) indicates that population intake is now 1% of energy and SACN advises that legislation to stimulate further reduction is unlikely to deliver additional public health benefit (Scientific Advisory Committee on Nutrition 2007e). However, a similar response is required by food operators (manufacturers and food service) in those countries where intakes remain high, in order to elicit a global impact. This point is emphasised in an update on *trans* fatty acids published by the World Health Organisation (Uauy *et al.* 2008).

Secondary analyses of the 2000/1 dataset for adults show that high consumers of total fat (>39%E) and saturates derive a greater proportion of their intake from cream, cheese, sausages, meat pies, chips, and crisps and savoury snacks compared to those consuming <35%E as fat. Also, plasma cholesterol levels in older age groups (55 and older in men and 65 and older in women) have fallen steadily over the past decade (in part owing to the widespread use of statins) (British Heart Foundation 2007). In 1986/7 amongst adults aged 19–64 years, only 13% of men and 10% of women had levels below the cut-off of 5.2 mmol/L. In 2000/1, this had risen to 41% of men and 25% of women. The proportion with very high levels (>7.8 mmol/L) had also fallen. In those over 65 years, in the mid-1990s, mean fat intakes were 35.7% of food energy in men

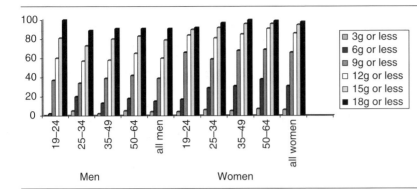

Figure 14.10: Percentage distribution of salt intake in men and women (g/day) estimated from total urinary sodium. Source: Scientific Advisory Committee on Nutrition (2007a).

and 36.1% in women, and saturates were 15% of food energy in both sexes. In this older age group, 34% of men and 24% of women in the free-living group and 62% of men and 43% of women in the institutionalised group had a plasma cholesterol level <5.2 mmol/L (Scientific Advisory Committee on Nutrition 2007a).

Based on estimates of sodium from 24-hour urine collections, average intakes of salt in 2000/1 in adults (19–64 years) had increased from 9 g/day in 1986/7 to 9.5 g/day overall (11 g/day in men and 8 g/day in women), well above the 6 g/day recommendation. Only 15% of men and 31% of women consumed less than 6 g/day (see Figure 14.10). Those aged 19–24 years were least likely to meet the target (2% men and 17% of women) (Scientific Advisory Committee on Nutrition 2007a). Data from the Health Survey for England, published by the Food Standards Agency in 2007, suggests that sodium intakes have fallen slightly over recent years. Furthermore, this trend seems to have continued according to data published in mid 2008, which shows that intakes are currently 9.0 g/day on average among adults. In men, intakes have fallen from 11 g to 10.2 g/day and in women from 8.1 g to 7.6 g/day (www.food.gov.uk/science).

14.5.3 Vitamins and minerals

Nutrient intake and nutritional status are both low for a number of essential vitamins and minerals, especially in older children, young adults and older people living in institutions. There is also evidence of marked differences in diet and nutritional status associated with economic status (receipt of benefits), and smoking (Scientific Advisory Committee on Nutrition 2007b). In the survey of adults conducted

in 2000/1 (Henderson, Gregory, Irving *et al.* 2003), intakes below the lower reference nutrient intake (LRNI) (which by definition are likely to be inadequate for most people) were reported for eight nutrients: vitamin A, riboflavin, iron, calcium, magnesium, potassium, zinc and iodine. Individuals with low intakes of one micronutrient were likely to have low intakes of the others. Low status was evident for thiamin, riboflavin, vitamins B_6 and B_{12}, vitamin C, folate, iron and vitamin D (Ruston *et al.* 2004), and again the variables were strongly associated with each other. A recent analysis (Scientific Advisory Committee on Nutrition 2007b) was undertaken to determine the dietary and non-dietary characteristics of those with intakes of vitamins and minerals classified as low (below the LRNI) or borderline (between the LRNI and the estimated average requirement, EAR) during the seven-day recording period. It also looked at the characteristics of those with low or marginal status for vitamins and minerals, and in addition to assessing the original data in these terms, a quintile analysis was performed. Both assessments revealed similar findings: those with low intakes/status were more likely to be smokers, living in a household in receipt of benefits and less likely to report taking supplements. Those with low vitamin D status reported being less physically active compared with those with adequate status, hence perhaps reducing their opportunities for skin synthesis of the vitamin. The analysis also confirmed that younger adults are more likely to have low intakes/status for some micronutrients than their older counterparts.

The picture for some nutrients is particularly concerning. Total iron intakes in girls and women of child-bearing age are low compared with the DRVs, with up to 50% of some age groups having intakes below the LRNIs. Status indices (haemoglobin and serum ferritin) suggest that a smaller proportion of females in the 11–49 age range have a lower status than is indicated by the consumption data, although there are still significant proportions of both males and females with low iron status (Scientific Advisory Committee on Nutrition 2007a). In the NDNS of older adults, there was a high prevalence of low iron status and low vitamin C status, especially in those living in institutions (Scientific Advisory Committee on Nutrition 2007a).

With regard to vitamin D, there is widespread evidence of poor status in the UK (see Section 14.3.2), and the impact of this on bone health is a cause for concern (see Chapter 4, Section 4.2.3). A recent discussion paper (Scientific Advisory Committee on Nutrition 2007c) highlights the likelihood that young women of childbearing age will begin pregnancy with low stores and notes the re-emergence of clinical vitamin D deficiency manifesting in rickets in UK children, predominantly those of African-Caribbean and South Asian origin. SACN has reiterated original Committee on Medical Aspects of Food Policy (COMA) advice for vitamin D supplementation of vulnerable groups: infants and young children, pregnant and breastfeeding women, older people, and black and ethnic minority groups. In the context of concern about the effect of sun exposure on skin cancer risk, there is urgent need for a clear recommendation on the length and intensity of sun exposure required to provide sufficient vitamin D.

The recent report from SACN on folate and disease prevention indicates that low or marginal folate status exists in 8% of young women aged 19–24 and 4% of those aged 25–34 years. Among older people over the age of 65, 16% of those in institutions and 8% of those who are free-living have low status (Scientific Advisory Committee on Nutrition 2006). In light of this, SACN has supported continued use of folic acid supplementation (400 μg per day) by women who may become pregnant and has recommended mandatory fortification of flour as the UK government's COMA did in 2000 (Department of Health 2000a). SACN's recommendation has now been supported by the Food Standards Agency, and whether or not this recommendation becomes policy will be decided by health ministers. One of the key issues that is still being considered is evidence about possible adverse effects of folic acid in those with early stage cancer (see Section 14.2.6).

SACN also highlighted the widespread prevalence of poor riboflavin status in the UK and the existence in the older population of vitamin B_{12} deficiency, which may affect 5–10% of individuals but is typically related to malabsorption (which becomes more common with ageing) rather than a dietary deficit (Scientific Advisory Committee on Nutrition 2006). Progression of B_{12} deficiency can have serious neural consequences and, to remove this risk, SACN recommends that the incidence and prevalence of low B_{12} status and appropriate management strategies should be assessed.

The quintile analysis revealed that those with the lowest intakes of the eight nutrients referred to above consumed a generally unbalanced diet compared with those with the highest intakes, characterised by consumption of significantly less of almost every food group, with some evidence of increased consumption of foods grouped as sugar, preserves and confectionery, and of savoury snacks. Other key indicators associated with lower nutrient status were lower consumption of fish and fish dishes, and fruit and vegetables (particularly fruit). The analysis also provides evidence that soft drinks (excluding fruit juice) may be replacing milk in the diets of those with low riboflavin intake (Scientific Advisory Committee on Nutrition 2007b). In addition, those with the lowest status for vitamin B_{12}, riboflavin, folate and vitamin C consumed less breakfast cereal (many of which are fortified).

A summary of progress in achieving the UK government's dietary recommendations is shown in Table 14.8.

14.5.4 Fluid intake

Adequate fluid intake is important for a number of reasons described in earlier sections (see Table 14.7 and Chapter 1, Section 1.5.5) and some beverages contribute nutrients (*e.g.* milk, fruit juice) and polyphenols (*e.g.* tea, coffee, wine), but beverages can also be a major source of energy and hence contribute to risk of obesity. Recommendations in the UK vary, but 6–8 glasses/mugs a day of liquid in combination with the water provided by food, which can be substantial, is generally considered adequate. In the US, beverages currently provide an average of 21% of energy intake (excluding children under two years) and this is of concern because beverages promote only weak satiety responses and elicit poor dietary energy compensation. With this

Table 14.8: Summary of achievement of dietary recommendations in the UK

Recommendation		Reason for the recommendation	Is the recommendation being met?	
Fruit and vegetables	At least 5 × 80 g portions/day	↓ risk some cancers, CVD and other chronic diseases	2.8 × 80 g portions/day in adults	×
Oil-rich fish	At least 1 × 140 g/week	↓ risk CVD	0.3 × 140 g portions/week among adults	×
Non-milk extrinsic sugars	<11% food energy (~60 g/day)	↓ risk dental caries	Up to 19% food energy across all population groups	×
Fat	Reduce to average of 35% food energy	↓ risk CVD and ↓ energy density of diets	Average 35% energy across the population	×
Saturates	Reduce to average of 11% food energy	↓ risk CVD and ↓ energy density of diets	Average 13% energy	×
NSP (fibre)	Average 18 g/day (adults)	To improve gastrointestinal health	15.2 g/day (♂), 12.6 g/day (♀)	×
Alcohol	3–4 units*/day (♂); 2–3 units*/day (♀)	Minimise risk of liver disease, CVD, cancers, injury from accidents and violence	60% (♂) exceed 44% (♀) exceed	×
Salt	Average 6 g/day (2.4 g/day sodium)	↓ risk hypertension and CVD	Average 9.5 g/day	×
Vitamins/Minerals	Dietary Reference Values	To promote optimum health and prevent deficiency	Low intakes seen for a number of these in various age groups	Not all
Energy intake	2500 kcal (♂) 2000 kcal (♀)	↓ risk of obesity, some cancers, CVD and type 2 diabetes	80–90% EAR	✓
Bodyweight	BMI 18.5–25 kg/m²		66% (♂) and 53% (♀) over BMI 25	×

BMI: body mass index; CVD: cardiovascular disease; EAR: estimated average requirement; ♂: male; ♀: female. *Half a pint of standard beer or lager provides 1 unit, a glass of wine provides about 2 units (www.eatwell.gov.uk).
Source: Adapted from Scientific Advisory Committee on Nutrition (2007d).

in mind, advice for US citizens has been published that suggests a beverage consumption pattern dominated by water and tea/coffee (unsweetened) (Popkin *et al.* 2006). They recommend a very substantial fluid intake (98 fl oz, about 3 L/day) in addition to water provided by food, which they estimate to be just under 900 ml/day on average. As a guide, allocation within this volume is: water (50 fl oz), tea or coffee (28 fl oz), low-fat milk (16 fl oz), fruit juice (4 fl oz). However, recognising that other beverages are also popular, an 'acceptable' pattern is also recommended, comprising: water (24 fl oz), tea or coffee (36 fl oz), low-fat milk

(6 fl oz), fruit juice (8 fl oz), non-calorically sweetened beverages (12 fl oz) and alcoholic beverages (12 fl oz). Alcoholic beverages can be dehydrating as they stimulate urine excretion. Although tea and coffee also have a mild diuretic effect, overall they make a useful contribution to fluid intake.

The justification for tea, for example, in the US recommendations is the association between intake of ≥3 cups/day of ordinary tea and modest reduction in risk of heart attack (Popkin *et al.* 2006; Stanner 2007). For cancer, there is solid evidence from animal studies of a beneficial effect of tea, but the picture is unclear for humans (Popkin *et al.* 2006).

In the UK, 77% of adults consume tea and average daily consumption is around two mugs (540 ml) (Henderson *et al.* 2002).

14.5.5 Dietary patterns

A principal components analysis of the NDNS was conducted to provide information on the characteristics of four different eating patterns (Scientific Advisory Committee on Nutrition 2007b). The 'healthy' pattern was characterised by higher consumption of fish/fish dishes and fruit/vegetables. People following this pattern were least likely to be smokers and were also most likely to take supplements. This pattern resulted in the highest-status levels for all variables except iron and the highest intakes of some of the nutrients. 'Traditional' dietary patterns yielded the highest mean intakes for the majority of the nutrients assessed and results for the status variables that were similar to, or lower than the 'healthy' pattern. Iron status was highest in the traditional pattern, which included higher consumption of a range of general food groups, including meat/meat products, cereals/cereal products, milk/ milk products and eggs. The 'unhealthy' pattern included higher consumption of soft drinks (excluding fruit juice) and savoury snacks, and was associated with the highest smoking prevalence and the greatest likelihood of receipt of benefits.

These new analyses suggest that micronutrient requirements are more likely to be met if a varied diet, typified by the eatwell plate model (see Section 14.7), is consumed. Fish/fish dishes and fruit/vegetables are key indicators and should be promoted; whereas regular consumption of large amounts of savoury snacks, confectionery and soft drinks could be displacing other foods rich in micronutrients from the diets of those with low micronutrient intakes and/or status. The analysis suggests that consideration should be given to promoting the replacement of some soft drinks with low-fat milks. High-priority groups for receiving targeted healthy eating advice are young adults, smokers and those living in households receiving benefits (Scientific Advisory Committee on Nutrition 2007b).

National cross-sectional survey data of this type suggest that the diets of older UK adults (50–64 years) are typically closer to the dietary recommendations than those of younger adults (<35 years) (See Chapter 1, Section 1.6.1). A particularly marked

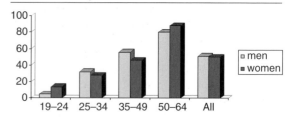

Figure 14.11: Consumption of oil-rich fish in adults aged 19–64 in 2000/1, g/week.
Source: Scientific Advisory Committee on Nutrition (2007b).

difference is seen with age for oil-rich fish consumption (Figure 14.11). In adults over 65 years, mean consumption of oil-rich fish was considerably lower at 12 g/week for men and 7 g/week for women who were free-living. For those in institutions, intakes were 4 g/week on average in both men and women. However, data on this group were collected in the mid-1990s and, since then, salmon has become cheaper and more readily available. Consumption of oil-rich fish was very low in children aged 4–18 years (5–10 g per week on average) (Scientific Advisory Committee on Nutrition 2007a).

One of the dietary patterns that has attracted particular interest is that associated with traditional Mediterranean eating habits, characterised by fruit and vegetables, olive oil, fish and red wine, and modest amounts of dairy products and meat. The EPIC elderly study has investigated the benefit of this type of diet in those over the age of 60 years and demonstrated that a modified diet (suitable for use across Europe by substituting unsaturated fatty acids for monounsaturates in the calculations) is associated with longer life expectancy (Trichopoulou *et al.* 2005). Recent evidence suggests that high vegetable (but not fruit) intake reduces the rate of cognitive decline in older adults (Kang *et al.* 2005; Morris *et al.* 2006). Kang and colleagues found the decline was slowest in subjects with the highest intakes of cruciferous vegetables (*i.e.* brassicas) and green leafy vegetables.

14.5.6 Socio-economic, regional and ethnic differences

In the NDNS surveys there were clear differences in the diets, nutrient intakes and nutritional status of people in lower compared to higher socio-economic status households (based on household receipt of benefits, social class and household income) (Scientific Advisory Committee on Nutrition 2007a). People in lower socio-economic status households had different dietary patterns, in particular lower consumption of fruits and vegetables (in adults, 2.1 portions a day for men and 1.9 a day for women in households receiving benefits, compared to 2.8 and 3.1 respectively in non-benefit households). Adults in households receiving benefits were also less likely to eat high-fibre breakfast cereals and oil-rich fish, and were more likely to eat whole milk, table sugar, burgers and kebabs, and meat pies. Findings in other age groups were similar. Adults in households receiving benefits were also more likely to have lower intakes and blood levels of many micronutrients, although this does not necessarily imply deficiency. For example, 53% of women aged 19–50 years living in benefit households had an iron intake from food sources that fell below the LRNI, compared to 29% of those in non-benefit households (Scientific Advisory Committee on Nutrition 2007a). There was also evidence of lower status, specifically vitamin C, folate, vitamin E and selenium for men and women, and carotenoids and vitamin D for women (Scientific Advisory Committee on Nutrition 2007a). Lower intakes of most vitamins have also been recorded for children and older people from manual home backgrounds (Scientific Advisory Committee on Nutrition 2007a).

There were also marked socio-economic differences in health, with health prospects of older people in lower socio-economic groups being typically poorer. As a result, age is not an automatic predictor of health or lifestyle.

Findings of a survey focusing specifically on low-income households, the Low Income Diet and Nutrition Survey (LIDNS), have recently been published (Nelson *et al.* 2007). In contrast to the earlier NDNS, the gap between the diets of people on low income and the rest of the population was not as great as expected and the study did not identify any direct link between dietary patterns and income, food access or cooking skills. Dietary patterns were much the same as in the general population, with room for improvement.

Generally, the NDNS surveys show few clear regional trends in dietary patterns, nutrient intake or nutritional status; this is partly because sample sizes for individual regions were sometimes too small for differences to reach statistical significance. However, there is some evidence of lower fruit and vegetable consumption in Scotland and to a lesser extent northern England, but this is not consistent across surveys. Regional differences in micronutrients (*e.g.* vitamin C and folate) were more apparent than for macronutrients (Scientific Advisory Committee on Nutrition 2007a), although the differences are less apparent in the more recent surveys.

The NDNS series is not sufficiently large to allow comparisons to be made among ethnic groups. However, special analyses within the Health Survey for England have focused on specific aspects of diet, *e.g.* fruit and vegetable intake (see Section 14.5.1).

14.6 Current trends in physical activity and the way forward

Physical activity is a key to predicting independence and mortality in later life. A report on physical activity from the UK's Chief Medical Officer (Department of Health 2004a) summarised the health benefits of leading a physically active life and highlighted the fact that in England alone the financial cost of inactivity (including the rising cost of treating related chronic disease) was £8.2 billion annually. The World Health Organization (2004b) has also called for increased physical activity levels in individuals and populations around the world.

Many organ systems can benefit from physical activity and increased fitness, for example the cardiovascular system (Buttriss and Hardman 2005; Miles 2007b) (see also Chapter 10, Section 10.8), muscle (Chapter 6, Section 6.10) and bones (Chapter 4, Section 4.2.14.1), and associated disease can be ameliorated or prevented, including CHD and colon cancer (Taylor *et al.* 2004) (see Chapter 10, Section 10.8 and Sections 14.2.6). Men and women who are physically active experience a lower risk of CVD in general and CHD in particular; it is never too late to change the habits of a lifetime. Stroke risk and hypertension also appear to be reduced (Buttriss and Hardman 2005; Barlow *et al.* 2006), as does the metabolic syndrome (LaMonte *et al.* 2005). Other benefits include improved weight control, lower blood pressure, and improved insulin sensitivity, blood lipid profile, endothelial function and glucose tolerance (Buttriss and Hardman 2005) (see Chapter 10, Section 10.8). There is also considerable evidence that regular physical activity protects against type 2 diabetes, the effect being independent of bodyweight (see Chapter 10, Section 10.8). As with CVD, there is some evidence of a dose-dependent response. Growing evidence supports the antidepressant effect of exercise and its role in improving emotional, cognitive, social and perceived physical function in older adults, and alleviating physical symptoms (Taylor *et al.* 2004). The psychology of physical activity has been reviewed by Biddle and Mutrie (2008).

There is evidence that age-related changes associated with the cardiovascular system (see Chapter 10, Section 10.8) can be reversed if physical activity levels are increased (*e.g.* by undertaking appropriate endurance training (Taylor *et al.* 2004)). Physical activity may also decrease risk of breast cancer in postmenopausal women and is an important component in the prevention and treatment of sarcopenia (Chapter 6, Section 6.10) and type 2 diabetes, possibly through an effect on insulin sensitivity.

Activity and fitness have been shown to be protective in every sub-group of the population. For example, in women aged 30–55, higher levels of physical activity were associated with reduced mortality rates at all levels of adiposity but did not eliminate the higher risk of death associated with obesity (Hu *et al.* 2004). Benefit has also been shown for older men and women (Blair 2007). Men aged 80 years and over who were in the highest fitness category had a lower death rate than unfit men who were 25 years younger, demonstrating just how powerful activity and fitness are as protective factors. A similar effect has been reported for preservation of functional capacity by moderate to high fitness levels (Huang *et al.* 1998; Larson *et al.* 2006; Blair 2007) and demonstrated that men and women over the age of 65 years who participated in a moderate level of activity at least three times a week had a 40% lower risk of developing dementia compared with sedentary individuals (Larson *et al.* 2006). Similarly L. Wang *et al.* (2006) reported a lower risk of dementia in those with higher physical activity performance scores.

It is well established from cross-sectional and cohort studies in sedentary populations that weight increases with age. However, even among the most active men and women who run regularly, bodyweight increases from year to year when exercise level remains constant (Williams and Wood 2006).

Disability and infirmity can be the result of disuse of muscle rather than the inevitable process of ageing. After the age of 60, muscle mass is lost at the rate of ~0.5–2% per year but this can be influenced by strengthening exercise programmes, and community-based exercise training for healthy older people can have profound effects in reversing muscle wasting and the accompanying functional deficit (see Chapter 6, Section 6.10). As with bone, the greater the muscle mass established earlier in life, the more there is to lose as ageing progresses without the loss substantially affecting function. Furthermore, physical activity, and in particular strength training, has been found to be effective in reducing the incidence of falls in older people (Taylor *et al.* 2004), which emphasises that different types of exercise benefit different body systems (aerobic exercise for the cardiovascular system, high-impact exercise for the skeleton and strength training to minimise muscle loss and hence falls). In older people, the type of activity chosen needs to take account of potential adverse effects on ageing joints. Regardless of body fat status, being physically active provides health benefits (see Figure 14.12) (C.D. Lee *et al.* 1999).

Current recommendations for physical activity, published in 2004, are shown in Table 14.9; more recent recommendations from the US and Canada are higher at 60 minutes of daily activity of moderate intensity, which is designed to promote weight

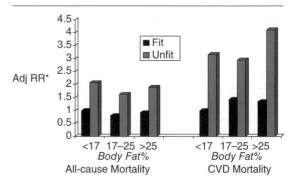

*Adjusted for age, exam year, smoking, alcohol and parental history.
Adj: adjusted; CVD: cardiovascular disease.

Figure 14.12: Relative risk (RR) for all-cause and CVD mortality in fit and unfit men by body fat categories.
Source: C.D. Lee *et al.* (1999).

Table 14.9: Recommendations for physical activity in the UK

Children	Children and young people should achieve a total of at least 60 minutes of at least moderate intensity activity each day. At least twice a week, this should include activities to improve bone health (activities that induce high physical stress on bones, *e.g.* running, skipping), muscle strength and flexibility.
Adults	At least 30 minutes of at least moderate intensity activity (*e.g.* brisk walking) on five or more days each week. Moderate intensity activity should lead to an increase in breathing rate, an increase in heart rate and a feeling of increased warmth, possibly accompanied by sweating. Shorter bouts of activity can be accumulated throughout the day and still count towards the 30-minute minimum. Different types of activity benefit different body systems: aerobic activity for the heart, weight-bearing activity for bones. To prevent obesity, many individuals will need to take at least 45–60 minutes of at least moderate intensity activity each day. In those who have lost weight, 60–90 minutes a day may be needed to prevent weight regain.
Older adults	As above and it's never too late to start.

Source: Department of Health (2004a).

Table 14.10: Proportion (%) achieving the current physical activity recommendations (at least 30 minutes of moderate intensity activity on five or more days a week) in England, by sex and age, 1997, 1998, 2003 and 2004

	All ages**	16–24	25–34	35–44	45–54	55–64	65–74	75 and over
Men								
1997	32	49	41	37	32	23	12	7
1998	34	53	45	41	34	30	14	6
2003	36	52	44	41	38	32	17	8
2004	37	56	46	41	37	32	18	8
Women								
1997	21	26	26	29	24	19	8	5
1998	21	28	28	28	25	18	9	3
2003 (weighted*)	24	30	29	30	31	23	13	3
2004 (weighted*)	25	32	30	32	30	20	14	4

*Weighted for non-response; **Adults aged 16 and over.
Source: British Heart Foundation (2006).
Similarly low levels of activity are found in most other European countries (see Table 14.11 for data for EU-15 countries), a notable exception being the Netherlands (British Heart Foundation 2005a).

maintenance and accrue health benefits such as enhanced quality of life, overall wellbeing and lower mortality rates (DHHS [US Department of Health and Human Services] & USDA [United States Department of Agriculture] 2005). The US/Canadian guidelines also recommend 60–90 minutes of moderate to vigorous activity a day for previously overweight adults in order to sustain weight loss. This includes everyday activities such as using the stairs, gardening and light housework.

In the UK, among adults aged 19–64, 60% of men and 70% of women are not taking sufficient physical activity to benefit their health (Ruston *et al.* 2004). Furthermore, activity levels fall with increasing age

(see Table 14.10) and 7 in 10 men and 8 in 10 women aged 75 years are inactive (Department of Health 2004a). Physical activity levels are greatly influenced by occupational activities but the majority of the population lead sedentary lives, with occupations that fall within the light or moderate categories. It should come as no surprise, then, that energy expenditure and activity levels have been declining and this makes recreational or opportunistic activity all the more important. For example, data from the national travel surveys show that the average distance walked per person per year has fallen from 255 miles in 1975/6 to 192 miles in 2003 and the distance cycled from 51 to 34 miles (National Statistics 2004).

Table 14.11: Self-reported physical activity levels, 2002, EU-15 countries: number of days in last week that moderate physical activity was taken (% of sample)

	None	1–3 days	4–6 days	7 days	Don't know
Austria	39	27	20	8	5
Belgium	38	24	18	18	3
Denmark	31	28	20	22	<1
Finland	36	33	16	15	1
France	53	27	9	10	1
Germany	29	30	24	15	3
Greece	38	23	12	27	<1
Ireland	46	22	17	14	2
Italy	50	26	10	12	2
Luxembourg	34	27	14	21	4
Netherlands	8	19	23	49	2
Portugal	26	19	18	31	6
Spain	51	20	14	13	2
Sweden	44	30	13	12	1
UK	43	28	14	15	<1
Total EU-15	**41**	**26**	**16**	**15**	**2**

Source: British Heart Foundation (2005a).

(Further information can be found at www.sustrans.org.uk.)

There are distinct socio-economic differences in activity patterns. For example, the proportion of men (adjusted for age) who walk as a leisure time activity is 38% higher in social class I than in social class V. In women, the levels in social class I are 67% higher than in class V (Department of Health 2004a). Similar trends are evident for sports participation. Furthermore, in both men and women, lower educational achievement predicts higher levels of inactivity. The prevalence of obesity in the Health Survey for England 2003 also reflects social class. Although prevalence is only slightly higher in men with manual (23%) vs. non-manual occupations (21%), there is a larger difference for women (manual 28% and non-manual 18%). The forecasts for 2010 predict a similar difference between manual and non-manual occupations (Zaninotto et al. 2006).

In the general population, 32% of men and 39% of women have low activity levels in the UK (Sproston and Mindell 2006). In ethnic minority groups in the same survey, low activity levels were particularly common among Bangladeshi and Pakistani men (both 51%) and Bangladeshi (68%) and Pakistani (52%) women (Sproston and Mindell 2006).

Activity levels in children are also a cause for concern. The NDNS of 4–18-year-olds revealed that, with the exception of very young children (aged 4–6 years), the majority are largely inactive (Gregory et al. 2000). About 40% of boys and 60% of girls aged 7–14 years spent less than one hour per day in activities of at least moderate intensity, and thus failed to meet the recommendation for young people (at least an hour each day). In 15–18-year-olds, the proportions rose to 56% of boys and 69% of girls. A study in Scotland revealed that a sedentary lifestyle is established during the preschool years (Reilly et al. 2004); at ages three and five years, almost 80% of the time (excluding sleeping at night) was spent in sedentary behaviour. These low activity levels are considered to be a major cause of the rising prevalence of obesity in children, which was 18.5% in 2–15-year-olds in 2004 (Health & Social Care Information Centre 2006) (Table 14.11).

There is evidence that high participation rates in interventions to increase physical activity among older adults can be achieved in the short term (<1 year). However, evidence for long-term effectiveness is generally absent (Taylor et al. 2004). Promotion of physical activity can also prolong independent living and this is a theme of the National Service Framework for Older People (see Section 14.7). Health professionals are ideally placed to encourage increased physical activity, and three levels of action for use in primary care have been identified: opportunistic advice, counselling, and exercise screening and programming (including exercise referral

Table 14.12: Benefits of physical activity in middle-aged and older people

Physiological	Immediate benefits	Regulation of blood glucose; stimulation of catecholamine activity; improved sleep
	Long-term effects	Improvements in cardiovascular function (aerobic/cardiovascular endurance exercise); maintenance of independence (resistive training/muscle strengthening); flexibility; maintenance of balance and coordination
Psychological	Immediate benefits	Enhanced relaxation; reduced stress and anxiety; enhanced mood state
	Long-term effects	Enhanced general wellbeing; improved mental health (*e.g.* depression and anxiety); cognitive improvements (*e.g.* delayed loss of reaction time; delayed loss of motor control and performance)
Social	Immediate benefits	Empowerment (*e.g.* maintenance of independence and self-sufficiency; enhanced social integration)
	Long-term effects	Enhanced integration; formation of new friendships; widened social networks; potential for enhanced intergenerational activity

Source: Based on World Health Organization (1996).

schemes) (Taylor *et al.* 2004). The benefits of physical activity are summarised in Table 14.12.

Given the importance of physical activity, the challenge is to recognise and overcome barriers to greater participation. The factors that contribute to low levels of physical activity are many and exert an influence across the lifespan. They include:

- reduced time allocated for physical activity at school;
- alternative options to active play (*e.g.* television, computer and video games, internet access);
- a declining need for physical activity in the home and the retail environment owing to labour-saving devices;
- a declining need for physical activity in the workplace owing to a change from an industrial to a service-based economy;
- lack of emphasis on opportunities for physical activity in community design and town planning, resulting in lack of safe, attractive, well-lit walking areas and cycle ways;
- transport systems dominated by cars;
- lack of prominence of stairs compared with escalators and lifts;
- perceived lack of time;
- lack of awareness of the importance of regular activity for health and of the amount and type required to be of benefit;
- lack of immediate reward, *e.g.* failure to lose weight;
- low tolerance of exercise owing to low fitness level or existing obesity;

- lack of motivation, low self-confidence or self-esteem.

Local authorities and town planners have an important role to play in helping people of all ages to gain the benefits of being more active, including through provision of appropriate sport and leisure facilities, but also by ensuring that pavements and recreational areas are of a suitable standard and that walking areas are well lit and maintained.

Recent research has demonstrated that for people in high-risk populations (*e.g.* those at risk of type 2 diabetes), there may be different determinants of physical activity participation and these need to be taken into account when identifying exercise programmes for individuals in primary and secondary care (Delahanty *et al.* 2006). Another challenge is to translate short-term gains into meaningful long-term changes in behaviour.

As to the way forward, a recent review (Fox and Hillsdon 2007) concludes that increased participation in sports is likely to be only a minor part of the solution without substantial investment in facilities and access to a well-thought-through strategy to overcome psychosocial barriers. Furthermore, although there appears to be limited scope for increasing energy expenditure at work or via domestic activities, active transport initiatives to and from work offer some scope. Reductions in cycling and walking are likely to have contributed to reductions in daily energy expenditure. Tackling these trends has potential for real benefit but requires major public campaigns in conjunction with other strategies to make walking, cycling and recreational activities more available and more appealing. Similar issues have been faced elsewhere in Europe and North America. Fox and Hillsdon emphasise that it is critical that physical activity becomes part of more comprehensive solutions to the obesity problem, which take impact on inequalities into account, rather than being viewed in isolation.

The National Institute for Health and Clinical Excellence (NICE) (www.nice.org.uk/Guidance/pH8#summary) has developed guidance aimed at professionals working for the Highways Agency, local authorities, the NHS, education and workplaces. The guidance considers adults and children and NICE has investigated the effectiveness of interventions across the broad social gradient that concern building design, urban planning, the natural environment, transport and policy (local and national) influencing physical activity through the environment. The primary aim is to recommend environmental interventions that are likely to increase physical activity across the population by incorporating activity into everyday life, increasing formal or informal recreational activity (including active play), and increasing active travel.

14.7 Recommendations: life-course strategies

Sections of this chapter have summarised the nutrition themes emerging from the deliberations of the Task Force members (Sections 14.3 and 14.4), and the context within which these themes are operating as demonstrated by morbidity trends (Section 14.2) and national nutrition and health survey data (Sections 14.5 and 14.6). These data indicate that while there is no need to change existing advice radically, there is an urgent need for changes in emphasis and for reaffirmation and repackaging of some existing recommendations.

The data presented in Sections 14.5 and 14.6 are largely cross-sectional. As yet it is unclear whether these data signify that people improve their diet with age, or that we are witnessing a cohort effect and the diets of younger adults, which are a cause for concern now, can be expected to continue to be relatively poor unless public health action is taken. Similarly, activity levels in young people today are lower than in the past. Again, a key question is whether these low activity levels are set to stay or even deteriorate further throughout life, or whether younger people

can be encouraged to become more active and so improve their long-term health prospects.

It is evident from the information presented in this Report that improvement of health in old age requires a life-course approach. This in turn needs a coordinated and multidisciplinary strategy, led by government in partnership with the food industry, the fitness industry, employers, local authorities, town planners, health professionals, health agencies, schools and the media.

As the basic guidelines for a healthy diet stay the same throughout the life-course, resources such as the eatwell plate model remain relevant for older people (Figure 14.13). This model is applicable to all healthy people aged over five years and provides a consistent set of messages about healthier eating habits throughout life. It shows the four main food groups that should make up the bulk of the diet in order to maintain health, but also illustrates that small amounts of foods high in fat and/or sugar can be part of a healthy diet.

For older people, there may be specific opportunities to develop 'functional' foods that target some of the specific nutrients identified earlier in this chapter (such as vitamin D, calcium, folate, vitamin B_{12}, fibre and long chain n-3 polyunsaturates). Such products may also be of relevance to younger adults who are already on a poor nutrition trajectory, which would benefit from improvement. But opportunities that will benefit the health of the population, regardless of age, also exist through continued product reformulation and innovation to reduce salt levels, improve fat and carbohydrate profile and ensure micronutrient density. If product reformulation is directed at mainstream products consumed by large proportions of the population it can have a considerable impact. In the UK, substantial reductions have been achieved in the sodium content of foods, including staple foods such as bread and breakfast cereals, as well as tinned vegetables, sauces, soups, processed meats and snack foods. Similarly, major progress has been made to eliminate or reduce *trans* fatty acids in spreads, baked goods, packet snack foods and products available in some high street fast food chains, via the adoption of alternative manufacturing processes that avoid the use of partially hydrogenated vegetable oils; average intakes in the UK have fallen to 1% of energy (Scientific Advisory Committee on Nutrition 2007e) and so are well below the recommended maximum of 2%

The eatwell plate

Use the eatwell plate to help you get the balance right. It shows how
much of what you eat should come from each food group.

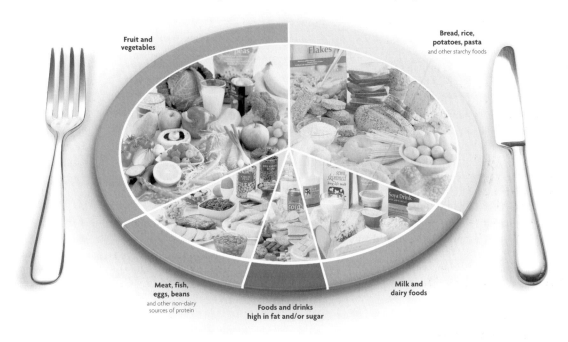

Figure 14.13: The Food Standards Agency's eatwell plate model.
Source: © Crown copyright material is reproduced with the permission of the Controller of HMSO and Queen's
Printer for Scotland.

of energy (and considerably lower than in Denmark
and New York City where legislative processes have
recently been applied). The UK government's Scientific Advisory Committee on Nutrition cautioned
against legislation to reduce population levels further
because such a reduction would be unlikely to deliver
a public health benefit and because of the likelihood
that such an approach might increase the quantity
of saturates in the national diet.

A strategy targeting saturates and energy density
is also being planned by the Food Standards Agency
(see Department of Health and Department of Children, Schools and Families 2008). However, for
some people, manipulation of the composition of
food may prove to be insufficient on its own and
targeted supplementation may be necessary (*e.g.*

folic acid for women of childbearing age and vitamin
D and vitamin B_{12} for older people).

Many opportunities exist for key sectors to work
together to make regular physical activity an easier
option for all age groups, by improving opportunities for walking and cycling in a relatively safe environment (see Chapter 16).

The following sections suggest some life-course
strategies that are linked to the findings presented in
earlier sections.

14.7.1 Children and young adults

Establishing good nutrition and activity patterns in
early life is very important in terms of future health.
Current trends in eating patterns and physical activ-

ity patterns among children and young adults are of concern (see Sections 14.5 and 14.6, and Table 14.8). These lifestyle patterns are directly associated with the increase in obesity among young people and the associated appearance of type 2 diabetes in obese adolescents. Concerns also exist about the rates of smoking in young people (in 2004 smoking rates in adults aged 20–24 were 36% in men and 29% in women) and the prevalence of heavy drinking, especially binge drinking (British Heart Foundation 2006). For example, 47% of young men and 39% of young women aged 16–24 drink more than the recommended daily benchmarks compared with 20% of men and 5% of women over the age of 65. Furthermore, 32% of men and 24% of women aged 16–24 drink heavily on at least one day a week. Action is needed if long-term health is to be nurtured.

Section 14.5 also alerts us to problems emerging in older children, *i.e.* poor vitamin D status that persists into adulthood, poor iron intakes and low levels of activity. In the UK, tackling childhood obesity trends and the eating habits of children are high on the political agenda, with targets for obesity prevention in the under 11s and the Department of Health's Obesity Prevention social marketing campaign targeting children and their parents launched in early 2007 (www.dh.gov.uk; Department of Health and Department of Children, Schools and Families 2008); banning of advertising of food and drink to children (www.ofcom.org.uk); the Healthy Start Initiative (www.healthystart.nhs.uk), that replaces the Welfare Foods Scheme; school fruit schemes and other school-based initiatives such as Food in Schools and the Healthy Schools Initiatives (www.healthyschools.gov.uk); initiatives such as the new school meals standards that came into force in England in September 2007 (www.schoolfoodtrust. org.uk) and had been preceded by the *Hungry for Success* initiative in Scotland (www.scotland.gov. uk); and active school travel and school sport initiatives.

However, much more should be done to address the poor eating and activity patterns in young adults, which are considered to be worse now than they have been in the past. Given the evidence of low intakes of some micronutrients, it is important that efforts to tackle energy intake in relation to obesity trends do not adversely affect intakes of essential micronutrients. Many young people have never learned to cook and this is now being addressed through nationwide initiatives that are establishing

school cookery clubs for children, *e.g.* the School Food Trust's *Let's Get Cooking* and the curriculum-focused *Licence to Cook* initiative from the Department for Children, Schools and Families. Awareness is now high of the need to act, but a concerted effort will be needed if trends are to change.

14.7.2 Middle-aged adults and healthy older people

Although we have yet to reach the time when personalised nutrition, based on our genetic inheritance, becomes the norm, it will be evident from the information presented in this Report that opportunities exist throughout life to help preserve good health into old age. Although such practices should ideally be adopted early in life and continued, it is never too late to start. Nutritional strategies and appropriate physical activity patterns are summarised in Sections 14.4–14.6. The importance of physical activity should not be underestimated. Simply expending energy through any activity may improve survival in older people, based on data from free-living high-functioning adults aged 70–82 (Manini *et al.* 2006). Lifestyle and leisure patterns of people in their 50s are surprisingly similar to those in their 30s and 40s. It is only when people pass 60 that age *per se* appears to impact on lifestyle activities, but age itself is no longer the predictor (Economic and Social Research Council 2000).

14.7.3 Older people at nutritional risk

Although life expectancy is increasing, many people spend their last years hampered by ill health and frailty. For older people, good nutrition has a valuable role to play in helping to maintain health and recovery from bouts of illness (see Chapter 11), particularly as many now live for 20 years or more beyond retirement age. There are approximately 410,000 older people in residential and nursing homes across the UK and the Food Standards Agency has published food-based guidelines for meals served to older people in residential care, together with sample menus (Food Standards Agency 2006) (www.food. gov.uk/healthiereating/ nutritioncommunity/care).

Under-nutrition is a common feature in the older population, with the extent of the problem being exacerbated by hospitalisation (Schenker 2003). For example, up to 50% of stroke patients are undernourished on admission (Ray *et al.* 2007) and require appropriate nutritional management. Furthermore, the impact of malnutrition on clinical outcome in hospitalised older people may be underestimated as many screening procedures require measurements of height and weight which often cannot be undertaken in sick older patients. The advantage of the Malnutrition Universal Screening Tool (MUST), which has been developed as a screening tool for adults in general, is that it can be used even if measurements of height and weight are unavailable. It has been shown to predict mortality and length of hospital stay in acutely ill older people (Stratton *et al.* 2006). MUST is a five-step screening tool to identify adults who are malnourished, at risk of malnutrition (under-nutrition) or obese. It includes management guidelines that can be used to develop a care plan (see www.bapen.org.uk).

When poor nutrition is identified, one option is to use food-based nutritional supplements to boost nutritional status (see Stanner 2005). A recent Cochrane Review of 49 trials (Milne *et al.* 2005) concluded that there is good evidence that supplementation can lead to a small weight gain, and there may also be beneficial effects on mortality rate, but many of the studies were of poor quality and as yet there is no clear evidence of improvements in clinical outcome. Micronutrient supplementation has also been investigated (see Chapter 11, Section 11.8.3) but benefits were generally evident only in those who were deficient in the nutrient(s) and effects were typically modest. A randomised controlled trial in Scotland (the MAVIS trial) found that routine multivitamin and mineral supplementation of older people living at home did not affect self-reported infection-related illness (Avenell, Campbell *et al.* 2005).

Owing to age-related reductions in the ability to absorb vitamin B_{12}, the need for B_{12} screening for older subjects with relevant symptoms has been highlighted, particularly in the context of the ability of folate sufficiency to mask the anaemia associated with vitamin B_{12} deficiency, thus allowing serious neurological repercussions associated with B_{12} deficiency to develop unchecked (Scientific Advisory Committee on Nutrition 2006) (see Section 14.5.3).

Adequate hydration is important for all age groups (see Section 14.5.4), but achieving this can be a particular problem in older people. Body water regulation relies on thirst to control water intake and there is evidence that this response is diminished in some older people and may contribute to severe dehydration (and related problems) and cognitive impairment (see Chapter 8) (Chernoff 1994). Some individuals, perhaps with functional impairments or frailty, may deliberately limit fluid intake perhaps because of difficulties associated with fetching a drink or to minimise the need to visit the toilet too often during the day, especially if they are prone to mild incontinence. Lack of easy access to drinks may be a common problem for institutionalised people who are dependent on carers. Symptoms of dehydration in older people include dry skin, swollen tongue, sunken eyeballs, elevated body temperature, mental confusion, decreased urine output and constipation. For healthy people of all ages in the UK, a fluid intake of 6–8 glasses or mugs (1.2 L) a day is recommended.

The NDNS of older people estimated that about 60% of those living in the community (rather than in residential homes and other care facilities) were overweight or obese, and one in six of the older people living in institutions were underweight (Finch *et al.* 1998). The Caroline Walker Trust (2004) subsequently produced practical guidance on providing food for older people in residential and nursing homes and through community meals services, such as meals on wheels and frozen meals services, and this has now been complemented by the food-based guidelines from the Food Standards Agency, mentioned earlier in this section.

A study in Scotland has focused on helping older people who live alone to eat well (Jones, Dewar and Donaldson 2005). The study found that low appetite was common among frail older participants, putting them at risk of malnutrition. They also identified a number of social and psychological factors that can help overcome poor appetite, including:

- eating with others, cooking for others, having a good quality meal cooked by someone else;
- eating food that looks appetising and smelling food as it is being cooked;
- getting out of the house and being active;
- having exposure to food ideas and foods in general;
- being supported to be spontaneous with food, *e.g.* being able to satisfy a particular increase in appetite or sudden desire for a particular food which is not at hand at home;
- support to address low mood or depression.

In assessing the care available locally to help ensure that nutritional needs are met, a number of quality indicators were identified, including: recognition of individuality, providing choice, accommodating personal tastes and preferences, appropriate timing of support, helping people to stay in control, ensuring care workers have appropriate nutritional knowledge and skills, provision of continuity, coordination and good communication. Jones, Dewar and Donaldson (2005) recommend a shift away from services that provide 'food as fuel' to services that focus on 'food as a route to wellbeing'.

A project in Newcastle funded by the Food Standards Agency has investigated the ability of a community-based, peer-led approach to help older people from socially deprived backgrounds to eat more healthily (Gibson 2007). The project involved the provision of a 20-week food club for older people (aged over 60 years) living in sheltered accommodation. Some participants reported a regained interest in cooking for themselves but the food clubs did not result in any change in knowledge of nutrition or food safety. Small dietary changes were reported at one year (*i.e.* slightly higher carbohydrate intake and non-significant increase in fruit intake). However, useful lessons learned from the project included:

- peer-led dietary interventions offer a social dimension and are well received by older people; their effectiveness warrants further investigation;
- it is possible to recruit and train older adults to become peer leaders;
- nutrition and food safety knowledge needs to be improved;
- optimistic bias needs to be addressed (participants believed their diet to be better than it was);
- dietary change may take time;
- older people do not necessarily have lots of spare time;
- the effect of improved access to small portions of fruit and vegetables (*e.g.* shared box schemes) on diet and health should be evaluated.

In March 2001, the Department of Health published the National Service Framework (NSF) for Older People, which set out a 10-year plan for action and reform to deliver higher quality services for older people, the expectations of which are set out below. As well as targeting clinicians, the plan also addressed other staff in health, social care services and the independent sectors.

In summary, the standards are focused on:

- identification and elimination of age discrimination in health and social care;
- importance of patient-centred care delivery services to individual needs;
- establishment of integrated continence and community equipment services;
- establishment of intermediary care services;
- improvements in the organisation of acute hospital-based care;
- prevention of strokes and improvements in stroke services;
- prevention of falls and appropriate treatment of people who fall;
- provision of a comprehensive mental health service for older people;
- promotion of good health in old age.

The NSF, and particularly progress with achieving these ambitions, has not been without its critics (House of Lords 2005). Perhaps as a result, the NSF was relaunched by the Department of Health (New Ambition for Old Age) (Department of Health 2006) and Living Well in Later Life (Commission for Healthcare Audit and Inspection 2006), with the announcement of a series of 10 programmes under three themes: dignity in care, joined-up care and healthy ageing, the latter being of particular relevance to the theme of this Task Force Report. Programme 9 focuses on promoting healthy ageing and its aims are to:

- improve physical fitness through encouraging and communicating the benefits of moderate regular physical activity for older people;
- overcome barriers to active life for older people through giving attention to equipment, foot care, oral health, continence care, low vision and hearing services;
- improve access to health care and health promotion services;
- extend healthy life expectancy through disease prevention and modifying health behaviour through life-checks and social marketing techniques.

The programme links in with the older people's component of the delivery of the White Paper *Choosing Health* and is said to be a key component of the delivery of the cross-government strategy for older people described in *Opportunity Age* (Department of Work and Pensions 2005), which aims to ensure that longer life is healthy and fulfilling, and that older people are full participants in society (www.dwp.gov.uk/opportunity_age). A report from the Social Exclusion Unit, *A Sure Start to Later Life – Ending Inequalities for Older People* (Office of Deputy Prime Minister 2006) has highlighted the need to promote wellbeing in later life by addressing poor health, poverty and social exclusion. A pilot programme to test the approach, *Link-Age Plus*, began in Spring 2006 (www.cabinetoffice.gov.uk/social_exclusion_task_force).

Physical activity is increasingly being seen as a key to good health and linked with reduced risk of diseases such as cancer, coronary heart disease, type 2 diabetes, osteoporosis, symptoms of osteoarthritis, sarcopenia and cognitive decline, as well as being important in the maintenance of a healthy bodyweight. In older people, physical activity is important in maintaining or improving mobility and improving functional capacity, hence facilitating independent living and helping to reduce anxiety and protecting against depression. For some older people, rising from a chair is difficult and getting up from the floor without help is impossible. The *Moving More Often* programme is an example of an initiative which aims to maintain and improve activity levels among frail older people (www.

bhfactive.org.uk). The campaign materials describe how:

- 20% of older women and 14% of older men do not have the physical flexibility to wash their hair comfortably;
- 47% of women aged 70–74 have insufficient leg muscle power to step on a bus without using their arms;
- 34% of men and 55% of women over the age of 80 are unable to walk for a quarter of a mile or more;
- Only 20% of women and 40% of men over the age of 80 are able to walk for 30 minutes or more.

Initiatives such as this have identified the importance of older people being involved directly with planning and delivery, and often involve peer-led programmes (*e.g. Someone Like Me* in the *Moving More Often* campaign) and cascade delivery. Many opportunities exist to develop provision to include the 65+ age group (*e.g.* dance and health initiatives and participation in cultural, sporting and leisure activities). The International Council for Active Ageing (ICAA) has produced a toolkit designed to help older adults initiate or return to a physical activity or fitness programme (www.icaa.cc/welcomeback.htm), and Help the Aged has produced a leaflet which offers practical advice to help prevent falling (www.helptheaged.org.uk).

14.8 Key points

- Life expectancy in the UK is currently increasing at the rate of ~two years for each decade that passes. This escalating demographic change can be expected to have profound consequences on all aspects of life.
- Nothing in this Report suggests that diet and lifestyle recommendations need to change radically, but there is need for changes in emphasis.
- Intakes of eight nutrients have been identified as problematic across the population: vitamin A, riboflavin, iron, calcium, magnesium, potassium, zinc and iodine. Additionally, there is evidence of low status of vitamin C, thiamin, riboflavin, B_6, B_{12}, D, folate and iron.

- Low nutrient status is widespread, affecting older children and young adults as well as older adults. Poor status is particularly evident in older people in residential care. There is plentiful evidence of low vitamin D status, particularly among young adults and older people in care.
- Low vitamin B_{12} status affects an estimated 5–10% of people over the age of 65 years and low folate status affects 16% of older people living in institutions.
- Such is the extent of these problems that a life-course approach to healthy ageing is essential; the extent of the challenge ahead should not be under-estimated.

Continued

- Fat intakes are now close to the 35% of energy target, but saturates and added sugars intakes remain higher than the targets.
- There is some evidence that sodium intakes may now be falling, but intakes are still well above the recommendation of 6 g salt/day.
- There has been considerable government-led effort to promote fruit and vegetables, but intakes still fall short of the 5+/day recommendation, with only 25% of adults achieving this. Intakes are particularly low in young men.
- Much more needs to be done to raise the profile of the importance of physical activity, which is a key predictor of independence in later life. It is never too late to start being more active.
- One of the key determinants of dietary variety in later life is retention of natural teeth, empha-

sising the importance of dental health throughout life.
- Adequate hydration is important at all ages, but is particularly important for older people who may become less able to recognise thirst.
- Over the past 5–10 years, a number of government initiatives have been put in place to promote healthy ageing among older people. It is important that these are monitored and evaluated to ensure that they are effective.
- There is ample opportunity for improvement in attitudes and behaviour in relation to healthy ageing, but a concerted effort will be required if progress is to be made, involving government, industry, employers, town planners, educators, health professionals, health agencies, the media and local authorities.

14.9 Key references

Finch S, Doyle W, Lowe C, *et al.* (1998) *National Diet and Nutrition Survey: People Aged 65 years and Over. Volume 1: Report of the Diet and Nutrition Survey.* London, Stationery Office.

Fox KR and Hillsdon M (2007) Physical activity and obesity. *Obesity Reviews*, **8**, 115–21.

House of Lords (2005) *Ageing: Scientific Aspects. Report from the Science and Technology Committee.* London, Stationery Office.

Kirkwood TBL (2006) Nutrition for a longer life. BNF Annual Lecture 2005. *Nutrition Bulletin*, **31(2)**, 88–92.

Miles L (2007b) Physical activity and health briefing paper. *Nutrition Bulletin*, **32**, 314–63.

Scientific Advisory Committee on Nutrition (2007a) The Nutritional Health of the Population SACN/07/14. www.sacn.gov.uk.

Scientific Advisory Committee on Nutrition (2007b) National Diet and Nutrition Survey: Adults 19–64 Years Further Analysis SACN/07/13. www.sacn.gov.uk.

Steele J, Sheiham A, Marcenes W and Walls A (1998) *National Diet and Nutrition Survey: People Aged 65 Years and Over. Volume 2: Report of the Oral Health Survey.* London, HMSO.

15
Conclusions of the Task Force

Improvements in health care and living conditions, together with a decrease in infant mortality, have contributed to a continued rise in average life expectancy and the ageing of the population worldwide. According to the national census of 2001, for the first time in the UK there are more people over the age of 60 years than under 16 years (Office for National Statistics 2001). Coping with this demographic change poses many challenges for society, especially for our health care system, as a large proportion of people aged over 60 suffer from chronic illnesses or disabilities. A focus on prevention and health maintenance is required to promote the concept of healthy ageing in order to relieve the social and economic costs of an ageing population and to enhance individual wellbeing; which is the situation in which people survive to an advanced age with their vigour, functional independence and quality of life maintained for as long as possible.

The ageing process involves progressive biological changes, resulting in a growing risk of chronic diseases, cognitive impairments, impairment of functions including mobility, sight and hearing, and an increased probability of dying. However, the rate of progression is variable and the process is malleable. Nevertheless, as we age, blood pressure and blood cholesterol concentrations usually rise, leading to increased risk of heart attack and stroke; glucose tolerance declines and insulin resistance increases, leading to diabetes; intraocular pressure can increase, leading to glaucoma and visual loss; and immune function deteriorates, resulting in increased risk of infection, poorer wound healing and slower recovery from illness. Loss of bone mass increases fracture risk, neuronal degeneration results in loss of

cognitive function and dementia, cartilage degeneration in arthritis, and muscle loss in functional weakness (Khaw 1997). This biological process of ageing reflects the interactions between our genetic inheritance and environmental influences. Huge variation in phenotype exists in people with the same genes, and gene expression and function is profoundly modified by environmental factors. Thus, while maximum life expectancy is probably genetically determined, the likelihood of reaching that maximum age in good health seems to be largely determined by environmental and lifestyle factors (Khaw 1997).

Many healthy lifestyle behaviours have been shown to be related to survival and health in older age and are therefore likely to contribute to healthy ageing. Risk of chronic disease is not only influenced by adult life experiences; risk factors often begin to take effect in early life. The intrauterine and early postnatal environment, for example, may programme basic metabolic processes and hence susceptibility to various conditions such as cardiovascular disease and type 2 diabetes in later life. In older groups, potential exists to reduce damage (*e.g.* from infections), increase protection against damage (*e.g.* by strengthening the immune system) or to prevent loss through lack of use (*e.g.* by remaining physically active). Improvements in lifestyle habits made at different stages of life can therefore impact on disease risk. In general, however, making such changes early in life and continuing these into older age is likely to be the most effective strategy for the prevention of diseases and disability. A life-course approach is therefore recognised as essential for the promotion of healthy ageing.

A better understanding of the regulation of ageing by modifiable factors such as nutrition and activity level will help to facilitate the development of targeted strategies for promoting successful ageing. This Task Force Report has reviewed evidence of the effect of ageing on the individual organ systems and described ways in which nutrition, physical activity and other lifestyle choices, applied throughout the life-course, can minimise or even negate the effects of the ageing process. The conclusions reached by the Task Force are presented below, in chapter order. The recommendations of the Task Force can be found in Chapter 16.

15.1 Chapter 1

- The trend of an increasing proportion of older adults and a decreasing proportion of children will continue in developed countries as well as spreading to less developed countries. The fastest-growing segment of the older population is amongst the oldest old – those aged 80 years and older, and in Great Britain there will be a growing proportion of older adults from non-white minority ethnic groups in this segment.
- While old age *per se* is not necessarily associated with poor health, the number of people reporting longstanding illness and disability increases with age. Older adults are also disproportionately affected by sensory impairments.
- Women tend to have a longer life expectancy than men, although in some countries this is changing. Life expectancy also varies by race; some ethnic groups are more susceptible to some chronic diseases.
- An ageing population impacts on health care spending and also has consequences in relation to the workforce and pensions.
- The energy, macronutrient and micronutrient requirements of older adults are not yet fully understood. The relevance of using a range of anthropometrical and biochemical measurements for older adults is unclear; much of the reference data for these measurements included few older adults.
- A number of surveys and studies in a range of countries have found that while older adults are generally well nourished, low intakes of fibre and a range of micronutrients have been found, especially in some sub-groups. Of particular concern is the number of older adults with low status of vitamin D, and of iron, folate and vitamin B_{12}.
- Food and nutritional intake (and therefore status) is influenced by a range of factors, including ill health, disease and disability, poor dentition, institutionalisation, socio-economic status, poverty and economic uncertainty.

15.2 Chapter 2

- The process of ageing is *not* genetically programmed. It appears to result from the accumulation of damage to cells and to the macromolecules within cells (especially DNA) cell.
- External factors that enhance cellular damage, such as stress and poor nutrition, are likely to speed up the ageing process. Both obesity and smoking are associated with a reduction in telomere length – a potential biological marker of the ageing process.
- As yet, there is limited understanding of the molecular mechanisms by which individual nutrients or other food constituents could affect the accumulation of the cellular and molecular damage responsible for ageing. However, antioxidant food components are likely to be protective and there is some evidence that nutrients (*e.g.* selenium) may enhance DNA repair.

15.3 Chapter 3

- The oral health status of older people is changing dramatically and rapidly with fewer older people being edentulous and a much larger proportion having some natural teeth.
- With natural teeth come the diseases associated with the dentate, notably tooth decay and periodontal (gum) disease.
- With increasing age the roots of teeth become exposed into the mouth. The root is made from dentine, which is softer and more susceptible to decay than the enamel of the crown of the tooth.
- Fluoride has a key role in helping to prevent disease, particularly in topical applications in older people. Community fluoridation schemes have a significant benefit for older dentate people because of the topical effect of an all-pervasive fluoride.

- Personal oral hygiene is a challenge for many older people as their dexterity and sight fail and the architecture of the mouth becomes more complex.
- There are minor changes in salivary flow with age, particularly in post-menopausal women. These are probably of limited clinical significance. However, reductions in salivary flow associated with disease of the glands or polypharmacy are a significant source of xerostomia (dry mouth) in older people, leading to tooth decay, tooth wear and difficulties in chewing and swallowing foods.
- Frequency of intake of simple carbohydrates is linked to tooth decay; this includes even small quantities of sugar used to sweeten drinks. This can be a problem when people are taking drugs with prolonged oral clearance, high-energy syrup food supplements and other forms of between-meal snacks.
- Chewing gum has a useful role in stimulating salivary flow and moderating the acidogenic response of dental plaque to sugars.
- Some micronutrients are important for oral mucosal health, notably the B vitamins and iron.
- Iron deficiency, alcohol and tobacco in various forms are all associated with oral cancer. Chewing tobaccos and quid particularly increases risk.
- The number and distribution of teeth influence food choice, with people who have few teeth tending to eat an 'unhealthy' diet low in fruit and vegetables and potentially higher in fat.
- Dental intervention alone has little impact on changing diet. However when teamed with tailored dietary advice a significant effect can be seen.
- Both the ability to taste and to smell deteriorate with age; this may also influence dietary selection. There is limited evidence of the benefits of taste enhancers (monosodium glutamate) in improving dietary intake in older people.
- Reductions in chewing efficiency, possibly linked with alterations in the availability of salivary mucin, result in older people with limited dentitions chewing food less efficiently, giving coarser particles in the food bolus prior to swallowing. Texture preferences change among older people, towards smooth, moist and slippery textures, rather than hard, crunchy or fibrous foods.

15.4 Chapter 4

- It is critical that the body is supplied with the nutrients required for the growth, mineralisation and repair of bone. Hence consumption of a balanced diet is crucial throughout the lifecycle.
- Adequate intakes of calcium and vitamin D are key for optimisation of peak bone mass attainment, reduction of postmenopausal bone loss and prevention of osteoporotic fractures.
- There is evidence of widespread vitamin D insufficiency, particularly in the vulnerable elderly and this urgently requires a public health strategy.
- Conflicting data exist for the effects of protein on the skeleton, with both high protein consumption (especially without a good calcium/alkali intake) and low protein intake (*e.g.* with respect to older people and vegan diets) being detrimental to bone. More long-term studies are required, as well as a meta-analysis of the evidence.
- There is evidence in the literature that low vitamin K intake and/or status is associated with low bone mass and increased fracture risk. Intervention studies, with fracture reduction as the clinical end-point are now needed required.
- There is support in the literature from a combination of observational, experimental, clinical and intervention studies of a positive link between fruit and vegetable consumption and bone health but more long-term intervention studies are required before firm conclusions can be drawn.
- Particular attention should be given to the benefits of impact-loading exercise (brisk walking, jogging, running, step aerobics, light gymnastics) for helping maintain a healthy skeleton. There is a positive relationship between weight-bearing exercise and bone mass in children and adults and being active may also protect against osteoporosis via effects on muscle strength, coordination, flexibility and balance.
- High sodium chloride (salt) intake is associated with an increase in urinary calcium excretion but there is limited data for a long-term adverse effect on bone. Further research in this area is urgently required.
- A high intake of vitamin A (from animal sources) may be associated with low bone mineral density and increased risk of osteoporotic fracture in certain populations. High consumption (>1500 μg retinol equivalents) should be avoided.

- At a cellular level vitamin C, B vitamins, copper, zinc and magnesium all have a role to play in skeletal development but specific mechanisms need to be identified.

15.5 Chapter 5

- Musculoskeletal pain and impairment are very common in older people; prevalence increases with age. This could be due to numerous age-related changes or result from the concomitant presence of several different diseases but is customarily attributed to joint disease (arthritis).
- Two main categories of arthritis exist: inflammatory arthropathies such as rheumatoid arthritis (RA) and gout, and age-related conditions such as osteoarthritis (OA). Inflammatory forms are characterised by chronic inflammation of the synovial lining of the joint; their aetiology is complex, involving both genetic susceptibility and environmental factors.
- Many different dietary manipulations have been tried to prevent or treat RA. While there is weak evidence to link high meat/protein diets, as well as those low in fish and fish oils, with an increased risk of acquiring RA, the data is conflicting and lacking in power. The bulk of the data and the most promising findings relate to the use of dietary fatty acid supplements to manipulate the inflammatory response in established arthritis. A review of 14 published randomised controlled trials concluded that there was evidence of a weak beneficial effect of fish oils (at levels of 2.7–4 g EPA and DHA/day).
- Gout is an inflammatory arthritis caused by crystals of uric acid. Obesity and alcohol intake, as well as diets rich in purines, are risk factors for this disease, and dietary manipulations to reduce them are a part of the disease management.
- In OA there are local areas of destruction and damage to the joint and related tissues, such as cartilage, which commonly affects the spine, hands, knees and hips. It is thought to be triggered by subtle abnormalities in joint loading.
- Risk factors for OA include increasing age and obesity, and genetics play a part. Weight reduction may be effective in reducing pain and disability in patients with knee OA but the link with obesity is not simply mechanical loading; systemic factors such as oestrogen, lipid or leptin metabolism are also thought to be important.
- A wide range of dietary supplements are also commonly used by those with OA despite a paucity of good evidence demonstrating a beneficial effect.

15.6 Chapter 6

- Skeletal muscle is required for a diverse range of essential metabolic functions in addition to the preservation of posture and mobility.
- Morbidity and mortality associated with sarcopenia affect a broad cross-section of older adults and are associated with a substantial economic cost to society. Actual prevalence and natural history are not clearly defined but up to one quarter of over 65 year olds and more than half of over 80 year olds are affected, with a greater incidence in women.
- Specific changes in muscle composition occur, specifically loss of type II fibres in proximal muscle groups and increase in type I collagen.
- Pro-inflammatory activation of the innate immune system, possibly triggered by mitochondrial DNA defects, has been put forward as the underlying cause of sarcopenia.
- Skeletal muscle demonstrates incipient insulin resistance with ageing even in individuals with no objective signs of glucose intolerance. There is some emerging evidence that n-3 polyunsaturates might have a protective effect.
- Anabolic triggers, such as protein-containing meals, are less effective in older individuals compared with young people.
- Protein requirements are not increased in older people.
- The benefits of regular (five times a week) exercise are not diminished in older muscle; exercise also enables maintenance of muscle mass and function. The benefits may be maximised if followed immediately by a protein-containing meal.
- Vitamin and mineral deficiencies are associated with reduced muscle mass but supplementation *per se* is of no additional value.

15.7 Chapter 7

- Skin signals health, appearance and attractiveness to our fellow human beings. It is composed of two main tissues: the outer epidermis and the deeper, collagen-rich dermis.

- The skin functions to maintain a robust barrier to the outside world and to prevent the desiccation of our bodies.
- Skin is relatively easily sampled and multiple, valuable *in vitro* cell research models have been developed and are available to study and investigate its properties.
- The skin ages in very characteristic ways giving rise to visible features such as wrinkling, uneven pigmentation and sagging. For this reason, maintaining a 'youthful' appearance is a major interest for consumers, and the cosmetic and food industries.
- Several biological ageing mechanisms have been proposed (*e.g.* photo-damage, oxidative damage, telomere shortening, neurological and physical stress, hormonal interactions) and each mechanism is currently the subject of many research investigations.
- Despite the very large number of supplement preparations that claim skin benefits, there are very few published placebo-controlled clinical trials using the products to test the claims. Many more placebo-controlled human studies are required to support food and supplement product claims.
- While the sun protection efficacy of dietary supplementation with β-carotene (>20 mg/day) and possibly other carotenoids is supported, the safety of higher doses of β-carotene (30 mg/day) in smokers is unacceptable. It seems likely that modest sun protection is provided by ingestion of combinations of ingredients such as carotenoids, *n*-3 fatty acids and vitamins C and E. However, whether dietary sun protection will give rise to measurable effects on skin ageing or other skin benefits remains to be tested in longer-term (>12-week) clinical studies.
- There are few human studies investigating the dietary effects of (non-vitamin) plant-derived ingredients on skin. Two non-carotenoid ingredient classes with potential are polyphenols including green tea extracts containing (-)-epigallocatechin-3-gallate, where animal studies suggest skin anti-cancer, anti-inflammatory and photo-protection benefits, and isoflavones with potential for sun protection and skin ageing benefits. There is great scope to explore the potential

of plant ingredients to positively influence skin properties and appearance.

- Poor nutrition adversely impacts wound healing. Therefore, it is not surprising that a proper balanced diet is recommended for optimal wound repair.
- Severe nutritional deficiencies (*e.g.* scurvy from vitamin C deficiency; pellagra from niacin deficiencies) that noticeably affect skin condition and skin ageing are now very rare in the developed world. However, the refinement of public health advice for optimal vitamin D bioavailability, either from balancing sun exposure with risk of photo-ageing and skin cancer or from fortified foods and supplements, requires more debate.

15.8 Chapter 8

- Stroke, dementia, Parkinson's disease and depression are common diseases affecting the brain in older people and account for most cases of disability in this age group. The incidence of these diseases increases exponentially with increasing age.
- Since the brain is dependent on a constant supply of oxygen and nutrients for optimum function, it is not surprising that these diseases have been linked with poor nutrition and with derangements in the blood supply to the brain.
- Observational studies have suggested that atherosclerotic vascular disease and nutritional factors may be relevant to the aetiology of cognitive impairment, dementia, Parkinson's disease and depression.
- Elucidation of the role of lifestyle modification and of nutrition for the prevention of dementia, Parkinson's disease or depression is complicated by the difficulty of distinguishing causal relationships associated with diet, or other aspects of lifestyle, from the consequences of having these diseases.
- Randomised trials of vascular risk factor modification or vitamin supplementation are required to assess if such treatment can prevent these diseases. These trials should initiate therapy before the onset of disease and include a sufficient number of participants to have adequate power to assess the effects of treatment.
- Randomised evidence for the effects on cognitive function of B-vitamins should be available on

about 20,000 of the 50,000 participants in the 12 large ongoing homocysteine-lowering trials for the prevention of cardiovascular events.

- Randomised trials assessing the effects of *n*-3 fatty acids on stroke, cognitive function and depression should be available in the next few years. Results are likely to confirm or refute the findings suggested in observational studies.

- Physical inactivity is a risk factor for cardiovascular disease. Cohort studies have also shown physical activity to be associated with better cognitive function and less cognitive decline in later life but there is little data available from randomised trials.

15.9 Chapter 9

- Good vision is essential to maintain quality of life and functional independence as people grow older. Refractive errors, cataracts, age-related macular degeneration (AMD), diabetic retinopathy and glaucoma are major problems resulting in vision loss which are progressively more common with ageing. For patients with diabetes the threat of vision loss through diabetic retinopathy is an added burden.

- Studies in the older population have consistently shown that about 50% of visual impairment is due to treatable conditions (*i.e.* cataract and refractive error). Refractive errors can be resolved by appropriate spectacle correction and cataract by a replacement lens. For other eye conditions treatment is not curative and in the case of macular degeneration has very limited effectiveness.

- Smoking is a major risk factor for cataract and macular degeneration. Older people who continue to smoke should be advised of the risk to their eyes. Smokers with early stages of AMD, or intermediate AMD or advanced AMD in one eye, are at high risk of disease progression. There is moderate evidence that high exposures to sunlight are associated with increased risk of cataracts and AMD. It would be prudent to recommend ocular protection (sunglasses, wide-brimmed hats) when outdoors in the middle of the day.

- Laboratory and animal studies have demonstrated the important role of antioxidants in the lens and retina. Epidemiological studies also provide evidence that high levels of antioxidants are protective against AMD and cataracts.

Although there is less consistency for individual antioxidants, the data from both animal and human studies suggest that vitamin C, and the carotenoids, lutein and zeaxanthein, play a critical role.

- Overall the evidence supports general dietary recommendations in older people especially for consumption of fruit and vegetables including:
  - at least five portions of fruit daily, especially those high in vitamin C such as citrus fruits, and
  - at least five portions of vegetables daily, especially those high in lutein and zeaxanthein such as spinach, kale, broccoli, red and orange peppers.

- Although the evidence is less robust, it is likely that consuming at least one portion of oily fish per week will reduce the risk of AMD.

- Vitamin supplements are of no proven benefit in the prevention of age-related eye disease. High dose multivitamin supplements with zinc are recommended for people with intermediate AMD in one or both eyes or advanced AMD in one eye.

- Along with many anti-ageing preparations, extravagant claims have been made for a range of products/supplements. Popular amongst these are bilberries and gingko biloba. Although the chemical properties of these compounds are consistent with a possible beneficial effect on physiological parameters, there is minimal evidence (if any) for benefit in humans.

- Overweight should be avoided, especially high abdominal adiposity or high waist:hip ratio.

- Recommendations apply to the majority of the older population. In sub-groups, such as by ethnicity or frailty, additional recommendations may be required if diets are low in key nutrients.

15.10 Chapter 10

- Cardiovascular disease (CVD), including coronary heart disease (CHD) and stroke, is the leading cause of morbidity and mortality in older men and women and those aged over 65 years represent an increasing proportion of the population treated for the condition.

- Ageing is clearly an important risk factor as the prevalence of CVD rises steeply with age and the outcome is more often fatal. This is thought to primarily reflect the length of time that people are exposed to the recognised risk factors.

- Scientific consensus exists on the importance of the main modifiable risk factors for the development of CVD. These include obesity, dyslipidaemia, hypertension, smoking, low levels of physical obesity and diabetes. Exposure to these risk factors in middle age predicts risk of premature death from CVD and risk in old age.

- The magnitude of the association between CVD and some of these factors (*e.g.* hypercholesterolaemia and hypertension) appears to decline when measured after the age of 65, although this may be due in part to difficulties of interpreting epidemiological studies in older populations (*e.g.* eliminating confounding factors such as co-morbidity). Nevertheless, the classical risk factors remain predictive of CVD in later life and large trials have demonstrated similar benefits from interventions such as antihypertensive and lipid-lowering drugs to those found in younger individuals. Due to the higher event rates, the absolute risk reduction yielded by preventive interventions is much greater in the older age segments of populations.

- The connection between CVD and more novel risk factors such as lipoprotein (a), homocysteine and oxidative stress in the elderly and the value of modifying them requires further investigation.

- As the risk factors that predict CVD in younger individuals remain relevant in older people for both primary and secondary prevention, dietary and lifestyle advice remains the same for the elderly as in middle age. Substantial evidence shows that diets incorporating non-hydrogenated unsaturated fatty acids as the predominant form of fat, whole-grains as the main form of carbohydrate, an abundance of fruits and vegetables, adequate *n*-3 fatty acids and not too much salt can offer significant protection against CVD. Such diets, together with regular physical activity, avoidance of smoking and maintenance of a healthy bodyweight, may prevent the majority of CVD in western populations.

- Whilst substantial evidence demonstrates physical activity to be effective in reducing CVD risk, the proportion of older people participating in regular activity is low. UK adults, including older people, are advised to accumulate at least 30 minutes of moderate-intensity activity (*e.g.* brisk walking) on at least five days a week. For many benefits to cardiovascular health, intensity can be traded for duration, provided that total energy expenditure remains high. Light- or moderate-intensity activities, which are often popular with older people, such as walking or gardening, can therefore be of benefit.

- The study of the interactions between nutritional and genetic factors is an emerging and important area of research, and has the potential to permit a more individual approach to dietary advice for CVD prevention.

- Because older people carry the greatest burden of CVD, risk factor interventions initiated or continued in later life can have considerable benefit. As CVD risk factors have multiplicative effects, a multifactorial approach is the best strategy for prevention. However, the greatest achievements will be gained from a life-course approach that considers the interacting roles of prenatal, childhood and adult life experiences in the prevention of adult CVD.

15.11 Chapter 11

- Aggressive immune and inflammatory responses are highly adaptive and have been selected through evolution. However, there are trade-offs between inflammation and fertility/fecundity. Further, whilst such responses may be beneficial acutely and at young ages, they tend to be maladaptive when chronic and at late ages.

- The immune system ages (immunosenescence); innate immune responses tend to be exaggerated, whilst humoral immunity is compromised. This leads to increased susceptibility to infectious diseases and cancers with age, and higher levels of inflammation.

- The immune system is not autonomous; it suffers from organismal ageing of its many compartments. But it also has to function in an ageing environment where the metabolic, trophic and regulatory contexts have changed and continue to change.

- 'Successful agers', such as high-functioning centenarians, have robust T-cell proliferative responses, potent natural killer cell function and low levels of inflammation.

- The rise in levels of inflammatory mediators with age is not solely due to dysregulations of the 'professional immune cells' but also due to increasing production from stromal cells, such as fibroblasts.

- The B-cell compartment and antibody production is less affected by age than the T-cell compartment. T-cell proliferative responses are compromised with age and probably skewed to a T1 (antibody production > cell-mediated immunity) profile.
- Natural killer cell functionality (kill of viral infected targets) declines with age.
- Macrophages become more activated with age, but are poorer at antigen presentation. Neutrophil function probably declines with age, contributing to more or poorly resolved infections.
- An 'immune risk profile' consisting of high CD8, low CD4, poor T-cell proliferative responses and cytomegalovirus seropositivity predicts morbidity and mortality.
- Polymorphisms which drive higher levels of inflammatory mediator production are associated with poor ageing trajectories.
- Inflammation is caused by the ageing process and by external factors such as sleep loss, postprandial responses, obesity, environmental toxicants and pollutants.
- Inflammation contributes to poor ageing outcomes, particularly by exacerbating insulin resistance and vascular dysfunction but probably also by leading directly to cancers.
- Controlling inflammation is beneficial in terms of a range of ageing outcomes. Improvements in insulin sensitivity and vascular function underpin many of the benefits.
- Diet and lifestyle interventions reduce acute and probably chronic inflammation. Fish oil, antioxidants and increasing physical activity (and weight loss) are all effective.
- Macronutrient or micronutrient deficiencies are detrimental to immune function and increase both the risk and severity of infections. Such deficiencies are common in the elderly due to poor diets associated with compromised dentition, hospitalisation and institutionalisation.
- There is no compelling evidence for the benefits of micronutrient supplementation on immune responses of those already replete. Indeed, there is evidence that it may be damaging. There is no evidence for the immune benefits of dietary interventions.

- There are no good randomised controlled trials in humans assessing the influence of dietary or lifestyle interventions on immunity as a function of age. The cost and duration of such studies is limiting and the ethics of performing such studies could be problematic.
- Redundancy and pleiotropy of the immune system makes it very challenging to design and perform nutritional interventions.
- With the exception of studies looking at macro- and micronutrient deficiency states and immune function, the result of animal model and particularly *in vitro* experiments are poorly transferable to human populations.

15.12 Chapter 12

- Recent studies suggest that, in older subjects (over 65 years), disorders of the gastrointestinal tract are the third most prevalent cause of visits to the GP.
- Gastro-oesophageal reflux disease (GERD) prevalence increases with age. GERD can lead to oesophagitis and in some instances to Barrett's oesophagus, which are risk factors for oesophageal adenocarcinoma. GERD is positively associated with body mass index.
- Incidence of oesophageal cancer (squamous cell carcinoma and adenocarcinoma) increases with age. It is not a very common malignancy but it has a poor prognosis. Adenocarcinoma of the oesophagus has increased dramatically over the last 40 years and is now the predominant form of oesophageal cancer in the US and UK. Smoking and high alcohol consumption are risk factors for squamous cell carcinoma. There is epidemiological evidence that high consumption of fruit and vegetables is protective for both types of cancer.
- The incidence of gastric and duodenal ulcers is increasing in old-aged populations worldwide, the main risk factors being use of non-steroidal anti-inflammatory drugs and *H. pylori* infection.
- The prevalence of atrophic change of the gastric mucosa generally increases with age, as does intestinal metaplasia and gastric carcinoma.
- In older people, atrophic gastritis is an important cause of poor vitamin B_{12} status.
- The crucial role of *H. pylori* in the development of chronic atrophic gastritis and gastric cancer

means antibiotic treatment is a primary means of prevention and therapy in infected subjects.

- A consistent association exists between gastric cancer risk and low intakes of fruit and vegetables, which has been attributed to intake of antioxidant micronutrients and vitamin C in particular.

- Studies in humans have not shown any age-related morphological changes in the small intestine in terms of surface structure, crypt depth, villous height, brush border and Brunner glands. Evidence for age-related changes in small intestinal hydrolases is limited and inconsistent.

- Diarrhoea is a significant worldwide problem; about 85% of deaths associated with diarrhoea in the developed world involve older people.

- There is evidence that the gut microflora of the colon alters with age, with an increase in species diversity and lower numbers of bifidobacteria. The implications for health have not been established. Prebiotics have been shown to increase the numbers of bifidobacteria, but there are few studies in older people.

- Probiotics show considerable promise as therapies for antibiotic associated diarrhoea and there is some evidence for efficacy of *S. boulardii* for *C. difficile* associated diarrhoea, although more extensive trials, particularly in older people, are needed in the latter area. Further studies are also required to investigate the role of prebiotics on antibiotic associated diarrhoea.

- Bowel dysfunction is a major problem for older people, especially constipation. The effect of adding dietary fibre to the diets of older people is variable but some studies report success, especially when fibre is combined with increased fluid intake. Insoluble fibre, such as wheat bran, appears to be more effective in increasing stool bulk than soluble fibre, resistant starch or prebiotics. A number of intervention trials have shown that probiotics relieve constipation in older subjects. In general, studies do not indicate that increased physical activity alleviates constipation.

- Diverticular disease is uncommon before the age of 40 years and incidence increases with age. There is an inverse relationship between dietary fibre intake and colonic diverticula and the principal treatment for diverticular disease is increased fibre intake. Consumption of 20–30 g of wheat bran per day is recommended for people with diverticular disease.

- Colorectal cancer incidence increases dramatically with age. In Europe, North America, Australia and New Zealand it is the second most common cancer after lung cancer in men and breast cancer in women. Epidemiological evidence suggests that diet plays a significant role in the aetiology of colorectal cancer. Processed meats, and to a lesser extent red meat, appear to be associated with a slightly elevated risk. Case-control studies indicate that increased vegetable intake is associated with reduced risk but a beneficial effect of fruit is less clear. Case-control and recent prospective studies indicate that high dietary fibre intakes are protective. Case-control and cohort studies have reported a significant protective effect of physical activity on colorectal cancer risk, with high levels of activity at work and leisure time throughout life appearing to carry the lowest risk (approximately 50% reduction). Recent prospective studies have indicated a significant effect of high body mass index or waist circumference on colon cancer risk, with the effects being more apparent in men than women.

15.13 Chapter 13

- The endocrine system is one of the major communication systems within the human body. Hormones are produced in one organ or cell and travel in the blood to a target organ or cell where they elicit a response.

- The endocrine system plays an important role in health and is involved in all of the body's functions. Hormonal imbalances and dysfunctions are associated with a number of diseases including chronic conditions such as diabetes, cardiovascular disease, obesity and some cancers.

- Older age appears to be associated with a number of changes to the endocrine system. These include a decrease in hormone secretion, a decrease in the sensitivity of the body's tissues to these hormones, and a change in hormone binding capacity/efficiency. Relatively little is known about hormones and ageing, especially with respect to different ethnic groups. However, there is now particular interest in some aspects of the endocrine system, *e.g.* the growth hormone/insulin-like growth factor-1 axis.

- Dietary treatment of type 2 diabetes has focused on modification of bodyweight and activity levels. A high-fibre diet, rich in fruits and vegetables, is advocated. More recently glycaemic index (GI) and glycaemic load (GL) have been included in some treatment plans, although the role of GI and GL in prevention of type 2 diabetes remains to be proven.
- The role of diet and physical activity in modulating hormonal changes is a relatively new area of research. Diets rich in plant foods are generally associated with a reduced risk of a range of chronic diseases. It has been suggested that plant-based diets might modulate disease risk through effects on steroid hormones but this remains to be proven.
- It has been suggested that because of their structural similarity to oestrogen, phytoestrogens may be beneficial in a number of hormonal-related conditions. However, evidence of their ability to reduce hot flushes in menopausal women remains conflicting and there is, as yet, insufficient evidence to draw conclusions about the effects of phytoestrogens in diabetes, colon cancer or breast cancer or bone health.
- There is growing evidence that the quality and quantity of dietary fat can affect hormones that may impact on a number of health outcomes, including insulin resistance, and perhaps even some cancers.
- It appears that protein and perhaps zinc may affect a number of hormones including growth hormone and insulin-like growth factor-I.

15.14 Chapter 14

- Life expectancy in the UK is currently increasing at the rate of ~two years for each decade that passes. This escalating demographic change can be expected to have profound consequences on all aspects of life.
- Nothing in this report suggests that diet and lifestyle recommendations need to change radically, but there is need for changes in emphasis.
- Intakes of eight nutrients have been identified as problematic across the population: vitamin A, riboflavin, iron, calcium, magnesium, potassium, zinc and iodine. Additionally, there is evidence of

low status of vitamin C, thiamin, riboflavin, B_6, B_{12}, D, folate and iron.
- Low nutrient status is widespread, affecting older children and young adults as well as older adults. Poor status is particularly evident in older people in residential care. There is widespread evidence of low vitamin D status (particularly among young adults and older people in care).
- Low vitamin B_{12} status affects an estimated 5–10% of people over the age of 65 years and low folate status affects 16% of older people living in institutions.
- Such is the extent of these problems that a life-course approach to healthy ageing is essential; the extent of the challenge ahead should not be underestimated.
- Fat intakes are now close to the 35% of energy target, but saturates and added sugars intakes remain higher than the targets.
- There is some evidence that sodium intakes may now be falling, but intakes are still well above the recommendation of 6 g salt/day.
- There has been considerable government-led effort to promote fruit and vegetables, but intakes still fall short of the 5+/day recommendation, with only 25% of adults achieving this. Intakes are particularly low in young men.
- Much more needs to be done to raise the profile of the importance of physical activity, which is a key predictor of independence in later life. It is never too late to start being more active.
- One of the key determinants of dietary variety in later life is retention of natural teeth, emphasising the importance of dental health throughout life.
- Adequate hydration is important at all ages, but is particularly important for older people who may become less able to recognise thirst.
- Over the past 5–10 years, a number of government initiatives have been put in place to promote healthy ageing among older people. It is important that these are monitored and evaluated to ensure that they are effective.
- There is ample opportunity for improvement in attitudes and behaviour in relation to healthy ageing, but a concerted effort will be required if progress is to be made, involving government, industry, employers, town planners, educators, health professionals, health agencies, the media and local authorities.

16
Recommendations of the Task Force

Life expectancy is increasing around the world and this is likely to have profound effects on many aspects of society, particularly if these extra years are to be associated with ill health. In the UK, lifespan is increasing at the rate of two years for every decade that passes (House of Lords 2005). Evidence linking dietary and lifestyle factors throughout the life-course with healthy ageing is emerging. However, a number of research challenges exist (Kirkwood 2006), and a higher priority needs to be given to these because of the increasing burden that diseases associated with ageing are likely to bring. A diversity of stakeholders have a role in addressing these challenges and a multidisciplinary approach will be essential, in terms of both the research agenda and the dissemination and implementation of findings.

It is, however, clear that a life-course approach is essential. Nutrition, for example, has a key role from early life (maternal nutrition and fetal metabolic programming), is important throughout childhood in relation to growth and development, and influences the maintenance of health in later life. It is also important to recognise the differences in the prevalence of different diseases and conditions among ethnic groups and to seek to understand the underlying causes of these differences (see Chapter 1, Section 1.3, and Chapter 14). Furthermore, action is needed to reduce high disease rates through health promotion, provision of information and appropriate targeting and application of health services.

Often due to their circumstances (wealthy vs. poor, urban vs. rural, reliance on public transport, disabilities, language difficulties), people experience differences in access to healthy foods and opportuni-

ties for regular physical activity. These need to be taken into account when planning local provision. Awareness and management of people's expectations (*e.g.* availability of traditional and familiar foods, affordable access to leisure facilities and adequate provision of public transport to shops) are also important.

This Task Force Report has evaluated evidence for the role of diet and lifestyle in promoting healthy ageing. Each chapter has identified specific areas that need to be addressed by further research and these are summarised in this chapter (Section 16.1.2). Using the available evidence on the associations between diet and lifestyle throughout the life-course and risk of age-related chronic diseases, general public health recommendations to help to promote healthy ageing are included for other key stakeholders, including health professionals, policy-makers, the food, pharmaceutical and supplement industries and local authorities (Section 16.2).

16.1 Recommendations for the research community

16.1.1 Ageing research in the UK

In 2005, The House of Lords Select Committee on Science and Technology undertook an inquiry to evaluate the current situation of ageing research in the UK. Among other findings, the inquiry emphasised the need for investment in research on ageing to be seen within the context of its potentially enormous societal returns and called for a more coordinated programme of multidisciplinary and longitudinal research to identify the mechanisms that provoke vulnerability to age-related disorders and effective ways in which individuals can be encouraged to adopt diet and lifestyle behaviours to reach old age in good health.

Although the arrangements for funding research on healthy ageing are still fragmented, there have been some recent improvements, such as the Strategic Promotion of Ageing Research Capacity (SPARC) initiative, supported by the Biotechnology and Biological Sciences Research Council (BBSRC) and the Economic and Social Research Council (ESRC) to encourage greater involvement of academics and researchers in issues associated with an ageing population, and the New Dynamics of Ageing programme co-funded by five UK Research Councils, including the Medical Research Council (MRC), BBSRC and ESRC, in conjunction with the Funders' Forum for Research on Ageing and Older People (FFRAOP). The EU-funded Framework Programmes have in the past included a minor focus on ageing. The European Technology Platform (*Food for Life*) has identified healthy ageing as an important theme and this has fed through to Framework Programme 7. The EU-funded ERA-AGE combines biologically oriented research programmes with sociologically focused programmes. The ERA-AGE database (www.shef.ac.uk/era-age) was launched in June 2006, and contains information about European research on ageing, research funding agencies, research programmes and research centres and institutes.

Consumer research carried out on behalf of BBSRC and MRC by Ipsos MORI (2006) revealed that the highest research priority associated with ageing from the public's perspective is research into the prevention of health problems associated with ageing. There was also support for research into managing such conditions and providing support and care. Opinion was divided on whether information campaigns about lifestyle changes that might slow down the ageing process are more important to fund than research into ageing. The vast majority of those surveyed believed the public should be consulted on funding decisions concerning research into ageing.

A recent workshop convened by the FFRAOP and Unilever developed a vision for action to promote the successful implementation of ageing research in the UK (Franco *et al.* 2007). Their recommendations called for a greater investment into

ageing research because of the immense gains to both the economy and society, in particular to the quality of life, productivity and self-sufficiency of the rapidly growing older population. They also highlighted the need to focus on early, reversible stages of lifestyle-related chronic diseases and for future efforts to embrace the role of genetics given the variability of responses of individuals to nutrients and lifestyles due to different polymorphisms.

16.1.2 Priorities for future research

A wealth of evidence implicates the substantial role of environmental (including lifestyle) factors in preventing many of the chronic diseases common at older ages. However, in relation to dietary factors, a number of general questions need to be considered including:

- How *exactly* does nutrition impact on the ageing process?
- Is there a role for nutritional supplements or functional foods?
- How do nutrition risk factors change with age?
- Can we develop better biomarkers of the ageing process to monitor the effects of nutrition?
- How do we change food intake patterns to deliver a healthier old age?

There is also a need to clarify the particular nutritional needs of the oldest old, the fastest growing age group of the population, and those with disabilities and diseases, which are common among older adults.

The study of the interactions between nutritional and genetic factors is an emerging and important area of research, and has the potential to permit a more individual approach to dietary advice for chronic disease prevention. However, further research is needed to develop robust biomarkers of the ageing process in humans which can be applied in both observational studies and in intervention studies designed to reduce the rate of biological ageing. Further work should also examine in detail how nutrition can impact, in particular in beneficial ways, on the networks for cell maintenance and repair. In order to gain the necessary level of understanding, a systems-biology approach is likely to be required.

This Task Force Report has also highlighted a number of specific areas for future research in relation to each of the individual organ systems considered in detail. These are summarised below.

16.1.2.1 The teeth and the oral cavity

- Further research is needed to determine the optimum combination of preventive strategies for dental caries, particularly in people with dry mouth; and the most effective methods for personal oral hygiene for older people with altered dental architecture.
- It remains to be clarified whether the alterations in nutrient uptake from foods in dentate compared with edentulous subjects are associated with their altered ability to chew foods.
- Studies should investigate the ability of dietary intervention/supplementation to influence the severity or progression of periodontal disease.
- Studies are also required to determine whether tailored dietary interventions delivered in a dental primary care setting can achieve meaningful and sustained changes in dietary patterns for patients whose ability to chew is compromised through lack of teeth.
- Other research questions that need to be addressed include whether edentulous people suffer greater levels of chronic disease and die earlier because of their altered dietary pattern; if taste enhancement can improve the perceived quality of foods for older people and, if it does, whether enhancers can be used in association with dietary intervention to bring about improvements in dietary quality and improvements in quality of life.
- It remains to be clarified whether reported changes in preferences for food texture are associated more with altered oral function than ageing.

16.1.2.2 Bone

- Standardised methodologies for measuring vitamin D status are needed, combined with assessment of the relationship between biochemical status and health outcomes.
- Longer-term studies of the effect of different dietary patterns, such as the Dietary Approaches to Stop Hypertension (DASH) diet, or specific types of fruit and vegetables on bone health markers (including fracture risk) are urgently needed. It remains to be established which nutrients or combination of nutrients may be respon-

sible for any beneficial effect (*e.g.* vitamins C and K, magnesium, carotenoids, fibre, phytonutrients, *etc.*).
- Long-term studies of the effects of protein and sodium intake on bone health are required.
- Intervention studies are needed to elucidate the effects of vitamin K intake/status on fracture reduction. The role of other micronutrients also remains to be clarified.
- Whether polyunsaturated fatty acids, particularly *n*-3 fatty acids, alter biochemical and molecular processes involved in bone modelling and bone cell differentiation warrants further research.
- Data are urgently required to characterise the key nutrient–gene interactions that are likely to affect bone health in both our younger and older population groups.
- The effects of different types of physical activity on fracture risk in older people should be investigated and work carried out to clarify the exact mechanism whereby mechanical loading affects bone.

16.1.2.3 The joints

- Given the importance of arthritis in older people, and the paucity of good evidence on how dietary factors influence risk, progression and symptom relief, there is an immediate need for much better studies to address this.
- Given the public's appetite for, and the belief in, dietary modulation, it is important that the scientific/medical community pushes for funding of better studies if only to counter the claims of the commercial suppliers, who may (wittingly or inadvertently) be selling ineffective products.
- Large studies are needed to consider diet–gene interactions, which may be very important in this area.

16.1.2.4 Skeletal muscle

- Further information is required about the natural history of sarcopenia and its underlying pathophysiology.
- Large-scale longitudinal studies are warranted to establish the true rates of muscle wasting in the UK, with subset analysis of ethnic and socioeconomic groups. Such a programme could identify further risk factors and confirm those currently hypothesised.

- Further research should clarify the cost/benefit ratios of exercise-based interventions. Supervised exercise programmes for the dependent elderly are associated with significant cost, particularly if domiciliary care is to be provided. However social care resource savings, through hospital admissions avoided or shortened, and independent-living, may substantially offset these costs.
- Basic molecular research is still required to elucidate further the causes of reduced muscle anabolism in ageing, in order to formulate alternative effective interventions.

16.1.2.5 The skin

- Further double-blind, placebo-controlled, clinical studies are required to investigate the ability of nutritional supplements and drinks to provide benefits for skin. Currently skin ageing benefits are best supported in the literature, but many other unsubstantiated claims are made.
- Several biological research areas show promise in elucidating the mechanisms of skin ageing and poor skin condition but require further investigation. Areas of current high interest in improving skin functioning include the role of mitochondria, biological effects of UV radiation, the skin's innate immune system, the ligand-activated nuclear hormone receptor classes including PPARα activation, and the recent discoveries that the neuroendocrine, stress and steroidogenesis pathways are operating in skin.
- Genome-wide association studies have recently become feasible following the sequencing of the human genome. It is now possible to use such technologies to identify the gene(s) that associate with complex human traits that have a genetic background: for example, pigmentation. Future research will depend more on the collection of DNA samples from high-quality clinical cohorts. A recent example of this approach has been the discovery that the filaggrin gene is linked to atopic dermatitis and ichthyosis vulgaris.

16.1.2.6 The brain

- Large-scale epidemiological evidence from prospective studies is required to assess the effects of specific dietary patterns and blood lipid and fatty acid profiles on risk of brain diseases, such as stroke, dementia, depression and Parkinsonism.

- Research is needed to evaluate brief diagnostic instruments for the assessment of cognitive function, depression and Parkinson's disease that would be feasible to use in large-scale studies.
- Large trials (and a meta-analysis of such trials) should be conducted to clarify the role of long chain n-3 fatty acids and α-linolenic acid in the prevention of cardiovascular disease and cognitive impairment.
- Large-scale trials (and meta-analysis of such trials) of B vitamins are required in people with prior cardiovascular disease to assess whether lowering homocysteine levels reduces the risk of cardiovascular disease and cognitive impairment. There is a need for further trials of vitamin B_{12} supplementation alone in older people.
- Randomised clinical trials to investigate the effect of physical activity programmes on risk of dementia in later life are warranted.

16.1.2.7 The eye

- There are few or no data on the prevalence of the major conditions leading to visual loss in ethnic minorities in the UK. Studies are required especially in those groups expected to be at high risk for certain eye conditions, such as myopia and glaucoma in people of Chinese origin, glaucoma in people of African origin and cataracts in people of south Asian origin.
- The association of diet and eye disease should be investigated for specific ethnic groups where patterns and types of food consumption differ from those of the majority of the population.
- In the light of important recent discoveries of the role of genetic factors in age-related eye conditions, especially age-related macular degeneration, further research is required to examine the effect of genetic variation on the association between diet and eye diseases (nutrigenetics).
- Further research is also required on other environment–nutrient interactions, for example the levels of antioxidants to protect the retina may depend on the levels of oxidative stress from sunlight exposure.
- Investigation of the role (if any) of dietary factors in the onset and progression of glaucoma.
- Further research is required to identify the effect of dietary intake of fatty acids, especially satu-

rates and *trans* fatty acids, on risk of age-related macular degeneration and cataracts.

16.1.2.8 The cardiovascular system

- The predictive role of cardiovascular disease risk factors is less clear at extreme ages and clarification is required regarding the likely benefits of treatments such as antihypertensives in the very elderly.
- There is a need to clarify desirable values of body mass index in the elderly and to determine if other indices, such as waist:hip ratio, are better at identifying older people at risk.
- Research is needed to provide more information about the relationship between novel risk factors and cardiovascular disease in the elderly, and the potential value of modifying them in later life.
- Further investigation of the link between oral health status, inflammatory and haemostatic markers and risk of cardiovascular disease is needed to determine if treatment of poor dental health can play a significant role in cardiovascular disease prevention.
- Further studies are needed to provide greater insight into the effects of low-fat diets (coupled with different sources of carbohydrate) and of different fatty acids on weight management and cardiovascular disease, and to identify the optimal amounts of monounsaturates and polyunsaturates and the optimal balance of *n*-3 and *n*-6 fatty acids in the diet.
- Further research is needed regarding the role of phytochemicals in cardiovascular disease prevention.
- Further studies are required to clarify the relationship between dietary protein (animal and plant) and blood pressure.
- Studies of diet–gene interactions in large population groups, in which subjects are recruited prospectively according to genotype, are required to determine the impact of genetic influences on individual responses to dietary change.
- Well-designed and evaluated studies are needed to gain a better understanding of the effect of altering lifestyle in the elderly on cardiovascular disease risk.
- Further research is needed to identify effective dietary interventions in later life.

- A better understanding of the intensity, frequency and duration of physical activity required to protect against cardiovascular disease in older populations is needed. This will allow specific recommendations, reflecting differences in age and functional ability, to be made.
- There is a need to identify ways of promoting physical activity as part of everyday life for older people.

16.1.2.9 The immune system

- The contribution and underlying mechanistic basis of the effects of inflammation on insulin resistance merit more attention.
- The mechanisms by which the gradual accrual of genomic damage are sensed and subsequently lead to age-related increases in inflammatory tone should be determined. This may lead to the identification of new intervention strategies.
- The contribution of low-level, sustained viral infections to poor ageing trajectories should be investigated.
- Short-term human models for modulation of both inflammation and broader immune functions need developing. These could be based on sleep deprivation, postprandial excursion or exercise as a starting point.
- The potentially detrimental effects of micronutrient supplementation of the 'replete' individual require further investigation; particularly given the very high penetration of these practices. Simple, rapid, inexpensive, accurate diagnostics for a range of micronutrients should be developed.
- Ever more thought needs to be given to the perennial problem of how to target appropriate interventions to those most in need; the elderly, vulnerable, isolated and members of low socioeconomic groups in our societies.

16.1.2.10 The gastrointestinal tract

- Further research is needed to identify effective dietary interventions throughout the life-course to help prevent a wide range of gastrointestinal disorders in later life.
- Impaired gastric motility with age appears to have consequences for malnutrition and other complications. There is a need to investigate the

aetiology of the disorder and to elucidate the nutritional factors involved.

- Further investigations are recommended to extend promising data suggesting that probiotics may suppress *H. pylori* and reduce inflammation in the gastric mucosa.
- Further investigations are needed into the health implications for older people of the changes in gut microflora composition with age and the potential for modifying such changes by dietary means (*e.g.* with pre- and probiotics).
- Research is needed to develop more effective dietary and lifestyle strategies for alleviating and preventing constipation in older people.
- Research is needed to validate potential biomarkers of cancer risk and to assess the potential for modifying them by diet and physical activity.
- Randomised controlled trials are required to provide greater insight into the role of specific dietary components in the aetiology and prevention of cancers of the gastrointestinal tract. Such trials will, however, need to employ validated biomarkers of disease, of which few are currently available.
- Further research is needed regarding the role of phytochemicals in reducing risk of gastrointestinal cancer. Primary prevention trials with validated biomarkers of risk are needed.
- Studies of diet–gene interactions in large population groups, in which subjects are recruited prospectively according to genotype, are required to determine the impact of genetic influences on individual responses to dietary change in gastrointestinal cancers.
- A better understanding of the intensity, frequency and duration of physical activity required to reduce cancer risk in older populations is needed.

16.1.2.11 *The endocrine system*

- The role of diet and physical activity in modulating hormonal changes is a relatively new area of research. Further work is needed to explore the effects of diet (including dietary patterns and specific components) and physical activity on the ageing endocrine system and the impact of dietary and lifestyle changes in relation to risk of disease and ill health in later life.

- The long-term effects on health of higher postprandial blood glucose concentrations within the normal range need to be investigated further.
- Well-designed studies are required to investigate the ability of phytoestrogens to reduce menopausal symptoms, especially given the consumer interest in alternative treatments and concerns about hormone replacement therapy.
- Further research is needed to investigate the effect of various nutrients on a number of hormones, including growth hormone and insulin-like growth factor-I, given the important role these hormones have in bone health and other body systems.

16.2 General recommendations to other key stakeholders

16.2.1 The food industry

Maintenance of health into old age requires a life-course approach, which includes a strong focus on healthy eating and increased physical activity levels. Consequently, there are numerous opportunities for the food industry to engage with this process. For older people, there may be specific opportunities to develop 'functional' foods that target some of the specific areas identified in this report (see Chapters 14 and 15). But opportunities to benefit the health of the population, regardless of age, also exist through continued product reformulation and innovation to reduce salt levels, improve fat and carbohydrate profiles and ensure micronutrient density. Also, within the scope of the new Regulation on the addition of vitamins and minerals to foods, which came into force in 2007, there is scope to tackle some of the micronutrient problems that clearly exist across the UK population. Many older people live alone and an appropriate range of products of a practical portion size is yet another area where the food industry can assist.

A strategic research agenda for 2007–20, which includes a focus on healthy ageing, has been developed under the auspices of a European Technology Platform, *Food for Life* (etp.ciaa.be/asp/home/welcome.asp). The working document published in April 2006 (and revised 2007, see below) outlines the many opportunities for the food industry to engage in research in this area, and presented a vision for improving population health (Figure 16.1), whereby

A vision for improving population health

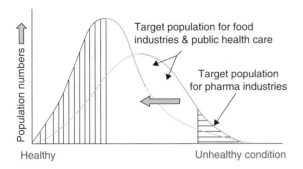

Figure 16.1: A schematic presentation of improving population health. Target areas of the food and pharmaceutical industries in public health.
Source: Green and van der Ouderaa (2003).
Reprinted by permission of Macmillan Publishers Ltd.

the food and pharmaceutical industries help to shift the population's health experience towards a more healthy profile. This vision focuses on helping to ensure that the increased longevity that many now experience is spent in better health rather than simply amounting to extra years in bad health.

16.2.2 Pharmaceutical and supplements industries

Although nutritionists recommend food rather than supplements as the main means of meeting nutritional requirements, it has long been recognised that some groups of the population benefit from targeted use of supplements, *e.g.* vitamin D and iron (see Chapter 4, Section 4.2.2.4). However, there is little evidence to support the widespread use of large-dose supplements in the general well-nourished population. Indeed, some studies with large-dose antioxidant supplements have demonstrated adverse effects on cancer risk, for example (see Chapter 14, Section 14.2.6), and the evidence for efficacy of the myriad of non-nutrient supplements now available in the high street and via the internet is often very poor indeed (see Chapter 5, Section 5.3.8.3). The recent Regulation on nutrition and health claims (1924/2006) which came into force in July 2007, is designed to safeguard consumers against unsubstantiated claims on foods, drinks and supplements. Associated with this Regulation and the partner Regulation on the addition of vitamins and minerals to foods

(1925/2006) is the setting of upper safe limits for individual vitamins and minerals (in relation to both foods and supplements) as a further protection for consumers. Specific legislation on food supplements (2002/46/EC) came into force in July 2002 and was implemented in England by the Food Supplements Regulation in 2003.

There is the potential that people looking for health-promoting strategies will be seduced by statements on products that seem to offer eternal youth. Tightening of legislation on health and nutrition claims by the European Commission is welcomed as this will help ensure that product claims are consistent with the evidence, but monitoring of the impact of the new Regulation will be important.

16.2.3 Policy-makers and law enforcers

Although a variety of government programmes are in place or in development focusing on major concerns such as obesity and diet in childhood, a need remains for these to be presented in a coordinated and joined-up manner. There is also a pressing need for evidence of progress in tackling the nutritional issues among older people identified almost 10 years ago. It is to be hoped that the relaunched National Service Framework will help with this.

At a European level, healthy ageing is a prominent component of the European Technology Platform, *Food for Life* (etp.ciaa.be/asp/home/welcome.asp), and a Strategic Research Agenda for 2007–20 was published in 2007. Details can be found in the 2007 annual report (ec.europa.eu/health/ph_determinants/life_style/nutrition/platform/docs/synopsis_commitments2007_en.pdf) and the second monitoring progress report (ec.europa.eu/health/ph_determinants/life_style/nutrition/platform/docs/eu_platform_2mon-framework_en.pdf). Another activity of relevance is the Diet and Physical Activity Platform (ec.europa.eu/health/ph_determinants/life_style/nutrition/platform/platform_en.htm).

As new regulations come into force (*e.g.* those on school meals that came into force in September 2007 in England), it is essential that their impact is monitored and evaluated. Similarly, in an era where use of health claims on foods and supplements is commonplace, it is important that the impact of the new EU Regulations referred to above is monitored and evaluated to ensure that claims are evidence-based and not misleading to consumers.

Most of the reference data used to establish energy and other nutrient requirements have used limited numbers of healthy older adults and very little representation from different ethnic groups. The UK Dietary Reference Values for Older Adults could be reviewed, taking into account the research findings accumulated since the early 1990s. With age-related changes in metabolism, advancing ill health and increased sensitivity to the effects of alcohol with age, specific advice for sensible limits for alcohol intake among older people may also be warranted.

16.2.4 Local authorities

Regardless of age, physical activity is one of the most effective ways of limiting the impact of ageing on functional capacity. Local authorities could do far more to encourage walking and cycling in both urban and rural settings by making walking an easier and less dangerous option in towns, by giving more priority to pedestrians and less to cars, and by providing better facilities for cyclists (which do not necessitate cycling on footpaths).

For older people in particular, unavailability or lack of access to amenities offering opportunities for social interactions (including shopping) and physical activity because of lack of suitable transport and/or concerns about personal safety can lead to a downward spiral of social isolation, reduced functional capacity, psychological decline and loss of independence. Effective and well-planned services to increase exercise in later life are essential to help deliver a number of milestones in the National Service Framework for Older People.

16.2.5 Health professionals and other educators

Links between healthy eating and healthy ageing need to be better understood by health professionals and educators and communicated to the public. Health professionals and educators have a pivotal role to play in ensuring that vulnerable groups at all levels of society are equipped with the information they need and empowered to make healthy diet and lifestyle choices. In particular, the lack of benefit of many nutrient supplements and other ageing products needs to be emphasised to the general population. There is a need for a much higher profile for 'ageing' in all its aspects, including lifestyle interventions, to ameliorate the adverse effects of ageing, in the training of doctors and other health professionals. Inclusion of nutrition updates in continued professional development activities would also be a way to help ensure that information passed on to patients and clients is evidence-based.

Oral health in later life is recognised to influence food choice and nutritional status. Preservation of natural teeth and provision of properly fitting dentures when natural teeth are absent are important in this respect. The current shortage of dentists in the UK and the impact of this on regular dental check-ups need to be remedied.

Health professionals should promote awareness of vision impairment in the older population. Appropriate action (*e.g.* media campaigns and advocacy) is required to ensure that health care practitioners and eye care providers are aware of the current unacceptably high levels of untreated conditions. Campaigns should also target older people and their carers to raise awareness of poor vision in later life and the potential for improving visual impairment through spectacle correction and cataract surgery.

Attention should be given to those whose socio-economic circumstances or health may make adherence to dietary and lifestyle recommendations difficult.

17
Healthy Ageing:
Answers to Common Questions

The purpose of this chapter is to summarise the key findings of this report in simple terms using a question-and-answer format. Many of the questions are commonly asked by journalists. While these are grouped under headings, they generally follow the same order as the chapters in the report.

17.1 The causes and consequences of our ageing population

Q1: Why is our population ageing?

Generally, people are now living much longer than in the past due to improvements in a range of factors, including decreased rates of infectious disease and improvements in sanitation as well as health care. There are also fewer children and young people because of the decrease in fertility rates, leading to an ageing population.

Q2: Is life expectancy likely to continue to increase over the next 20 years?

Life expectancy has been steadily increasing for some time and is showing no sign of slowing down (see Chapter 1, Figure 1.2 and Chapter 14, Figure 14.3). It is increasing by about two years for each decade that passes. It has more than doubled over the past century in some parts of the world and it is estimated that by 2010 there will be twice as many people aged over 65 years in Europe than there were in 1960. So, assuming circumstances remain the same, it may continue to increase. However, a key factor in this will be whether the increased preva-

lence of chronic conditions now being seen in adolescents and young people, such as obesity and type 2 diabetes, will begin to impact on the longevity of the younger generations.

Q3: What are the most common causes of ill health in old age?

Chronic illnesses affecting the musculoskeletal system, the heart and the circulatory system are the most common causes of ill health in older people, and the prevalence of each increases with age. In some cases, one sex is more likely to be affected than the other. For example, arthritis and rheumatism are more common in women than men. Statistics show that a substantial number of people, even in middle age, have their quality of life impaired by potentially preventable illness. This emphasises the importance of a life-course approach to healthy ageing.

Q4: What are the likely consequences of an ageing population on health costs?

Although life expectancy has increased, these extra years are not always spent in good health. The number of people reporting long-standing illness increases with age, as does disability. An ageing population will lead to increased health care costs as a disproportionate amount of public funds are spent on older adults. Conversely, 'savings' may be made from the decreased proportion of money spent on education.

17.2 The effect of ageing on diet and nutritional needs

Q5: What effect does ageing have on nutritional needs?

Because ageing is often associated with ill health, the true nutritional needs of ageing are not well understood. For example, it is thought that energy requirements decrease with age due to older people being less active and because of changes to body composition. However, research in this area is not conclusive.

Q6: Are dietary recommendations different for older people compared with younger adults?

Many dietary recommendations do not differ between younger and older adults. In the UK, micronutrient requirements are the same for 51-year-olds as for 71-year-olds, with the exception of vitamin D (where a supplement is recommended for those over 65) (see Chapter 1, Section 1.5.4 for more information). However, as further information is gathered, this may change.

Q7: What are the common nutritional concerns in relation to older people today?

As with other age groups in the UK, a relatively high proportion of older adults are obese or overweight. But there are also some older adults who are underweight. This is worrying as undernutrition can affect a range of functions and increase the risk of some diseases as well as delay recovery from illness. Low vitamin D status is common among older adults in the UK (see Chapter 1, Section 1.6.3.2; Chapter 4, Section 4.2.3 and Chapter 14, Section 14.3.2). Vitamin D is made from the action of sunlight on skin, but as we get older our bodies become less efficient at making vitamin D and some older people remain indoors most of the time. This is why a supplement is recommended for older adults.

Markers of some other nutrients have also been found to be low. Low iron, vitamin C, folate, thiamin, riboflavin and vitamin B_{12} status have been found in surveys of older adults.

Q8: Are some groups more likely to have a poor diet than others?

Older adults with no or few natural teeth tend to eat a more restricted range of foods, probably because of difficulties with chewing. Another determinant of diet, regardless of age, is socio-economic status. Older people from manual households, for example, have been shown to have lower intakes of some nutrients compared to those in non-manual households.

People living in institutions tend to have poorer intakes, as well as lower nutritional status, of a number of nutrients compared to those older adults who live in the community but there are many reasons why this may be the case, not just poor diet. For example, people in institutions may be ill and may be taking more medication which could influence their diet, their nutritional status or their nutrient requirements.

Factors such as bereavement, depression and illness can also limit appetite and motivation and therefore impact on nutritional status.

Q9: Many older adults are taking medications. Can these affect nutritional status?

A range of medications can change the sense of smell and taste, and affect food intake and therefore influence nutritional status. Medication can also influence nutritional status in other ways, for example by affecting the absorption of the nutrient.

Many older adults also take herbal medicines and dietary supplements. Some of these can interact with medication. For example, gingko biloba may interact with aspirin.

17.3 Impact of genes vs. environmental factors on life expectancy

Q10: Are we programmed to die – is senescence programmed in our genes?

There is no active genetic programming for ageing in the sense that genes do not exist that have specifically evolved to cut short our lives. Although it is widely believed that such programming does exist, perhaps to prevent species from overcrowding their environments, we know that this does not make evolutionary sense. Ageing is rarely seen in natural populations and would have been very rare in our distant evolutionary ancestors. So there was neither need to evolve genes for ageing in order to control population size, nor is it conceivable that natural selection could have driven the active evolution of a process that is never normally seen. Instead, it is now believed that because survival in the wild is limited by high levels of death from extrinsic factors (predation, accident, starvation or disease) there was no pressure to evolve the high levels of maintenance and repair that might be required for biological immortality. This is known as the disposable soma theory (see Chapter 2, Section 2.2).

Q11: What are the main factors that influence length of life?

Genes exert some influence on longevity through their effect in regulating the level of molecular and cellular maintenance. It has been shown that genes account for about a quarter of what determines length of life. Since the genetic settings of maintenance systems are insufficient to prevent damage from accumulating, there are several factors that can modulate the rate at which damage accumulates, which in turn has an effect on the length of time taken before the damage is revealed as age-related frailty, disability, disease and eventually mortality. These include nutrition, lifestyle, housing and education, as well as an essential element of chance.

Q12: Can the right nutrition in terms of quantity and quality help?

Severe under-nutrition can leave the body unable to power the mechanisms essential for cellular maintenance. Similarly, excess nutrition can over-burden physiological systems resulting in obesity and consequent stresses on cellular systems, which contribute to premature development of a range of age-associated conditions. In some animals, notably rodents, there is a range of nutrition, known as calorie restriction, which actually shifts the body towards increasing its maintenance which it appears to do by shutting down investments in fertility and reproduction. There is no evidence that such calorie restriction works in humans and some have argued that it is highly unlikely, on scientific grounds, that

it will do so. The quality of nutrition appears to be important for healthy longevity, although at present the mechanisms through which this works are not well understood and remain a matter of hypothesis.

Q13: At what age does nutrition begin to have an impact on the prospects for healthy longevity?

The damage that contributes to eventual ageing accumulates in our bodies throughout the life-course, beginning in the womb. There is evidence that fetal under-nutrition can predispose an individual to increased risk of adverse health outcomes in middle and later life, which some have argued results from some kind of metabolic programming. Such an effect, if it is general, will act in addition to the direct effects of nutrition on the rate of accumulation of cellular and molecular damage.

Q14: Is how we look a good guide to ageing? In other words, if someone looks older than their years, are they likely to have a shorter life?

The idea that looking older or younger than one's chronological age is an indicator of underlying biological age has some support, although the connection is far from being firmly established. It is likely that an accelerated appearance of ageing will be due to the early accumulation of the same kinds of damage that underpin changes within the body. As better biomarkers of ageing are developed, it will become possible to establish this connection more clearly. There is little evidence that covering up the signs of early ageing will have any deeper effect, although it is plausible that an improved self-image may result in improved psychological wellbeing, which may in turn have systemic health benefits.

17.4 Ageing and oral health

Q15: Is there an association between ageing and oral health?

Currently, many older people have no natural teeth and rely on dentures for chewing. Having no teeth is not an inevitable part of ageing and the high proportion of older people who have lost their teeth reflects historical patterns of dental care and, in particular in the UK, the advent of the NHS and a need to manage a substantial disease burden quickly. This resulted in tooth extraction rather than conservation (which was much more time-consuming in the 1950s and 1960s and there were fewer options available). Some age-related changes occur in the mouth which can affect oral health, for example increased exposure of root dentine making new surfaces accessible for decay, altered salivary flow and composition, and reductions in taste (see Chapter 3). However, in healthy older people these changes have little clinical significance.

Q16: What is dental decay and how is it influenced by diet?

Tooth decay is a consequence of the interaction between bacteria growing on the surface of teeth in dental plaque and sugars. The bacteria use the sugars as food but the waste product from that process is acidic and the acid causes the tooth to lose mineral content and soften. The mouth has good mechanisms to re-harden the surface of the tooth but they can be overwhelmed if sugars are consumed too frequently during the day or night. Tooth decay is the result of these repair mechanisms being overwhelmed with progressive damage initially to the surface of the tooth and subsequently beneath that surface.

Q17: Are there any differences in the type of decay seen in older adults compared with the young?

As people get older the root of the tooth becomes exposed close to the gum margin. There are two mineralised tissues that make up a tooth: enamel, which covers the crown; and dentine, which forms the core of the crown and the whole of the root. Dentine is not as highly mineralised as enamel and, as a consequence, is more at risk from acid attack and decay. Thus root caries occur more frequently in older people because they are more likely to have exposed tooth roots and there is also some evidence of an increased rate of decay among the very old. It is not clear what causes this increased rate of decay but it is likely to be a combination of reduced defence (probably related to the quantity and quality of

saliva present) and increased risk of damage (through deteriorating oral cleanliness).

Q18: What can be done to decrease dental decay, especially in older adults?

Tooth decay is preventable. There are two key messages for preventing decay. First, reduce the severity of damage to the tooth by reducing the frequency of intakes of sugars. This includes the use of sugar in tea and coffee. Ideally, sugar should be consumed on fewer than five occasions throughout the day. Second, bolster the mouth's defence mechanisms by using a fluoride containing toothpaste. Nearly all toothpastes contain fluoride and have a beneficial effect. There are some high-concentration pastes that are specifically designed for older people who are at risk of tooth decay.

There are some groups, including those with a dry mouth, those who wear a part-denture in either jaw or people who have particular difficulty brushing their teeth, who are at increased risk of decay. Such individuals should seek specialist advice on how to prevent decay from occurring.

Q19: Can diet and other lifestyle factors influence oral health?

Oral health is not just about teeth and sugar, there are other dietary components which harm the teeth, particularly dietary acids (*e.g.* soft and alcoholic drinks, fruit and fruit juices and pickled foods) if consumed in large quantities. The integrity of the soft tissues which line the mouth is also vital for comfort and function. These can be affected by inadequate intake of some vitamins (notably the B vitamins) and also in people who have anaemia.

The single most harmful lifestyle factor for the mouth is tobacco use. People who smoke are at increased risk of tooth decay, gum disease and oral cancer. The risk of oral cancer is particularly acute in people who use smokeless tobacco products to chew or hold in their mouths, either in the form of raw tobacco or mixed to form a quid with nuts and leaves (betel and areca nut quids).

Alcohol intake can also be associated with harm to the mouth, either because of its acidity causing damage to the teeth or as a risk factor for oral cancer. When smoking and elevated alcohol consumption are combined, the risks are particularly acute.

Good oral hygiene, use of fluoride toothpaste, regularly chewing sugar-free gum (which stimulates saliva flow) and opting for sugar-free snacks and drinks will help to protect teeth into old age.

Q20: Is chewing important?

There is some evidence that chewing is not required, as a result of modern food preparation, to allow the stomach to digest foods. However, chewing remains important to facilitate the release of tastes from food and to prepare the food for swallowing. People who do not, or cannot, chew their food well are at increased risk of choking.

Q21: How will older adults with chewing problems be affected?

People who can't chew very well tend to alter what they choose to eat to allow them to cope in a social context with eating foods. So they opt for things that are easy to chew and swallow and avoid things that are hard to chew or have a hard or sharp/crunchy texture. The consequence of these choices is often a reduced intake of fruits and vegetables and dietary fibre. There is also a tendency for people to prepare their food in different ways, eating cooked things rather than raw, for example. There are some circumstances when this is good, for example carotene is more bioavailable from cooked carrot than raw. But there are others where over-cooking destroys micronutrients or the nutrients are localised in a food close to the skin and so are removed if the food is peeled.

Q22: What happens to saliva flow with age?

There is a widespread belief that saliva flow diminishes with age. This is incorrect as recent studies on healthy older people show either no change or a small reduction which would have a negligible practical effect. However, there are a number of diseases (*e.g.* diabetes) which occur more commonly in older people and in which dry mouth is part of the presentation of the disease. Furthermore, and probably of much greater significance, there is a wide variety of drugs used to treat age-related diseases that cause a dry mouth as a side-effect of their therapeutic action. People who take lots of different drugs are particularly

likely to have a reduced salivary flow as a consequence. If older people taking such medications experience a dry mouth most of the day, they should seek advice from their dentist.

Q23: What are the effects of dry mouth on oral health in older adults?

Dry mouth can be a very distressing condition. Saliva has a number of roles in the mouth:

- It is a lubricant for chewing and swallowing food and talking.
- It is critical in helping to prevent tooth decay. Saliva is a very good remineralising solution helping to counter the effects of acids in the diet or of sugars being metabolised into acid by dental plaque causing tooth decay.
- It contains a number of non-specific defence mechanisms which help to protect the integrity of the oral mucosa.
- It contains enzymes that start to break down starches in foods to sugars as part of the digestive process.

People with a dry mouth have an increased risk of dental decay, wear of the teeth and oral mucosal disease, and they have difficulty chewing and swallowing foods and talking.

Q24: What happens to our senses of taste and smell as we age?

Ageing causes reductions in the ability to detect both taste and smell which can obviously influence an individual's enjoyment of food (see Chapter 3, Section 3.4). There is some evidence to suggest that the use of flavour enhancement (with monosodium glutamate) may help to limit this effect and improve both people's ability to taste and, as a consequence, their enjoyment of foods.

17.5 Ageing and bone health

Q25: Are we in an epidemic of osteoporosis?

Yes, global estimates for 2006 are that 1 in 3 women and 1 in 10 men aged 55 years and over will suffer from osteoporosis in their lifetime. In the US, 10 million Americans have osteoporosis with costs estimated at $17.9 billion annually. In the UK, three million people are affected and the estimated costs for Europe are in excess of €13.9 billion annually. This is likely to get even worse when the World Health Organization's estimations are taken into account. By 2050, it is believed that there will be 6.26 million hip fractures worldwide (compared with 1.66 million in 1990) and that 1 in 4 people living in the UK will be aged 65 years and over.

Q26: What is the best way of assessing an individual's bone health?

Currently, the clinical diagnosis of osteoporosis can only be undertaken by dual X-ray absorptiometry (DXA). Bone mineral density data are expressed as absolute bone mineral density (g/cm^2) and defined either as the number of standard deviations (SDs) from the mean of age-matched controls (known as the z-score) or the number of SDs from the young normal mean (known as the t-score). The World Health Organization's diagnostic criteria for osteoporosis is based on t-scores, with a t-score value of less than −1.0 being defined as osteopenic (decreased bone mineral density, but not as severe as osteoporosis) and a t-score of less than −2.5 being referred to as osteoporotic (a low bone mass which increases the risk of fractures).

Although there is a growing appreciation of the value of measurements of markers of bone turnover and quantitative ultrasound as a screening tool for fracture risk, the World Health Organization's definition of osteoporosis is only applicable to bone mineral density measurements using DXA.

17.6 Effect of nutrient intake/status on bone health

Q27: Do we have a marker for calcium nutrition status?

There is no functional marker for calcium nutrition status because blood calcium levels are maintained within very narrow limits (90–110 mg/L) because of the important role that calcium plays in regulating metabolic function. Calcium is essential for cellular structure, intercellular and intracellular metabolic function, and signal transmission, muscle contractions, including heart muscle, nerve function, activities of enzymes and normal clotting of blood. Blood calcium levels are therefore tightly regulated by three hormones (calcitriol, calcitonin and parathyroid hormone). As a result, blood measurements of calcium have little association with calcium intake. Urinary calcium also appears to be a poor intake marker.

Q28: Is there a problem in the UK of vitamin D insufficiency and is this impacting on bone health?

Currently we do not have a reference nutrient intake (RNI) for vitamin D in the UK for the 4–64 year age group, as it is considered that we get enough vitamin D from sunlight. However, this needs to be urgently addressed given the findings of national surveys that have indicated that vitamin D deficiency is a common problem (24% of men and 28% of women in the 19–24 year age groups have blood levels of <25 nmol/L) (see Chapter 4, Section 4.2.3; Chapter 1, Section 1.6.3.2 and Chapter 14, Section 14.3.2 for further information). The current level used to signify deficiency is <25 nmol/L but additional functions for vitamin D are emerging and some experts are suggesting that the cut-off should be far higher (closer to 75 nmol/L). Data just published from the large 1958 British birth cohort has also shown vitamin D deficiency to be common (25-hydroxyvitamin D levels <25, <40 and <75 nmol/L were found in 15.5%, 46.6% and 87.1% of the population respectively). Vitamin D is critical to bone and essential for calcium absorption. There are also good data to show that vitamin D is key to obtaining an optimal peak bone mass (the maximal bone mass achieved by midlife), and is involved in post-menopausal bone loss and skeletal integrity in our ageing population.

Q29: Could increasing fruit and vegetable consumption help prevent osteoporosis?

Potentially yes, but results from randomised controlled trials (where intakes of fruit and vegetables are well above the recommended five a day) are urgently needed before any conclusive statements can be made. There is growing agreement from those working in the field (from a combination of observational, experimental, clinical and intervention studies) that a positive link exists between fruit and vegetable consumption and indices of bone health. There is a variety of mechanisms which might explain this, not least the potential role that the skeleton may play in acid-base homeostasis (see

Chapter 4, Section 4.2.6). Natural, pathological and experimental states of acid loading/acidosis have been associated with high levels of calcium being lost in the urine and negative calcium balance, and there is good evidence of the detrimental effects of 'acid' on bone mineral. Alternatively other identified (*e.g.* vitamin K, phytoestrogens) or unidentified 'dietary' components may explain the positive associations found between fruit and vegetable consumption and bone health. More research is urgently required.

Q30: Is vitamin K a critical nutrient for bone health?

Yes. There are at least three vitamin K-dependent proteins present in bone and cartilage: osteocalcin, matrix Gla protein and proteins. Specifically, osteocalcin is the most abundant non-collagenous protein in bone and is a well-recognised marker of bone formation. Evidence demonstrates that the vitamin K requirement for carboxylation of osteocalcin is not met by usual dietary intakes, but that carboxylation readily responds to vitamin K supplementation. There is good evidence which supports a link between vitamin K insufficiency and osteoporosis with low circulating vitamin K concentrations in osteoporotic patients, and that circulating GluOC (under-carboxylated osteocalcin) is an independent risk predictor of bone fractures. Furthermore, low vitamin K consumption or impaired vitamin K status is associated with a higher risk of hip fracture among older women and men, a lower bone mass in older women and men, and an increased bone turnover in girls.

Q31: Does salt cause osteoporosis?

There is currently insufficient information to say whether salt influences osteoporosis risk. High salt intakes are certainly associated with increases in urinary calcium loss. However, the data with respect to salt and bone markers are inconclusive and it is suggested that increased urinary losses are counteracted by increased absorption in the gastrointestinal tract. In a recent supplementation study, urinary excretion of de-oxypyridinoline (a valid marker of bone breakdown/loss) was found to be higher in postmenopausal women on a high-salt diet compared to a low-salt diet, but no difference was seen in the premenopausal women. In the DASH-sodium

trial, the DASH diet (low in fat, rich in fruit and vegetables and including low-fat dairy foods) (see Chapter 4, Section 4.2.6.2), compared with the control diet, was found to significantly reduce both bone formation (by measurement of the marker osteocalcin) and bone loss (by measurement of the marker CTx), but sodium intake did not significantly affect markers of bone metabolism. Further research is urgently required.

Q32: Is vitamin A detrimental to the skeleton?

Vitamin A refers to a family of essential, fat-soluble compounds called retinoids. Retinol is the principal dietary form of vitamin A. The main natural sources of vitamin A are provided by animal foods such as liver, meat, milk products, eggs and fatty fish. In addition, some foods are fortified with vitamin A. Cod-liver oil also contains high levels of vitamin A. There are about 600 or so carotenoids, with approximately 10% of these having provitamin A activity (*i.e.* they can be used as a source of vitamin A by the body). Vitamin A is necessary for normal bone growth. However, intakes of vitamin A >1500 mg of retinol equivalents have been associated with lower bone mineral density and higher fracture risk in populations in the US and Sweden but not the UK. In both these countries, dairy products and cereals are generally fortified with vitamin A and hence habitual intake of vitamin A is likely to be much higher than in the UK. It should be noted, however, that high doses of pure cod-liver oil can provide as much as 1200 mg retinol equivalents of vitamin A in a 10 ml dose. In 2006 the UK Scientific Advisory Committee on Nutrition in the UK recommended that, as a precaution, those regularly eating liver (a rich source of vitamin A) should not take supplements containing retinol and that groups at increased risk of osteoporosis, such as postmenopausal women and older people, should limit consumption of liver and supplements containing retinol (*e.g.* cod-liver oil).

17.7 Ageing and joint health

Q33: What is arthritis, how common is it and what causes it?

Over 200 forms of arthritis exist but relatively few are common. Those more common forms fall into two categories: those that involve inflammation of joints, such as rheumatoid arthritis and gout, and age-related conditions, such as osteoarthritis. The inflammatory forms together affect about 1 person in 100. They often begin at a relatively young age and remain throughout life. Osteoarthritis is far more common, affecting about 10 in 100 people aged over 65 years.

Inflammatory forms are characterised by chronic inflammation of the synovial lining of the joint, and both genetic and environmental factors are involved. Osteoarthritis is thought to be triggered by subtle abnormalities in joint loading, which result in localised damage to joint and related tissue.

Q34: Can diet influence the development or treatment of arthritis?

Relatively little is known about the role, if any, of diet in the development of arthritis (see Chapter 5). There is weak evidence linking a diet low in fish/fish oils with an increased risk of acquiring the disease, but the data are inconsistent and lacking in strength. The most promising evidence is in the use of fatty acid supplements, such as fish oils, in the treatment of the symptoms of existing rheumatoid arthritis, at levels of 2.7–4 g/day of eicosapentaenoic acid (EPA) and docosahexaenoic acid (DHA) (*i.e.* similar to those levels linked to heart health benefit) (see Q70).

With regard to osteoarthritis, this is often associated with overweight. Weight loss may be effective in reducing pain and disability in osteoarthritis of the knee.

Q35: How strong is the evidence for other dietary supplements?

A wide range of supplements are on offer and commonly used. A recent patient survey (knee osteoarthritis) in the UK found that 15.9% were taking glucosamine and 5.4% were taking chondroitin. By comparison, 38.2% were taking cod-liver oil and 45.5% and 42.5% respectively taking non-steroid anti-inflammatory drugs and paracetamol (see Chapter 5, Table 5.3). A similar picture exists in the US, where more is spent on natural remedies for osteoarthritis (mostly dietary, including glucosamine, chondroitin and S-adenosylmethionine) than for any other condition. Other products include ginger extracts, vitamin supplements (vitamin C and

D) and avocado-soybean. However, the data to support the use of such remedies are at best weak and often inadequate. Recent trials and meta-analyses suggest that glucosamine and chondroitin probably have little or no greater efficacy than a placebo. Unlike rheumatoid arthritis, there is almost no rationale for the use of cod-liver (or other fish) oils in osteoarthritis, despite their widespread use. There is a limited amount of evidence to support modest symptomatic benefit with avocado-soybean (oil extracts) and S-adenosylmethionine, and somewhat less for ginger extracts. With regard to vitamins, supportive data are currently lacking.

Q36: What about alcohol and caffeine?

Most studies investigating the role of alcohol, coffee or caffeine and the risk of arthritis have not supported any association. Gout is the exception: alcohol intake is a risk factor for gout and reduced intake can aid disease management.

Q37: What about specific types of diet – can these offer symptom relief?

There is very little evidence to support many of the popular diets that sufferers adopt in the hope of attenuating their symptoms. As many of these encourage avoidance of common foods (*e.g.* meat, dairy products, citrus fruits), it is important to ensure that diets do not become nutritionally unbalanced. There is some very weak evidence that a vegan diet may be beneficial to those with rheumatoid arthritis and a Mediterranean-style diet (see Q92) may also offer some sufferers symptom relief. A sub-group of rheumatoid arthritis sufferers may benefit from an elimination diet, followed by a reintroduction phase, to identify 'culprit' foods, but this approach should be undertaken with medical supervision and preferably the input of a dietitian. Elemental diets (formulas of amino acids, sugars, vitamins and minerals) are very restrictive and hence impractical long term, and are therefore an inappropriate option.

Q38: Is osteoarthritis preventable?

Prevention would require major changes in current behaviour across society, including maintenance of healthy weight throughout adult life, less risk of joint injury and far greater physical activity levels. In the current climate, this seems unrealistic.

17.8 Ageing and muscle loss

Q39: Why is preservation of skeletal muscle important for older people?

Skeletal muscle has many important functions, both mechanical and metabolic (see Chapter 6). Maintenance of posture, protection of internal organs and mobility are the key mechanical roles enabling older people to continue activities of daily living and thus independence. As 75% of total lean body mass, muscle also functions as a metabolic factory, detoxifying excess and hence toxic amino acids, stabilising blood glucose and providing amino acids for DNA production, wound healing and energy generation. Muscle also plays a role in maintaining the body's immunity by generating molecules which activate the immune system. Age-related muscle loss can lead to failure of these diverse functions, rendering people immobile and dependent, and at increased risk of infection and disease.

Q40: What are the characteristic changes in skeletal muscle which occur with ageing?

By the age of 60 years, muscle mass and strength decline at an increasing rate due to atrophy of muscle fibres, change in fibre type composition, loss and regeneration of neural supply, increase in muscle collagen and increase in intramuscular fat deposition. The underlying cellular mechanisms for these alterations are unclear; however older muscle is definitely less responsive to the growth stimulant effect of feeding and may be less responsive to exercise than young muscle.

Q41: What measures should be adopted throughout life to optimise and retain muscle mass and strength?

Regular physical activity (at least 30 minutes of moderate intensity five times for per week) (see Q98 and Chapter 14, Section 14.6) and avoidance of both smoking and heavy alcohol consumption will optimise muscle mass during younger life and thus reduce the risk of sarcopenia (loss of skeletal muscle). This is of particular importance to people with sed-

entary occupations. High-risk groups such as those with other illnesses, prolonged periods of immobility or history of corticosteroid usage should be targeted with intensive exercise programmes during immediate convalescence and encouraged to continue higher levels of exercise throughout life. When periods of immobility can be predicted (*e.g.* prior to elective surgery), individuals should undergo intensive physical training to counteract the negative effects of immobility.

Q42: Which nutritional strategies are of most importance, are there particular at-risk groups and is there a role for nutraceuticals?

There are no specific dietary recommendations that are of established benefit to prevent muscle loss (sarcopenia) although eating a diet which is low in saturated fatty acids and rich in carbohydrates with a low glycaemic index from an early age is likely to reduce the risk of developing diabetes, which is associated with accelerated muscle wasting. Nutraceuticals which have a direct advantage in sarcopenia have yet to be identified. However, research is ongoing and may yet identify a specific nutritional strategy for sarcopenia management in the future.

Q43: Does the type of physical activity matter?

Pure resistance exercise is more anabolic than pure endurance exercise, but it should be noted that most exercise activities encompass variable degrees of both types of exercise and thus there is often no clear distinction between the two types. This said, the most appropriate type of physical activity should be determined by an individual's aptitude and preferences so that activity levels are maintained over the decades. It is clear, however, that protein-containing foods should be taken immediately after all forms of exercise to have the most effect.

Q44: What measures can be implemented to reduce muscle loss in the elderly?

To preserve muscle mass and function through to the ninth and tenth decades of life, muscle must be used frequently and supplied with essential nutrients. Structured, supervised exercise programmes are essential. When planning resources for such a programme, provision must be made for the house-bound, whether due to infirmity or lack of confidence, as this group stands to benefit the most. Motivation and support of younger age groups through education programmes encouraging physical activity, and avoidance of smoking and excessive alcohol consumption, facilitate prevention of muscle loss by increasing muscle bulk in younger life, thus minimising the impact of ageing. Screening for mineral and vitamin deficiencies and arranging for meals (providing protein) immediately after physical activity should also be considered, particularly in at-risk populations such as those in hospitals and nursing homes.

17.9 Ageing and skin damage

Q45: What happens to skin as we age?

The processes of photo-ageing (sun-induced ageing) compared to intrinsic (natural) ageing are somewhat different. In photo-ageing sunlight, particularly UVA and UVB, damages and inflames the skin leading to destruction of collagen in the dermis, which provides the supporting scaffold for the epidermis (the outermost layer of skin). The dermal damage is never completely repaired and the end result over many years is disorganised, fragmented and degraded collagen and elastin (the latter gives rise to elastosis). This is manifest visibly as wrinkling and sagging respectively. In intrinsic ageing the skin tends to thin with age, particularly the dermis. This process is particularly marked in women after the menopause. The effect of thinning skin is to make wrinkling more likely and to give the skin a fragile, translucent appearance.

Q46: Can anything be done to slow down skin ageing?

Yes. The majority of the visible signs of skin ageing in the middle-aged to older person are due to the accumulated effects of photo-damage, especially from damage that occurred early in life. Acute episodes of sunburn should be avoided completely. A high-quality sun cream that blocks both UVB and UVA radiation should be used, taking particular care to cover all parts of the exposed skin. Appropriate clothing and wearing a sunhat to minimise acute sun exposure are very important as well. As a sec-

ondary line for the prevention of sun damage, the skin's natural ability to absorb and deal with sunlight may be improved modestly by a diet higher in carotenoids, fish oils and vitamins, A, C and E (see Chapter 7).

Smoking should be completely avoided. In smokers over time, characteristic smokers' wrinkles develop giving the region of cheek around the mouth a 'shrivelled prune' appearance.

Prolonged environmental (*e.g.* wind, rain and a physically hard lifestyle) and chronic psychological stress also lead to visible skin ageing over time; such types of stress are best avoided.

Q47: Do older people need different dietary advice from younger people in relation to their skin?

In general, no. The universal advice of eating a good, balanced diet containing at least five portions of fruit and vegetables a day is satisfactory for skin health at all ages. However, some nutrients may help specific sub-optimal skin conditions; not only for skin problems arising from vitamin deficiency but also for benefits in relation to sun protection. This is particularly true to promote wound healing in the elderly (Chapter 7, Section 7.10). There is a very strong need for older people to maintain vitamin D sufficiency (made in skin, rather than needed by skin) for optimum body health (Chapter 4 and Chapter 7, Section 7.5).

Q48: How much sun exposure do I need to make sufficient vitamin D for good health?

The amount of UVB exposure required to make a sufficiency of vitamin D has been estimated as ~25% of the minimal erythemal dose per day over 40% of the body area (Holick 2004; Grant and Holick 2005). The minimal erythemal dose is the minimum UVB dose required to induce skin redness after 24 hours. Typically, there is sufficient UVB radiation to generate vitamin D from 10 am to 3 pm during spring, summer and autumn. For pale skin, the required UVB dose is estimated as 4–10 minutes' exposure a day in the summer noonday sun, while for Black Africans the exposure time may be up to 80 minutes. Many factors influence effective UVB exposure, including latitude and season, atmospheric conditions, indoor lifestyle, cultural factors, skin colour and sunscreen use. In the known absence of sufficient vitamin D from the diet, particularly in at-risk communities with darker pigmented skin living at higher latitudes (*i.e.* further away from the equator), the promotion of the generation of adequate vitamin D naturally via limited sun exposure around the midday hours in summer is a sensible recommendation.

Q49: How efficacious are topical products compared to oral products?

That depends entirely on the parameter being measured or the condition being treated. For example, for sun protection, topical products containing sunscreens, if applied correctly, can provide much better sun protection with an SPF >50 compared to oral ingredients providing an SPF of only 2–4. However, topical products can often be incorrectly applied, leaving gaps on the skin which burn. With oral delivery, the protection may be low but the protection provided is long-lasting and uniform. For a generalised nutrient deficiency or skin condition, oral delivery is clearly going to be a better approach than topical, assuming the oral route is effective in treating the disorder. In addition, oral delivery is to be preferred for deep skin delivery (*e.g.* using an antibiotic to treat a tissue infection). In contrast, topical products can be very effective for the treatment of localised problems (*e.g.* dry skin). It may be hypothesised that some disorders such as aged skin from excessive sun exposure are best treated by a combination of topical and dietary approaches.

17.10 Effect of lifestyle factors on stroke and cognitive function in later life

Q50: Are older people more likely to suffer from stroke than younger people?

Advanced age is one of the most significant risk factors for stroke. In the UK, 97% of strokes occur in people aged 55 and older, and 81% occur in those over the age of 75 (British Heart Foundation 2006). The severity of an event and a person's risk of dying from stroke also increases with age. This is because ageing is associated with important risk factors for stroke including atherosclerosis ('furring' of the arteries) and hypertension (high blood pressure) (see Chapter 8, Section 8.2).

Q51: What are the most important lifestyle determinants of blood pressure?

A number of lifestyle factors can help to prevent or treat high blood pressure, for example, not smoking, being physically active, maintaining a healthy bodyweight, drinking alcohol in moderation, if at all, and eating a balanced and varied diet. Eating a diet that is low in fat (particularly saturates) and sodium (salt) and that includes low-fat dairy products has been shown to lower blood pressure in people with hypertension. Reducing stress may also be of benefit.

Q52: What is homocysteine?

Homocysteine is an amino acid that is normally in the blood. High levels of homocysteine have been associated with several disease states including heart disease, stroke, age-related cognitive decline, dementia and Alzheimer's disease. However, it is uncertain whether these associations are causal, *i.e.* whether a raised amount of homocysteine is a cause of the disease.

Q53: Can homocysteine levels be lowered by diet?

Several of the B vitamins are involved in homocysteine metabolism (folic acid, vitamin B_6, vitamin B_{12} and riboflavin) and supplementation with these vitamins, particularly folic acid, can lower homocysteine levels. The results of ongoing randomised trials are awaited, however, to determine whether supplementation with B vitamins can prevent cardiovascular disease or have any effect on cognitive decline. Homocysteine levels are higher in current smokers than in non-smokers and in people who consume very high amounts of coffee, but are lower in individuals who are moderate alcohol drinkers.

Q54: Can antioxidant supplements help to reduce the risk of stroke or Alzheimer's disease?

As a diet that contains plenty of fruit and vegetables appears to protect against stroke and Alzheimer's disease, there has been a lot of interest in the role of the antioxidant nutrients (vitamins E and C and β-carotene) found in these foods. Free radical damage has been implicated as a factor in the development of these age-related conditions and antioxidant nutrients are important in the body's defence system. However, large trials administering antioxidant vitamins have not shown any beneficial effects on stroke or cognitive function.

Q55: Can oil-rich fish reduce the risk of dementia?

Oil-rich fish have recently hit the headlines for their potential role in preventing dementia because they contain a type of polyunsaturated fatty acid known as omega-3. However, a recent review concluded that data are not sufficient to draw any strong conclusions about their effects either on cognitive function in normal ageing or on the incidence or treatment of dementia (Issa *et al.* 2006). However, it is advisable to include at least one portion of oil-rich fish in the diet each week to protect against heart disease and stroke (see Q70).

Q56: Can drinking alcohol or coffee help preserve cognitive function in old age?

Excessive alcohol consumption, particularly binge drinking, has been associated with an increased risk of dementia, as well as stroke. However, there is some evidence that the benefits of moderate alcohol consumption (up to 3–4 units a day for men and 2–3 for women) may extend beyond heart disease (see Q72) to ischaemic stroke, Alzheimer's disease and vascular dementia. These findings are still tentative, as there are well-recognised problems in trying to measure people's alcohol consumption. It is also unclear if any benefit should be ascribed to alcohol itself or to other constituents in alcoholic drinks (*e.g.* polyphenols in wine).

Low doses of caffeine have been suggested to enhance cognitive function, which has been attributed to its ability to affect neurotransmitters in the brain. For example, caffeine can stimulate nerve cells to take up more choline, which is needed for the formation of acetylcholine, a chemical used to transmit impulses between the nerve cells in the brain. Some studies have reported people who drink coffee to have reduced risk of Alzheimer's disease in later life, but large prospective studies of the relationship between caffeine intake and Alzheimer's disease are needed to support these findings. High doses of caffeine should be avoided as they can cause side-effects in vulnerable people.

Q57: Is there a link between aluminium and Alzheimer's disease?

Aluminium is toxic at high levels at which it can cause neurological damage. Some studies have linked aluminium to increased risk of Alzheimer's disease, for example, by reporting a high aluminium content in the brains of Alzheimer's sufferers or suggesting that the disease is more common in areas where water supplies contain a lot of aluminium. However, recent studies in which the brains of people with Alzheimer's disease have been carefully compared with brains of those without the condition failed to find any difference in aluminium levels. It has also been pointed out that the amount of aluminium in water supplies is minute compared with dietary sources. The common medical and scientific opinion is, therefore, that evidence for a causal relationship is lacking.

Q58: Can being physically active help people maintain their cognitive function as they age?

Yes, being physically active in older age may improve blood flow to the brain and reduce the risk of stroke, dementia and cognitive decline. This includes activities such as gardening and walking, which are often popular with older people. Being active also enhances mood, self-esteem and wellbeing and has many other health benefits in later life (see Q97).

17.11 Vision problems in ageing adults

Q59: What aspects of vision are impaired during ageing?

The most common aspect of impaired vision during ageing is the inability to focus on close objects and this is easily corrected by spectacles. Increasing cloudiness of the lens (opacification) with ageing also causes blurred vision and glare problems. Age-related damage to the retina (the membrane at the back of the eye) and age-related macular degeneration, although less common than lens opacification, cause problems when looking straight ahead or reading.

Q60: What are the main causes of visual impairment in older people?

Near- or long-sightedness, cataracts (partial or complete clouding of the lens), age-related macular degeneration (damage to the retina of the eye), diabetic retinopathy (a complication of diabetes) and glaucoma (related to high pressure inside the eye which damages the optic nerve and leads to vision loss) are the main causes of vision impairment or loss, and are progressively more common with ageing. For patients with diabetes the threat of vision loss through diabetic retinopathy is an added burden.

17.12 Nutrition and lifestyle factors and the ageing eye

Q61: Can antioxidants prevent or alleviate cataract and age-related macular degeneration, and if so which are the most important?

Laboratory and animal studies have demonstrated the important role of antioxidants in the lens and retina. Epidemiological studies also provide evidence that high intakes of antioxidants are protective against age-related macular degeneration and cataract (see Chapter 9, Sections 9.5.2 and 9.5.4). Although there is less consistency for individual antioxidants, the data from both animal and human studies suggest that vitamin C, and the carotenoids, lutein and zeaxanthein, play a critical role.

Q62: What recommendations can be made for optimal nutrient intake to prevent onset of age-related eye disease?

Overall, the evidence supports general dietary recommendations for older people, especially for the consumption of fruit and vegetables. Older people should be advised to eat fruit, especially those high in vitamin C such as citrus fruits, and vegetables, especially those high in lutein and zeaxanthein, such as spinach, kale, broccoli and red and orange peppers. Although the evidence is less robust, it is likely that consuming at least one portion of oil-rich fish each week will help reduce the risk of age-related macular degeneration. Other dietary recommenda-

tions in older people for optimal health should also be followed.

Q63: Are supplements indicated in the elderly to prevent or alleviate eye disease?

Vitamin supplements are of no proven benefit in the prevention of age-related eye disease. High-dose multivitamin supplements with zinc are recommended for people with intermediate age-related macular degeneration in one or both eyes or advanced age-related macular degeneration in one eye.

Along with many anti-ageing preparations, extravagant claims have been made for benefit for a range of products and supplements. Popular among these are blue/purple fruits and gingko biloba. Although the chemical properties of these compounds are consistent with a possible beneficial effect on a range of physiological parameters, there is minimal (if any) evidence for most products for their effects in humans.

Q64: Are there any other factors that increase or decrease risk of eye disease in older people?

Smoking is a major risk factor for cataract and age-related macular degeneration. Older people who continue to smoke should be advised of the risk to their eyes. Smokers with early stage age-related macular degeneration, or intermediate or advanced age-related macular degeneration in one eye, are at high risk of disease progression.

There is moderate evidence that high exposure to sunlight is associated with increased risk of cataracts and age-related macular degeneration. It would be prudent to recommend protecting eyes with sunglasses and wide-brimmed hats when outdoors in the middle of the day.

Overweight should be avoided, especially excess fat accumulation around the middle (stomach) area.

17.13 Ageing and cardiovascular disease

Q65: Why is ageing associated with increased risk of cardiovascular disease?

Older people are more likely to suffer from cardiovascular diseases primarily because atherosclerosis, or the 'furring up' of the arteries associated with heart disease, is a gradual process that takes place over many years. Increased years of life provide a longer period of exposure to the important risk factors, such as high blood pressure and high blood cholesterol levels, and time for any damage to develop.

Q66: Are the risk factors in middle age the same as those in later life?

Yes, the main risk factors for cardiovascular disease, such as being obese, having high blood pressure or abnormal lipid levels, smoking, being physically inactive or having type 2 diabetes, are similar in later life as for younger people. So the dietary and lifestyle advice to protect against heart disease remains the same.

Q67: Is there any point changing lifestyle once you've reached 65 or has the damage already been done?

It is unlikely that you will reverse years of damage by changing your habits late in life, but you can still reduce your risk of suffering from a heart attack or stroke by improving your diet, being more physically active and giving up smoking after the age of 65. But you will gain most benefit by adopting healthy lifestyle and dietary habits throughout the whole life-course.

Q68: Can't we give older people drugs to prevent heart disease and strokes?

A few years ago there was considerable media interest in the suggestion from some leading scientists that giving people over the age of 55 a 'polypill' containing a cocktail of drugs (statins, β-blockers and aspirin) and folic acid could help to prevent most cases of heart disease and stroke. This led to a lot of controversy about how much benefit this would bring, with many doctors concerned about the cost-effectiveness and possible side-effects of such a strategy and that offering a pill might discourage people from making lifestyle changes. A healthy diet and active lifestyle are a better option as they can confer the same benefits for cardiovascular disease but also help to protect against other conditions, such as cancer and diabetes.

17.14 Effect of diet and lifestyle on risk of cardiovascular disease

Q69: Can vitamin supplements reduce the risk of heart disease or stroke in later life?

Intervention trials have not supported the notion that vitamin supplements (vitamins E and C and β-carotene) provide the same protection against heart disease and stroke as increasing fruit and vegetable intake. This might be because it is the cocktail effect of the many substances present in whole fruit and vegetables that confer the health properties or that the substances tested are not those responsible.

Q70: What types of fat are beneficial in reducing heart disease risk and what are their main sources?

Omega-6 (or *n*-6) polyunsaturates, found primarily in vegetable oils (sunflower, corn and soya bean) and spreads made from these, lower 'bad' LDL-cholesterol levels, which are associated with heart disease. Monounsaturates also appear to lower LDL-cholesterol levels and may have other cardio-protective benefits. These fatty acids are found in olive oil, rapeseed oil and walnut oil, as well as meat and dairy products, and are a feature of Mediterranean-style diets (see Q92), which seem to protect against heart disease. The long-chain omega-3 (or *n*-3) polyunsaturates found in oil-rich fish such as salmon, pilchards, sardines, mackerel, trout and fresh tuna can also reduce the risk of deaths from heart disease and stroke (see Chapter 10, Section 10.7.3.6), particularly in people who have already suffered a heart attack. At least one portion of oil-rich fish is generally recommended weekly to reduce risk of heart disease (see Chapter 10, Table 10.3).

Q71: What types of fat should be limited and what are their sources?

To keep your heart healthy it is crucial to eat the right fats and to lower the intake of all fats. Reducing the amount of saturates in the diet is important in reducing blood cholesterol levels. The main sources of saturates in the UK diet are fat spreads (*e.g.* butter, hard margarine, lard) and products made from them (*e.g.* pastry and baked goods), hydrogenated vegetable oils, fatty meat and meat products, and dairy products made from whole milk. High intakes of *trans* fatty acids, found in hard margarine and in those processed foods, cakes and biscuits made using partially hydrogenated vegetable oils, can also have a detrimental effect on blood cholesterol levels and increase the risk of heart disease. Some experts have, therefore, advocated elimination of industrially produced *trans* fatty acids from the diet through voluntary agreement with the food industry or by legislation. In the UK, intake of *trans* fatty acids has fallen considerably in recent years and is now at or below 1% dietary energy intake (*i.e.* well below the recommended maximum level of 2%). This is due to the decision made by food manufacturers to remove these fats in light of emerging evidence (see Chapter 14). A similar response is now required by food companies operating in those countries where intakes remain high.

Q72: Can drinking alcohol protect against heart disease and are some types of drinks better than others?

Regular consumption of a moderate amount of alcohol (around two units a day) can reduce risk of heart disease in middle and old age. The benefit seems to be associated with the alcohol in the drinks, rather than the type of drink. Many investigators have claimed that red wine is particularly beneficial due to the presence of flavonoids, which may act as antioxidants in the body, but this remains to be substantiated. Consuming larger amounts of alcohol increases the risk of accidents, high blood pressure, haemorrhagic (bleeding) stroke, liver cirrhosis and some types of cancer.

Q73: What is an ideal bodyweight?

Being overweight is a well-established risk factor for heart disease and risk generally increases when body mass index (defined as weight in kilograms divided by the square of height in metres) rises above 25 and is greatly increased if it rises about 30.

The distribution of fat in the body also influences the risk of heart disease. People with excessive abdominal fat (central obesity) are at greater risk and, as we age, fat tends to accumulate around this area of the body. An increased risk to health is associated with a waist circumference of >94 cm (37 inches) in men and >80 cm (32 inches) in women. A substantial risk to health is associated with a waist circumference of >102 cm (40 inches) in men and >88 cm (35 inches) in women.

17.15 Ageing and the immune system

Q74: How is the immune system organised?

The first line of defence is non-specific and provided by the 'innate immune system', which distinguishes between dangerous pathogens and harmless molecules on which the body depends. Specialised immune cells (*e.g.* neutrophils, monocytes, macrophages and natural killer cells) are involved alongside more generalised cell types, such as cells lining the blood vessels (endothelial cells) that participate by producing chemical mediators and cell surface markers (see Chapter 11, Section 11.1). The second line of defence is the more powerful and flexible 'adaptive immune response' and provides immunological surveillance via the continuous circulation of T lymphocytes (T-cells) and B lymphocytes (B-cells). The adaptive immune system has a 'memory' based on past experience that resides within T- and B-cells, which enables it to recognise specific 'foreign' proteins (antigens) and to elicit a rapid response to disable them. Communication within the immune system occurs via cell-to-cell contact and production of specialised chemical messengers (cytokines).

Q75: Does the immune system deteriorate with age?

Yes. With ageing there is an increased incidence and severity of infectious disease, cancer and autoimmunity (in which the body's immune system is tricked into attacking its own cells). Antibody production to vaccinations and infections diminishes with age. Our immune system is less able to kill viral infected cells and cancerous cells. Our scavenger cells are less able to chase down and kill pathogens. The level of chronic inflammation brought about by over-production of pro-inflammatory cytokines (which are central to immune system communication) also increases with age and contributes to immune cell dysfunction.

Q76: What is chronic inflammation? Which conditions might this play a role in?

The process of inflammation is designed to protect us against acute damage from infections, cuts and burns, for example. However, inflammation needs to be well controlled. Problems arise when inflammation is not turned off after doing its job and becomes longstanding/unresolved (*i.e.* chronic). Examples include rheumatoid arthritis and chronic bronchitis, where inflammation is out of control. Chronic inflammation is a feature of advancing age and contributes to muscle and bone loss, diabetes, cardiovascular diseases and cognitive decline. Overall, chronic inflammation contributes to frailty and compromised function. The majority of those over the age of 55 in Europe and North America already have chronic low-grade inflammation, underlying the progress of chronic degenerative diseases such as cardiovascular disease, insulin resistance and type 2 diabetes.

Q77: Do long-term diet and lifestyle play a role in protecting immune function?

People with the genetic predisposition to produce low levels of inflammatory cytokines seem to be more likely to live to an old age, and so it has been suggested that control of the pro-inflammatory response to ageing (the chronic inflammation associated with excess production of inflammatory cytokines) may provide a route to healthy ageing. The suggested mechanisms include improvements in insulin sensitivity and vascular function. The most consistent evidence to date concerns long chain *n*-3 (omega 3) fatty acids, antioxidants such as vitamin E, weight loss and increased physical activity, but much more research is required before conclusions can be drawn.

Q78: Can nutrient deficiencies contribute to impairment of the immune system in later life?

The majority of older people who eat a healthy, balanced diet, such as described by the Food Standards Agency's Eatwell plate model (www.eatwell.gov.uk) (Chapter 14, Figure 14.13), and have a reasonable appetite are unlikely to become deficient in key nutrients. However, in later life nutrient intake may be compromised because of mobility issues, poor dentition, social isolation or bereavement, institutionalisation or illness. Protein- and energy-deficient diets and various micronutrient deficiencies are detrimental to the immune system and increase the risk and severity of infections. Micronutrient deficiencies are common among vulnerable older people (see Q8) and correction of deficiencies in nutritionally compromised people improves markers of immune function, although effects are typically modest.

Q79: Should older people take vitamin and mineral supplements to protect against infections?

There is currently no evidence to support the routine use of micronutrient supplementation to improve immune function in well-nourished people. However, individuals who have poor diets or low status of particular micronutrients are likely to benefit from dietary improvement. But individuals who already have good intakes and status of these nutrients are very unlikely to benefit from supplementation and may actually do themselves some harm as demonstrated in a study providing smokers with β-carotene (see Chapter 10, Section 10.7.6.2). Ideally, deficiencies are best addressed through dietary means (whole foods rather than supplements) via which it is very unlikely that any adverse reactions will be provoked.

17.16 Ageing and the digestive system

Q80: What are the major changes that occur in the gastrointestinal tract as a consequence of ageing?

A number of changes can occur to the gastrointestinal tract with ageing which can impact on its function. For example, older people are also more likely to suffer from reflux of the stomach juice into the oesophagus (gullet), which can lead to inflammation of the oesophagus (oesophagitis) and changes in the cells of the lining. In some people this can develop into cancer. Changes in muscle activity in the gut also increase the prevalence of constipation in older people. Recent studies suggest that in older subjects (over 65 years), disorders of the gastrointestinal tract are the third most prevalent cause of consultation with GPs.

Q81: Does the absorption of nutrients, for instance vitamins and minerals, decline with age and, if so, are supplements indicated in the elderly?

Malnourishment of older people is of concern, particularly in hospitals and long-term care facilities. Many factors contribute to this including poor dentition, medication, psychological and social issues. Although there is some evidence from animal experiments that nutrient absorption declines with age, data from human studies suggest that the small intestine and pancreas undergo few clinically and nutritionally significant changes with ageing. Unequivocal evidence for loss of digestive or absorptive capacity with ageing in the absence of disease is scanty. Absorption of vitamin B_{12} is often impaired in older people usually as a consequence of reduced gastric acid secretion from atrophic gastritis or the use of medications. It has been recommended that general supplementation with vitamin B_{12} of >50 µg/day should be considered. There is also some evidence of decreased calcium absorption in older women (>75 years).

Q82: What aspects of diet and lifestyle may have a beneficial effect on gut health in later life?

The maintenance of a healthy bodyweight, increased consumption of fruit and vegetables and avoidance of smoking and excess alcohol intake can help to reduce the risk of gastric reflux and oesophageal cancer. Antibiotic therapy is important in the treatment of *Helicobacter pylori* infection and can therefore help to reduce the risk of gastric and duodenal ulcers and stomach cancer. A high intake of fruit and vegetables and avoidance of large amounts of salt and highly salted foods can help to prevent cancer of the stomach.

Increasing the amount of fibre in the diet, particularly insoluble fibre, and being physically active can help to protect against constipation and diverticular disease. Probiotics supplied via yogurts or fermented milks may help relieve constipation (see Q83).

In relation to colorectal cancer, a diet rich in a diversity of fruit and vegetables and fibre (including that from whole-grain cereals and pulses), with small or moderate amounts of red meat and moderate amounts of low-fat dairy products (as a source of calcium), is likely to be protective. Being physically active, not drinking to excess and maintaining a healthy bodyweight are also very important in the prevention of this type of cancer. Milk and calcium probably protect against colon cancer and there is limited evidence suggesting protection from non-starchy vegetables, fruit, folate-rich foods, fish and vitamin D.

Q83: Can probiotics prevent or delay age-related changes in the gut and are there any strains that are particularly beneficial?

There is some evidence that certain *Lactobacillus* strains can help in the treatment of *Helicobacter pylori* infections (which can cause peptic ulcers) in adults and reduce inflammation of the lining of the stomach (the gastric mucosa) when used in combination with antibiotics (See Chapter 12, Section 12.3.4.1). For example, a specific strain of lactobacillus, *Lactobacillus johnsonii* La1, showed inhibitory effects on *Helicobacter pylori* in infected subjects and in a randomised trial of 53 subjects with this infection, those patients receiving *Lactobacillus johnsonii* La1 (in addition to antibiotic therapy) showed significant, though modest, decreases in their level of *Helicobacter pylori*, inflammation of the lower part of the stomach and activity of the inflammation in the stomach. Similar results were obtained with another strain called *Lactobacillus gasseri* LG21 in 31 patients with *Helicobacter pylori* infections. LG21 suppressed *Helicobacter pylori* colonisation of the gastric mucosa and reduced mucosal inflammation.

Probiotics supplied in yogurts or fermented milks may help relieve constipation (see Chapter 12, Section 12.5.2.1). A large study (350 healthy older subjects) tested the effect of yogurt containing *Bifidobacterium animalis* DN-173-010 on transit time through the gut. There was a significant, dose-related reduction in the time food stayed in the gut (the transit time) with the effect lasting 2–6 weeks after the two-week period of consumption ceased. A commercially available mixture of *Lactobacillus rhamnosus* LC705 and *Propionibacter freundreichii* JS brought about a 24% increase in defaecation frequency in a group of older subjects.

Probiotics are also effective in alleviating antibiotic-associated diarrhoea which is common in hospitalised older patients (see Chapter 12, Section

12.4.4). The protective effect is strain-specific with *Saccharomyces boulardii*, *Lactobacillus rhamnosus GG* and *Lactobacillus casei* DN114001 being particularly beneficial. There is also some evidence that *Saccharomyces boulardii* and *Lactobacillus casei* DN114001 are protective against *Clostridium difficile* infections.

17.17 Ageing and hormones

Q84: What is the endocrine system?

The endocrine system comprises organs and other tissues that produce chemical messengers called hormones to allow communication between and within different organ systems, and to regulate function (see Chapter 13). Some organs, such as the heart and gastrointestinal tract, have a number of functions including hormone production, while others such as the pituitary gland are dedicated endocrine glands. Hormonal regulation of processes such as reproduction involves a hierarchy of responses delivered via special trophic hormones (typically produced in the pituitary gland) and coordinated by the hypothalamus.

There are three classes of hormones: amine hormones, which contain nitrogen and are made from the amino acids tyrosine and tryptophan (*e.g.* the thyroid hormone, thyroxine); peptide hormones (*e.g.* insulin); and lipid-derived hormones such as the sex hormones and activated vitamin D. Hormone secretion is controlled in a number of ways, including the presence of another hormone (*e.g.* a tropic hormone), by nerve response or by a nutrient or ion that the hormone regulates (*e.g.* the response to glucose of insulin).

Q85: How do hormones contribute to health? What about disease?

Because hormones are messengers they have an important role to play in health. In fact, hormones interact with most of the other organ systems and therefore contribute to a number of important functions, including growth, digestion and absorption, immunity, bone health, blood pressure and stress responses.

Endocrine problems can lead to a large number of diseases and disorders, some of which are very rare and some of which are more common. For example, hormonal factors have been identified as risk factors for a number of cancers, including cancers of the breast and ovary. While hormone abnormalities causing obesity are rare, obesity and hormones interact in a number of other ways. Body fat produces a number of factors (*e.g.* messengers known as adipokines which typically act locally) that are active in the body and can influence its metabolism in very specific ways by binding to receptors within or on the surface of cells. Hormones are important in another chronic condition, diabetes. There are two different types of diabetes: type 1, where there is partial or complete inability to produce the hormone insulin; and type 2, where not enough insulin can be produced or the body is less responsive to it.

Q86: Does ageing affect the endocrine system?

While our knowledge of the effect of ageing on the endocrine system is not comprehensive, ageing appears to be associated with some changes. These may be due to a decrease in the ability to produce hormones and hormone receptors may also become less responsive. There is a relatively good understanding of the effect of ageing on certain sex hormones, especially those associated with the menopause. The prevalence of type 2 diabetes increases with age; while the mechanisms are not fully understood, it is generally thought that ageing is associated with a decrease in the number of cells in the pancreas that produce insulin. Ageing also seems to affect hormones associated with feeding, bone health, stress and the thyroid gland. Hormonally related changes to circadian rhythms, which establish the body's biological clock, have also been suggested to occur with ageing. These are suggested to be associated with disturbed sleep patterns, depression and dementia, all of which are more common in older people.

Q87: Can diet and physical activity influence the endocrine system?

Diet and physical activity can influence the endocrine system, but this is a relatively new area of research. It has been demonstrated that diet and activity are important in the prevention and treatment of diabetes, with inactivity and overweight known to decrease insulin sensitivity. There has been interest in low glycaemic index (GI) and low glycaemic load (GL) diets (focusing on foods which are digested and absorbed more slowly than a standard food, usually white bread or glucose). While these diets have been shown to be useful in treatment of diabetes, their role in diabetes prevention is not yet clear.

There are many other areas where the evidence is less clear-cut or more limited. While chronic energy (calorie) restriction has been shown to slow down the ageing process in a variety of species, it is not known if this is true for humans (see Q12). Prolonged calorie restriction could be associated with negative consequences, including effects on libido and fertility, strength and/or stamina, and wound healing. Other areas which require further investigation include the role that nutrients have on a number of hormones, especially those important for bone health and the effect of plant-based diets on steroid hormones.

17.18 Dietary and lifestyle advice to promote healthy ageing

Q88: Which current dietary and lifestyle patterns are of particular concern in terms of their likely impact on the health and life expectancy of the populations of developed countries?

Although there have been improvements in various aspects of diet in recent years – for example we are eating less fat, saturates, *trans* fats and salt and consuming more fruit and vegetables – there is still room for improvement (see Chapter 14, Section 14.5). Although energy intakes have been falling over recent decades, so have levels of physical activity, and the reality is that many of us are expending less energy than we are consuming. As a direct result, the prevalence of obesity, the metabolic syndrome and related conditions such as type 2 diabetes is soaring, with huge implications for health care costs and the life expectancy of future generations. There is also evidence of widespread micronutrient insufficiency (*e.g.* vitamin D).

Q89: What advice can be followed throughout life to enhance the likelihood of a healthier old age?

The advice is all about moderation and variety in what we eat and drink, not smoking and being far

more active in our everyday lives than most of us are currently. The crucial message is the need to be more active (see Q96 and Q97 and Chapter 14, Section 14.6) as well as eating more healthily, because when these two are combined, the risk of developing type 2 diabetes, for example, can be halved.

Q90: Which dietary and lifestyle factors influence the risk of cancer in later life?

Tobacco use is the factor that carries the most risk, but diet, physical activity and maintenance of a healthy bodyweight are important too (see Chapter 14, Section 14.2.6). It has been recognised for some time that a high fruit and vegetable intake is associated with lower cancer risk at some sites, although the effect now seems to be less strong than originally thought. The importance of being active and avoiding becoming obese are now recognised as of particular importance, for example in reducing the chance of developing colon cancer (see Q82). Other factors have also been identified (*e.g.* moderation in alcohol intake, high fibre intake).

Q91: Can childhood diet significantly affect health in old age?

The nutrients provided during childhood influence growth, development and bodyweight, and these in turn can influence health during childhood (*e.g.* response to infection and ability to concentrate in school) and health in later life (*e.g.* bone health, reproductive health and risk factors for chronic disease such as blood pressure, blood lipids, insulin sensitivity). It is essential that a life-course approach to healthy ageing is adopted; it is important not to wait until retirement age.

Q92: Will eating a Mediterranean diet improve life expectancy?

Much is said in the media about the benefits of a Mediterranean diet (see Q37 and Q70). It is sometimes taken for granted that this relates to the type of food we eat during our summer holiday in the sun but in reality the attributes under the microscope are the more traditional features of Mediterranean cuisine, which rely heavily on large amounts of fruit and vegetables, olive oil as the main source of fat, fish, bread, pulses, some meat and dairy products, and a distinctive meal pattern, focusing on a large meal consumed in the afternoon often with some wine. This dietary pattern was also accompanied by lots of physical activity associated with work, and of course a warm climate. Whilst it is not that easy to import the traditional way of life in the Mediterranean region to northern Europe, we can take some lessons from it and modify the fatty acid profile of our diet to make it more unsaturated, increase consumption of fish, fruit and vegetables, and become more physically active. These features have all been shown to help reduce risk of chronic diseases.

Q93: Can supplements or fortified foods help to ensure a healthy life expectancy?

The expectation that antioxidant supplements can benefit risk of cardiovascular disease and cancer has, on balance, not been demonstrated. Indeed, in some cases, supplementation actually increased risk (*e.g.* lung cancer among smokers and asbestos workers). This finding has resulted in considerable caution in recommending supplements, and most nutritionists prefer to advocate diet as the route of choice, although there are exceptions to the rule. For example, fish oils have proved to be a useful source of long chain *n*-3 fatty acids for those who don't like oil-rich fish, and supplements are recommended for vulnerable groups, for example folic acid for women of child-bearing age, iron for women with heavy menstrual losses, vitamin D for young children, pregnant women and older (especially housebound) people, and calcium for those at high risk of osteoporosis. Fortified foods may also have a role to play; for example for those people who don't like oil-rich fish, foods with added long chain *n*-3 fatty acids can be a useful option and some foods, such as margarine and bread, are already fortified by law (with vitamins A and D, and iron, thiamin, niacin and calcium respectively). Functional foods, for example those with added fibre or prebiotics, may also be of benefit.

Q94: Which dietary factors can help to preserve mental function in later life?

Dementia is expected to become increasingly common as lifespan increases. Recent research is beginning to throw some light on ways in which decline in mental function can be delayed (see Section 17.10). One of the dietary factors of interest is vitamin B_{12}; many older people have biochemical evidence of low vitamin B_{12} status and this increases with age, from 5% at age 65 to 20% at age 80. It is of concern that B_{12} deficiency may go unnoticed in countries with mandatory folic acid fortification because folate can mask B_{12} deficiency as it shares some of the functions of B_{12} (but cannot influence deterioration in neurological function). Studies are also examining the effect of long chain *n*-3 fatty acids on cognition. Low doses of the stimulant caffeine may also enhance cognitive function and vitamin D deficiency has been implicated in low mood and impaired cognitive performance. Cognitive decline has also been slowed through regular physical activity.

Q95: Why is it important to stay hydrated and what drinks are best to do this?

Adequate hydration is important for concentration, bowel function, kidney function and skin appearance, and some beverages also contribute protein (*e.g.* milk), vitamins and minerals (*e.g.* milk, fruit juices) and polyphenols (*e.g.* tea, coffee, wine). Recommendations vary but, typically in the UK climate, 6–8 glasses/mugs per day (about 1.2 litres) are recommended *in addition* to the water provided via food, which can be substantial. Many beverages provide energy (calories) and so can contribute to the risk of obesity. Drinks such as water, tea (without sugar) and milk are the best choices between meals, while sugar-containing drinks should be kept to mealtimes to protect teeth from decay (see Chapter 3).

Q96: Do older people still need to be physically active?

Physical activity has benefits for people of all ages, including older people. Physical activity can have an important impact on energy balance as well as providing opportunities for social interaction. Strength training in particular is important for older adults to maintain muscle strength. In the UK, all adults are advised to have at least 30 minutes of moderate activity at least five times a week (see Q98). Older adults should also aim to stay mobile (current thinking is 'use it or lose it').

Q97: Why is being physically active so important?

Regular physical activity benefits the heart and circulation; muscle strength and function; joint flexibility and bone strength; cognitive decline and risk of dementia; mood and general wellbeing. Risk of cardiovascular disease and type 2 diabetes is reduced, as is risk of some cancers (*e.g.* breast cancer in postmenopausal women and colon cancer), and leading an active life helps maintain a healthy bodyweight. Furthermore, overweight people who remain fit have a lower all-cause and cardiovascular mortality rate than their unfit counterparts. Benefit is evident at all ages, for example men aged 80 and over who have kept fit have a lower death rate than unfit men 25 years younger. It's never too late to start being more active, although the earlier we start the better. For example, among older people, fitness and strength training can build muscle and help protect against falls.

Q98: How much physical activity should older people aim for and what forms of physical activity are safe for older people?

The recommendations for older adults are the same as for younger adults: at least 30 minutes of at least moderate-intensity activity (*e.g.* brisk walking) on at least five days a week. The good news is that the 30 minutes can be made up of several shorter periods of activity provided it is sufficient to increase heart rate and lead to a feeling of increased warmth, possibly accompanied by sweating. To prevent obesity, many individuals will need to take at least 60–90 minutes each day. Ideally, the type of activity should be varied: aerobic activity for the heart, weight-bearing activity for bones, activity to increase flexibility and muscle strength. The type of activity suitable for older people will be determined by fitness level and mobility: some 75-year-olds are still keen hill walkers while others are largely confined to a wheelchair, so the activity must be determined by functional capacity. Those who have previously led sedentary lives should start gradually, but even light activity on most days, such as walking, can reap rewards.

For those who have led very sedentary lives into old age, it can be harmful to engage in vigorous activity because of increased injury and heart attack risk. Types of physical activity with lower intensities (walking, cycling or gardening) are often preferable. Although older people should aim to meet the recommendation for physical activity for younger adults, even light activities conducted almost daily (≥ 5 times per week) may have substantial benefits for cardiovascular risk profile in this age group. They may also result in improvements in many physical and psychological parameters (Department of Health 2004a).

17.19 Dietary interventions and policies

Q99: What types of interventions are most successful in improving nutritional intake amongst older people in the community?

Poor appetite is common among frail older people, putting them at risk of malnutrition. Appetite can often be stimulated by eating and cooking with others (smelling food that is being cooked or being offered food that is attractively presented), getting out of the house and being active, being stimulated with new ideas about food, having the opportunity to satisfy a particular increase in appetite or sudden desire for a food (particularly when it is not readily available at home).

Q100: Are current policies targeting the health of older people adequate?

No. In 1998, the National Diet and Nutrition Survey of people over the age of 65 identified a number of nutritional issues which have yet to be fully addressed, for example poor vitamin D status and a high prevalence of low intakes of essential nutrients (see Chapter 14, Section 14.5). Recent evidence has added to concerns about the vitamin D status of the population and the prevalence of low folate and vitamin B_{12} status has been highlighted. The National Service Framework established in 2001 has been heavily criticised by a House of Lords Committee and subsequently re-focused. However, it still lacks a specific focus on some of the major issues identified in this Task Force Report.

Glossary

1,25 hydroxyvitamin D or 1,25 $(OH)_2$ D_3: The active form of the vitamin which is involved in calcium homeostasis.

25 hydroxyvitamin D (25 OHD): The main circulating vitamin D metabolite and the best indicator of clinical status.

Aberrant: Abnormal.

Absolute difference in risk (absolute risk reduction): The difference in risk of a particular event between two groups.

Achalasia: An oesophageal motility disorder in which the smooth muscle layer of the oesophagus has impaired peristalsis and the lower oesophageal sphincter fails to relax properly in response to swallowing.

Achlorhydria or hypochlorhydria: Occurs when gastric acid levels are either absent or low in the stomach.

Acquired immunity: An immune reaction involving lymphocytes that is specific to any given antigen that gives rise to immunological memory.

Actinic: Sun-induced.

Adenocarcinoma: A form of carcinoma that originates in glandular tissue.

Adenosine triphosphate (ATP): The energy store for all cell processes. The breakdown of ATP to ADP (adenosine diphosphate) or AMP (adenosine monophosphate) releases phosphate groups and usable energy in the cell.

Adipokines: A group of cytokines (cell to cell signalling proteins) secreted by cells in adipose tissue.

Adipose tissue: Tissue found under the skin and around the body organs that is composed of fat-storing cells.

Aerobic glycolysis: The main energy-releasing pathway leading to ATP formation; it occurs in the mitochondria.

Age composition: The proportionate number of children, young adults, middle-aged adults and older adults.

Age-related macular degeneration (AMD): Damage to and/or loss of the photoreceptors in the macula region of the retina. Age-related macular degeneration results in decreased central vision and, in advanced cases, blindness.

Agnosia: Loss of the ability to recognise objects, persons, sounds, shapes or smells, although the specific sense is not defective and there is no significant memory loss. Agnosia is usually associated with a brain injury or neurological illness.

Alpha linolenic acid: An n-3 polyunsaturated fatty acid (C18:3), rich sources of which include walnuts, rapeseed, walnut, soya and blended vegetable oils. Some is also found in green leafy vegetables.

Amyloids: Insoluble fibrous protein aggregations sharing specific structural traits.

Anaerobes: Organisms that do not require oxygen for growth.

Andropause: Male menopause.

Antibodies: Proteins found in blood or other bodily fluids of vertebrates used by the immune system to identify and neutralise foreign objects, such as bacteria and viruses.

Antioxidant: A compound that prevents or protects against the damage that could be caused by the oxidation of molecules such as fatty acids, proteins and DNA.

Aphasia: A loss of the ability to produce and/or comprehend language, due to injury to brain areas specialised for these functions.

Apolipoprotein E (apoE): Occurs in all types of lipoproteins and is thought to be involved in the conversion of very low-density lipoproteins to intermediate-density lipoproteins and the removal of low-density lipoproteins from the circulation.

Apoptosis: Programmed cell death ('suicide').

Apraxia: A neurological disorder characterised by a loss of the ability to execute or carry out purposeful movements, despite having the desire and physical ability to perform them.

Arthropathy: A disease of a joint.

Atherogenic: Having the capacity to start or accelerate the process of atherogenesis or the formation of lipid deposits in the arteries.

Atherosclerosis: The process in which fatty and fibrous deposits cause thickening and hardening of the arterial walls.

Atrophic gastritis: Chronic inflammation of the stomach mucosa leading to loss of gastric glandular cells and their eventual replacement by intestinal and fibrous tissues. It impairs stomach secretion of essential substances such as hydrochloric acid, digestive enzymes and intrinsic factor and leads to digestive problems, vitamin B_{12} deficiency and megaloblastic anaemia. It can be caused by persistent infection with *Helicobacter pylori* or can be autoimmune in origin.

Axons: Long fibres that carry signals away from the cell body of a neuron or nerve cell.

Basal metabolic rate (BMR): The amount of energy required to maintain physiological equilibrium while lying at rest in the fasted state; can also be measured using indirect calorimetry.

B-cell: A white blood cell (lymphocyte) that matures in the bone marrow, produces antibodies and plays a large role in the humoral immune response. B-cells may be found in the bone marrow and in the blood circulation (*cf.* T-cell).

Betaine (trimethylglycine): Found in several tissues in humans. It is involved in homocysteine metabolism as an alternative methyl donor and is used in the treatment of homocystinuria in humans.

Blood pressure: A measure of the force that the circulating blood exerts on the walls of the main arteries. The pressure wave transmitted along the arteries with each heartbeat is felt as the pulse –

the highest (**systolic**) pressure is created by the heart contracting, and the lowest (**diastolic**) pressure is measured as the heart fills.

Body mass index (BMI): An index of obesity calculated as weight in kilograms divided by the square of height in metres $(w \div h^2)$.

Bolus: The aggregate of chewed food particles, brought together by the tongue and bound together with saliva prior to swallowing.

Bone mineral density: A measure used to assess bone density and determine fracture risk for osteoporosis.

Calcitonin: Hormone secreted by the thyroid gland to decrease the concentration of calcium in the blood (*cf.* parathyroid hormone).

Carcinoma: Malignant cancer that arises from epithelial cells.

Cardiovascular disease: A disease of the heart or circulation. This broad term encompasses coronary heart disease, peripheral vascular disease and stroke.

Case-control study: A study that compares people with a disease or condition ('cases') to another group of people from the same population who don't have that disease or condition ('controls').

Cataract: A clouding of the normally clear lens caused by change in structure, which restricts the amount of light entering the eye, thus impairing vision.

Catecholamines: Amines derived from the amino acid tyrosine, including adrenaline (epinephrine), noradrenaline (norepinephrine) and dopamine, which act as hormones or neurotransmitters.

Cell-mediated immunity: Also known as delayed-type hypersensitivity, this is an immune response that depends on the activation of macrophages, natural killer cells, antigen-specific cytotoxic T-lymphocytes and cytokines via T-cells rather than the action of antibodies derived from B-cells (*cf.* humoral immunity, B-cell).

Central obesity: Accumulation of fat around the abdominal (stomach) region (also known as abdominal obesity, upper-body obesity or 'apple' body shape). This is associated with an elevated risk of cardiovascular disease and type 2 diabetes.

Chemokines: A family of cytokines involved in a wide variety of processes including acute and chronic types of inflammation, infectious diseases and cancer.

Cholecystokinin: A hormone that stimulates the contraction of the gallbladder with release of bile and the secretion of pancreatic enzymes into the small intestine.

Cholesterol: A fat-like substance found in the bloodstream as well as in bodily organs and nerve fibres. Most cholesterol in the body is made by the liver. It is an essential constituent of cells, but when present in excess becomes a key component in the development of atherosclerosis.

Chondroitin: A polysaccharide which is a polymer of galactosamine and glucuronic acid. Chondroitin sulphate is a component of cartilage and the organic matrix of bone, and has been used extensively in treatment of osteoarthritis, but there is currently little evidence to support its efficacy.

Chromosomes: A single large macromolecule of DNA. They are the physically organised form of DNA in a cell nucleus.

Cobalamin: Vitamin B_{12}.

Coeliac disease: An autoimmune disorder of the small bowel caused by a reaction to gliadin, a gluten protein found in wheat, barley and rye.

Collagen: Found in the connective tissue and provides strength, resilience and support to skin and cartilage.

Commensal: Living in a relationship in which one organism derives food or other benefits from another organism without hurting or helping it. Commensal bacteria are part of the normal flora in the mouth.

Confidence interval: This is the range of values within which we can be 95% sure that the true answer lies when we estimate something with some uncertainty, though this description is only approximate. Wide confidence intervals reflect a lot of uncertainty about the value and arise from small sample sizes and/or large variability.

Conjugated linoleic acid (CLA): A series of isomers of the fatty acid linoleic acid found predominantly in the meat and milk of ruminant animals.

Cornea: The clear, transparent outer portion of the front of the eye that provides most of the eye's focusing power.

Coronary heart disease (CHD) (ischaemic heart disease): Heart disease resulting from the build-up of fatty deposits in the lining of the coronary arteries. It may cause angina (stiffening of the arterial walls), a heart attack or sudden death.

Cortisol: The body's primary stress hormone.

C-peptide: A peptide which is made when proinsulin is split into insulin and C-peptide. Proinsulin splits when it is released from the pancreas into the blood in response to a rise in blood glucose levels.

C-reactive protein: A plasma protein that rises in the blood with inflammation.

Crown: That portion of the tooth which is covered by enamel and is usually exposed as a result of tooth eruption in early life.

Cytokines: Small, hormone-like proteins released by leukocytes, endothelial cells and other cells to promote an inflammatory immune response to an injury. Interleukins, interferons, and some growth factors are examples of cytokines.

Dehydroepiandrosterone (DHEA): A natural steroid prohormone produced from cholesterol by the adrenal glands, the gonads, adipose tissue, brain and in the skin. DHEA is the precursor of androstenedione, which can undergo further conversion to produce the androgen testosterone and the oestrogens oestrone and oestradiol.

Dementia: The progressive decline in cognitive function due to damage or disease in the brain beyond what might be expected from normal ageing.

Dental caries (tooth decay): Damage to the structures of teeth caused by certain types of acid-producing bacteria in the presence of fermentable carbohydrates such as sucrose, fructose, and glucose.

Dental erosion: Damage to teeth resulting from chemical dissolution of the protective enamel by acid not of bacterial origin.

Dental implant: An artificial tooth root placed in the bone of the jaw surgically to act as a means of tooth replacement. Commonly made from titanium.

Dental pulp: The collective term for nerves, blood vessels and connective tissues which are contained within the dentine and which provide a tooth with a nerve supply and nutrition.

Dentate: Having one or more remaining natural teeth.

Dentine: The core of the tooth, covered by enamel on the crown of the tooth, but exposed into the mouth if the gum recedes and the roots become visible with increasing age and/or gum disease.

Dermis: The layer of the skin that lies just below the epidermis on most of the body. It is largely made up of collagen (fibrous or connective) tissue. The dermis protects the body from mechanical injury, binds water, stores water, maintains temperature and carries nerves to detect sensation and feeling.

Diabetic retinopathy: A complication of diabetes that is caused by changes in the blood vessels of the retina. It is a leading cause of blindness.

Dietary reference value (DRV): Ranges of figures, published by the UK Department of Health in 1991, designed to assess the nutritional adequacy of the diets of groups of people in the UK.

Diet-induced thermogenesis (DIT): The energy required for digestion and for forming tissue reserves of fat, glycogen and protein following a meal.

Disposable soma theory: A theory proposed by Professor Thomas Kirkwood to ascribe an evolutionary framework to understand the existence of, and variations in, the universal process of ageing. It proposes that individuals should invest in the maintenance and repair of their body or soma in relation to their expected life history objectives.

Diverticular disease/diverticulosis: The presence of diverticula (small pouches in the wall of the digestive tract) that bulge outward through weak spots in the colon wall.

DNA: An abbreviation for deoxyribonucleic acid, the molecule that contains the genetic code for all life forms except for a few viruses. It consists of two intertwined chains (double helix) made up of nucleotides.

Docosahexaenoic acid (DHA): A long chain *n-3* (omega-3) fatty acid that is abundant in oil-rich fish (see also eicosapentaenoic acid) and is associated with heart health.

Drug–nutrient interaction: An interaction between a drug and a nutrient within the body that influences the effect of either the drug, the nutrient, or both.

Duodenum: The first part of the small intestine where most chemical digestion takes place.

Dysgeusia: Altered taste perception.

Dyslipidaemia: An abnormal concentration in the blood of one or more lipids, such as an elevated low-density lipoprotein (LDL) cholesterol level or a depressed high-density lipoprotein (HDL) cholesterol level.

Dysplasia: An abnormality in the maturation of cells within a tissue. It is often indicative of abnormal proliferation of cells in a tissue or organ.

Edentulous: Having no natural teeth.

Eicosanoids: Signalling molecules derived from omega-3 (*n-3*) or omega-6 (*n-6*) fatty acids. They exert complex control over many bodily systems, especially in inflammation, immunity and as messengers in the central nervous system. Eicosanoids derived from *n-6* fatty acids are generally pro-inflammatory, whilst those derived from *n-3* fatty acids are much less so.

Eicosapentaenoic acid (EPA): A long chain *n-3* (omega-3) fatty acid that is abundant in oil-rich fish (see also docosahexaenoic acid).

Enamel: The hard calcified tissue that covers and protects the outside of the crown of the tooth.

Endothelium: The membrane lining various vessels and cavities of the body, including the heart and blood vessels.

Enterocyte: A type of epithelial cell of the superficial layer of the small and large intestine tissue. These cells can help break up molecules for onward transport of the resultant constituents.

Epidermis: The outermost layer of the skin. The epidermis contains keratinocytes (cells that make keratin) and melanocytes (cells that make pigment), as well as other specialised cells.

Epigallocatechin-3-gallate: A flavonoid of the catechin family found particularly in tea.

Epigenetics: The study of heritable changes in gene function that occur without a change in the DNA sequence.

Erythema: Redness of the skin as a result of a widening of the small blood vessels near its surface.

Estimated average requirement (EAR): An estimate of the average requirement or need for food energy or a nutrient. Some people will need less than the average and some people will need more.

Extrinsic ageing: Damage caused by external factors, such as exposure to UV radiation.

Fecundity: Generally refers to the ability to reproduce.

Fibrinogen: The soluble, circulating precursor of the insoluble blood clotting protein, fibrin.

Fibroblast: A large flat cell in connective tissue that secretes collagen and elastic fibres.

Flavonoid: The most numerous of the polyphenolic compounds found in plants.

Fluorapatite: An apatite crystal in which fluoride has replaced some of the hydroxyl ions. It is a member of the family of minerals that make up the basic structure of bones and teeth.

Folate: A B vitamin found in green leafy vegetables (especially sprouts, spinach, green beans, peas), potatoes, fruit (especially oranges) and milk. A synthetic form (folic acid) is also found in some fortified foods (*e.g.* breakfast cereals, bread, yeast extract) and in vitamin supplements.

Free radicals: Highly reactive, short-lived molecules which promote oxidative damage by reacting with cell constituents, such as fatty acids, proteins and DNA.

Fructooligosaccharides: Molecules containing from two to ten units of the simple sugar, fructose. These can act as prebiotics, stimulating the growth of a beneficial intestinal flora.

Gene: A segment of a DNA molecule that contains information for making a protein or, sometimes, an RNA molecule.

Genetic: Inherited.

Genome: All of an organism's genetic material.

Genotype: The genetic constitution (the genome) of a cell, an individual or an organism. The genotype is distinct from its expressed features, or phenotype.

Ghrelin: A hormone that stimulates appetite.

Glaucoma: An eye disease, related to high pressure inside the eye, which damages the optic nerve and leads to vision loss. Glaucoma affects peripheral, or side, vision and is a leading cause of blindness because of an absence of symptoms in the early stages.

Glucagon-like peptide-1 (GLP-1):   A peptide cleaved from proglucagon. The major source of GLP-1 in the body is the intestinal L cell that secretes GLP-1 as a gut hormone.

Glucocorticoids: A class of steroid hormones characterised by an ability to bind with the cortisol receptor and trigger similar effects.

Gluconeogenesis: The generation of glucose from non-sugar carbon substrates like pyruvate, lactate, glycerol and glucogenic amino acids (primarily alanine and glutamine).

Glucosamine: An amino sugar which is a precursor for glycosaminoglycans, a major component of joint cartilage. Oral glucosamine is often used in the treatment of osteoarthritis, although evidence for its effectiveness is currently lacking.

Glucose-dependent insulinotrophic polypeptide (GIP):   A peptide synthesised by cells in the gastrointestinal tract, which stimulates insulin secretion.

Glycaemic index: A scale for evaluating foods, based on the rate at which sugar is absorbed into the bloodstream after eating a specific food.

Glycaemic load: A measure to assess the total glycaemic effect of a food or diet which is the product of its dietary glycaemic index and total carbohydrate content.

Glycolysis: The breakdown of glucose to pyruvate yielding energy (ATP).

Goblet cells: Mucus-secreting columnar epithelial cells located in the respiratory system and intestines.

Gout: A disturbance of uric acid metabolism, characterised by painful inflammation of the joints, especially of the feet and hands, and arthritic attacks resulting from elevated levels of uric acid in the blood and the deposition of urate crystals around the joints. The condition can become chronic and result in deformity.

Gram-negative bacteria: Bacteria that do not retain crystal violet dye in a Gram stain test.

Growth hormone (or somatotrophin):   A hormone that stimulates cell growth and reproduction.

Heat shock proteins: Proteins which help other proteins to fold properly and which also recognise molecules altered by stress and mark them for destruction.

***Helicobacter pylori*:**   A Gram-negative bacterium that infects various areas of the stomach and duodenum, infection with which can lead to peptic ulcers, gastritis and possibly cancer.

High-density lipoprotein (HDL):   Lipoproteins that transport cholesterol from cells to the liver, where they are degraded or repackaged. HDLs are responsible for removing excess cholesterol from the blood, preventing a build-up of cholesterol on the artery walls and are therefore referred to as 'good' cholesterol. High levels of HDL-cholesterol are associated with low risk of CHD.

Homocysteine: A sulphydryl amino acid derived from the metabolic conversion of methionine, which is dependent on vitamins (folate, B_{12}, and B_6) as cofactors or co-substrates.

Homocystinuria: A congenital disease in which an affected individual is unable to metabolise or utilise methionine properly. The main features of the condition are abnormality of the lens of the eye, mental retardation, fair complexion, fair hair and a high cheek colour.

Humoral immunity: The immediate response to an antigen which triggers antibody production, produced in the cells of the B lymphocyte lineage (B-cell). This is distinct from cell-mediated immunity, which involves white blood cells and is a delayed response to an antigen (*cf.* cell-mediated immunity).

Hypermethylation: Abnormally increased methylation observed in the promoter regions of some genes during ageing and in disease. It is associated with silencing (switching off) of the gene.

Hypertension: Elevated blood pressure (usually defined as a blood pressure of 140/90 mmHg or above).

Hypochlorhydria: *See* achlorhydria.

Hypothalamus: Region of the brain that links the nervous system with the endocrine system via the pituitary gland.

Immunosenescence: The ageing of the immune system.

Impaired glucose tolerance (IGT): A state that is borderline to diabetes and associated with elevated risk of cardiovascular disease.

***In vitro*:** From the Latin meaning 'in glass'. The term is applied to biological processes studied experimentally in isolation from the organism, as distinct from *in vivo*, which refers to the study of processes in the living organism (*cf. in vivo*).

***In vivo*:** Observations carried out inside the living body of animals, including man (*cf. in vitro*).

Incidence: The rate at which new events occur in a population, *i.e.* the number of new cases of a disease in a specific period of time, divided by the total population at risk of getting the disease during that period (*cf.* prevalence).

Inflammation: The reaction of the body to an injury, for example resulting from trauma, infection or chemicals. In response, local blood vessels dilate, increasing blood flow to the injured site, and white blood cells invade the affected tissue engulfing bacteria or other foreign bodies. The process causes a characteristic up-regulation of cytokines.

Innate (or natural) immunity: Natural non-specific host defences.

Insulin resistance: A condition in which the body's cells are less responsive (or sensitive) to the action of insulin. This causes more insulin to be released by the pancreas, resulting in an excess amount of insulin circulating in the blood. This metabolic abnormality underlies type 2 diabetes.

Insulin resistance syndrome: A set of heart disease risk factors, which have been found to occur together causing a substantial increase in the risk of a heart attack (also known as Syndrome X, Reaven's syndrome and metabolic syndrome).

Insulin-like growth factor (IGF): A hormone that promotes growth whose chemical structure is similar to insulin. While insulin primarily affects the body's metabolic system (energy delivery and use), IGF helps regulate cell growth.

Interferons: Proteins released by cells in response to viral infection, which activate the synthesis and secretion of antiviral proteins.

Interleukins: Molecules made by leukocytes that are involved in signalling between cells of the immune system.

Intrinsic ageing: The continuous natural ageing process which causes the slow irreversible degeneration of tissue and affects almost all body organs.

Irritable bowel syndrome: A functional bowel disorder characterised by abdominal pain and changes in bowel habits that are not associated with any abnormalities seen on routine clinical testing.

Isoflavones: Plant compounds found in legumes, especially soya beans, that may have positive effects against cancer and heart disease (*e.g.* genistein).

Keratinocytes: Also called squamous cells. The primary cell types found in the epidermis, the outer layer of skin.

Langerhans cells: Dendritic cells abundant in epidermis.

Lean body mass: The remainder of body mass after accounting for adipose tissue.

Leptin: A hormone produced by the ob (obese) gene and secreted by fat tissue that acts on the brain to regulate appetite and has a central role in fat metabolism.

Ligands: An atom, molecule, group, or ion that is bound to a central atom of a molecule, forming a complex.

Lipoprotein (a) or Lp(a): A lipoprotein particle similar to low-density lipoprotein cholesterol with an attached protein. Studies have suggested an association between elevated blood levels of Lp(a) and an increased risk of heart disease.

Low-density lipoprotein (LDL): The particles that deliver cholesterol to tissues where it is needed for membrane structure or to manufacture steroid hormones and bile acids. Too much LDL-cholesterol in the blood leads to a build-up of cholesterol (referred to as plaques) in the artery walls. These build-ups can eventually lead to ischaemia and thrombosis, by impeding adequate perfusion of the tissues with blood carrying oxygen. If this blockage is to the muscle of the heart, this may result in a heart attack. This is why LDL-cholesterol is referred to as 'bad' cholesterol. A high-fat diet can result in raised LDL-cholesterol levels in the blood.

Lower reference nutrient intake (LRNI): The amount of a nutrient that is adequate for only 2.5% of a population group, those who have low needs. A regular intake at this level is therefore inadequate to meet the needs of most people (see also reference nutrient intake).

Lymphocytes: A population of white blood cells, of which T-cells, B-cells and natural killer cells are subpopulations.

Macrophage: A large white blood cell that has scavenger properties and normally collects at infection sites to remove foreign bodies. It is also involved in the development of atherosclerotic lesions.

Macula: An oval yellow spot near the centre of the retina of the human eye. It contains special light-sensitive cells for high acuity vision.

Magnetic resonance imaging (MRI): A non-invasive method using nuclear magnetic resonance to render images of the inside of an object. It is primarily used in medical imaging to demonstrate pathological or other physiological alterations of living tissues.

Mast cells: A large cell in connective tissue consisting of granules that release histamine and heparin during allergic reactions.

Mastication: The process of chewing by which food is mashed and crushed as the first step of digestion.

Maté: A caffeinated drink prepared by steeping dry leaves (and twigs) of yerba maté (a species of holly native to subtropical South America) in hot water. When drunk as traditionally in parts of South America, scalding hot through a metal straw, it is a probable cause of oesophageal cancer (probably as a result of epithelial damage resulting from the heat and not from the herb itself).

Melanocytes: A cell in the epidermal layer of the skin that produces the dark brown or black pigment melanin.

Meta-analysis: A discipline that reviews critically and combines statistically the results of previous research in an attempt to summarise the totality of the evidence relating to a particular medical issue.

Metabolomics: The study of the entire complement of metabolites in the cell including those involved in metabolic regulation and fluxes.

Metaplasia: A process by which cells change from one cell type to another usually in response to an abnormal stimulus.

Methylation: The attachment of or substitution with a methyl group.

Minimal erythemal dose: The minimum UVB dose required to induce skin redness after 24 hours.

Mitochondria: Membrane-enclosed organelles, found in most eukaryotic cells. Mitochondria are sometimes described as 'cellular power plants', because they generate most of the cell's supply of ATP, used as a source of chemical energy.

Mitosis: The process in which a cell duplicates its chromosomes to generate two identical cells.

Monocyte: A type of white blood cell that circulates in the blood. Monocytes are transformed into macrophages in the artery wall.

Mucosa: The lining of various body cavities that are exposed to the external environment and internal organs. The mucosa is covered in epithelium and involved in absorption and secretion.

Mutation: A change in a DNA sequence.

Myopia: Nearsightedness. A refractive condition wherein light focuses in front of the retina, which results in far vision being blurred. Concave or 'minus' lenses are prescribed for myopia.

***n*-3 (or omega-3) polyunsaturates:** Fatty acids with their first double bond at the third carbon atom from the methyl end ($-CH_3$) of the molecule. These include alpha linolenic acid (C18:3) (rich sources of which include walnuts; rapeseed, walnut, soya & blended vegetable oils), eicosapentaenoic acid

(C20:5) and docosahexaenoic acid (C22:6) (the main sources of which are oil-rich fish) (see also eicosapentaenoic acid, docosahexaenoic acid) (*cf.* *n*-6 polyunsaturates).

n-6 (or omega-6) polyunsaturates: Fatty acids with their first double bond at the sixth carbon atom from the methyl end ($-CH_3$) of the molecule. These are the typical fatty acids of vegetables oils (*e.g.* sunflower, corn and soyabean) and spreads made from these (*cf. n*-3 polyunsaturates).

Natural killer cell: A lymphocyte that kills targets such as certain tumour cells.

Neutrophil: A type of white blood cell that can act as a phagocyte. Neutrophils are the most numerous cell type in the bloodstream and the major cell type found in acute inflammatory lesions.

Non-communicable disease: A disease which is not infectious. Such diseases, which include diabetes, cardiovascular disease and cancer, may result from genetic or lifestyle factors. Those resulting from lifestyle factors are sometimes called diseases of affluence.

Non-milk extrinsic sugars: Sugars not naturally present in fruit or milk.

Nucleosomes: Structural units of chromatin consisting of DNA wrapped around octets of histone proteins.

Nucleotide: A building block of DNA or RNA. It includes one base, one phosphate molecule, and one sugar molecule (deoxyribose in DNA, ribose in RNA).

Nutraceutical: A merging of 'nutrition' and 'pharmaceutical' which refers to foods claimed to have a medicinal effect on human health. Such foods are also called functional foods.

Nutrigenomics: The study of molecular relationships between nutrition and the response of genes, with the aim of extrapolating how such subtle changes can affect human health.

Odds ratio: A ratio used in epidemiological studies (in particular case-control studies) to compare the odds of an event occurring in an exposed versus non exposed group, or in an intervention versus control group.

Oesophagitis: Inflammation of the lining of the oesophagus resulting from reflux of the acid contents of the stomach into the oesophagus.

Oestrogens: A group of steroid compounds that function as the primary female sex hormone.

Older person: Defined in this report as a person aged 65 years or older.

Oldest old: Defined in this report as those aged 80 years or over.

Oligosaccharide: A carbohydrate molecule composed of 3–20 monosaccharides (simple sugars).

Oncogene: A modified gene, or a set of nucleotides that codes for a protein and is believed to cause cancer.

Oncogenesis: The process through which tumours develop.

Osteoarthritis (OA): The most common form of arthritis in which the cartilage that covers and acts as a cushion inside the joints becomes damaged in weight-bearing areas of the joint. As the bone surfaces become less well protected by cartilage, the sufferer experiences pain upon weight bearing, including walking and standing.

Osteoblast: A type of bone cell responsible for bone formation. Bone mass is maintained by a balance between the activity of osteoblasts that form bone and osteoclasts that break it down (*cf.* osteoclast).

Osteoclast: A type of bone cell involved in bone resorption (bone loss/removal) (*cf.* osteoblast).

Osteomalacia: A disease in adults that results from a deficiency in vitamin D or problems with the metabolism of this vitamin. It is characterised by softening of the bones, resulting from defective bone mineralisation. Signs include pain, weakness and fragility of the bones.

Osteopenia: A decrease in bone mineral density that can be a precursor condition to osteoporosis.

Osteoporosis: A metabolic bone disease which has two predominant characteristics – low bone mass and micro-architectural deterioration of bone tissue. Both factors lead to enhanced bone fragility and a consequent increase in fracture risk.

Oxidative stress: A condition in which the production of oxidants and free radicals exceeds the body's ability to inactivate them.

p53/p21/pRb system: A consortium of proteins which contribute to regulation of the cell cycle and which help protect the genome against damage.

Paneth cells: Specialised cells of the small intestine that release antibacterial substances and engage in phagocytosis. They regulate the small intestinal flora population.

Parathyroid hormone: Hormone secreted by the parathyroid glands to increase the concentration of calcium in the blood (*cf.* calcitonin).

Peak bone mass: The maximum bone mass achieved by midlife. The age at which peak bone mass is achieved varies between different regions of the skeleton and different populations.

Periodontal disease (periodontitis): A gum disease that causes inflammation of gums, ligaments and bone structure or loss of the bone supporting teeth. Can lead to tooth loss.

Peristalsis: The rhythmic contraction of smooth muscles to propel contents through the digestive tract.

Pernicious anaemia: A form of megaloblastic anaemia due to vitamin B_{12} deficiency. Usually occurs due to impaired absorption of vitamin B_{12}.

Peroxisome proliferator-activated receptors (PPARs): Members of the nuclear hormone receptor family.

Phagocytosis: A process whereby cells engulf and destroy foreign material, *e.g.* bacteria, cells, cell debris and other small particles. Cells that act in this way are called phagocytes.

Phytoestrogens: Chemicals produced by plants that act like oestrogens in mammalian cells.

Plaque: A soft and sticky substance that accumulates on the teeth from food debris and bacteria.

Pleiotropy: The phenomenon in which a single gene determines two or more apparently unrelated characteristics of the same organism.

Poly (ADP-ribose) polymerase (PARP): A protein involved in a number of cellular processes involving mainly DNA repair and programmed cell death.

Polymorphism: The existence of variation of a genetic characteristic in a population that is too common to be due merely to new mutation. A polymorphism must have a frequency of at least 1% in the population.

Polyphenols: A group of chemical substances found in plants, characterised by the presence of more than one phenol group per molecule. Polyphenols are generally further subdivided into tannins, and phenylpropanoids such as lignins and flavonoids.

Polyunsaturates (polyunsaturated fatty acids): Fatty acids containing two or more double bonds; common in vegetable oils (see also *n*-3 polyunsaturates *n*-6 polyunsaturates) (*cf.* saturates).

Posterior subcapsular opacities: A type of cataract in the eye.

Prevalence: This is a measure of the total number of existing cases of a disease or condition at a particular point in time (or during some specified time period). Prevalence is usually expressed as a percentage of the total population, or per 1000, 10,000, or 100,000 people (*cf.* incidence).

Primary prevention: Measures taken to prevent someone from developing a disease (*e.g.* modifying the diet to reduce coronary risk before there are signs of heart disease).

Promoter: A nucleotide sequence within the non-transcribed region of the DNA of a gene that regulates the process of transcription.

Prospective (follow-up, cohort or longitudinal) study: Data on exposure are first collected and subjects are followed up for the development of a given condition or outcome. A randomised controlled trial, for example, is always prospective.

Prostaglandins: A type of eicosanoid. These hormone-like substances participate in a wide range of body functions. They have several actions as inflammatory mediators, particularly those derived from the *n*-6 fatty acid, arachidonic acid, such as prostaglandin E_2.

Proteomics: The study of proteomes (the full cellular content of proteins).

Psoriasis: A chronic skin condition characterised by inflamed, red, raised areas that develop a scaly appearance.

Randomised controlled trial (RCT): In a randomised controlled trial, participants are assigned by chance to receive either an experimental or control treatment. Both groups are followed up for a specified time and the effects of the intervention on a specific outcome (*e.g.* serum cholesterol level, death rates) are analysed. The idea behind the randomised controlled trial is that when it is done properly, the effect of a treatment can be studied in groups of people who are the same at the outset and treated the same way except for the intervention being studied. Any differences then seen in the groups at the end can be attributed to the difference in treatment alone, and not to bias or chance.

Reactive oxygen species (ROS): A collective term that includes free radicals of oxygen and non-radical derivatives of oxygen such as hydrogen peroxide and singlet oxygen.

Reference nutrient intake (RNI): The amount of a nutrient that is enough for almost every individual (97.5% of the population), even those with high needs. If an individual is regularly consuming the RNI he/she is unlikely to be deficient (*cf.* lower reference nutrient intake).

Relative risk: The likelihood of an adverse health outcome in people exposed to a particular risk, compared with people who are not exposed. For example, if people who smoke for a certain time are on average 15 times more likely to develop lung cancer than those who do not smoke, their relative risk is 15.

Rete pegs: A series of finger-like structures which project up from the dermis.

Retina: The nerve layer that lines the back of the eye, which senses light and creates impulses that travel through the optic nerve to the brain.

Retinoids: A class of chemical compounds that are related chemically to vitamin A.

Retinol: Vitamin A.

Rheumatoid arthritis (RA): This is traditionally considered a chronic, inflammatory autoimmune disorder that causes the immune system to attack the joints. It is a disabling and painful inflammatory condition which can lead to substantial loss of mobility due to pain and joint destruction.

Rickets: A softening of the bones in children potentially leading to fractures and deformity. The predominant cause is a vitamin D deficiency, but lack of adequate calcium in the diet may also lead to rickets.

Risk factor/risk marker: Characteristics found to be related to the subsequent occurrence of disease.

Root: That portion of the tooth which is usually associated with supporting the tooth in bone but becomes exposed into the mouth with gum recession. The root is comprised of dentine.

Rosacea: A common skin condition characterised by redness and broken blood vessels.

Sarcopenia: The degenerative loss of skeletal muscle that occurs in a wide variety of chronic clinical conditions and with ageing. This loss of mass reduces the performance of muscles.

Saturates (saturated fatty acids): Fatty acids containing no carbon–carbon double bonds, typical of 'hard' fats and animal fats (*cf.* polyunsaturates).

Sebaceous glands: Glands in the skin that secrete oil to the surface of the skin.

Secondary prevention: Measures taken to limit the effects or progression of disease once it has occurred.

Senescence: In biology, this is the combination of processes of deterioration which follow the period of development of an organism.

Skeletal muscle: A type of striated muscle, usually attached to the skeleton and used for movement.

Somatotrophes: Cells in the anterior pituitary that produce growth hormone.

Squames: Flattened, scale-like, dead keratinised cells periodically shed from the surface of the skin.

Squamous cell carcinoma: A form of cancer that can occur in many different organs, including the skin, mouth, oesophagus, prostate, lungs and cervix.

Statins: A group of drugs that reduce the concentration of low-density lipoprotein (LDL) cholesterol in the blood.

Stroke (cerebrovascular disease): Damage to part of the brain resulting from a breakdown in the blood supply (ischaemia) or haemorrhage.

Subcutaneous: Beneath the skin.

Superoxide dismutase: The enzyme that converts superoxide radicals ($O_2^{\cdot-}$) into hydrogen peroxide (H_2O_2).

Synovitis: Inflammation of a synovial membrane around a joint. Synovitis is usually painful, particularly when the joint is moved. The joint usually swells due to fluid collection. Synovitis occurs in several forms of arthritis as well as lupus, gout and other conditions.

Systems biology approach: The study of the interactions between the components of *biological systems*, and how these interactions give rise to the function and behaviour of that system.

T-cell: A type of white blood cell (lymphocyte) that matures in the thymus and plays a central role in cell-mediated immunity. They are essential for various aspects of immunity, especially in combating viral infections and cancers. T-cells may be found in the thymus, lymph nodes and blood circulation (*cf.* B-cell).

Telomeres: Specialised repeated DNA sequences on the ends of chromosomes that protect the chromosomes from degradation.

Thrombosis: The pathological condition in which a blood clot blocks an artery or vein and stops the blood flow through it.

Thymus: An organ located behind the sternum, just over the heart, where T-cells mature.

Thyroxine: The major hormone secreted by the thyroid gland which is involved in controlling the rate of metabolic processes in the body and influencing physical development.

Tocopherols: Forms of vitamin E.

***Trans* fatty acids:** Unsaturated fatty acids have some of their carbon atoms in their 'backbone' joined by double bonds, and can exist in two different geometric forms – the *cis* and *trans* forms. In *trans* fatty acids the two hydrogen atoms are spatially on opposite sides of the double bond. *Trans* fatty acids occur naturally in small amounts in foods produced from ruminant animals, such as meat and dairy products but most of the *trans* fatty acids in the diet are produced during the hydrogenation (hardening) process that converts vegetable oils into solid fats. They have, therefore, been found predominantly in hard margarines, processed foods, cakes and biscuits. However, in recent years in the UK, the food industry has acted voluntarily to reduce substantially the levels present in food.

Transcription factors: Proteins that help synthesise RNA using a DNA template. NF-κB protein and AP-1 protein are two well-known transcription factors.

Translation: The stage where mRNA guides the assembly of the polypeptide chain that results in protein synthesis.

Triglyceride (or triacylglycerol): The major type of fat in the diet. Triglycerides comprise three fatty acids attached to a glycerol backbone. They are also present in the bloodstream.

Trophic hormones: Hormones that regulate the activity of various other endocrine glands.

Tumorigenesis: Tumour development.

Tumour necrosis factor alpha (TNFα): A cytokine produced by many types of leukocyte, named after its ability to kill tumour cells in tissue culture. It modifies the response of many cells and causes inflammation and has been implicated in the pathology of a wide range of chronic inflammatory conditions including heart disease.

Ultraviolet radiation: Electromagnetic radiation of shorter wavelength than visible light but longer than X-rays, the most common source being the sun. Ultraviolet radiation can be divided in three bands: UVA (320–400 nM), UVB (280–320 nM) and UVC (100–280 nM). Of these, the combination of UVA and UVB is responsible for the tanning process.

Unami: The fifth taste modality described as the taste of savoury or blandness.

UV exposure: Exposure to the sun's ultraviolet rays associated with premature ageing (photo-ageing), skin cancer, cataracts and other eye disorders and immune system damage.

Visual acuity: A measurement of the ability to discern characters at a given distance.

Xenobiotic: A chemical compound, such as a drug or pesticide, that is foreign to the body of a living organism.

Xerostomia: The medical term for a dry mouth due to a lack of saliva.

Zinc finger: A protein domain containing a zinc atom that can bind to DNA.

References

Abbott R, Curb J, Rodriguez B, *et al.* (2002) Age-related changes in risk factor effects on the incidence of coronary heart disease. *Annals of Epidemiology*, **12**, 173–81.

Abdulla A, Jones P and Pearce V (1999) Leg cramps in the elderly: prevalence, drug and disease associations. *International Journal of Clinical Practice*, **53**, 494–6.

Abelow BJ, Holford TR and Insogna KL (1992) Cross-cultural association between dietary animal protein and hip fracture: a hypothesis. *Calcified Tissue International*, **50**, 14–18.

Abercrombie M, Flint MH and James DW (1956) Wound contraction in relation to collagen formation in scorbutic guinea-pigs. *Journal of Embryology and Experimental Morphology*, **4**, 167.

Aboderin I, Kalache A, Ben-Shlomo Y, *et al.* (2002) *Life Course Perspective on Coronary Heart Disease, Stroke and Diabetes. Key Issues and Implications for Policy and Research.* Geneva, World Health Organization.

Abrams SA (2003) Normal acquisition and loss of bone mass. *Hormone Research*, **60 (Suppl 3)**, 71–6.

Abrams SA (2005) Calcium supplementation during childhood: long-term effects on bone mineralization. *Nutrition Reviews*, **63**, 251–5.

Ackermann R and Munroe P (1996) Bacteremic urinary tract infection in older people. *Journal of the American Geriatric Society*, **44**, 927–33.

Adamo ML and Farrar RP (2006) Resistance training, and IGF involvement in the maintenance of muscle mass during the aging process. *Ageing Research Reviews*, **5**, 310–31.

Administration on Aging (2003) *A Statistical Profile of Older Americans aged 65+.* Washington, Administration on Aging.

Afting E, Bernhardt W, Jansen R and Rothig H-J (1981) Quantitative importance of non-skeletal muscle Nt-methylhistidine and creatinine in human urine. *Biochemical Journal*, **220**, 449–52.

Agency for Healthcare Research and Quality. www.ahrq.gov/ppip/50plus/index.htm. Accessed 8 February 2005.

Age-Related Eye Disease Study (2001) Risk factors associated with age-related nuclear and cortical cataract: a case-control study in the Age-Related Eye Disease Study, AREDS Report No. 5. *Ophthalmology*, **108**, 1400–8.

Age-Related Eye Disease Study Research Group (2001) A randomized, placebo-controlled, clinical trial of high-dose supplementation with vitamins C and E, beta carotene, and zinc for age-related macular degeneration and vision loss: AREDS report no. 8. *Archives of Ophthalmology*, **119**, 1417–36, 1439–52.

Agudelo CA and Wise CM (2001) Gout: diagnosis, pathogenesis, and clinical manifestations. *Current Opinion in Rheumatology*, **13**, 234–9.

Aiba Y, Suzuki N, Kabir AM, *et al.* (1998) Lactic acid-mediated suppression of *Helicobacter pylori* by the oral administration of *Lactobacillus salivarius* as a probiotic in a gnotobiotic murine model. *American Journal of Gastroenterology*, **93**, 2097–101.

Akeel R, Nilner M and Nilner K (1992) Masticatory efficiency in individuals with natural dentition. *Swedish Dental Journal*, **16**, 191–8.

Alaluf S, Heinrich U, Stahl W, *et al.* (2002) Dietary carotenoids contribute to normal human skin color and UV photosensitivity. *Journal of Nutrition*, **132**, 399–403.

Alaluf S, Muir-Howie H, Hu H-L, *et al.* (2000) Atmospheric oxygen accelerates the induction of a post-mitotic phenotype in human fibroblasts: the key protective role of glutathione. *Journal of Nutrition*, **66**, 147–55.

Albandar J (2005) Epidemiology and risk factors of periodontal diseases. *Dental Clinics of North America*, **49**, 517–32.

Albanes D, Heinonen O, Taylor P, *et al.* (1996) Alpha-tocopherol and beta-carotene supplements and lung cancer incidence in the alpha-tocopherol, beta-carotene cancer prevention study: effects of baseline characteristics and study compliance. *Journal of the National Cancer Institute*, **88**, 1560–80.

Albers R, Antoine J-M, Bourdet-Sicard R, *et al.* (2005) Markers to measure immunomodulation in human nutrition intervention studies. *British Journal of Nutrition*, **94**, 452–81.

Albert C, Campos H, Stampfer M, *et al.* (2002) Blood levels of long-chain *n*-3 fatty acids and the risk of sudden death. *New England Journal of Medicine*, **346**, 1113–18.

Alberts DS, Martinez ME, Roe DJ, *et al.* (2000) Lack of effect of a high-fiber cereal supplement on the recurrence of colorectal adenomas. Phoenix Colon Cancer Prevention Physicians' Network. *New England Journal of Medicine*, **342**, 1156–62.

Albina JE, Gladden P and Walsh WR (1993) Detrimental effects of an omega-3 fatty acid-enriched diet on wound healing. *Journal of Parenteral & Enteral Nutrition*, **17**, 519–21.

Aldoori WH, Giovannucci EL, Rimm EB, *et al.* (1995) A prospective study of alcohol, smoking, caffeine, and the risk of symptomatic diverticular disease in men. *Annals of Epidemiology*, **5**, 221–8.

Alessi C (1988) Constipation and faecal impaction in the long-term care patient. *Clinical Geriatric Medicine*, **4**, 571–88.

Alexander C (2004) Idiopathic osteoarthritis: time to change paradigms? *Skeletal Radiology*, **33**, 321–4.

Aljada A, Mohanty P, Ghanim H, *et al.* (2004) Increase in intranuclear nuclear factor kappaB and decrease in inhibitor kappaB in mononuclear cells after a mixed meal: evidence for a proinflammatory effect. *American Journal of Clinical Nutrition*, **79**, 682–90.

Allen NE, Appleby PN, Davey GK, *et al.* (2002) The associations of diet with serum insulin-like growth factor I and its main binding proteins in 292 women meat-eaters, vegetarians, and vegans. *Cancer Epidemiology, Biomarkers & Prevention*, **11**, 1441–8.

Allen NE, Roddam AW, Allen DS, *et al.* (2005) A prospective study of serum insulin-like growth factor-1 (IGF-1), IGF-II, IGF-binding protein-3 and breast cancer risk. *British Journal of Cancer*, **92**, 1283–7.

Allison D, Gallagher D, Heo M, *et al.* (1997) Body mass index and all-cause mortality among people age 70 and over: the Longitudinal Study of Aging. *International Journal of Obesity and Related Metabolic Disorders*, **21**, 424–31.

Alm L, Humble D, Ryd-Kjellen E and Setterberg G (1983) The effect of an acidophilus milk in the treatment of constipation in hospitalized geriatric patients. *Nutrition and Intestinal Flora*. Ed. B. Hallgen. Stockholm, Almqvist & Eiksell International: 131–8.

Alpha-Tocopherol Beta-Carotene Cancer Prevention Study Group (1994) The effect of vitamin E and beta carotene on the incidence of lung cancer and other cancers in male smokers. The Alpha-Tocopherol, Beta Carotene Cancer Prevention Study Group. *New England Journal of Medicine*, **330**, 1029–35.

Altman R (1991) Classification of disease: osteoarthritis. *Seminars in Arthritis and Rheumatism*, **20 (Suppl 2)**, 40–7.

Altman R and Marcussen K (2001) Effects of a ginger extract on knee pain in patients with osteoarthritis. *Arthritis and Rheumatism*, **44**, 2531–8.

American Cancer Society (2004) *Cancer Facts and Figures*. Atlanta, GA, American Cancer Society.

American Dietetic Association (2000) Position of the American Dietetic Association: Nutrition, aging, and the continuum of care. *Journal of the American Dietetic Association*, **100**, 580–95.

American Heart Association (2006) Diet and Lifestyle Recommendations Revision 2006: A scientific statement from the American Heart Association Nutrition Committee. *Circulation*, **114**, 82–96.

Amoh Y, Li L, Campillo R, *et al.* (2005) Implanted hair follicle stem cells form Schwann cells that support repair of severed peripheral nerves. *Proceedings of the National Academy of Sciences of the United States of America*, **102**, 17734–8.

Amundsen L, Haugum B and Andersson H (2003) Changes in blood cholesterol and sterol metabolites after intake of products enriched with oat bran concentrate within a controlled diet. *Scandinavian Journal of Nutrition*, **47**, 68–74.

Andersen J (2003) Muscle fibre type adaptation in the elderly human muscle. *Scandinavian Journal of Medicine and Science in Sports*, **13**, 40–7.

Andersen J, Terzis G and Kryger A (1999) Increase in the degree of coexpression of myosin heavy chain isoforms in skeletal muscle fibers of the very old. *Muscle Nerve*, **22**, 449–54.

Andersen L, Tufekovic G, Zebis M, *et al.* (2005) The effect of resistance training combined with timed ingestion of protein on muscle fiber size and muscle strength. *Metabolism*, **54**, 151–6.

Anderson J, Johnstone B and Cook-Newell M (1995) Meta-analysis of the effects of soy protein intake on serum lipids. *New England Journal of Medicine*, **333**, 276–82.

Anderson R, Blair S, Cheskin L and Bartlett S (1997) Encouraging patients to become more physically active: the physician's role. *Annals of Internal Medicine*, **127**, 395–400.

Andres E, Kaltenbach G, Perrin AE, *et al.* (2002) Food-cobalamin malabsorption in the elderly. *American Journal of Medicine*, **113**, 351–2.

Ansari MS and Gupta NP (2004) Lycopene: a novel drug therapy in hormone refractory metastatic prostate cancer. *Urologic Oncology*, **22**, 415–20.

Appel L, Miller ER, Jee S, *et al.* (2000) Effect of dietary patterns on serum homocysteine: results of a randomized, controlled feeding study. *Circulation*, **102**, 852–7.

Appel L, Moore T, Obarzanek E, *et al.* (1997) A clinical trial of the effects of dietary patterns on blood pressure. DASH Collaborative Research Group. *New England Journal of Medicine*, **336**, 1117–24.

Applegate W, Miller S, Elam J, *et al.* (1992) Nonpharmacologic intervention to reduce blood pressure in older patients with mild hypertension. *Archives of Internal Medicine*, **152**, 1162–6.

Archimandritis A, Souyioultzis S, Katsorida M and Tzivras M (1998) *Clostridium difficile* colitis associated with a 'triple' regimen, containing clarithromycin and metronidazole, to eradicate *Helicobacter pylori*. *Journal of Internal Medicine*, **243**, 251–3.

Arck PC, Slominski A, Theoharides TC, *et al.* (2006) Neuroimmunology of stress: skin takes center stage. *Journal of Investigative Dermatology*, **126**, 1697–704.

Arden NK, Baker J, Hogg C, *et al.* (1996) The heritability of bone mineral density, ultrasound of the calcaneus and hip axis length: a study of postmenopausal twins. *Journal of Bone & Mineral Research*, **11**, 530–4.

AREDS (2000) Risk factors associated with age-related macular degeneration. A case-control study in the age-related eye disease study: age-related eye disease study report number 3. Age-Related Eye Disease Study Research Group. *Ophthalmology*, **107**, 2224–32.

Arnal M, Mosoni L, Boirie Y, *et al.* (1999) Protein pulse feeding improves protein retention in elderly women. *American Journal of Clinical Nutrition*, **69**, 1202–8.

Arnal M, Mosoni L, Boirie Y, *et al.* (2000) Protein feeding pattern does not affect protein retention in young women. *Journal of Nutrition*, **130**, 1700–4.

Asaka M, Kato M, Kudo M, *et al.* (1996) Atrophic changes of gastric mucosa are caused by *Helicobacter pylori* infection rather than aging: studies in asymptomatic Japanese adults. *Helicobacter*, **1**, 52–6.

Asano T and McLeod RS (2002) Dietary fibre for the prevention of colorectal adenomas and carcinomas. *Cochrane Database of Systematic Reviews*, CD003430.

Ashcroft GS, Dodsworth J, van Boxtel E, *et al.* (1997) Estrogen accelerates cutaneous wound healing associated with an increase in TGF-beta1 levels. *Nature Medicine*, **3**, 1209–15.

Asia Pacific Cohort Studies Collaboration (2003) Cholesterol, coronary heart disease, and stroke in the Asia Pacific region. *International Journal of Epidemiology*, **32**, 563–72.

Astrup A, Buemann B, Flint A and Raben A (2002) Low-fat diets and energy balance: how does the evidence stand in 2002? *Proceedings of the Nutrition Society*, **61**, 299–309.

Augood C, Fletcher A, Bentham G, *et al.* (2004) Methods for a population-based study of the prevalence of and risk factors for age-related maculopathy and macular degeneration in elderly European populations: the EUREYE study. *Ophthalmic Epidemiology*, **11**, 117–29.

Augood C, Vingerling JR, de Jong PTVM, *et al.* (2006) Prevalence of age-related maculopathy in older Europeans: The EUREYE Study. *Archives of Ophthalmology*, **124**, 529–35.

Augustin LS, Franceschi S, Jenkins DJA, *et al.* (2002) Glycemic index in chronic disease: a review. *European Journal of Clinical Nutrition*, **56**, 1049–71.

Aust O, Stahl W, Sies H, *et al.* (2005) Supplementation with tomato-based products increases lycopene, phytofluene, and phytoene levels in human serum and protects against UV-light-induced erythema. *International Journal for Vitamin & Nutrition Research*, **75**, 54–60.

Austad SN (1997) Comparative aging and life histories in mammals. *Experimental Gerontology*, **32**, 23–38.

Australian Bureau of Statistics (2002) *National Health Survey – Summary of Results*. Canberra, Australia Bureau of Statistics.

Avenell A, Campbell M, Cook J, *et al.* (2005) Effect of multivitamin and multimineral supplements on morbidity from infections in older people (MAVIS trial). *British Medical Journal*, **331**, 324–7.

Avenell A, Gillespie WJ, Gillespie LD and O'Connell DL (2005) Vitamin D and vitamin D analogues for preventing fractures associated with involutional and postmenopausal osteoporosis. *Cochrane Database of Systematic Reviews*, CD000227.

Axelsson P, Paulander J and Lindhe J (1998) Relationship between smoking and dental status in 35-, 50-, 65-, and 75-year-old individuals. *Journal of Clinical Periodontology*, **25**, 297–305.

Ayabe T, Ashida T, Kohgo Y and Kono T (2004) The role of Paneth cells and their antimicrobial peptides in innate host defense. *Trends in Microbiology*, **12**, 394–8.

Babb P, Butcher H, Church J and Zealey L (2006) *Social Trends No. 36*. Basingstoke, Palgrave Macmillan.

Babraj J, Cuthbertson D, Smith K, *et al.* (2005) Collagen synthesis in human musculoskeletal tissues and skin. *American Journal Of Physiology-Endocrinology & Metabolism*, **289**, E864–9.

Bachmann O, Dahl D, Brechtel K, *et al.* (2001) Effects of intravenous and dietary lipid challenge on intramyocellular lipid content and the relation with insulin sensitivity in humans. *Diabetes Care*, **50**, 2579–84.

Backett-Milburn KC, Wills WJ, Gregory S and Lawton J (2006) Making sense of eating, weight and risk in the early teenage years: views and concerns of parents in poorer socio-economic circumstances. *Social Science & Medicine*, **63**, 624–35.

Baigent C, Keech A, Kearney P, *et al.* (2005) Efficacy and safety of cholesterol-lowering treatment: prospective meta-analysis of data from 90,056 participants in 14 randomised trials of statins. *Lancet*, **366**, 1267–78.

Bailey AJ (1978) Collagen and elastin fibres. *Journal of Clinical Pathology – Supplement (Royal College of Pathologists)*, **12**, 49–58.

Bajaj P, Bajaj P, Braven-Neilson T and Arendt-Neilson L (2001) Osteoarthritis and its association with muscle hyperalgesia: an experimental controlled study. *Pain*, **93**, 107–14.

Bajekal M (2002) *Health Survey for England 2000: Care Homes and Their Residents*. London, Stationery Office.

Bajekal M and Prescott A (2003) *Health Survey for England 2001: Disability*. London, Stationery Office.

Bajekal M, Primatesta P and Prior G (2003) *Health Survey for England 2000: Fruit and Vegetable Consumption*. London, Stationery Office.

Baker F, Picton D, Blackwood S, *et al.* (2002) Blinded comparison of folic acid and placebo in patients with ischemic heart disease: an outcome trial. *Circulation*, **106**, A3642.

Balagopal P, Ljungqvist O and Nair K (1997) Skeletal muscle myosin heavy-chain synthesis rate in healthy humans. *American Journal of Physiology-Endocrinology & Metabolism*, **35**, E45–E50.

Balagopal P, Rooyackers O, Adey D, *et al.* (1997) Effects of aging on *in vivo* synthesis of skeletal muscle myosin heavy-chain and sarcoplasmic protein in humans. *American Journal of Physiology-Endocrinology & Metabolism*, **36**, E790–E800.

Balkwill F and Mantovani A (2001) Inflammation and cancer: back to Virchow? *Lancet*, **357**, 539–45.

Bannerman E, Magarey A and Daniels L (2001) Evaluation of micronutrient intakes of older Australians: The National Nutrition Survey – 1995. *Journal of Nutrition, Health and Aging*, **5**, 243–7.

Bannerman E, Reilly J, MacLennan W, *et al.* (1997) Evaluation of validity of British anthropometric reference data for assessing nutritional status of elderly people in Edinburgh: cross-sectional study. *British Medical Journal*, **315**, 338–41.

Baracos V (2005) Personal communication.

Barbieri M, Ferrucci L, Ragno E, *et al.* (2003) Chronic inflammation and the effect of IGF-1 on muscle strength and power in older persons. *American Journal of Physiology-Endocrinology & Metabolism*, **284**, E481–7.

Barbul A and Purtill WA (1994) Nutrition in wound healing. *Clinics in Dermatology*, **12**, 133–40.

Barbul A, Thysen B, Rettura G, *et al.* (1978) White cell involvement in the inflammatory, wound healing, and immune actions of vitamin A. *Journal of Parenteral & Enteral Nutrition*, **2**, 129–38.

Barger-Lux MJ and Heaney RP (2002) Effects of above average summer sun exposure on serum 25-hydroxyvitamin D and calcium absorption. *Journal of Clinical Endocrinology & Metabolism*, **87**, 4952–6.

Barker D (1998) *Mothers, Babies and Health in Later Life*. London, Churchill Livingstone.

Barker DJ, Shiell AW, Barker ME and Law CM (2000) Growth in utero and blood pressure levels in the next generation. *Journal of Hypertension*, **18**, 843–6.

Barker DJP, Eriksson JG, Forsen T and Osmond C (2002) Fetal origins of adult disease: strength of effects and biological basis. *International Journal of Epidemiology*, **31**, 1235–9.

Barker ME, McCloskey E, Saha S, *et al.* (2005) Serum retinoids and beta-carotene as predictors of hip and other fractures in elderly women. *Journal of Bone & Mineral Research*, **20**, 913–20.

Barker W and Mullooly J (1980) Impact of epidemic type A influenza in a defined adult population. *American Journal of Epidemiology*, **112**, 798–813.

Barkin R, Barkin S and Barkin D (2005) Perception, assessment, treatment and management of pain in the elderly. *Clinics in Geriatric Medicine*, **21**, 465–91.

Barlow CE, LaMonte MJ, Fitzgerald SJ, *et al.* (2006) Cardiorespiratory fitness is an independent predictor of hypertension incidence among initially normotensive healthy women. *American Journal of Epidemiology*, **163**, 142–50.

Barnes E and Edwards N (2005) Treatment of osteoarthritis. *Southern Medical Journal*, **98**, 205–9.

Baron JA, Beach M, Mandel JS, *et al.* (1999) Calcium supplements for the prevention of colorectal adenomas. Calcium Polyp Prevention Study Group. *New England Journal of Medicine*, **340**, 101–7.

Baron JA, Bertram JS, Britton G, *et al.* (1998) *IARC Handbooks of Cancer Prevention: Carotenoids*. Lyon, IARC.

Bartali B, Salvini S, Turrini A, *et al.* (2003) Age and disability affect dietary intake. *Journal of Nutrition*, **133**, 2868–73.

Barthelman M, Bair WB, 3rd, Stickland KK, *et al.* (1998) (-)-Epigallocatechin-3-gallate inhibition of ultraviolet B-induced AP-1 activity. *Carcinogenesis*, **19**, 2201–4.

Bass SL, Naughton G, Saxon L, *et al.* (2007) Exercise and calcium combined results in a greater osteogenic effect than either factor alone: A blinded randomized placebo-controlled trial in boys. *Journal of Bone and Mineral Research*, **22**, 458–64.

Bassey E and Harries U (1993) Normal values for hand-grip strength in 920 men and women aged over 65 years, and longitudinal changes over 4 years in 620 survivors. *Clinical Science (Lond)*, **84**, 331–7.

Bassey EJ and Ramsdale SJ (1994) Increase in femoral bone density in young women following high-impact exercise. *Osteoporosis International*, **4**, 72–5.

Bassey EJ, Rothwell MC, Littlewood JJ and Pye DW (1998) Pre- and postmenopausal women have different bone mineral density responses to the same high-impact exercise. *Journal of Bone & Mineral Research*, **13**, 1805–13.

Basta G, Lazzerini G, Massaro M, *et al.* (2002) Advanced glycation end products activate endothelium through signal-transduction receptor RAGE: a mechanism for amplification of inflammatory responses. *Circulation*, **105**, 816–22.

Basu HN and Liepa GU (2002) Arginine: a clinical perspective. *Nutrition in Clinical Practice*, **17**, 218–25.

Bates C, Schneede J, Mishra G, *et al.* (2003) Relationship between methylmalonic acid, homocysteine, vitamin B$_{12}$ intake and status and socio-economic indices, in a subset of participants in the British National Diet and Nutrition Survey of people aged 65 y and over. *European Journal of Clinical Nutrition*, **57**, 349–57.

Bates C, Thane C, Prentice A and Delves H (2002) Selenium status and its correlates in a British national diet and nutrition survey: people aged 65 years and over. *Journal of Trace Elements in Medicine and Biology*, **16**, 1–8.

Bates CJ, Prentice A, Jackson LV, *et al.* (2000) *National Diet and Nutrition Survey: Young People aged 4 to 18 Years. Volume 1: Report of the Diet and Nutrition Survey.* London, Stationery Office.

Bateson P, Barker D, Clutton-Brock T, *et al.* (2004) Developmental plasticity and human health. *Nature*, **430**, 419–21.

Baulieu EE, Thomas G, Legrain S, *et al.* (2000) Dehydro-epiandrosterone (DHEA), DHEA sulfate, and aging: Contribution of the DHEage study to a sociobiomedical issue. *Proceedings of the National Academy of Sciences of the United States of America*, **97**, 4279–84.

Baum B and Bodner L (1983) Aging and oral motor function: Evidence for altered function among older persons. *Journal of Dental Research*, **62**, 2–6.

Baum BJ, Ship JA and Wu A (1992) Salivary gland function and aging: a model for studying the interaction of aging and systemic disease. *Critical Reviews in Oral Biology & Medicine*, **4**, 53–64.

Baumgartner R, Koehler K, Gallagher D, *et al.* (1998) Epidemiology of sarcopenia among the elderly in New Mexico. *American Journal of Epidemiology*, **147**, 755–63.

Bavdekar A, Yajnik C, Fall C, *et al.* (2000) The insulin resistance syndrome (IRS) in eight-year-old Indian children: small at birth, big at 8 years or both? *Diabetes Care*, **48**, 2422–9.

Beatty S, Boulton M, Henson D, *et al.* (1999) Macular pigment and age related macular degeneration. *British Journal of Ophthalmology*, **83**, 867–77.

Beatty S, Koh H, Phil M, *et al.* (2000) The role of oxidative stress in the pathogenesis of age-related macular degeneration. *Survey of Ophthalmology*, **45**, 115–34.

Beaufrere B and Morio B (2000) Fat and protein redistribution with aging: metabolic considerations. *European Journal of Clinical Nutrition*, **54 (Suppl 3)**, S48–53.

Beck A and Ovesen L (1998) At which body mass index and degree of weight loss should hospitalized elderly patients be considered at nutritional risk? *Clinical Nutrition*, **17**, 195–8.

Beck MA, Levander OA and Handy J (2003) Selenium deficiency and viral infection. *Journal of Nutrition*, **133**, 1463S–7S.

Beharka AA, Meydani M, Wu D, *et al.* (2001) Interleukin-6 production does not increase with age. *Journals of Gerontology Series A-Biological Sciences & Medical Sciences*, **56**, B81–8.

Beiqing L, Carle K and Whisler R (1997) Reduction in the activation of ERK and JNK are associated with decreased IL-2 production in T cells from elderly humans stimulated by the TcWCD3 complex and costimulatory signals. *Cellular Immunology*, **182**, 79–88.

Beisel W (1982) Single nutrients and immunity. *American Journal of Clinical Nutrition*, **35**, 417–68.

Belch J (1990) Fish oil and rheumatoid arthritis: does a herring a day keep the rheumatologist away? *Annals of the Rheumatic Diseases*, **49**, 71–2.

Bennet W, Connacher A, Scrimgeour C, Jung R and Rennie M (1990) Euglycemic hyperinsulinemia augments amino acid uptake by human leg tissue during hyperaminoacidemia. *American Journal of Physiology – Endocrinology and Metabolism*, **259**, E185–94.

Bennett FC and Ingram DM (1990) Diet and female sex hormone concentrations: an intervention study for the type of fat consumed. *American Journal of Clinical Nutrition*, **52**, 808–12.

Bennett G and Talley NJ (2002) Irritable bowel syndrome in the elderly. *Best Practice & Research: Clinical Gastroenterology*, **16**, 63–76.

Benton D (2002) Selenium intake, mood and other aspects of psychological functioning. *Nutritional Neuroscience*, **5**, 363–74.

Benton D and Cook R (1991) The impact of selenium supplementation on mood. *Biological Psychiatry*, **29**, 1092–8.

Beral V and Million Women Study Collaborators (2003) Breast cancer and hormone-replacement therapy in the Million Women Study. *Lancet*, **362**, 419–27.

Berbert A, Dondo C, Almendra C, *et al.* (2005) Supplementation of fish oil and olive oil in patients with rheumatoid arthritis. *Nutrition*, **21**, 131–6.

Beresford SAA, Johnson KC, Ritenbaugh C, *et al.* (2006) Low-fat dietary pattern and risk of colorectal cancer: the Women's Health Initiative Randomized Controlled Dietary Modification Trial. *Journal of the American Medical Association*, **295**, 643–54.

Berglund G (2002) Anthropometry, physical activity and cancer of the breast and colon. *Nutrition and Lifestyle:*

Opportunities for Cancer Prevention. E. Riboli and R. Lambert. Lyon, IARC Scientific Publications, **156**, 237–41.

Bergman EA, Massey LK, Wise KJ and Sherrard DJ (1990) Effects of dietary caffeine on renal handling of minerals in adult women. *Life Sciences*, **47**, 557–64.

Bermudez O, Falcon L and Tucker K (2000) Intake and food sources of macronutrients among older Hispanic adults: association with ethnicity, acculturation, and length of residence in the United States. *Journal of the American Dietetic Association*, **100**, 665–73.

Berneburg M, Plettenberg H, Medve-Konig K, *et al.* (2004) Induction of the photoaging-associated mitochondrial common deletion *in vivo* in normal human skin. *Journal of Investigative Dermatology*, **122**, 1277–83.

Berry RJ and Bronson FH (1992) Life history and bioeconomy of the house mouse. *Biological Reviews of the Cambridge Philosophical Society*, **67**, 519–50.

Berstein E and Murasko D (1998) Effect of age on cytokine production in humans. *Age*, **21**, 137–51.

Berthelemy P, Bouisson M, Vellas B, *et al.* (1992) Postprandial cholecystokinin secretion in elderly with protein-energy undernutrition. *Journal of the American Geriatrics Society*, **40**, 365–9.

Bhasin S, Storer TW, Berman N, *et al.* (1997) Testosterone replacement increases fat-free mass and muscle size in hypogonadal men. *Journal of Clinical Endocrinology & Metabolism*, **82**, 407–13.

Biasi D, Carletto A, Dell'Agnola C, *et al.* (1996) Neutrophil migration, oxidative metabolism, and adhesion in elderly and young subjects. *Inflammation*, **20**, 673–81.

Biddle SJH and Mutrie N (2008) *Psychology of Physical Activity: Determinants, Well-being and Intervention.* London, Routledge.

Bień B, Wojszel B, Polityňska B and Wilmańska J (1999) *COPE: Background Report on Poland.* Bialystok, Medical University of Bialystok.

Bierhaus A, Schiekofer S, Schwaninger M, *et al.* (2001) Diabetes-associated sustained activation of the transcription factor nuclear factor-kappaB. *Diabetes*, **50**, 2792–808.

Bierhaus A, Wolf J, Andrassy M, *et al.* (2003) A mechanism converting psychosocial stress into mononuclear cell activation. *Proceedings of the National Academy of Sciences of the United States of America*, **100**, 1920–5.

Bijnen F, Caspersen C, Feskens E, *et al.* (1998) Physical activity and 10-year mortality from cardiovascular diseases and all causes: The Zutphen Elderly Study. *Archives of Internal Medicine*, **158**, 1499–505.

Bingham S (2006) The fibre-folate debate in colo-rectal cancer. *Proceedings of the Nutrition Society*, **65**, 19–23.

Bingham SA, Day NE, Luben R, *et al.* (2003) Dietary fibre in food and protection against colorectal cancer in the European Prospective Investigation into Cancer and Nutrition (EPIC): an observational study. *Lancet*, **361**, 1496–501.

Bingham SA, Norat T, Moskal A, *et al.* (2005) Is the association with fiber from foods in colorectal cancer confounded by folate intake? *Cancer Epidemiology, Biomarkers & Prevention*, **14**, 1552–6.

Birt DF, Mitchell D, Gold B, *et al.* (1997) Inhibition of ultraviolet light induced skin carcinogenesis in SKH-1 mice by apigenin, a plant flavonoid. *Anticancer Research*, **17**, 85–91.

Bischoff-Ferrari HA, Dawson-Hughes B, Willett WC, *et al.* (2004) Effect of vitamin D on falls: a meta–analysis. *Journal of the American Medical Association*, **291**, 1999–2006.

Bischoff–Ferrari HA, Giovannucci E, Willett WC, *et al.* (2006) Estimation of optimal serum concentrations of 25–hydroxyvitamin D for multiple health outcomes. *American Journal of Clinical Nutrition*, **84**, 18–28.

Bischoff-Ferrari HA, Willett WC, Wong JB, *et al.* (2005) Fracture prevention with vitamin D supplementation. *Journal of the American Medical Association*, **293**, 2257–64.

Bjorntorp P (2002) Alterations in the ageing corticotropic stress-response axis. *Novartis Foundation Symposium*, **242**, 46–58; discussion 65.

Blair S (2007) Physical inactivity: a major public health problem. *Nutrition Bulletin*, **32**, 113–17.

Blair S and Wei M (2000) Sedentary habits, health, and function in older women and men. *American Journal of Health Promotion*, **15**, 1–8.

Blair S, Kohl H, Barlow C, *et al.* (1995) Changes in physical fitness and all-cause mortality: a prospective study of healthy and unhealthy men. *Journal of the American Medical Association*, **273**, 1093–8.

Blanc S, Schoeller D, Bauer D, *et al.* (2004) Energy requirements in the eighth decade of life. *American Journal of Clinical Nutrition*, **79**, 303–10.

Blaut M, Collins MD, Welling GW, *et al.* (2002) Molecular biological methods for studying the gut microbiota: the EU human gut flora project. *British Journal of Nutrition*, **87 (Suppl 2)**, S203–11.

Blottiere HM, Buecher B, Galmiche J-P and Cherbut C (2003) Molecular analysis of the effect of short-chain fatty acids on intestinal cell proliferation. *Proceedings of the Nutrition Society*, **62**, 101–6.

Boelsma E, Hendriks HF and Roza L (2001) Nutritional skin care: health effects of micronutrients and fatty acids. *American Journal of Clinical Nutrition*, **73**, 853–64.

Boelsma E, van de Vijver LPL, Goldbohm RA, *et al.* (2003) Human skin condition and its associations with nutrient concentrations in serum and diet. *American Journal of Clinical Nutrition*, **77**, 348–55.

Bogden J, Bendich A, Kemp F, *et al.* (1994) Daily micro-nutrient supplements enhance delayed-hypersensitivity skin test responses in older people. *American Journal of Clinical Nutrition*, **60**, 437–47.

Bogden J, Oleske J, Lavenhar M, *et al.* (1988) Zinc and immunocompetence in elderly people: effects of zinc supplementation for 3 months. *American Journal of Clinical Nutrition*, **48**, 655–63.

Bogden J, Oleske J, Lavenhar M, *et al.* (1990) Effects of one year of supplementation with zinc and other micro-nutrients on cellular immunity in the elderly. *Journal of the American College of Nutrition*, **9**, 214–25.

Boirie Y, Gachon P, Cordat N, *et al.* (2001) Differential insulin sensitivities of glucose, amino acid, and albumin metabolism in elderly men and women. *Journal of Clinical Endocrinology and Metabolism*, **86**, 638–44.

Bolton-Smith C, McMurdo MET, Paterson CR, *et al.* (2007) Two-year randomized controlled trial of vitamin K1 (phylloquinone) and vitamin D3 plus calcium on the bone health of older women. *Journal of Bone & Mineral Research*, **22**, 509–19.

Bonaa K, Njolstad I, Ueland P, *et al.* (2006) Homocysteine lowering and cardiovascular events after acute myocardial infarction. *New England Journal of Medicine*, **354**, 1578–88.

Bonafe M, Olivieri F, Cavallone L, *et al.* (2001) A gender-dependent genetic predisposition to produce high levels of IL-6 is detrimental for longevity. *European Journal of Immunology*, **31**, 2357–61.

Bonar BD, McColgan B, Smith DF, *et al.* (2000) Hypo-thyroidism and aging: the Rosses' survey. *Thyroid*, **10**, 821–7.

Bonithon-Kopp C, Kronborg O, Giacosa A, *et al.* (2000) Calcium and fibre supplementation in prevention of colorectal adenoma recurrence: a randomised intervention trial. European Cancer Prevention Organisation Study Group. *Lancet*, **356**, 1300–6.

Bonjour JP, Ammann P, Chevalley T, *et al.* (2003) Nutritional aspects of bone growth: an overview. *Nutritional Aspects of Bone Health*. Ed. SA New and JP Bonjour. Cambridge, Royal Society of Chemistry: 111–28.

Bonjour JP, Theintz G, Buchs B, *et al.* (1991) Critical years and stages of puberty for spinal and femoral bone mass accumulation during adolescence. *Journal of Clinical Endocrinology & Metabolism*, **73**, 555–63.

Bonora E, Kiechl S, Willeit J, *et al.* (1998) Prevalence of insulin resistance in metabolic disorders: the Bruneck Study. *Diabetes*, **47**, 1643–9.

Booth SL, Broe KE, Gagnon DR, *et al.* (2003) Vitamin K intake and bone mineral density in women and men. *American Journal of Clinical Nutrition*, **77**, 512–16.

Borrego F, Alonso M, Galiani M, *et al.* (1999) NK phenotypic markers and IL2 response in NK cells from elderly people. *Experimental Gerontology*, **34**, 253–65.

Bortolotti M, Frada G, Vezzadini P, *et al.* (1987) Influence of gastric acid secretion on interdigestive gastric motor activity and serum motilin in the elderly. *Digestion*, **38**, 226–33.

Boucher N, DufueDuchesne T, Vicaut E, *et al.* (1998) CD28 expression in cell aging and human longevity. *Experimental Gerontology*, **33**, 267–82.

Bourne GH (1944) Effect of vitamin C deficiency on experimental wounds: tensile strength and histology. *Lancet*, **1**, 688–92.

Bova LM, Sweeney MH, Jamie JF and Truscott RJ (2001) Major changes in human ocular UV protection with age. *Investigative Ophthalmology and Visual Science*, **42**, 200–5.

Bowman L and Armitage J (2002) Diabetes and impaired glucose tolerance: a review of the epidemiological and trial evidence for their role in cardiovascular risk. *Seminars in Vascular Medicine*, **2**, 383–9.

Bowser PA, Nugteren DH, White RJ, *et al.* (1985) Identification, isolation and characterization of epidermal lipids containing linoleic acid. *Biochimica et Biophysica Acta*, **834**, 419–28.

Boyle P and Langman JS (2000) ABC of colorectal cancer: Epidemiology. *British Medical Journal*, **321**, 805–8.

Braam LAJLM, Knapen MHJ, Geusens P, *et al.* (2003) Vitamin K1 supplementation retards bone loss in post-menopausal women between 50 and 60 years of age. *Calcified Tissue International*, **73**, 21–6.

Brachet P, Chanson A, Demigné C, *et al.* (2004) Age-associated B vitamin deficiency as a determinant of chronic diseases. *Nutrition Research Reviews*, **17**, 55–68.

Bradbury J, Thomason JM, Jepson NJ, *et al.* (2006) Nutrition counseling increases fruit and vegetable intake in the edentulous. *Journal of Dental Research*, **85**, 463–8.

Braegger CP and Nadal D (1994) Clarithromycin and pseudomembranous enterocolitis. *Lancet*, **343**, 241–2.

Brandt K, Doherty M and Lohmander S (2003) *Osteoarthritis*. Oxford, Oxford University Press.

Brann DW and Mahesh VB (2005) The aging reproductive neuroendocrine axis. *Steroids*, **70**, 273–83.

Brash DE and Havre PA (2002) New careers for antioxidants. *Proceedings of the National Academy of Sciences of the United States of America*, **99**, 13969–71.

Brass LM (2004) Hormone replacement therapy and stroke: clinical trials review. *Stroke*, **35**, 2644–7.

Bratthall D (2006) WHO Oral Health Country/Area Profile Programme. www.whocollab.od.mah.se/index.html. Accessed May 2006.

Bray G, Lovejoy J, Smith S, *et al.* (2002) The influence of different fats and fatty acids on obesity, insulin resistance and inflammation. *Journal of Nutrition*, **132**, 2488–91.

Breeze E, Clarke R, Shipley M, *et al.* (2006) Cause-specific mortality in old age in relation to body mass index in middle age and in old age: follow-up of the Whitehall cohort of male civil servants. *International Journal of Epidemiology*, **35**, 169–78.

Briefel RR, Bialostosky K, Kennedy-Stephenson J, *et al.* (2000) Zinc intake of the US population: findings from the third National Health and Nutrition Examination Survey, 1988–1994. *Journal of Nutrition*, **130**, 1367S–73S.

Brierley EJ, Johnson MA, Lightowlers RN, *et al.* (1998) Role of mitochondrial DNA mutations in human aging: implications for the central nervous system and muscle. *Annals of Neurology*, **43**, 217–23.

British Cardiac Society, British Hyperlipidaemia Association and British Hypertension Society (1998) Joint British recommendations on prevention of coronary heart disease in clinical practice. *Heart*, **80 (Suppl 2)**, S1–S29.

British Heart Foundation (2005a) *European Cardiovascular Disease Statistics*. London, British Heart Foundation.

British Heart Foundation (2005b) www.bhf.org.uk. Accessed 27 October 2005.

British Heart Foundation (2006) *Coronary Heart Disease Statistics*. London, British Heart Foundation.

British Heart Foundation (2007) *Coronary Heart Disease Statistics*. British Heart Foundation/Department of Public Health, Oxford.

British Nutrition Foundation (1999) *Obesity. The Report of the British Nutrition Foundation Task Force*. London, Blackwell Science.

British Nutrition Foundation (2001) *Selenium and Health*. London, British Nutrition Foundation.

British Nutrition Foundation (2003a) *Plants: Diet and Health*. Ed. G. Goldberg. Oxford, Blackwell Science.

British Nutrition Foundation (2003b) *Soya and Health*. London, British Nutrition Foundation.

British Nutrition Foundation (2005) *Cardiovascular Disease: Diet, Nutrition and Emerging Risk Factors*. The Report of the British Nutrition Task Force. Ed. S. Stanner. Oxford, Blackwell Publishing.

British Nutrition Foundation (2008) *The Evidence for the Cholesterol-Lowering Effects of Plant Stanol Esters*. London, British Nutrition Foundation.

Brodsky IG, Balagopal P and Nair KS (1996) Effects of testosterone replacement on muscle mass and muscle protein synthesis in hypogonadal men – a clinical research center study. *Journal of Clinical Endocrinology & Metabolism*, **81**, 3469–75.

Brown L, Rimm EB, Seddon JM, *et al.* (1999) A prospective study of carotenoid intake and risk of cataract extraction in US men. *American Journal of Clinical Nutrition*, **70**, 517–24.

Brown L, Rosner B, Willett W and Sacks F (1999) Cholesterol lowering effects of dietary fibre: a meta-analysis. *American Journal of Clinical Nutrition*, **69**, 30–42.

Brown LM, Blot WJ, Schuman SH, *et al.* (1988) Environmental factors and high risk of esophageal cancer among men in coastal South Carolina. *Journal of the National Cancer Institute*, **80**, 1620–5.

Brown SA, Coimbra M, Coberly DM, *et al.* (2004) Oral nutritional supplementation accelerates skin wound healing: a randomized, placebo-controlled, double-arm, crossover study. *Plastic & Reconstructive Surgery*, **114**, 237–44.

Browner W, Kahn A, Ziv E, *et al.* (2004) The genetics of human longevity. *The American Journal of Medicine*, **117**, 851–60.

Brucher BL, Stein HJ, Bartels H, *et al.* (2001) Achalasia and esophageal cancer: incidence, prevalence, and prognosis. *World Journal of Surgery*, **25**, 745–9.

Bruckdorfer K (2005) Oxidative Stress. *Cardiovascular Disease: Diet, Nutrition and Emerging Risk Factors*. Ed. S. Stanner. Oxford, Blackwell Publishing: 78–99.

Brustman BA (1986) Impact of exposure to fluoride-adequate water on root surface caries in elderly. *Gerodontics*, **2**, 203–7.

Bruun JM, Helge JW, Richelsen B and Stallknecht B (2006) Diet and exercise reduce low-grade inflammation and macrophage infiltration in adipose tissue but not in skeletal muscle in severely obese subjects. *American Journal of Physiology – Endocrinology & Metabolism*, **290**, E961–7.

Bryan J, Calvaresi E and Hughes D (2002) Short-term folate, vitamin B-12 or vitamin B-6 supplementation slightly affects memory performance but not mood in women of various ages. *Journal of Nutrition*, **132**, 1345–56.

Brynes AE, Mark Edwards C, Ghatei MA, *et al.* (2003) A randomised four-intervention crossover study investigating the effect of carbohydrates on daytime profiles of insulin, glucose, non-esterified fatty acids and triglycerides in middle-aged men. *British Journal of Nutrition*, **89**, 207–18.

Brzozowski AM, Pike AC, Dauter Z, *et al.* (1997) Molecular basis of agonism and antagonism in the oestrogen receptor. *Nature*, **389**, 753–8.

Bucciarelli LG, Wendt T, Rong L, *et al.* (2002) RAGE is a multiligand receptor of the immunoglobulin superfamily: implications for homeostasis and chronic disease. *Cellular & Molecular Life Sciences*, **59**, 1117–28.

Buclin T, Cosma M, Appenzeller M, *et al.* (2001) Diet acids and alkalis influence calcium retention in bone. *Osteoporosis International*, **12**, 493–9.

Buhling A, Radun D, Muller WA and Malfertheiner P (2001) Influence of anti-Helicobacter triple-therapy with metronidazole, omeprazole and clarithromycin on intestinal microflora. *Alimentary Pharmacology & Therapeutics*, **15**, 1445–52.

Buisine MP, Devisme L, Degand P, *et al.* (2000) Developmental mucin gene expression in the gastroduodenal tract and accessory digestive glands. II. Duodenum and liver, gallbladder, and pancreas. *Journal of Histochemistry & Cytochemistry*, **48**, 1667–76.

Bulpitt C, Beckett N, Cooke J, *et al.* (2003) Results of the pilot study for the Hypertension in the Very Elderly Trial. *Journal of Hypertension*, **21**, 2249–50.

Bunout D, Barrera G, Hirsch S, *et al.* (2004) Effects of a nutritional supplement on the immune response and cytokine production in free-living Chilean elderly. *Journal of Parental and Enteral Nutrition*, **28**, 348–54.

Burdge G, Finnegan Y, Minihane A, *et al.* (2003) Effect of altered dietary *n*-3 fatty acid intake upon plasma lipid acid composition, conversion of [13C] alpha-linolenic acid to longer-chain fatty acids and partitioning towards beta-oxidation in older men. *British Journal of Nutrition*, **90**, 311–21.

Burkle A, Beneke S, Brabeck C, *et al.* (2002) Poly(ADP-ribose) polymerase-1, DNA repair and mammalian longevity. *Experimental Gerontology*, **37**, 1203–5.

Burr M, Ashfield-Watt P, Dunstan F, *et al.* (2003) Lack of benefit of dietary advice to men with angina: results of a controlled trial. *European Journal of Clinical Nutrition*, **52**, 193–200.

Burr M, Gilbert J, Holliday R, *et al.* (1989) Effects of changes in fat, fish and fibre intake on death and myocardial reinfarction: diet and reinfarction trial (DART). *Lancet*, **ii**, 757–61.

Bursell SE and King GL (1999) Can protein kinase C inhibition and vitamin E prevent the development of diabetic vascular complications? *Diabetes Research and Clinical Practice*, **45**, 169–82.

Burt BA, Eklund SA and Loesche WJ (1986) Dental benefits of limited exposure to fluoridated water in childhood. *Journal of Dental Research*, **65**, 1322–5.

Butler JV, Mulkerrin EC and O'Keeffe ST (2002) Nocturnal leg cramps in older people. *Postgraduate Medical Journal*, **78**, 596–8.

Buttriss J (2005) A public health approach to cardiovascular disease risk reduction. *Cardiovascular Disease: Diet, Nutrition and Emerging Risk Factors*. Ed. S. Stanner. Oxford, Blackwell Publishing: 245–65.

Buttriss J and Hardman A (2005) Physical activity: Where are we now? *Cardiovascular Disease: Diet, Nutrition and Emerging Risk Factors*. Ed. S. Stanner. Oxford, Blackwell Publishing: 234–44.

Buttriss J and Korpela R (2002) *Enzyme Defects and Food Intolerance*. Oxford, Blackwell Science.

B-Vitamin Treatment Trialists' Collaboration (2006) Homocysteine-lowering trials for prevention of cardiovascular events: a review of the design and power of the large randomized trials. *American Heart Journal*, **151**, 282–7.

Caffrey BB and Jonsson HT, Jr. (1981) Role of essential fatty acids in cutaneous wound healing in rats. *Progress in Lipid Research*, **20**, 641–7.

Cai D, Spence L and Weaver C (2003) Soy isoflavones and bone health. *Nutritional Aspects of Bone Health*. Ed. S. New and J. P. Bonjour. Cambridge, Royal Society of Chemistry: 421–38.

Cakman I, Kirchner H and Rink L (1997) Reconstitution of interferon production by zinc supplementation of leucocyte of elderly individuals. *Journal of Interferon and Cytokine Research*, **13**, 15–20.

Cakman I, Rohwer J, Schutz R, *et al.* (1996) Dysregulation between TH1 and TH2 T cell subpopulations in the elderly. *Mechanisms of Ageing & Development*, **87**, 197–209.

Calder PC (2002) Dietary modification of inflammation with lipids. *Proceedings of the Nutrition Society*, **61**, 345–58.

Caldwell MD, Jonsson HT and Othersen HB, Jr. (1972) Essential fatty acid deficiency in an infant receiving prolonged parenteral alimentation. *Journal of Pediatrics*, **81**, 894–8.

Campbell AJ, Busby WJ and Horwath CC (1993) Factors associated with constipation in a community based sample of people aged 70 years and over. *Journal of Epidemiology & Community Health*, **47**, 23–6.

Campbell D, Hall M, Barker D, *et al.* (1996) Diet in pregnancy and the offspring's blood pressure 40 years later. *British Journal of Obstetrics and Gynaecology*, **103**, 273–80.

Campbell W, Crim M, Dallal G, *et al.* (1994) Increased protein requirements in elderly people: new data and retrospective reassessments. *American Journal of Clinical Nutrition*, **60**, 501–9.

Campbell WW, Trappe TA, Wolfe RR and Evans WJ (2001) The recommended dietary allowance for protein may not be adequate for older people to maintain skeletal muscle. *Journals of Gerontology Series A – Biological Sciences & Medical Sciences*, **56**, M373–80.

Campisi J (1997) Aging and cancer: the double-edged sword of replicative senescence. *Journal of the American Geriatrics Society*, **45**, 482–8.

Campisi J (1998) The role of cellular senescence in skin aging. *Journal of Investigative Dermatology Symposium Proceedings*, **3**, 1–5.

Canalis E and Delany AM (2002) Mechanisms of glucocorticoid action in bone. *Annals of the New York Academy of Sciences*, **966**, 73–81.

Cancer Research UK (2007) UK oesophageal cancer statistics. http://info.cancerresearchuk.org/cancerstats/types/oesophagus. Accessed 23 April 2007.

Cao SX, Dhahbi JM, Mote PL and Spindler SR (2001) Genomic profiling of short- and long-term caloric restriction effects in the liver of aging mice. *Proceedings of the National Academy of Sciences of the United States of America*, **98**, 10630–5.

Cappola AR, Xue QL, Ferrucci L, *et al.* (2003) Insulin-like growth factor I and interleukin-6 contribute synergistically to disability and mortality in older women. *Journal of Clinical Endocrinology & Metabolism*, **88**, 2019–25.

Capri M, Salvioli S, Sevini F, *et al.* (2006) The genetics of human longevity *Annals of the New York Academy of Sciences*, **1067**, 252.

Carmen W, Sowers M, Hawthorne V and Weissfeld L (1994) Obesity as a risk factor for osteoarthritis of the hand and wrist. *American Journal of Epidemiology*, **39**, 119–29.

Caroline Walker Trust (2004) *Eating Well for Older People: Practical and Nutritional Guidelines for Food in Residential and Nursing Homes and for Community Meals*. Abbots Langley, The Caroline Walker Trust.

Carrieri G, Marzi E, Olivieri F, *et al.* (2004) The G/C 915 polymorphism of transforming growth factor B1 is associated with human longevity: a study in Italian centenarians. *Aging Cell*, **3**, 443.

Carroccio A, Montalto G, Cavera G and Notarbatolo A (1998) Lactose intolerance and self-reported milk intolerance: relationship with lactose maldigestion and nutrient intake. Lactase Deficiency Study Group. *Journal of the American College of Nutrition*, **17**, 631–6.

Cartwright A (2002) Nutritional assessment as part of wound management. *Nursing Times*, **98**, 62–3.

Caruso C, Candore G, Cigna D, *et al.* (1996) Cytokine production pathway in the elderly. *Immunologic Research*, **15**, 84–90.

Casas J, Bautista L, Smeeth L, *et al.* (2005) Homocysteine and stroke: evidence on a causal link from mendelian randomisation. *Lancet*, **365**, 224–32.

Cashman K and Flynn A (2003) Sodium effects on bone and calcium metabolism. *Nutritional Aspects of Bone Health*. Ed. SA New and JP Bonjour. Cambridge, Royal Society of Chemistry: 267–90.

Cassidy A (2003) Cereals, nuts and pulses. *Plants: Diet and Health*. Ed. G. Goldberg. Oxford, Blackwell Science: 134–46.

Cassidy A, Albertazzi P, Lise Nielsen I, *et al.* (2006) Critical review of health effects of soyabean phytooestrogens in post-menopausal women. *Proceedings of the Nutrition Society*, **65**, 76–92.

Castelletto R, Munoz N, Landoni N, *et al.* (1992) Pre-cancerous lesions of the oesophagus in Argentina: prevalence and association with tobacco and alcohol. *International Journal of Cancer*, **51**, 34–7.

Castle S, Uyemura K, Wong W, *et al.* (1997) Evidence of enhanced type 2 immune response and impaired upregulation of a type 1 response in frail elderly nursing home residents. *Mechanisms of Ageing & Development*, **94**, 7–16.

Castle SC, Uyemura K, Crawford W, *et al.* (1999) Age-related impaired proliferation of peripheral blood mononuclear cells is associated with an increase in both IL-10 and IL-12. *Experimental Gerontology*, **34**, 243–52.

Cauley J, Petrini A, LaPorte R, *et al.* (1987) The decline of grip strength in the menopause: relationship to physical activity, estrogen use and anthropometric factors. *Journal of Chronic Disease*, **40**, 115–20.

Cawthon RM, Smith KR, O'Brien E, *et al.* (2003) Association between telomere length in blood and mortality in people aged 60 years or older. *Lancet*, **361**, 393–5.

Cazzola R, Russo-Volpe S, Miles E, *et al.* (2007) Age- and dose-dependent effects of an eicosapentaenoic acid-rich oil on cardiovascular risk factors in healthy male subjects. *Atherosclerosis*, **193**, 159–67.

Cesarini JP, Michel L, Maurette JM, *et al.* (2003) Immediate effects of UV radiation on the skin: modification by an antioxidant complex containing carotenoids. *Photodermatology, Photoimmunology & Photomedicine*, **19**, 182–9.

Chadwick B and Pendry L (2004) Non-carious dental conditions. *Children's Dental Health 2003*. London, Office for National Statistics: 5.

Chae CU, Lee RT, Rifai N and Ridker PM (2001) Blood pressure and inflammation in apparently healthy men. *Hypertension*, **38**, 399–403.

Chainani-Wu N (2002) Diet and oral, pharyngeal, and esophageal cancer. *Nutrition & Cancer*, **44**, 104–26.

Chakravarti B and Abraham GN (1999) Aging and T-cell-mediated immunity. *Mechanisms of Ageing & Development*, **108**, 183–206.

Chan L-N (2002) Drug-nutrient interaction in clinical nutrition. *Current Opinion in Clinical Nutrition and Metabolic Care*, **5**, 327–32.

Chandra RK, Hambreaus L, Purl S, *et al.* (1993) Immune responses of healthy volunteers given supplements of zinc or selenium. *FASEB Journal*, **7**, A723.

Chang AM and Halter JB (2003) Aging and insulin secretion. *American Journal of Physiology – Endocrinology & Metabolism*, **284**, E7–12.

Chapman IM (2004) Endocrinology of anorexia of ageing. *Best Practice & Research Clinical Endocrinology & Metabolism*, **18**, 437–52.

Chapuy MC, Arlot ME, Duboeuf F, *et al.* (1992) Vitamin D3 and calcium to prevent hip fractures in the elderly women. *New England Journal of Medicine*, **327**, 1637–42.

Chard J and Dieppe P (2001) Glucosamine for osteoarthritis: magic, hype or confusion? *British Medical Journal*, **322**, 1439–40.

Chard J, Tallon D and Dieppe P (2000) Epidemiology of research into interventions for the treatment of osteoarthritis of the knee joint. *Annals of the Rheumatic Diseases*, **59**, 414–18.

Chasan-Taber L, Willett WC, Seddon JM, *et al.* (1999a) A prospective study of vitamin supplement intake and cataract extraction among US women. *Epidemiology*, **10**, 679–84.

Chasan-Taber L, Willett WC, Seddon JM, *et al.* (1999b) A prospective study of carotenoid and vitamin A intakes and risk of cataract extraction in US women. *American Journal of Clinical Nutrition*, **70**, 509–16.

Chattopadhyay B and Al-Zahawi M (1983) Septicaemia and its unacceptably high mortality in the elderly. *Journal of Infection*, **7**, 134–8.

Chauncey HH, Muench ME, Kapur KK and Wayler AH (1984) The effect of the loss of teeth on diet and nutrition. *International Dental Journal*, **34**, 98–104.

Chavance M, Herbeth B, Fournier C, *et al.* (1989) Vitamin status, immunity and infections in an elderly population. *European Journal of Clinical Nutrition*, **43**, 827–35.

Chavance M, Herbeth B, Lemoine A and Zhu BP (1993) Does multivitamin supplementation prevent infections in healthy elderly subjects? A controlled trial. *International Journal for Vitamin & Nutrition Research*, **63**, 11–16.

Chernoff R (1994) Thirst and fluid requirements. *Nutrition Reviews*, **52**, S3–5.

Chernoff R (1995) Effects of age on nutrient requirements. *Clinics in Geriatric Medicine*, **11**, 641–51.

Chevalley T, Rizzoli R, Hans D, *et al.* (2005) Interaction between calcium intake and menarcheal age on bone mass gain: an eight-year follow-up study from prepuberty to postmenarche. *Journal of Clinical Endocrinology & Metabolism*, **90**, 44–51.

Chicago Dietetic Association (2000) *The South Suburban Dietetic Association and the Dietitians of Canada. Manual of Clinical Dietetics.* Chicago, American Dietetic Association.

Chiuve S, Giovannucci E, Hankinson S, *et al.* (2005) Alcohol intake and methylenetetrahydrofolate reductase polymorphism modify the relation of folate intake to plasma homocysteine. *American Journal of Clinical Nutrition*, **82**, 155–62.

Chivot M (2005) Retinoid therapy for acne. A comparative review. *American Journal of Clinical Dermatology*, **6**, 13–19.

Cho E, Hung S, Willett WC, *et al.* (2001) Prospective study of dietary fat and the risk of age-related macular degeneration. *American Journal of Clinical Nutrition*, **73**, 209–18.

Cho E, Seddon JM, Rosner B, *et al.* (2004) Prospective study of intake of fruits, vegetables, vitamins, and carotenoids and risk of age-related maculopathy. *Archives of Ophthalmology*, **122**, 883–92.

Cho E, Smith-Warner SA, Spiegelman D, *et al.* (2004a) Dairy foods, calcium, and colorectal cancer: a pooled analysis of 10 cohort studies. *Journal of the National Cancer Institute*, **96**, 1015–22.

Cho E, Smith-Warner SA, Ritz J, *et al.* (2004b) Alcohol intake and colorectal cancer: a pooled analysis of 8 cohort studies. *Annals of Internal Medicine*, **140**, 603–13.

Cho E, Stampfer MJ, Seddon JM, *et al.* (2001) Prospective study of zinc intake and the risk of age-related macular degeneration. *Annals of Epidemiology*, **11**, 328–36.

Chobanian A, Bakris G, Black H, *et al.* (2003) Seventh report of the Joint National Committee on prevention, detection, evaluation and treatment of high blood pressure: the JNC 7 report. *Journal of the American Medical Association*, **289**, 2560–72.

Choi H (2005) Dietary risk factors for rheumatic diseases. *Current Opinions in Rheumatology*, **17**, 141–6.

Choi SW and Mason JB (2000) Folate and carcinogenesis: an integrated scheme. *Journal of Nutrition*, **130**, 129–32.

Cholesterol Treatment Trialists' (CTT) Collaboration (2005) Efficacy and safety of cholesterol-lowering treatment: prospective meta-analysis of data from 90 056 participants in 14 randomised trials of statins. *Lancet*, **366**, 1267–78.

Chow WH, Blot WJ, Vaughan TL, *et al.* (1998) Body mass index and risk of adenocarcinomas of the esophagus and gastric cardia. *Journal of the National Cancer Institute*, **90**, 150–5.

Christen W, Glynn R, Sperduto R, Chew E and Buring J (2004) Age-related cataract in a randomized trial of beta-carotene in women. *Ophthalmic Epidemiology*, **11**, 401–12.

Christen WG (1999) Antioxidant vitamins and age-related eye disease. *Proceedings of the Association of American Physicians*, **111**, 16–21.

Christen WG, Ajani UA, Glynn RJ, *et al.* (1999) Prospective cohort study of antioxidant vitamin supplement use and the risk of age-related maculopathy. *American Journal of Epidemiology*, **149**, 476–84.

Christen WG, Manson JE, Glynn RJ, *et al.* (2003) A randomized trial of beta carotene and age-related cataract in US physicians. *Archives of Ophthalmology*, **121**, 372–8.

Christensen R, Astrup A and Bliddal H (2005) Weight loss: the treatment of choice for knee osteoarthritis? A randomized trial. *Osteoarthritis Cartilage*, **13**, 20–7.

Chumlea W and Sun S (2004) The availability of body composition reference data for the elderly. *Journal of Nutrition, Health and Aging*, **8**, 76–82.

Church TS, Barlow CE, Earnest CP, *et al.* (2002) Associations between cardiorespiratory fitness and C-reactive protein in men. *Arteriosclerosis, Thrombosis & Vascular Biology*, **22**, 1869–76.

Chylack LT, Jr., Brown NP, Bron A, *et al.* (2002) The Roche European American Cataract Trial (REACT): a randomized clinical trial to investigate the efficacy of an oral antioxidant micronutrient mixture to slow progression of age-related cataract. *Ophthalmic Epidemiology*, **9**, 49–80.

Chylack LT, Jr., Leske M, McCarthy D, *et al.* (1989) Lens opacities classification system II (LOCS II). *Archives of Ophthalmology*, **107**, 991–7.

Ciccocioppo R, Di Sabatino A, Luinetti O, *et al.* (2002) Small bowel enterocyte apoptosis and proliferation are increased in the elderly. *Gerontology*, **48**, 204–8.

Clark R and Kupper T (2005) Old meets new: the interaction between innate and adaptive immunity. *Journal of Investigative Dermatology*, **125**, 629–37.

Clark R, Feleke G, Din M, *et al.* (2000) Nutritional treatment for acquired immunodeficiency virus-associated wasting using beta-hydroxy beta-methylbutyrate, glutamine, and arginine: a randomized, double-blind, placebo-controlled study. *Journal of Parenteral and Enteral Nutrition*, **24**, 133–9.

Clarke R (2005a) Homocysteine. *Cardiovascular Disease: Diet, Nutrition and Emerging Risk Factors. A British Nutritional Foundation Task Force Report.* Ed. S. Stanner. London, Blackwell Publishing: 147–60.

Clarke R (2005b) Homocysteine-lowering trials for prevention of heart disease and stroke. *Seminars in Vascular Medicine*, **5**, 215–22.

Clarke R (2006) Vitamin B_{12}, folic acid and the prevention of dementia. *New England Journal of Medicine*, **354**, 2817–19.

Clarke R, Daly L, Robinson K, *et al.* (1991) Hyperhomocysteinemia: an independent risk factor for vascular disease. *New England Journal of Medicine*, **324**, 1149–55.

Clarke R, Emberson JR, Breeze E, *et al.* (2008) Biomarkers of inflammation predict both vascular and nonvascular mortality in older men. *European Heart Journal*, **29**, 800–9.

Clarke R, Emberson JR, Parish S, *et al.* (2007) Cholesterol fractions and apolipoproteins as risk factors for heart disease mortality in older men. *Archives of Internal Medicine*, **167**, 1373–8.

Clarke R, Frost C, Collins R, *et al.* (1997) Dietary lipids and blood cholesterol: quantitative meta-analysis of metabolic ward studies. *British Medical Journal*, **314**, 112–17.

Clarke R, Grimley Evans J, Schneede J, *et al.* (2004) Vitamin B_{12} and folate deficiency in later life. *Age & Ageing*, **33**, 34–41.

Clarke R, Harrison G, Richards S and Vital Trial Collaborative Group (2003) Effect of vitamins and aspirin on markers of platelet activation, oxidative stress and homocysteine in people at high risk of dementia. *Journal of Internal Medicine*, **254**, 67–75.

Clarke R, Lewington L, Youngman P, *et al.* (2002) Underestimation of the importance of blood pressure and cholesterol for coronary heart disease mortality in old age. *European Heart Journal*, **23**, 286–93.

Clarke R, Refsum H, Birks J, *et al.* (2003) Screening for vitamin B12 and folate deficiency in older people. *American Journal of Clinical Nutrition*, **77**, 1241–7.

Clarke R, Shipley M, Lewington S, *et al.* (1999) Underestimation of risk associations due to regression dilution in long-term follow-up of prospective studies. *American Journal of Epidemiology*, **150**, 341–53.

Clarke R, Smith A, Jobst K, *et al.* (1998) Folate, vitamin B12, and serum total homocysteine levels in confirmed Alzheimer disease. *Archives of Neurology*, **55**, 1449–55.

Clegg DO, Reda DJ, Harris CL, *et al.* (2006) Glucosamine, chondroitin sulfate and the two in combination for painful knee osteoarthritis. *New England Journal of Medicine*, **354**, 795–808.

Clements DM, Oleesky DA, Smith SC, *et al.* (2005) A study to determine plasma antioxidant concentrations in patients with Barrett's oesophagus. *Journal of Clinical Pathology*, **58**, 490–2.

Clemons TE, Milton RC, Klein R, *et al.* (2005) Risk factors for the incidence of Advanced Age-Related Macular Degeneration in the Age-Related Eye Disease Study (AREDS). AREDS report no. 19. *Ophthalmology*, **112**, 533–9.

Clowes JA, Riggs BL and Khosla S (2005) The role of the immune system in the pathophysiology of osteoporosis. *Immunological Reviews*, **208**, 207–27.

Clydesdale GJ, Dandie GW and Muller HK (2001) Ultraviolet light induced injury: immunological and inflammatory effects. *Immunology & Cell Biology*, **79**, 547–68.

Coburn SP, Slominski A, Mahuren JD, *et al.* (2003) Cutaneous metabolism of vitamin B-6. *Journal of Investigative Dermatology*, **120**, 292–300.

Cockayne S, Adamson J, Lanham-New S, *et al.* (2006) Vitamin K and the prevention of fractures: systematic review and meta-analysis of randomized controlled trials. *Archives of Internal Medicine*, **166**, 1256–61.

Coenen C, Wegener M, Wedmann B, *et al.* (1992) Does physical exercise influence bowel transit time in healthy young men? *American Journal of Gastroenterology*, **87**, 292–5.

Coffey M, Reidy A, Wormald R, *et al.* (1993) Prevalence of glaucoma in the west of Ireland. *British Journal of Ophthalmology*, **77**, 17–21.

Coggan AR, Spina RJ, King DS, *et al.* (1992) Histochemical and enzymatic comparison of the gastrocnemius muscle of young and elderly men and women. *Journal of Gerontology*, **47**, B71–6.

Cohen BE, Gill G, Cullen PR and Morris PJ (1979) Reversal of postoperative immunosuppression in man by vitamin A. *Surgery, Gynecology & Obstetrics*, **149**, 658–62.

Cohen HJ, Pieper CF, Harris T, *et al.* (1997) The association of plasma IL-6 levels with functional disability in community-dwelling elderly. *Journals of Gerontology Series A-Biological Sciences & Medical Sciences*, **52**, M201–8.

Collins AR, Harrington V, Drew J, *et al.* (2003) Nutritional modulation of DNA repair in a human intervention study. *Carcinogenesis*, **24**, 511–15.

Combaret L, Dardevet D, Rieu I, *et al.* (2005) A leucine-supplemented diet restores the defective postprandial inhibition of proteasome-dependent proteolysis in aged rat skeletal muscle. *Journal of Physiology*, **569**, 489–99.

Combination Pharmacotherapy and Public Health Research Working Group (2005) Combination pharmacotherapy for cardiovascular disease. *Annals of Internal Medicine*, **143**, 593–9.

Commission for Healthcare Audit and Inspection (2006) *Living Well in Later Life. A Review of Progress against the National Service Framework for Older People.* London, Commission for Healthcare Audit and Inspection.

Congdon N, O'Colmain B, Klaver CC, *et al.* (2004) Causes and prevalence of visual impairment among adults in the United States. *Archives of Ophthalmology*, **122**, 477–85.

Congdon N, Vingerling JR, Klein BE, *et al.* (2004) Prevalence of cataract and pseudophakia/aphakia among adults in the United States. *Archives of Ophthalmology*, **122**, 487–94.

Congdon NG and West KP, Jr. (1999) Nutrition and the eye. *Currents Opinions in Ophthalmology*, **10**, 464–73.

Connor MJ (1986) Retinoid stimulation of epidermal differentiation *in vivo*. *Life Sciences*, **38**, 1807–12.

Consensus Development Conference (1991) Prophylaxis and treatment of osteoporosis. *Osteoporosis International*, **1**, 114–17.

Cooper C, Barker DJ and Wickham C (1988) Physical activity, muscle strength, and calcium intake in fracture of the proximal femur in Britain. *British Medical Journal*, **297**, 1443–6.

Cooper C, McAlindon T, Snow S, *et al.* (1994) Mechanical and constitutional risk factors for symptomatic knee osteoarthritis: differences between medial tibiofemoral and patellofemoral disease. *Journal of Rheumatology*, **21**, 307–13.

Cooper C, Snow S, McAlindon T, *et al.* (2000) Risk factors for the incidence and progression of radiographic knee osteoarthritis. *Arthritis and Rheumatism*, **43**, 995–1000.

Coppack S, Mohamed-Ali V and Karpe F (2005) Metabolic syndrome: insulin resistance, obesity, diabetes mellitus, hypertension, physical activity and genetic factors. *Cardiovascular Disease: Diet, Nutrition and Emerging Risk Factors*. Ed. S Stanner. Oxford, Blackwell Publishing: 22–49.

Coppen A and Bailey J (2000) Enhancement of the antidepressant action of fluoxetine by folic acid: a randomised, placebo controlled trial. *Journal of Affective Disorders*, **60**, 121–30.

Coppin RJ, Wicke DM and Little PS (2005) Managing nocturnal leg cramps – calf-stretching exercises and cessation of quinine treatment: a factorial randomised controlled trial. *British Journal of General Practice*, **55**, 186–91.

Cordain L, Lindeberg S, Hurtado M, *et al.* (2002) Acne vulgaris: a disease of Western civilization. *Archives of Dermatology*, **138**, 1584–90.

Corre S, Mekideche K, Adamski H, *et al.* (2006) *In vivo* and *ex vivo* UV-induced analysis of pigmentation gene expressions. *Journal of Investigative Dermatology*, **126**, 916–18.

Correa P (1991) The epidemiology of gastric cancer. *World Journal of Surgery*, **15**, 228–34.

Correa P (1992) Human gastric carcinogenesis: a multistep and multifactorial process – First American Cancer Society Award Lecture on Cancer Epidemiology and Prevention. *Cancer Research*, **52**, 6735–40.

Correa P, Malcom G, Schmidt B, *et al.* (1998) Review article: Antioxidant micronutrients and gastric cancer. *Alimentary Pharmacology & Therapeutics*, **12 (Suppl 1)**, 73–82.

Cosgrove M, Franco OH, Granger SP, *et al.* (2007) Dietary nutrient intakes and skin-ageing appearance among middle-aged American women. *American Journal of Clinical Nutrition*, **86**, 1225–31.

Cossarizza A, Ortolani C, Monti D and Franceschi C (1997) Cytometric analysis of immunosenescence. *Cytometry*, **27**, 297–313.

COT (2003) Committee on Toxicity of Chemicals in Food, Consumer Products and the Environment. COT Statement on Fluorine in The 1997 Total Diet Study. www.food.gov.uk/multimedia/pdfs/fluoride.pdf.

Cotsarelis G, Sun TT and Lavker RM (1990) Label-retaining cells reside in the bulge area of pilosebaceous unit: implications for follicular stem cells, hair cycle, and skin carcinogenesis. *Cell*, **61**, 1329–37.

Cottrell DA, Blakely EL, Johnson MA, *et al.* (2001) Cytochrome C oxidase deficient cells accumulate in the hippocampus and choroid plexus with age. *Neurobiology of Aging*, **22**, 265–72.

Creamer O, Lethbridge-Cejku M and Hochberg M (1999) Determinants of pain severity in knee osteoarthritis: effect of demographic and psychosocial variables using 3 pain measures. *Journal of Rheumatology*, **26**, 1785–92.

Cree M, Newcomer B, Katsanos C, *et al.* (2004) Intramuscular and liver triglycerides are increased in the elderly. *Journal of Clinical Endocrinology and Metabolism*, **89**, 3864–71.

Crilly RG, Anderson C, Hogan D and Delaquerriere-Richardson L (1988) Bone histomorphometry, bone mass, and related parameters in alcoholic males. *Calcified Tissue International*, **43**, 269–76.

Cruickshanks KJ, Klein R and Klein BE (1993) Sunlight and age-related macular degeneration. The Beaver Dam Eye Study. *Archives of Ophthalmology*, **111**, 514–18.

Cruickshanks KJ, Klein R, Klein BE and Nondahl DM (2001) Sunlight and the 5-year incidence of early age-related maculopathy: the beaver dam eye study. *Archives of Ophthalmology*, **119**, 246–50.

Cumming RG, Mitchell P and Smith W (2000) Diet and cataract: the Blue Mountains Eye Study. *Ophthalmology*, **107**, 450–6.

Cummings J (2004) Alzheimer's disease. *New England Journal of Medicine*, **351**, 56–67.

Cummings JH and Bingham SA (1998) Diet and the prevention of cancer. *British Medical Journal*, **317**, 1636–40.

Cummings JH and Macfarlane GT (1991) The control and consequences of bacterial fermentation in the human colon. *Journal of Applied Bacteriology*, **70**, 443–59.

Cummings JH, Bingham SA, Heaton KW and Eastwood MA (1992) Fecal weight, colon cancer risk, and dietary intake of nonstarch polysaccharides (dietary fiber). *Gastroenterology*, **103**, 1783–9.

Cummings JH, Hill MJ, Jenkins DJ, *et al.* (1976) Changes in fecal composition and colonic function due to cereal fiber. *American Journal of Clinical Nutrition*, **29**, 1468–73.

Curcio CA, Owsley C and Jackson GR (2000) Spare the rods, save the cones in aging and age-related maculopathy. *Investigative Ophthalmology and Visual Science*, **41**, 2015–18.

Curran JE, Jowett JBM, Elliott KS, *et al.* (2005) Genetic variation in selenoprotein S influences inflammatory response. *Nature Genetics*, **37**, 1234–41.

Cushman M, Arnold AM, Psaty BM, *et al.* (2005) C-reactive protein and the 10-year incidence of coronary heart disease in older men and women: the cardiovascular health study. *Circulation*, **112**, 25–31.

Cuthbertson D, Smith K, Babraj J, *et al.* (2005) Anabolic signaling deficits underlie amino acid resistance of wasting, aging muscle. *FASEB Journal*, **19**, 422–4.

D'Aiuto F, Parkar M, Nibali L, *et al.* (2006) Periodontal infections cause changes in traditional and novel cardiovascular risk factors: results from a randomized controlled clinical trial. *American Heart Journal*, **151**, 977–84.

D'Avanzo B, La Vecchia C, Talamini R and Franceschi S (1996) Anthropometric measures and risk of cancers of the upper digestive and respiratory tract. *Nutrition & Cancer*, **26**, 219–27.

Dahl WJ, Whiting SJ, Healey A, *et al.* (2003) Increased stool frequency occurs when finely processed pea hull fiber is added to usual foods consumed by elderly residents in long-term care. *Journal of the American Dietetic Association*, **103**, 1199–202.

Dalais FS, Ebeling PR, Kotsopoulos D, *et al.* (2003) The effects of soy protein containing isoflavones on lipids and indices of bone resorption in postmenopausal women. *Clinical Endocrinology (Oxford)*, **58**, 704–9.

Danesh J, Wheeler J, Hirschfield G, *et al.* (2004) C-reactive protein and other circulating markers of inflammation in the prediction of coronary heart disease. *New England Journal of Medicine*, **350**, 1387–97.

Dangour AD, Clemens F, Elbourne D, *et al.* (2006) A randomised controlled trial investigating the effect of n-3 long-chain polyunsaturated fatty acid supplementation on cognitive and retinal function in cognitively healthy older people: the Older People and n-3 Long-chain Polyunsaturated Fatty Acids (OPAL) study protocol [ISRCTN72331636]. *Nutrition Journal*, **5**, 20.

Dangour AD, Sibson VL and Fletcher AE (2004) Micronutrient supplementation in later life: limited evidence for benefit. *Journals of Gerontology Series A – Biological Sciences & Medical Sciences*, **59**, 659–73.

Daniell HW (1979) Simple cure for nocturnal leg cramps. *New England Journal of Medicine*, **301**, 216.

Dankner R, Chetrit A, Lubin F and Sela B (2004) Lifestyle habits and homocysteine levels in an elderly population. *Aging Clinical and Experimental Research*, **16**, 437–42.

Dantzer R, Wollman E, Vitkovic L and Yirmiya R (1999) Cytokines and depression: fortuitous or causative association? *Molecular Psychiatry*, **4**, 328–32.

Darvin ME, Gersonde I, Meinke M, *et al.* (2005) Non-invasive *in vivo* determination of the carotenoids beta-carotene and lycopene concentrations in the human skin using the Raman spectroscopic method. *Journal of Physics D: Applied Physics*, **38**, 2696–700.

Darzins P, Mitchell P and Heller RF (1997) Sun exposure and age-related macular degeneration. An Australian case-control study. *Ophthalmology*, **104**, 770–6.

Das N, Thompson JR, Patel R and Rosenthal AR (1990) The prevalence of age related cataract in the Asian community in Leicester: a community based study. *Eye*, **4**, 723–6.

Dawson-Hughes B, Dallal GE, Krall EA, *et al.* (1990) A controlled trial of the effect of calcium supplementation on bone density in postmenopausal women. *New England Journal of Medicine*, **323**, 878–83.

Dawson-Hughes B, Harris SS, Krall EA and Dallal GE (1997) Effect of calcium and vitamin D supplementation on bone density in men and women 65 years of age or older. *New England Journal of Medicine*, **337**, 670–6.

Dawson-Hughes B, Heaney RP, *et al.* (2005) Estimates of optimal vitamin D status. *Osteoporosis International*, **16**, 713–16.

Daynes RA and Jones DC (2002) Emerging roles of PPARs in inflammation and immunity. *Nature Reviews Immunology*, **2**, 748–59.

De Groot C, van Staveren W and de Graaf C (2000) Determinants of macronutrient intake in elderly people. *European Journal of Clinical Nutrition*, **54 (Suppl 3)**, S70–6.

de la Fournierre F, Ferry M, Crockaert X, *et al.* (1997) Deficiente en vitamin B12 et état dementie: étude épidemiologique muticentrique et thérapeutique. *Essai preliminaire. Semanatique Hop*, **73**, 133–40.

de Lau L, Koudstaal P, Witteman J, *et al.* (2006) Dietary folate, vitamin B12, and vitamin B6 and the risk of Parkinson disease. *Neurology*, **67**, 315–18.

de Lorgeril M, Renaud S, Mamelle N, *et al.* (1994) Mediterranean alpha-linolenic acid-rich diet in secondary prevention of coronary heart disease. *Lancet*, **343**, 1454–9.

de Magalhaes JP (2004) From cells to ageing: a review of models and mechanisms of cellular senescence and their impact on human ageing. *Experimental Cell Research*, **300**, 1–10.

de Mendonca A and Maia L (2002) Does caffeine protect against Alzheimer's disease? *European Journal of Neurology*, **9**, 377–82.

De Schryver AM, Keulemans YC, Peters HP, *et al.* (2005) Effects of regular physical activity on defecation pattern in middle-aged patients complaining of chronic constipation. *Scandinavian Journal of Gastroenterology*, **40**, 422–9.

DeBlack SS (2003) Cigarette smoking as a risk factor for cataract and age-related macular degeneration: a review of the literature. *Optometry*, **74**, 99–110.

DEFRA (2001) National Food Survey 2000. London, Stationery Office. statistics.defra.gov.uk/esg/publications/nfs/default.asp.

Dekker P, Parish WE and Green MR (2005) Protection by food-derived antioxidants from UV-A1-induced photodamage, measured using living skin equivalents. *Photochemistry & Photobiology*, **81**, 837–42.

Delahanty LM, Conroy MB, Nathan DM and Diabetes Prevention Program Research Group (2006) Psychological predictors of physical activity in the diabetes prevention program. *Journal of the American Dietetic Association*, **106**, 698–705.

Delcourt C, Carriere I, Delage M, *et al.* (2003) Associations of cataract with antioxidant enzymes and other risk factors: the French Age-Related Eye Diseases (POLA) Prospective Study. *Ophthalmology*, **110**, 2318–26.

Delcourt C, Carriere I, Delage M, *et al.* (2006) Plasma lutein and zeaxanthin and other carotenoids as modifiable risk factors for age-related maculopathy and cataract: the POLA Study. *Investigative Ophthalmology and Visual Science*, **47**, 2329–35.

Delcourt C, Carriere I, Ponton-Sanchez A, *et al.* (2001) Light exposure and the risk of age-related macular degeneration: the Pathologies Oculaires Lieés à l'Age (POLA) study. *Archives of Ophthalmology*, **119**, 1463–8.

Delcourt C, Cristol JP, Leger CL, *et al.* (1999) Associations of antioxidant enzymes with cataract and age-related macular degeneration. The POLA Study. Pathologies Oculaires Lieés à l'Age. *Ophthalmology*, **106**, 215–22.

Delcourt C, Cristol JP, Tessier F, *et al.* (1999) Age-related macular degeneration and antioxidant status in the POLA study. POLA Study Group. Pathologies Oculaires Lieés à l'Age. *Archives of Ophthalmology*, **117**, 1384–90.

Delcourt C, Cristol JP, Tessier F, *et al.* (2000) Risk factors for cortical, nuclear, and posterior subcapsular cataracts: the POLA study. Pathologies Oculaires Lieés à l'Age. *American Journal of Epidemiology*, **151**, 497–504.

Delcourt C, Dupuy AM, Carriere I, *et al.* (2005) Albumin and transthyretin as risk factors for cataract: the POLA study. *Archives of Ophthalmology*, **123**, 225–32.

Delcourt C, Michel F, Colvez A, *et al.* (2001) Associations of cardiovascular disease and its risk factors with age-related macular degeneration: the POLA study. *Ophthalmic Epidemiology*, **8**, 237–49.

Demetriou AA, Levenson SM, Rettura G and Seifter E (1985) Vitamin A and retinoic acid: induced fibroblast differentiation in vitro. *Surgery*, **98**, 931–4.

Demling RH and DeSanti L (1999) Involuntary weight loss and the nonhealing wound: the role of anabolic agents. *Advances in Wound Care*, **12**, 1–14; quiz 5–6.

den Heijer T, Vermeer S, Clarke R, *et al.* (2003) Homocysteine and brain atrophy on MRI of non-demented elderly. *Brain*, **126**, 170–5.

Deng HW, Chen WM, Recker S, *et al.* (2000) Genetic determination of Colles' fracture and differential bone mass in women with and without Colles' fracture. *Journal of Bone & Mineral Research*, **15**, 1243–52.

Dennett NS, Barcia RN and McLeod JD (2002) Age associated decline in CD25 and CD28 expression correlate with an increased susceptibility to CD95 mediated apoptosis in T cells. *Experimental Gerontology*, **37**, 271–83.

Dennison E and Cooper C (2007) Lifestyle and constitutional risk factors. In: *Managing Osteoporosis*. Ed. S. A. Lanham-New, T. O'Neill, R. Morris, D. Skeleton and A. Sutcliffe. Oxford, Clinical Publishing: 69–80.

Dentino AN, Pieper CF, Rao MK, *et al.* (1999) Association of interleukin-6 and other biologic variables with depression in older people living in the community.

Journal of the American Geriatrics Society, **47**, 6–11.

Deon D, Ahmed S, Tai K, *et al.* (2001) Cross-talk between IL-1 and IL-6 signaling pathways in rheumatoid arthritis synovial fibroblasts. *Journal of Immunology*, **167**, 5395–403.

Department of Health (1991) *Dietary Reference Values for Food Energy and Nutrients for the United Kingdom. Report of the Panel on Dietary Reference Intakes of the Committee on Medical Aspects of Food Policy.* London, HMSO.

Department of Health (1992) *Report on Health and Social Subjects 43. The Nutrition of Elderly People.* London, HMSO.

Department of Health (1994) *Nutritional Aspects of Cardiovascular Disease.* London, HMSO.

Department of Health (1998a) *Nutrition and Bone Health: with Particular Reference to Calcium and Vitamin D. Report on Health and Social Sciences Subjects 49.* London, HMSO.

Department of Health (1998b) *Nutritional Aspects of the Development of Cancer.* London, Stationery Office.

Department of Health (2000a) *Folic Acid and the Prevention of Disease.* London, Stationery Office.

Department of Health (2000b) *National Service Framework for Coronary Heart Disease.* London, Department of Health.

Department of Health (2001) *National Service Framework for Older People.* London, Department of Health.

Department of Health (2003) *Health Survey for England.* London, HMSO.

Department of Health (2004a) *At Least Five a Week. Evidence on the Impact of Physical Activity and its Relationship to Health. A Report from the Chief Medical Officer.* London, Department of Health.

Department of Health (2004b) *Choosing a Better Diet, a Food and Health Action Plan.* London, Department of Health.

Department of Health (2004c) *The National Service Framework for Coronary Heart Disease: Winning the War on Heart Disease.* London, Department of Health.

Department of Health (2005) *Choosing Better Oral Health: An Oral Health Plan for England.* London, Stationery Office.

Department of Health (2006) *A New Ambition for Old Age: Next Steps in Implementing the National Service Framework for Older People.* www.dh.gov.uk.

Department of Health and Department of Children, Schools and Families (2008) *Healthy Weight, Healthy Lives: A Cross-Government Strategy for England.* www.dh.gov.uk/publications.

Department of Health and Human Services. www.health.gov/dietaryguidelines/dga2005/document/html/chapter4.htm.

Department of Work and Pensions (2005) *Opportunity Age.* www.dwp.gov.uk/opportunity_age (accessed August 11 2008).

Derave W, Eijnde B, Ramaekers M and Hespel P (2005) No effects of lifelong creatine supplementation on sarcopenia in senescence-accelerated mice (SAMP8). *American Journal Of Physiology-Endocrinology & Metabolism*, **289**, E272–E7.

Dergal J, Gold J, Laxer D, *et al.* (2002) Potential interactions between herbal medicines and conventional drug therapies used by older adults attending a memory clinic. *Drugs & Aging*, **19**, 879–86.

Desai M, Pratt L, Lentzner H and Robinson K (2001) Trends in vision and hearing among older Americans. *Ageing Trends No.2.* Hyattsville, MD, National Centre for Health Statistics.

Destro C, Maggi S and Crepaldi G (2003) Epidemiology of gastrointestional disorders in the elderly. In: *Aging and the Gastrointestional Tract.* Ed. A. Pilotto, P. Malfertheiner and P. Holt. Basel, Karger Press: 1–11.

Desvergne B and Wahli W (1999) Peroxisome proliferator-activated receptors: nuclear control of metabolism. *Endocrine Reviews*, **20**, 649–88.

Devaraj S and Jialal I (2000) Alpha tocopherol supplementation decreases serum C-reactive protein and monocyte interleukin-6 levels in normal volunteers and type 2 diabetic patients. *Free Radical Biology & Medicine*, **29**, 790–2.

Devareddy L, Khalil DA, Smith BJ, *et al.* (2006) Soy moderately improves microstructural properties without affecting bone mass in an ovariectomized rat model of osteoporosis. *Bone*, **38**, 686–93.

Devine A, Rosen C, Mohan S, *et al.* (1998) Effects of zinc and other nutritional factors on insulin-like growth factor I and insulin-like growth factor binding proteins in postmenopausal women. *American Journal of Clinical Nutrition*, **68**, 200–6.

Dhahbi JM, Kim H-J, Mote PL, *et al.* (2004) Temporal linkage between the phenotypic and genomic responses to caloric restriction. *Proceedings of the National Academy of Sciences of the United States of America*, **101**, 5524–9.

DHHS (US Department of Health and Human Services) & USDA (United States Department of Agriculture) (2005). Dietary Guidelines for Americans 2005. www.health.gov/dietaryguidelines/dga2005/document.

Di Lorenzo G, Balistreri CR, Candore G, *et al.* (1999) Granulocyte and natural killer activity in the elderly. *Mechanisms of Ageing & Development*, **108**, 25–38.

di Minno G and Mancini M (1992) Drugs affecting plasma fibrinogen levels. *Cardiovascular Drugs & Therapy*, **6**, 25–7.

di Stefano M, Veneto G, Malservisi S, *et al.* (2001) Lactose malabsorption and intolerance in the elderly. *Scandinavian Journal of Gastroenterology*, **36**, 1274–8.

Dickerson J, New S and Massey L (2003) Alcohol and caffeine: effects on osteoporosis risk. *Nutritional Aspects of Bone Health*. Ed. S. A. New and J. P. Bonjour. Cambridge, Royal Society of Chemistry: 439–50.

Dieppe P (1999) Subchondral bone should be the main target for the treatment of pain and disease progression in osteoarthritis. *Osteoarthritis Cartilage*, 7, 325–6.

Dieppe P and Brandt K (2003) What is important in treating osteoarthritis: Whom should we treat and how should we treat them? *Rheumatic Diseases Clinics of North America*, 29, 687–716.

Dieppe P and Lohmander S (2005) Pathogenesis and management of pain in osteoarthritis. *Lancet*, 365, 965–73.

Dieppe P and Tobias J (1998) Bone and joint ageing. *Geriatric Medicine and Gerontology*. 5th edition. Ed. R. Tallis, H. Fillit and J. Brocklehurst. Edinburgh and London, Churchill Livingstone: 1131–6.

Dillon J (1994) UV-B as a pro-aging and pro-cataract factor. *Documenta ophthalmologica. Advances in Ophthalmology*, 88, 339–44.

Dirks A and Leeuwenburgh C (2006) Caloric restriction in humans: potential pitfalls and health concerns. *Mechanisms of Ageing & Development*, 127, 1–7.

Dixon KM, Deo SS, Wong G, *et al.* (2005) Skin cancer prevention: a possible role of 1,25dihydroxyvitamin D3 and its analogs. *Journal of Steroid Biochemistry & Molecular Biology*, 97, 137–43.

Dixon L, Winkleby M and Radimer K (2001) Dietary intakes and serum nutrients differ between adults from insufficient and food-sufficient families: Third National Health and Nutrition Examination Survey, 1988–1994. *Journal of Nutrition*, 131, 1232–46.

Dobson CM (2002) Getting out of shape. *Nature*, 418, 729–30.

Dodds MW, Hsieh SC and Johnson DA (1991) The effect of increased mastication by daily gum-chewing on salivary gland output and dental plaque acidogenicity. *Journal of Dental Research*, 70, 1474–8.

Dodds MW, Johnson DA and Yeh CK (2005) Health benefits of saliva: a review. *Journal of Dentistry*, 33, 223–33.

Donahue R, Abbott R, Reed D and Yano K (1988) Physical activity and coronary heart disease in middle-aged and elderly men: the Honolulu Heart Program. *American Journal of Public Health*, 78, 683–5.

Dorrens J and Rennie MJ (2003) Effects of ageing and human whole body and muscle protein turnover. *Scandinavian Journal of Medicine & Science in Sports*, 13, 26–33.

Dowd PS and Heatley RV (1984) The influence of undernutrition on immunity. *Clinical Science*, 66, 241–8.

Downs JM, Clearfield S, Weis S, *et al.* (1998) Primary prevention of acute coronary events with lovastatin in men and women with average cholesterol levels: results of AFCAPS/TexCAPS. Air Force/Texas Coronary Atherosclerosis Prevention Study. *Journal of the American Medical Association*, 279, 1615–22.

Drake A and Walker B (2004) The intergenerational effects of fetal programming: non-genomic mechanisms for the inheritance of low birth weight and cardiovascular risk. *Journal of Endocrinology*, 180, 1–16.

Drake AJ, Smith A, Betts PR, Crowne EC and Shield JPH (2002) Type 2 diabetes in obese white children. *Archives of Disease in Childhood*, 86, 207–8.

Draser BS (1988) The bacterial flora of the intestine. In: *The role of the Gut Flora in Toxicity and Cancer*. Ed. I. R. Rowland. London, Academic Press: 23–8.

Dreher F, Gabard B, Schwindt DA and Maibach HI (1998) Topical melatonin in combination with vitamins E and C protects skin from ultraviolet-induced erythema: a human study *in vivo*. *British Journal of Dermatology*, 139, 332–9.

Dreon D and Krauss R (1997) Diet–gene interactions in human lipoprotein metabolism. *Journal of the American College of Nutrition*, 16, 313–24.

Drucker DJ (2003) Glucagon-like peptides: regulators of cell proliferation, differentiation, and apoptosis. *Molecular Endocrinology*, 17, 161–71.

Dubey RK, Imthurn B, Zacharia LC and Jackson EK (2004) Hormone replacement therapy and cardiovascular disease: what went wrong and where do we go from here? *Hypertension*, 44, 789–95.

Dukas L, Willett WC and Giovannucci EL (2003) Association between physical activity, fiber intake, and other lifestyle variables and constipation in a study of women. *American Journal of Gastroenterology*, 98, 1790–6.

Dunger D, Ong K, Huxtable S, *et al.* (1998) Association of the INS VNTR with size at birth. ALSPAC Study Team. Avon Longitudinal Study of Pregnancy and Childhood. *Nature Genetics*, 19, 98–100.

Dunn AL, Marcus BH, Kampert JB, *et al.* (1999) Comparison of lifestyle and structured interventions to increase physical activity and cardiorespiratory fitness: a randomized trial. *Journal of the American Medical Association*, 281, 327–34.

Dunn-Walters DK, Banerjee M and Mehr R (2003) Effects of age on antibody affinity maturation. *Biochemical Society Transactions*, 31, 447–8.

Durga J, van Boxtel MPJ, Schouten EG, *et al.* (2007) Effect of 3-year folic acid supplementation on cognitive function in older adults in the FACIT trial: a randomised, double blind, controlled trial. *Lancet*, 369, 208–16.

Eberlein-Konig B, Placzek M and Przybilla B (1998) Protective effect against sunburn of combined systemic ascorbic acid (vitamin C) and d-alpha-tocopherol (vitamin E). *Journal of the American Academy of Dermatology*, 38, 45–8.

Ebrahim S and Davey Smith G (1996) *Health Promotion in Older People for the Prevention of Coronary Heart Disease and Stroke*. London, Health Education Authority.

Economic and Social Research Council (2000) *Fit and Fifty?* Swindon, ESRC.

Edelstein SL and Barrett-Connor E (1993) Relation between body size and bone mineral density in elderly men and women. *American Journal of Epidemiology*, **138**, 160–9.

Edward M (1986) Ascorbate induced changes in glycosaminoglycan synthesis and distribution of normal and SV40-transformed fibroblasts. *Journal of Cell Science*, **85**, 217–29.

Efron DT and Barbul A (1998) Modulation of inflammation and immunity by arginine supplements. *Current Opinion in Clinical Nutrition & Metabolic Care*, **1**, 531–8.

Egger G, Liang G, Aparicio A and Jones PA (2004) Epigenetics in human disease and prospects for epigenetic therapy. *Nature*, **429**, 457–63.

Egger G, Wolfenden K, Pares J and Mowbray G (1991) 'Bread: it's a great way to go'. Increasing bread consumption decreases laxative sales in an elderly community. *Medical Journal of Australia*, **155**, 820–1.

Ehrmann DA (2005) Polycystic ovary syndrome. *New England Journal of Medicine*, **352**, 1223–36.

Eisman JA (1999) Genetics of osteoporosis. *Endocrine Reviews*, **20**, 788–804.

Elia M, Ritz P and Stubbs R (2000) Total energy expenditure in the elderly. *European Journal of Clinical Nutrition*, **54 (Suppl 3)**, S92–S103.

Elias PM (2005) Stratum corneum defensive functions: an integrated view. *Journal of Investigative Dermatology*, **125**, 183–200.

El-Kadiki A and Sutton AJ (2005) Role of multivitamins and mineral supplements in preventing infections in elderly people: systematic review and meta-analysis of randomised controlled trials. *British Medical Journal*, **330**, 871–4.

Elliott A, Smith B, Penny K, *et al.* (1999) The epidemiology of chronic pain in the community. *Lancet*, **354**, 1248–52.

Elliott P (2003) Protein intake and blood pressure in cardiovascular disease. *Proceedings of the Nutrition Society*, **62**, 495–504.

Elliott P, Stamler J, Nichols R, *et al.* (1996) Intersalt revisited: further analyses of 24 hour sodium excretion and blood pressure within and across populations. Intersalt Cooperative Research Group. *British Medical Journal*, **312**, 1249–53.

Ellis FR, Holesh S and Ellis JW (1972) Incidence of osteoporosis in vegetarians and omnivores. *American Journal of Clinical Nutrition*, **25**, 555–8.

Elmets CA, Singh D, Tubesing K, *et al.* (2001) Cutaneous photoprotection from ultraviolet injury by green tea polyphenols. *Journal of the American Academy of Dermatology*, **44**, 425–32.

Emahazion T, Jobs M, Howell WM, *et al.* (1999) Identification of 167 polymorphisms in 88 genes from candidate neurodegeneration pathways. *Gene*, **238**, 315–24.

Enattah NS, Sahi T, Savilahti E, *et al.* (2002) Identification of a variant associated with adult-type hypolactasia. *Nature Genetics*, **30**, 233–7.

Engeset D, Alsaker E, Lund E, *et al.* (2006) Fish consumption and breast cancer risk. The European Prospective Investigation into Cancer and Nutrition (EPIC). *International Journal of Cancer*, **119**, 175–82.

England S and Seifter S (1986) The biochemical functions of ascorbic acid. *Annual Review of Nutrition*, **6**, 365–406.

Engstrom C, Loeb G, Reid J, Forrest W and Avruch L (1991) Morphometry of the human thigh muscles. A comparison between anatomical sections and computer tomographic and magnetic resonance images. *Journal of Anatomy*, **176**, 139–56.

Erden-Inal M, Sunal E and Kanbak G (2002) Age-related changes in the glutathione redox system. *Cell Biochemistry & Function*, **20**, 61–6.

Erens B, Primatesta P and Prior GE (2001) *Health Survey for England: The Health of Minority Ethnic Groups 1999*. London, Stationery Office.

Eriksson J, Forsen T, Tuomilehto J, *et al.* (1999) Catch-up growth in childhood and death from coronary heart disease: longitudinal study. *British Medical Journal*, **318**, 427–31.

Ernst E (2003) Avocado-soybean unsaponifiables (ASU) for osteoarthritis – a systematic review. *Clinical Rheumatology*, **22**, 285–8.

Ershler WB and Keller ET (2000) Age-associated increased interleukin-6 gene expression, late-life diseases, and frailty. *Annual Review of Medicine*, **51**, 245–70.

Ershler WB, Sun WH, Binkley N, *et al.* (1993) Interleukin-6 and aging: blood levels and mononuclear cell production increase with advancing age and in vitro production is modifiable by dietary restriction. *Lymphokine & Cytokine Research*, **12**, 225–30.

Ervin R and Kennedy-Stephenson J (2002) Mineral intakes of elderly adult supplement and non-supplement users in the Third Health and Nutrition Examination Survey. *Journal of Nutrition*, **132**, 3422–7.

Eskelinen A and Santalahti J (1992) Natural cartilage polysaccharides for the treatment of sun-damaged skin in females: a double-blind comparison of Vivida and Imedeen. *Journal of International Medical Research*, **20**, 227–33.

Esmarck B, Andersen J, Olsen S, *et al.* (2001) Timing of postexercise protein intake is important for muscle hypertrophy with resistance training in elderly humans. *Journal of Physiology*, **535**, 301–11.

Esposito K, Marfella R, Ciotola M, *et al.* (2004) Effect of a Mediterranean-style diet on endothelial dysfunction and markers of vascular inflammation in the metabolic syndrome: a randomized trial. *Journal of the American Medical Association*, **292**, 1440–6.

Esposito K, Nappo F, Giugliano F, *et al.* (2003) Effect of dietary antioxidants on postprandial endothelial dysfunction induced by a high-fat meal in healthy subjects. *American Journal of Clinical Nutrition*, **77**, 139–43.

Esposito K, Nappo F, Marfella R, *et al.* (2002) Inflammatory cytokine concentrations are acutely increased by hyperglycemia in humans: role of oxidative stress. *Circulation*, **106**, 2067–72.

Essen B, Jansson E, Henriksson J, *et al.* (1975) Metabolic characteristics of fibre types in human skeletal muscle. *Acta Physiologica Scandinavica*, **95**, 153–65.

European Food Safety Authority (2004) Opinion of the Scientific Panel on Dietetic Products, Nutrition and Allergies on a request from the Commission related to the presence of *trans* fatty acids in foods and the effect on human health of the consumption of *trans* fatty acids. (Request N° EFSA-Q-2003-022), www.efsa.eu.int/science/nda/nda_opinions/588_en.html.

Eurostat (2004) *Living Conditions in Europe – Statistical Pocketbook.* Luxembourg, European Communities.

Eussen S, deGroot L, Joosten L, *et al.* (2006) Effect of oral vitamin B-12 with or without folic acid on cognitive function in older people with mild vitamin B-12 deficiency: a randomized, placebo-controlled trial. *American Journal of Clinical Nutrition*, **84**, 361–70.

Evans CE, Chughtai AY, Blumsohn A, *et al.* (1997) The effect of dietary sodium on calcium metabolism in premenopausal and postmenopausal women. *European Journal of Clinical Nutrition*, **51**, 394–9.

Evans J, Rooney C, Ashwood F, *et al.* (1996) Blindness and partial sight in England and Wales: April 1990–March 1991. *Health Trends*, **28**, 5–12.

Evans JR (2002) Antioxidant vitamin and mineral supplements for age-related macular degeneration. *Cochrane Database of Systematic Reviews,* CD000254.

Evans JR, Fletcher AE and Wormald RP (2004) Causes of visual impairment in people aged 75 years and older in Britain: an add-on study to the MRC Trial of Assessment and Management of Older People in the Community. *British Journal of Ophthalmology*, **88**, 365–70.

Evans JR, Fletcher AE, Wormald RP, *et al.* (2002) Prevalence of visual impairment in people aged 75 years and older in Britain: results from the MRC trial of assessment and management of older people in the community. *British Journal of Ophthalmology*, **86**, 795–800.

Evans W and Cyr-Campbell D (1997) Nutrition, exercise, and healthy aging. *Journal of the American Dietetic Association*, **97**, 632–8.

Evenson K, Rosamond W, Cai J, *et al.* (2002) Influence of retirement on leisure-time physical activity: The Atherosclerosis Risk in Communities Study. *American Journal of Epidemiology*, **155**, 692–9.

Expert Panel on Detection, Evaluation and Treatment of High Blood Cholesterol in Adults (2001) Executive summary of the Third Report of the National Cholesterol Education Program (NCEP). Expert Panel on Detection, Evaluation, and Treatment of High Blood Cholesterol in Adults (Adult Treatment Panel III). *Journal of the American Medical Association*, **285**, 2486–97.

Eye Disease Case-Control Study Group (1992) Risk factors for neovascular age-related macular degeneration. *Archives of Ophthalmology*, **110**, 1701–8.

Eye Disease Case-Control Study Group (1993) Antioxidant status and neovascular age-related macular degeneration. Eye Disease Case-Control Study Group. *Archives of Ophthalmology*, **111**, 104–9.

Fair J (2003) Cardiovascular risk factor modification: is it effective in older adults? *Journal of Cardiovascular Nursing*, **18**, 161–8.

Fall C (2005) Fetal and maternal nutrition. In: *Cardiovascular Disease: Diet, Nutrition and Emerging Risk Factors.* Ed. S. Stanner. Oxford, Blackwell Publishing: 177–95.

Falsey RA (2000) Epidemiology of infectious disease. In: *Oxford Textbook of Geriatric Medicine.* Ed. J. Grimley Evans, T. Franklin Williams, B. Lynn Beattie, J.-P. Michel and G. K. Wilcock. Oxford, Oxford University Press: 55–64.

Fam AG (2005) Gout: excess calories, purines, and alcohol intake and beyond. Response to a urate-lowering diet. *Journal of Rheumatology*, **32**, 773–7.

FAO/WHO (2002) Guidelines for the Evaluation of Probiotics in Food. Report of a Joint FAO/WHO Working Group on Drafting Guidelines for the Evaluation of Probiotics in Food.

FAO/WHO/UNU (2004) Human Energy Requirements. Report of a Joint FAO/WHO/UNU Expert Consultation. Accessed 13 January 2005.

Faraday MM (2006) Stress revisited. A methodological and conceptual history. *Nutrients, Stress, and Medical Disorders.* Ed. S. Yehuda and D. I. Mostofsky. Totowa, NJ, Humana Press: 3–19.

Farrell JH (1956) The effect of mastication on the digestion of food. *British Dental Journal*, **100**, 149–55.

Farrell JH (1957) Partial dentures in the restoration of masticatory efficiency. *Dental Practitioner and the Dental Record*, **7**, 375–9.

Farrell M, Gibson S, McMeekan J and Helme R (2000) Pain and hyperalgesia in osteoarthritis of the hands. *Journal of Rheumatology*, **27**, 441–7.

Fayet G, Rouche A, Hogrel J, *et al.* (2001) Age-related morphological changes of the deltoid muscle from 50 to

79 years of age. *Acta Neuropathologica (Berlin)*, **101**, 358–66.

Fearon ER and Vogelstein B (1990) A genetic model for colorectal tumorigenesis. *Cell*, **61**, 759–67.

Federal Interagency Forum on Ageing-Related Statistics (2004) Older Americans 2000: Key Indicators of Well-being. www.agingstats.gov/chartbook2000/healthstatus.html. Accessed 7 October 2004.

Fehervari Z and Sakaguchi S (2004) CD4+ Tregs and immune control. *Journal of Clinical Investigation*, **114**, 1209–17.

Feinberg C, Hawkins S, Weinkauf R and Marriott R (2006) Clinical improvement to photodamaged facial skin with cosmetic PPAR lipids in Japanese subjects. *Journal of the American Academy of Dermatology*, **54 (Suppl)**, AB101.

Feinle-Bisset C, Vozzo R, Horowitz M and Talley NJ (2004) Diet, food intake, and disturbed physiology in the pathogenesis of symptoms in functional dyspepsia. *American Journal of Gastroenterology*, **99**, 170–81.

Feldman HA, Longcope C, Derby CA, *et al.* (2002) Age trends in the level of serum testosterone and other hormones in middle-aged men: longitudinal results from the Massachusetts Male Aging study. *Journal of Clinical Endocrinology & Metabolism*, **87**, 589–98.

Feldman M, Cryer B, McArthur KE, *et al.* (1996) Effects of aging and gastritis on gastric acid and pepsin secretion in humans: a prospective study. *Gastroenterology*, **110**, 1043–52.

Feldman RS, Kapur KK, Alman JE and Chauncey HH (1980) Aging and mastication: changes in performance and in the swallowing threshold with natural dentition. *Journal of American Geriatric Society*, **28**, 97–103.

Felley C and Michetti P (2003) Probiotics and *Helicobacter pylori*. *Best Practice & Research: Clinical Gastroenterology*, **17**, 785–91.

Felson D (2005) The sources of pain in knee osteoarthritis. *Current Opinion in Rheumatology*, **17**, 624–8.

Felson D and Zhang Y (1998) An update on the epidemiology of knee and hip osteoarthritis with a view to prevention. *Arthritis and Rheumatism*, **41**, 1343–55.

Felson D, Lawrence R, Dieppe P, *et al.* (2000) Osteoarthritis: new insights. Part 1: the disease and its risk factors. *Annals of Internal Medicine*, **133**, 635–46.

Ferguson FG, Wikby A, Maxson P, *et al.* (1995) Immune parameters in a longitudinal study of a very old population of Swedish people: a comparison between survivors and nonsurvivors. *Journals of Gerontology Series A – Biological Sciences & Medical Sciences*, **50**, B378–82.

Ferlay J, Bray F, Pisani P and Parkin DM (2004) GLOBOCAN (2002) *Cancer Incidence, Mortality and Prevalence Worldwide*. Lyon, IARC Press.

Fernandes J (2002) Nutrition and health – recommendations of the Health Council of the Netherlands regarding energy, protein, fats and carbohydrate. *Nederlands Tijdschrift voor Geneeskunde*, **146**, 2226–9.

Fernández-Gutiérrez B, Jover JA, De Miguel S, *et al.* (1999) Early lymphocyte activation in elderly humans: impaired T and T-dependent B cell responses. *Experimental Gerontology*, **34**, 217–29.

Ferrannini E, Camastra S, Gastaldelli A, *et al.* (2004) Beta-cell function in obesity: effects of weight loss. *Diabetes*, **53 (Suppl 3)**, S26–33.

Ferri CP, Prince M, Brayne C, *et al.* (2005) Global prevalence of dementia: a Delphi consensus study. *Lancet*, **366**, 2112–17.

Ferrigno L, Aldigeri R, Rosmini F, *et al.* (2005) Associations between plasma levels of vitamins and cataract in the Italian-American Clinical Trial of Nutritional Supplements and Age-Related Cataract (CTNS): CTNS Report No. 2. *Ophthalmic Epidemiology*, **12**, 71–80.

Ferrucci L, Corsi A, Lauretani F, *et al.* (2005) The origins of age-related proinflammatory state. *Blood*, **105**, 2294–9.

Ferrucci L, Harris TB, Guralnik JM, *et al.* (1999) Serum IL-6 level and the development of disability in older persons. *Journal of the American Geriatrics Society*, **47**, 639–46.

Ferrucci L, Penninx BWJH, Volpato S, *et al.* (2002) Change in muscle strength explains accelerated decline of physical function in older women with high interleukin-6 serum levels. *Journal of the American Geriatrics Society*, **50**, 1947–54.

Feskanich D, Singh V, Willett WC and Colditz GA (2002) Vitamin A intake and hip fractures among postmenopausal women. *Journal of the American Medical Association*, **287**, 47–54.

Finch CE and Crimmins EM (2004) Inflammatory exposure and historical changes in human life-spans. *Science*, **305**, 1736–9.

Finch CE and Kirkwood TBL (2000) *Chance, Development, and Aging*. New York, Oxford University Press.

Finch S, Doyle W, Lowe C, *et al.* (1998) *National Diet and Nutrition Survey: People Aged 65 years and Over. Volume 1: Report of the Diet and Nutrition Survey*. London, Stationery Office.

Finkelstein JA and Schiffman SS (1999) Workshop on taste and smell in the elderly: an overview. *Physiology & Behavior*, **66**, 173–6.

Fioravanti M, Ferrario E, Massaia M, *et al.* (1997) Low folate levels in the cognitive decline of elderly patients and the efficacy of folate as a treatment for improving memory deficits. *Archives of Gerontology and Geriatrics*, **26**, 1–13.

Fischer CP, Hiscock NJ, Penkowa M, *et al.* (2004) Supplementation with vitamins C and E inhibits the release of interleukin-6 from contracting human skeletal muscle. *Journal of Physiology*, **558**, 633–45.

Fisher MA, Taylor GW and Tilashalski KR (2005) Smokeless tobacco and severe active periodontal disease, NHANES III. *Journal of Dental Research*, **84**, 705–10.

FitzGerald R, Murray B and Walsh D (2004) The emerging role of dairy proteins and bioactive peptides in nutrition and health. *Journal of Nutrition*, **134**, 980S–8S.

Flood V, Smith W, Wang JJ, *et al.* (2002) Dietary antioxidant intake and incidence of early age-related maculopathy: the Blue Mountains Eye Study. *Ophthalmology*, **109**, 2272–8.

Food and Nutrition Board. Institute of Medicine (1997) *Dietary Reference Intakes for Calcium, Magnesium, Phosphorus, Vitamin D and Fluoride.* Washington, DC, National Academy Press.

Food and Nutritional Board. Institute of Medicine (2002) Dietary reference intakes for energy, carbohydrate, fiber, fat, fatty acids, cholesterol, protein, and amino acids, Appendix E: Dietary intake data from the Continuing Survey of Food Intakes by Individuals (CSFII) 1994–1996, 1998. In: *Dietary Reference Intakes and Recommended Dietary Allowances.* Washington DC, National Academic Press.

Food Standards Agency (2002) *McCance and Widdowson's The Composition of Foods,* Sixth summary edition. Cambridge, Royal Society of Chemistry.

Food Standards Agency (2002) Sweeteners Regulations. www.food.gov.uk/foodindustry/regulation/foodlawguidebranch/foodlawguidech04/foodlawsweetner.

Food Standards Agency (2006) *Food Served to Older People in Residential Care.* London, Food Standards Agency.

Forbes G (1999) Longitudinal changes in adult fat-free mass: influence of body weight. *American Journal of Clinical Nutrition*, **70**, 1025–31.

Ford I and Norrie J (2002) The role of covariates in estimating treatment effects and risk in long-term clinical trials. *Statistics in Medicine*, **21**, 2899–908.

Forette F, Seux M, Staessen J, *et al.* (1998) Prevention of dementia in randomised double-blind placebo-controlled Systolic Hypertension in Europe (Syst-Eur) trial. *Lancet*, **352**, 1347–51.

Forsen T, Eriksson J, Tuomilehto J, *et al.* (1997) Mother's weight in pregnancy and coronary heart disease in a cohort of Finnish men: follow-up study. *British Medical Journal*, **315**, 837–40.

Forsen T, Erikkson J, Tuomilehto J, *et al.* (2000) The fetal and childhood growth of persons who develop type 2 diabetes. *Annals of Internal Medicine*, **133**, 176–82.

Forsey RJ, Thompson JM, Ernerudh J, *et al.* (2003) Plasma cytokine profiles in elderly humans. *Mechanisms of Ageing & Development*, **124**, 487–93.

Foster RK and Marriott HE (2006) Alcohol consumption in the new millennium – weighing up the risks and benefits for our health. *Nutrition Bulletin*, **31**, 286–331.

Fox KR and Hillsdon M (2007) Physical activity and obesity. *Obesity Reviews*, **8**, 115–21.

Foy MM, Kim JJ, Shors TJ and Thompson RF (2006) Neurobiological foundations of stress. *Nutrients, Stress, and Medical Disorders.* Ed. S. Yehuda and D. I. Mostofsky. Totowa, NJ, Humana Press: 37–65.

Franceschi C, Bonafe M, Valensin S, *et al.* (2000) Inflammaging. An evolutionary perspective on immunosenescence. *Annals of the New York Academy of Sciences*, **908**, 244–54.

Franceschi C, Olivieri F, Marchegiani F, *et al.* (2005) Genes involved in immune response/inflammation, IGF1/insulin pathway and response to oxidative stress play a major role in the genetics of human longevity: the lesson of centenarians. *Mechanisms of Ageing & Development*, **126**, 351–61.

Franco B (2006) Androgens and breast cancer. *International Journal of Gynecologic Cancer*, **16 (Suppl 2)**, 493.

Franco OH, Kirkwood TBL, Powell JR, *et al.* (2007) Ten commandments for the future of ageing research in the UK: a vision for action. *BMC Geriatrics*, **7**, 10.

Freeman H, Lemoyne M and Pare P (2002) Coeliac disease. *Best Practice & Research: Clinical Gastroenterology*, **16**, 37–49.

Freund-Levi Y, Eriksdotter-Jonhagen M, Cederholm T, *et al.* (2006) Omega-3 fatty acid treatment in 174 patients with mild to moderate Alzheimer disease: OmegAD study: a randomized double-blind trial. *Archives of Neurology*, **63**, 1402–8.

Freyssenet D, Berthon P, Denis C, *et al.* (1996) Effect of a 6-week endurance training programme and branched-chain amino acid supplementation on histomorphometric characteristics of aged human muscle. *Archives of Physiology and Biochemistry*, **104**, 157–62.

Frezza EE, Wachtel MS and Chiriva-Internati M (2006) Influence of obesity on the risk of developing colon cancer. *Gut*, **55**, 285–91.

Friedenreich C, Norat T, Steindorf K, *et al.* (2006) Physical activity and risk of colon and rectal cancers: the European prospective investigation into cancer and nutrition. *Cancer Epidemiology, Biomarkers & Prevention*, **15**, 2398–407.

Friedman DS, Wilson MR, Liebmann JM, *et al.* (2004) An evidence-based assessment of risk factors for the progression of ocular hypertension and glaucoma. *American Journal of Ophthalmology*, **138**, S19–31.

Friedman DS, Wolfs RC, O'Colmain BJ, *et al.* (2004) Prevalence of open-angle glaucoma among adults in the United States. *Archives of Ophthalmology*, **122**, 532–8.

Friedmann PS, Cooper HL and Healy E (2005) Peroxisome proliferator-activated receptors and their relevance to dermatology. *Acta Dermato-Venereologica*, **85**, 194–202.

Friguet B (2002) Protein repair and degradation during aging. *The Scientific World Journal*, **2**, 248–54.

Frontera W, Hughes V, Fielding R, *et al.* (2000) Aging of skeletal muscle: a 12-yr longitudinal study. *Journal of Applied Physiology*, **88**, 1321–6.

Frost G, Leeds A, Trew G, *et al.* (1998) Insulin sensitivity in women at risk of coronary heart disease and the effect of a low glycemic diet. *Metabolism: Clinical & Experimental*, **47**, 1245–51.

Frost G, Wilding J and Beecham J (1994) Dietary advice based on the glycaemic index improves dietary profile and metabolic control in type 2 diabetic patients. *Diabetic Medicine*, **11**, 397–401.

Frost HM (1987) Bone 'mass' and the 'mechanostat': a proposal. *Anatomical Record*, **219**, 1–9.

Frost HM (1992) The role of changes in mechanical usage set points in the pathogenesis of osteoporosis. *Journal of Bone & Mineral Research*, **7**, 253–61.

Frost NA, Sparrow JM, Durant JS, *et al.* (1998) Development of a questionnaire for measurement of vision-related quality of life. *Ophthalmic Epidemiology*, **5**, 185–210.

Fuchs CS, Giovannucci EL, Colditz GA, *et al.* (1999) Dietary fiber and the risk of colorectal cancer and adenoma in women. *New England Journal of Medicine*, **340**, 169–76.

Fuchs CS, Willett WC, Colditz GA, *et al.* (2002) The influence of folate and multivitamin use on the familial risk of colon cancer in women. *Cancer Epidemiology Biomarkers & Prevention*, **11**, 227–34.

Fuchs J and Kern H (1998) Modulation of UV-light-induced skin inflammation by D-alpha-tocopherol and L-ascorbic acid: a clinical study using solar simulated radiation. *Free Radical Biology & Medicine*, **25**, 1006–12.

Fuller N, Sawyer M, Coward W, *et al.* (1996) Components of total energy expenditure in free-living elderly men (over 75 years of age): measurement, predictability and relationship to quality-of-life indices. *British Journal of Nutrition*, **75**, 161–73.

Fung T, Willett W, Stampfer M, *et al.* (2001) Dietary patterns and the risk of coronary heart disease in women. *Archives of Internal Medicine*, **161**, 1857–62.

Funk JL, Frye JB, Oyarzo JN, *et al.* (2006) Efficacy and mechanism of action of turmeric supplements in the treatment of experimental arthritis. *Arthritis & Rheumatism*, **54**, 3452–64.

Fure S (2004) Ten-year cross-sectional and incidence study of coronal and root caries and some related factors in elderly Swedish individuals. *Gerodontology*, **21**, 130–40.

Gadek JE, DeMichele SJ, Karlstad MD, *et al.* (1999) Effect of enteral feeding with eicosapentaenoic acid, gamma-linolenic acid, and antioxidants in patients with acute respiratory distress syndrome. Enteral Nutrition in ARDS Study Group. *Critical Care Medicine*, **27**, 1409–20.

Gale C, Martyn C, Kellingray S, *et al.* (2001) Intrauterine programming of adult body composition. *Journal of Clinical Endocrinology and Metabolism*, **86**, 267–72.

Gale CR, Hall NF, Phillips DI and Martyn CN (2001) Plasma antioxidant vitamins and carotenoids and age-related cataract. *Ophthalmology*, **108**, 1992–8.

Gale CR, Hall NF, Phillips DI and Martyn CN (2003) Lutein and zeaxanthin status and risk of age-related macular degeneration. *Investigative Ophthalmology and Visual Science*, **44**, 2461–5.

Gallagher D, Ruts E, Visser M, *et al.* (2000) Weight stability masks sarcopenia in elderly men and women. *American Journal Of Physiology-Endocrinology & Metabolism*, **279**, E366–75.

Gallagher D, Visser M, De Meersman R, *et al.* (1997) Appendicular skeletal muscle mass: effects of age, gender, and ethnicity. *Journal of Applied Physiology*, **83**, 229–39.

Gallistl S, Sudi K, Cvirn G, Muntean W and Borkenstein M (2001) Effects of short-term energy restriction and physical training on haemostatic risk factors for coronary heart disease in obese children and adolescents. *International Journal of Obesity*, **25**, 529–32.

Gangarosa RE, Glass RI, Lew JF and Boring JR (1992) Hospitalizations involving gastroenteritis in the United States, 1985: the special burden of the disease among the elderly. *American Journal of Epidemiology*, **135**, 281–90.

Gangemi S, Basile G, Merendino RA, *et al.* (2003) Increased circulating Interleukin-18 levels in centenarians with no signs of vascular disease: another paradox of longevity? *Experimental Gerontology*, **38**, 669–72.

Garland CF, Garland FC, Gorham ED, *et al.* (2006) The role of vitamin D in cancer prevention. *American Journal of Public Health*, **96**, 252–61.

Garmyn M, Ribaya-Mercado JD, Russel RM, Bhawan J and Gilchrest BA (1995) Effect of beta-carotene supplementation on the human sunburn reaction. *Experimental Dermatology*, **4**, 104–11.

Garnero P, Arden NK, Griffiths G, *et al.* (1996) Genetic influence on bone turnover in postmenopausal twins. *Journal of Clinical Endocrinology & Metabolism*, **81**, 140–6.

Garrigues V, Galvez C, Ortiz V, *et al.* (2004) Prevalence of constipation: agreement among several criteria and evaluation of the diagnostic accuracy of qualifying symptoms and self-reported definition in a population-based survey in Spain. *American Journal of Epidemiology*, **159**, 520–6.

Garssen J and van Loveren H (2001) Effects of ultraviolet exposure on the immune system. *Critical Reviews in Immunology*, **21**, 359–97.

Ge K, Xue A, Bai J and Wang S (1983) Keshan disease – an endemic cardiomyopathy in China. *Virchows Archiv – A, Pathological Anatomy & Histopathology*, **401**, 1–15.

Geleijnse J, Giltay E, Grobbee D, *et al.* (2002) Blood pressure response to fish oil supplementation: metaregression analysis of randomized trials. *Journal of Hypertension*, **20**, 1493–9.

Gems D and Partridge L (2001) Insulin/IGF signalling and ageing: seeing the bigger picture. *Current Opinion in Genetics & Development*, **11**, 287–92.

General Household Survey (2004) www.statistics.gov.uk.

Gerli R, Monti D, Bistoni O, *et al.* (2000) Chemokines, sTNF-Rs and sCD30 serum levels in healthy aged people and centenarians. *Mechanisms of Ageing & Development*, **121**, 37–46.

Gey K, Puska P, Jordan P and Moser U (1991) Inverse correlation between plasma vitamin E and mortality from ischemic heart disease in cross-cultural epidemiology. *American Journal of Clinical Nutrition*, **53**, 326S–34S.

Gharzi A, Reynolds AJ and Jahoda CAB (2003) Plasticity of hair follicle dermal cells in wound healing and induction. *Experimental Dermatology*, **12**, 126–36.

Ghezzi EM and Ship JA (2003) Aging and secretory reserve capacity of major salivary glands. *Journal of Dental Research*, **82**, 844–8.

Ghezzi EM, Lange LA and Ship JA (2000) Determination of variation of stimulated salivary flow rates. *Journal of Dental Research*, **79**, 1874–8.

Ghezzi EM, Wagner-Lange LA, Schork MA, *et al.* (2000) Longitudinal influence of age, menopause, hormone replacement therapy, and other medications on parotid flow rates in healthy women. *The Journals of Gerontology, Series A, Biological Sciences and Medical Sciences*, **55**, M34–42.

Giacconi R, Cipriano C, Albanese F, *et al.* (2004) The -174G/C polymorphism of IL-6 is useful to screen old subjects at risk for atherosclerosis or to reach successful ageing. *Experimental Gerontology*, **39**, 621–8.

Giacconi R, Cipriano C, Muti E, *et al.* (2005) Novel -209A/G MT2A polymorphism in old patients with type 2 diabetes and atherosclerosis: relationship with inflammation (IL-6) and zinc. *Biogerontology*, **6**, 407–13.

Gibbons LW, Mitchell TL, Wei M, Blair SN and Cooper KH (2000) Maximal exercise test as a predictor of risk for mortality from coronary heart disease in asymptomatic men. *American Journal of Cardiology*, **86**, 53–8.

Gibson GR and Roberfroid MB (1995) Dietary modulation of the human colonic microbiota: introducing the concept of prebiotics. *Journal of Nutrition*, **125**, 1401–12.

Gibson GR and Wang X (1994) Regulatory effects of bifidobacteria on the growth of other colonic bacteria. *Journal of Applied Bacteriology*, **77**, 412–20.

Gibson S (2007) Peer-led approaches to dietary change: report of the Food Standards Agency seminar held on 19 July 2006. *Public Health Nutrition*, **10**, 980–8.

Giguere V (1994) Retinoic acid receptors and cellular retinoid binding proteins: complex interplay in retinoid signaling. *Endocrine Reviews*, **15**, 61–79.

Gillis S, Kozak R, Durante M and Weksler ME (1981) Immunological studies of aging. Decreased production of and response to T cell growth factor by lymphocytes from aged humans. *Journal of Clinical Investigation*, **67**, 937–42.

Ginaldi L, De Martinis M, D'Ostilio A, *et al.* (1999) The immune system in the elderly: III. Innate immunity. *Immunologic Research*, **20**, 117–26.

Ginaldi L, De Martinis M, D'Ostilio A, *et al.* (2001) Changes in the expression of surface receptors on lymphocyte subsets in the elderly: quantitative flow cytometric analysis. *American Journal of Hematology*, **67**, 63–72.

Ginaldi L, Di Benedetto CM and de Martinis M (2005) Osteoporosis, inflammation and ageing. *Immunity & Ageing*, **2**, 14.

Giovannucci E, Pollak M, Liu Y, *et al.* (2003) Nutritional predictors of insulin-like growth factor I and their relationships to cancer in men. *Cancer Epidemiology, Biomarkers & Prevention*, **12**, 84–9.

Giovannucci E, Rimm EB, Ascherio A, *et al.* (1995) Alcohol, low-methionine – low-folate diets, and risk of colon cancer in men. *Journal of the National Cancer Institute*, **87**, 265–73.

Giovannucci E, Stampfer MJ, Colditz GA, *et al.* (1993) Folate, methionine, and alcohol intake and risk of colorectal adenoma. *Journal of the National Cancer Institute*, **85**, 875–84.

Giovannucci E, Stampfer MJ, Colditz GA, *et al.* (1998) Multivitamin use, folate, and colon cancer in women in the Nurses' Health Study. *Annals of Internal Medicine*, **129**, 517–24.

Girodon F, Galan P, Monget AL, *et al.* (1999) Impact of trace elements and vitamin supplementation on immunity and infections in institutionalized elderly patients: a randomized controlled trial. MIN. VIT. AOX. geriatric network. *Archives of Internal Medicine*, **159**, 748–54.

GISSI–Prevenzione Investigators (1999) Dietary supplementation with *n*-3 polyunsaturated fatty acids and vitamin E after myocardial infarction: results from the GISSI – Prevenzione trial. *Lancet*, **354**, 447–55.

Globocan (2002) www-dep.iarc.fr/globocan/database.htm, IARC.

Gluckman PD and Hanson MA (2004a) Living with the past: evolution, development, and patterns of disease. *Science*, **305**, 1733–6.

Gluckman PD and Hanson MA (2004b) The developmental origins of the metabolic syndrome. *Trends in Endocrinology & Metabolism*, **15**, 183–7.

Glynn RJ, Christen WG, Manson JE, *et al.* (1995) Body mass index. An independent predictor of cataract. *Archives of Ophthalmology,* **113**, 1131–7.

Glynn SA, Albanes D, Pietinen P, *et al.* (1996) Colorectal cancer and folate status: a nested case-control study among male smokers. *Cancer Epidemiology Biomarkers & Prevention,* **5**, 487–94.

Godar DE (2001) UV doses of American children and adolescents. *Photochemistry & Photobiology,* **74**, 787–93.

Godar DE, Urbach F, Gasparro FP and van der Leun JC (2003) UV doses of young adults. *Photochemistry & Photobiology,* **77**, 453–7.

Godar DE, Wengraitis SP, Shreffler J and Sliney DH (2001) UV doses of Americans. *Photochemistry & Photobiology,* **73**, 621–9.

Goff L, Bell J, So P, Dornhorst A and Frost G (2005) Veganism and its relationship with insulin resistance and intramyocellular lipid. *European Journal of Clinical Nutrition,* **59**, 291–8.

Goldberg J, Flowerdew G, Smith E, *et al.* (1988) Factors associated with age-related macular degeneration. An analysis of data from the first National Health and Nutrition Examination Survey. *American Journal of Epidemiology,* **128**, 700–10.

Goldberg RB (2006) Lifestyle interventions to prevent type 2 diabetes. *Lancet,* **368**, 1634–6.

Gollnick P, Piehl K, Saubert C, *et al.* (1972) Diet, exercise, and glycogen changes in human muscle fibers. *Journal of Applied Physiology,* **33**, 421–5.

Gon Y, Hashimoto S, Hayashi S, *et al.* (1996) Lower serum concentrations of cytokines in elderly patients with pneumonia and the impaired production of cytokines by peripheral blood monocytes in the elderly. *Clinical & Experimental Immunology,* **106**, 120–6.

Gonzalez CA, Jakszyn P, Pera G, *et al.* (2006a) Meat intake and risk of stomach and esophageal adenocarcinoma within the European Prospective Investigation Into Cancer and Nutrition (EPIC). *Journal of the National Cancer Institute,* **98**, 345–54.

Gonzalez CA, Pera G, Agudo A, *et al.* (2006b) Fruit and vegetable intake and the risk of stomach and oesophagus adenocarcinoma in the European Prospective Investigation into Cancer and Nutrition (EPIC-EURGAST). *International Journal of Cancer,* **118**, 2559–66.

Gonzalez S, Astner S, An W, *et al.* (2003) Dietary lutein/zeaxanthin decreases ultraviolet B-induced epidermal hyperproliferation and acute inflammation in hairless mice. *Journal of Investigative Dermatology,* **121**, 399–405.

Goodman GE, Thornquist MD, Balmes J, *et al.* (2004) The Beta-Carotene and Retinol Efficacy Trial: incidence of lung cancer and cardiovascular disease mortality during 6-year follow-up after stopping beta-carotene and retinol supplements. *Journal of the National Cancer Institute,* **96**, 1743–50.

Goodpaster B, He J, Watkins S and Kelley D (2001) Skeletal muscle lipid content and insulin resistance: evidence for a paradox in endurance-trained athletes. *Journal of Clinical Endocrinology and Metabolism,* **86**, 5755–61.

Goodpaster B, Park S, Harris T, *et al.* (2006) The loss of skeletal muscle strength, mass, and quality in older adults: the health, aging and body composition study. *Journals of Gerontology Series A – Biological Sciences & Medical Sciences,* **61**, 1059–64.

Goodson WH, III and Hunt TK (1988) Wound healing and nutrition. *Nutrition and Metabolism in Patient Care.* Ed. J. M. Kinney, K. N. Jeejeebhoy, G. L. Hill and O. E. Owen. Philadelphia, WB Saunders: 635–42.

Goodwin JS and Garry PJ (1983) Relationship between megadose vitamin supplementation and immunological function in a healthy elderly population. *Clinical & Experimental Immunology,* **51**, 647–53.

Goodwin JS and Garry PJ (1988) Lack of correlation between indices of nutritional status and immunologic function in elderly humans. *Journal of Gerontology,* **43**, M46–9.

Gorczynski RM, Cinader B, Ramakrishna V, *et al.* (1997) An antibody specific for interleukin-6 reverses age-associated changes in spontaneous and induced cytokine production in mice. *Immunology,* **92**, 20–5.

Gorse GJ, Thrupp LD, Nudleman KL, *et al.* (1984) Bacterial meningitis in the elderly. *Archives of Internal Medicine,* **144**, 1603–7.

Gosling P, Rothe HM, Sheehan TM and Hubbard LD (1995) Serum copper and zinc concentrations in patients with burns in relation to burn surface area. *Journal of Burn Care & Rehabilitation,* **16**, 481–6.

Goulding A (2003) Nutritional strategies for prevention and treatment of osteoporosis in populations and individuals. In: *Nutritional Aspects of Bone Health.* Ed. S. A. New and J. P. Bonjour. Cambridge, Royal Society of Chemistry: 709–32.

Goulding A and Grant A (2007) Nutritional strategies to optimize bone health throughout the life course. In: *Managing Osteoporosis.* Ed. S. A. Lanham-New, T. O'Neill, R. Morris, D. Skeleton and A. Sutcliffe. Oxford, Clinical Publishing: 3–20.

Government Office for Science (2007) *Tackling Obesities: Future Choices. Project Report* (www.foresight.gov.uk).

Graat JM, Schouten EG and Kok FJ (2002) Effect of daily vitamin E and multivitamin-mineral supplementation on acute respiratory tract infections in elderly persons: a randomized controlled trial. *Journal of the American Medical Association,* **288**, 715–21.

Grace PB, Taylor JI, Low Y-L, *et al.* (2004) Phytoestrogen concentrations in serum and spot urine as biomarkers for dietary phytoestrogen intake and their relation to breast cancer risk in European prospective investigation of cancer and nutrition – Norfolk. *Cancer Epidemiology, Biomarkers & Prevention,* **13**, 698–708.

Grant AM, Avenell A, Campbell MK, *et al.* (2005) Oral vitamin D$_3$ and calcium for secondary prevention of low-trauma fractures in elderly people (Randomised Evaluation of Calcium Or vitamin D, RECORD): a randomised placebo-controlled trial. *Lancet*, **365**, 1621–8.

Grant WB and Holick MF (2005) Benefits and requirements of vitamin D for optimal health: a review. *Alternative Medicine Review*, **10**, 94–111.

Gray A, Feldman HA, McKinlay JB and Longcope C (1991) Age, disease, and changing sex hormone levels in middle-aged men: results of the Massachusetts Male Aging Study. *Journal of Clinical Endocrinology & Metabolism*, **73**, 1016–25.

Green MR and van der Ouderaa F (2003) Nutrigenomics: where next for the food industry? *Pharmacogenomics Journal*, **3(4)**, 191–3.

Green MR, Basketter DA, Couchman JR and Rees DA (1983) Distribution and number of epidermal growth factor receptors in skin is related to epithelial cell growth. *Developmental Biology*, **100**, 506–12.

Green T, Venn B, Skeaff C and Williams S (2005) Serum vitamin B12 concentrations and atrophic gastritis in older New Zealanders. *European Journal of Clinical Nutrition*, **59**, 205–10.

Greenberg JA, Dunbar CC, Schnoll R, *et al.* (2007) Caffeinated beverage intake and the risk of heart disease mortality in the elderly: a prospective analysis. *American Journal of Clinical Nutrition*, **85**, 392–8.

Greenlee RT, Murray T, Bolden S and Wingo PA (2000) Cancer statistics, 2000. *CA: A Cancer Journal for Clinicians*, **50**, 7–33.

Greenlund LJS and Nair KS (2003) Sarcopenia – consequences, mechanisms, and potential therapies. *Mechanisms of Ageing & Development*, **124**, 287–99.

Greeves J, Cable N, Luckas M, *et al.* (1997) Effects of acute changes in oestrogen on muscle function of the first dorsal interosseus muscle in humans. *Journal of Physiology*, **500**, 265–70.

Gregory J, Lowe S, Bates CJ, *et al.* (2000) *National Diet and Nutrition Survey: Young People Aged 4 to 18 years. Volume 1: Report of the Diet and Nutrition Survey.* London, Stationery Office.

Greig C, Botella J and Young A (1993) The quadriceps strength of healthy elderly people remeasured after eight years. *Muscle Nerve*, **16**, 6–10.

Griffith JD, Comeau L, Rosenfield S, *et al.* (1999) Mammalian telomeres end in a large duplex loop. *Cell*, **97**, 503–14.

Griffiths CE, Russman AN, Majmudar G, *et al.* (1993) Restoration of collagen formation in photodamaged human skin by tretinoin (retinoic acid). *New England Journal of Medicine*, **329**, 530–5.

Grimaldi LM, Casadei VM, Ferri C, *et al.* (2000) Association of early-onset Alzheimer's disease with an interleukin-1alpha gene polymorphism. *Annals of Neurology*, **47**, 361–5.

Grimble RF (2003) Inflammatory response in the elderly. *Current Opinion in Clinical Nutrition & Metabolic Care*, **6**, 21–9.

Grinnell F, Rocha LB, Iucu C, *et al.* (2006) Nested collagen matrices: a new model to study migration of human fibroblast populations in three dimensions. *Experimental Cell Research*, **312**, 86–94.

Gronemeyer H and Laudet V (1995) Transcription factors 3: nuclear receptors. *Protein Profile*, **2**, 1173–308.

Grose R and Werner S (2002) An aPPARently protective mechanism for keratinocytes in wounded skin. *Trends in Molecular Medicine*, **8**, 149–51.

Gross G, Jaccaud E and Huggett A (1997) Analysis of the content of the diterpenes cafestol and kahweol in coffee brews. *Food Chemistry and Toxicology*, **35**, 547–54.

Grossmann M, Nakamura Y, Grumont R and Gerondakis S (1999) New insights into the roles of ReL/NF-kappa B transcription factors in immune function, hemopoiesis and human disease. *International Journal of Biochemistry & Cell Biology*, **31**, 1209–19.

Grubben M, Boers G, Blom H, *et al.* (2000) Unfiltered coffee increases plasma homocysteine concentrations in healthy volunteers: a randomised trial. *American Journal of Clinical Nutrition*, **71**, 480–4.

Grube K and Burkle A (1992) Poly(ADP-ribose) polymerase activity in mononuclear leukocytes of 13 mammalian species correlates with species-specific lifespan. *Proceedings of the National Academy of Sciences of the United States of America*, **89**, 11759–63.

Guerre-Millo M (2004) Adipose tissue and adipokines: for better or worse. *Diabetes and Metabolism*, **30**, 13–19.

Guillet C, Zangarelli A, Gachon P, *et al.* (2004) Whole body protein breakdown is less inhibited by insulin, but still responsive to amino acid, in nondiabetic elderly subjects. *Journal of Clinical Endocrinology and Metabolism*, **89**, 6017–24.

Gunne HJ (1985) Masticatory efficiency and dental state. A comparison between two methods. *Acta Odontologica Scandinavic*, **43**, 139–46.

Guo L, LaDu MJ and Van Eldik LJ (2004) A dual role for apolipoprotein e in neuroinflammation: anti- and pro-inflammatory activity. *Journal of Molecular Neuroscience*, **23**, 205–12.

Guo S, Roche A, Chumlea W, *et al.* (2000) Statistical effects of varying sample sizes on the precision of percentile estimates. *American Journal of Human Biology*, **12**, 64–74.

Guralnik J, Eisenstaedt R, Ferrucci L, *et al.* (2004) Prevalence of anemia in persons 65 years and older in the United States: evidence for a high rate of unexplained anemia. *Blood*, **104**, 2263–8.

Hager K, Machein U, Krieger S, *et al.* (1994) Interleukin-6 and selected plasma proteins in healthy persons of different ages. *Neurobiology of Aging*, **15**, 771–2.

Hagfors L, Leanderson P, Skoldstam L *et al.* (2003) Antioxidant intake, plasma antioxidants and oxidative stress in a randomised controlled parallel, Mediterranean dietary intervention study on patients with rheumatoid arthritis. *Nutrition Journal*, **2**, 1475–91.

Haigis M and Guarente L (2006) Mammalian sirtuins – emerging roles in physiology, aging, and calorie restriction. *Genes and Development*, **20**, 2913–21.

Haley-Zitlin V and Richardson A (1993) Effect of dietary restriction on DNA repair and DNA damage. *Mutation Research*, **295**, 237–45.

Halioua L and Anderson JJ (1989) Lifetime calcium intake and physical activity habits: independent and combined effects on the radial bone of healthy premenopausal Caucasian women. *American Journal of Clinical Nutrition*, **49**, 534–41.

Hall G and Phillips TJ (2005) Estrogen and skin: the effects of estrogen, menopause, and hormone replacement therapy on the skin. *Journal of the American Academy of Dermatology*, **53**, 555–68.

Hallbook T and Lanner E (1972) Serum-zinc and healing of venous leg ulcers. *Lancet*, **2**, 780–2.

Halpern GM, Prindiville T, Blankenburg M, *et al.* (1996) Treatment of irritable bowel syndrome with Lacteol Fort: a randomized, double-blind, cross-over trial. *American Journal of Gastroenterology*, **91**, 1579–85.

Hampel H, Abraham NS and El-Serag HB (2005) Meta-analysis: obesity and the risk for gastroesophageal reflux disease and its complications. *Annals of Internal Medicine*, **143**, 199–211.

Hankey CR, Cullen A, Wynne *et al.* (1993) Non-starch polysaccharide/dietary fibre supplementation using small meals in long-stay frail elderly patients. *European Journal of Clinical Nutrition*, **47**, 521–3.

Hankinson SE and Eliassen AH (2007) Endogenous estrogen, testosterone and progesterone levels in relation to breast cancer risk. *Journal of Steroid Biochemistry and Molecular Biology*, **106**, 24–30.

Hankinson SE, Stampfer MJ, Seddon JM, *et al.* (1992) Nutrient intake and cataract extraction in women: a prospective study. *British Medical Journal*, **305**, 335–9.

Hanley K, Komuves LG, Bass NM, *et al.* (1999) Fetal epidermal differentiation and barrier development *in vivo* is accelerated by nuclear hormone receptor activators. *Journal of Investigative Dermatology*, **113**, 788–95.

Hannaford PC, Selvaraj S, Elliott AM, *et al.* (2007) Cancer risk among users of oral contraceptives: cohort data from the Royal College of General Practitioners' oral contraception study. *British Medical Journal*, **335**, 651.

Hannan MT, Felson DT, Dawson-Hughes B, *et al.* (2000a) Risk factors for longitudinal bone loss in elderly men and women: the Framingham Osteoporosis Study. *Journal of Bone & Mineral Research*, **15**, 710–20.

Hannan MT, Tucker KL, *et al.* (2000b) Effect of dietary protein on bone loss in elderly men and women: the Framingham Osteoporosis Study. *Journal of Bone & Mineral Research*, **15**, 2504–12.

Hara M, Tanaka K and Hirota Y (2005) Immune response to influenza vaccine in healthy adults and the elderly: association with nutritional status. *Vaccine*, **23**, 1457–63.

Harbottle A and Birch-Machin MA (2006) Real-time PCR analysis of a 3895 bp mitochondrial DNA deletion in nonmelanoma skin cancer and its use as a quantitative marker for sunlight exposure in human skin. *British Journal of Cancer*, **94**, 1887–93.

Harman D (1956) Aging: a theory based on free radical and radiation chemistry. *Journal of Gerontology*, **11**, 298–300.

Harman S, Metter E, Tobin J, *et al.* (2001) Longitudinal effects of aging on serum total and free testosterone levels in healthy men. Baltimore Longitudinal Study of Aging. *Journal of Clinical Endocrinology and Metabolism*, **86**, 724–31.

Harper EJ (1998) Changing perspectives on aging and energy requirements: aging and digestive function in humans, dogs and cats. *Journal of Nutrition*, **128**, 2632S–5S.

Harris TB, Ferrucci L, Tracy RP, *et al.* (1999) Associations of elevated interleukin-6 and C-reactive protein levels with mortality in the elderly. *American Journal of Medicine*, **106**, 506–12.

Harrison DE and Archer JR (1989) Natural selection for extended longevity from food restriction. *Growth, Development, & Aging*, **53**, 3.

Hartwig M (1995) Immune ageing and Alzheimer's disease. *Neuroreport*, **6**, 1274–6.

Hartwig M and Steinmann G (1994) On a causal mechanism of chronic thymic involution in man. *Mechanisms of Ageing & Development*, **75**, 151–6.

Hascall V and Kuettner KE (2002) *The Many Faces of Osteoarthritis*. Basel, Birkhauser Verlag.

Hasegawa Y, Sawada M, Ozaki N, *et al.* (2000) Increased soluble tumor necrosis factor receptor levels in the serum of elderly people. *Gerontology*, **46**, 185–8.

Hassan A and Gordon CM (2007) Polycystic ovary syndrome update in adolescence. *Current Opinion in Pediatrics*, **19**, 389–97.

Hasten D, Pak-Loduca J, Obert K and Yarasheski K (2000) Resistance exercise acutely increases MHC and mixed muscle protein synthesis rates in 78–84 and 23–32 yr olds. *American Journal Of Physiology-Endocrinology & Metabolism*, **278**, E620–6.

Hata TR, Scholz TA, Ermakov IV, *et al.* (2000) Non-invasive raman spectroscopic detection of carotenoids in human skin. *Journal of Investigative Dermatology*, **115**, 441–8.

Hathcock JN, Shao A, Vieth R and Heaney R (2007) Risk assessment for vitamin D. *American Journal of Clinical Nutrition*, **85**, 6–18.

Hattersley A, Beards F, Ballantyne E, *et al.* (1998) Mutations in the glucokinase gene of the fetus result in reduced birth weight. *Nature Genetics*, **19**, 268–70.

Haugaard SB, Madsbad S, Hoy C-E and Vaag A (2006) Dietary intervention increases n-3 long-chain polyunsaturated fatty acids in skeletal muscle membrane phospholipids of obese subjects. Implications for insulin sensitivity. *Clinical Endocrinology*, **64**, 169–78.

Hauner H (2002) Insulin resistance and the metabolic syndrome – a challenge of the new millennium. *European Journal of Clinical Nutrition*, **56 (Suppl 1)**, S25–9.

Hauner H (2005) Secretory factors from human adipose tissue and their functional role. *Proceedings of the Nutrition Society*, **64**, 163–9.

Havel PJ (2004) Update on adipocyte hormones: regulation of energy balance and carbohydrate/lipid metabolism. *Diabetes*, **53 (Suppl 1)**, S143–51.

Haveman-Nies A, de Groot L and van Staveren W (2003) Dietary quality, lifestyle factors and healthy ageing in Europe: the SENECA study. *Age & Ageing*, **32**, 427–34.

Hawkes C (2006) Olfaction in neurodegenerative disorder. *Advances in Oto-rhino-laryngology*, **63**, 133–51.

Hawkes W and Hornbostel L (1996) Effects of dietary selenium on mood in healthy men living in a metabolic research unit. *Biological Psychiatry*, **39**, 121–8.

Hayward LM, Burden ML, Burden AC, *et al.* (2002) What is the prevalence of visual impairment in the general and diabetic populations: are there ethnic and gender differences? *Diabetic Medicine*, **19**, 27–34.

He K, Rimm E, Merchant A, *et al.* (2002) Fish consumption and risk of stroke in men. *Journal of the American Medical Association*, **288**, 3130–6.

Health & Social Care Information Centre (2005) Health Survey for England 2004 – Updating of Trend Tables to include 2004 data. www.ic.nhs/pubs.

Health & Social Care Information Centre (2006) Health Survey for England 2004. Updating of Trend Tables to Include Childhood Obesity Data. www.ic.nhs.uk/pubs.

Heaney RP, Dowell MS, Dawson-Hughes B, *et al.* (2003) Calcium absorption varies within the reference range for serum 25-hydroxyvitamin D. *Journal of the American College of Nutrition*, **22**, 142–6.

Heart Outcomes Prevention Evaluation (HOPE) Study Investigators (2000) Effects of an angiotensin converting enzyme inhibitor, ramipril, on cardiovascular events in high-risk patients. *New England Journal of Medicine*, **342**, 145–53.

Heart Protection Study (2002) MRC/BHF Heart Protection Study of antioxidant vitamin supplementation in 20,536 high-risk individuals: a randomised placebo-controlled trial. *Lancet*, **360**, 23–33.

Heavey PM, McKenna D and Rowland IR (2004) Colorectal cancer and the relationship between genes and the environment. *Nutrition & Cancer*, **48**, 124–41.

Heijnen ML, van Amelsvoort JM, Deurenberg P and Beynen AC (1998) Limited effect of consumption of uncooked (RS2) or retrograded (RS3) resistant starch on putative risk factors for colon cancer in healthy men. *American Journal of Clinical Nutrition*, **67**, 322–31.

Heilbronn LK and Clifton PM (2002) C-reactive protein and coronary artery disease: Influence of obesity, caloric restriction and weight loss. *Journal of Nutritional Biochemistry*, **13**, 316–21.

Heilbronn LK, de Jonge L, Frisard MI, *et al.* (2006) Effect of 6-month calorie restriction on biomarkers of longevity, metabolic adaptation, and oxidative stress in overweight individuals: a randomized controlled trial. *Journal of the American Medical Association*, **295**, 1539–48.

Heinrich U, Gartner C, Wiebusch M, *et al.* (2003) Supplementation with beta-carotene or a similar amount of mixed carotenoids protects humans from UV-induced erythema. *Journal of Nutrition*, **133**, 98–101.

Helisalmi S, Hiltunen M, Valonen P, *et al.* (1999) Promoter polymorphism (-491A/T) in the APOE gene of Finnish Alzheimer's disease patients and control individuals. *Journal of Neurology*, **246**, 821–4.

Helliwell TR, Wilkinson A, Griffiths RD, *et al.* (1998) Muscle fibre atrophy in critically ill patients is associated with the loss of myosin filaments and the presence of lysosomal enzymes and ubiquitin. *Neuropathology & Applied Neurobiology*, **24**, 507–17.

Henderson CD, Black HS and Wolf JE, Jr. (1989) Influence of omega-3 and omega-6 fatty acid sources on prostaglandin levels in mice. *Lipids*, **24**, 502–5.

Henderson L, Gregory J and Swan G (2002) *The National Diet & Nutrition Survey: Adults aged 19 to 64 Years. Volume 1: Types and Quantities of Foods Consumed.* London, Stationery Office.

Henderson L, Gregory J, Irving K and Swan G (2003) *The National Diet and Nutrition Survey: Adults Aged 19–64 Years. Volume 2: Energy, Protein, Carbohydrate, Fat and Alcohol Intake.* London, Stationery Office.

Henderson L, Gregory J, Irving K, *et al.* (2003) *The National Diet and Nutrition Survey: Adults Aged 19–64 Years. Volume 3: Vitamin and Mineral Intake and Urinary Analysis.* London, Stationery Office.

Henrotin Y, Sanchez C, Deberg M, *et al.* (2003) Avocado/soybean unsaponifiables increase aggrecan synthesis and reduce catabolic and proinflammatory mediator production by human osteoarthritic chondrocytes. *Journal of Rheumatology*, **30**, 1825–34.

Henzel JH, DeWeese MS and Lichti EL (1970) Zinc concentrations within healing wounds. Significance of postoperative zincuria on availability and requirements during tissue repair. *Archives of Surgery*, **100**, 349–57.

Herraiz L, Rahman A, Parker R and Roe D (1994) The role of beta-carotene supplementation in prevention of photosuppression of cellular immunity in elderly men. *FASEB Journal*, **8**, A423.

Herraiz LA, Hsieh WC, Parker RS, *et al.* (1998) Effect of UV exposure and beta-carotene supplementation on delayed-type hypersensitivity response in healthy older men. *Journal of the American College of Nutrition*, **17**, 617–24.

Herrmann W, Quast S, Ullrich M, *et al.* (1999) Hyperhomocysteinemia in high-aged subjects: relation of B-vitamins, folic acid, renal function and the methylenetetrahydrofolate reductase mutation. *Atherosclerosis*, **144**, 91–101.

Heuberger RA, Mares-Perlman JA, Klein R, *et al.* (2001) Relationship of dietary fat to age-related maculopathy in the Third National Health and Nutrition Examination Survey. *Archives of Ophthalmology*, **119**, 1833–8.

Heuser MD and Adler WH (1997) Immunological aspects of aging and malnutrition: consequences and intervention with nutritional immunomodulators. *Clinics in Geriatric Medicine*, **13**, 697–715.

Heydari AR, You S, Takahashi R, *et al.* (1996) Effect of caloric restriction on the expression of heat shock protein 70 and the activation of heat shock transcription factor 1. *Developmental Genetics*, **18**, 114–24.

Heymsfield S, Lohman T, Wang Z and Going S (2005) *Human Body Composition.* 2nd edition. Champaign, IL, Human Kinetics.

Hickson M, D'Souza AL, Muthu N, *et al.* (2007) Use of probiotic *Lactobacillus* preparation to prevent diarrhoea associated with antibiotics: randomised double blind placebo controlled trial. *British Medical Journal*, **335**, 80–3.

Higgins PD and Johanson JF (2004) Epidemiology of constipation in North America: a systematic review. *American Journal of Gastroenterology*, **99**, 750–9.

Hightower KR (1994) A review of the evidence that ultraviolet irradiation is a risk factor in cataractogenesis. *Documenta ophthalmologica. Advances in Ophthalmology*, **88**, 205–20.

Hightower KR (1995) The role of the lens epithelium in development of UV cataract. *Current Eye Research*, **14**, 71–8.

Hill MJ (1988) Gut flora and cancer in humans and laboratory animals. In: *The Role of the Gut Flora in Toxicity and Cancer*. Ed. I. R. Rowland. London, Academic Press: 461–502.

Hill MJ (1995) The normal gut bacterial flora. In: *The Role of Gut Bacteria in Human Toxicology and Pharmacology*. Ed. M. J. Hill. London, Taylor & Francis: 3–17.

Hin H, Clarke R, Sherliker P, *et al.* (2006) Clinical relevance of low serum vitamin B_{12} concentrations in older people: Banbury B12 study. *Age & Ageing*, **35**, 416–22.

Hines L, Stampfer M, Ma J, *et al.* (2001) Genetic variation in alcohol dehydrogenase and the beneficial effect of moderate alcohol consumption on myocardial infarction. *New England Journal of Medicine*, **344**, 549–55.

Ho E (2004) Zinc deficiency, DNA damage and cancer risk. *Journal of Nutritional Biochemistry*, **15**, 572–8.

Hobbs K, Mascali J, Klemm D and Borish L (1996) Contribution of interleukin (IL)-10 promoter polymorphism to allergic inflammation. *Journal of Allergy & Clinical Immunology*, **97**, 714.

Hodge W, Barnes D, Schachter HM, *et al.* (2005) Effects of omega-3 fatty acids on eye health. Summary. *Evidence Report/Technology Assessment.* Rockville, MD, Agency for Healthcare Research and Quality.

Hodgson J, Burke V, Beilin L and Puddey I (2005) Increased protein intake from lean red meat lowers blood pressure in hypertensive men and women. *Fifteenth European Meeting on Hypertension,* Abstract No. 635.

Hoffmann JC and Zeitz M (2002) Small bowel disease in the elderly: diarrhoea and malabsorption. *Best Practice & Research: Clinical Gastroenterology*, **16**, 17–36.

Hofman MA and Swaab DF (2006) Living by the clock: the circadian pacemaker in older people. *Ageing Research Reviews*, **5**, 33–51.

Hogg R and Chakravarthy U (2004) AMD and micronutrient antioxidants. *Current Eye Research*, **29**, 387–401.

Hogstrom M, Nordstrom P and Nordstrom A (2007) *n*-3 Fatty acids are positively associated with peak bone mineral density and bone accrual in healthy men: the NO_2 Study. *American Journal of Clinical Nutrition*, **85**, 803–7.

Hoidrup S, Gronbaek M, Gottschau A, *et al.* (1999) Alcohol intake, beverage preference, and risk of hip fracture in men and women. Copenhagen Centre for Prospective Population Studies. *American Journal of Epidemiology*, **149**, 993–1001.

Holben D and Smith A (1999) The diverse role of selenium within selenoproteins: a review. *Journal of the American Dietetic Association*, **99**, 836–43.

Holbrook TL and Barrett-Connor E (1993) A prospective study of alcohol consumption and bone mineral density. *British Medical Journal*, **306**, 1506–9.

Holick MF (2000) Microgravity-induced bone loss – will it limit human space exploration? *Lancet*, **355**, 1569–70.

Holick MF (2004) Sunlight and vitamin D for bone health and prevention of autoimmune diseases, cancers, and cardiovascular disease. *American Journal of Clinical Nutrition*, **80**, 1678S–88S.

Holick MF (2007) Vitamin D deficiency. *New England Journal of Medicine*, **357**, 266–81.

Holliday R (1987) The inheritance of epigenetic defects. *Science*, **238**, 163–70.

Holliday R (1989) Food, reproduction and longevity: is the extended lifespan of calorie-restricted animals an evolutionary adaptation? *Bioessays*, **10**, 125–7.

Hollingworth W, Todd C and Parker M (1995) The cost of treating hip fractures in the twenty-first century. *Journal of Public Health Medicine*, **17**, 269–76.

Hollman PC and Katan MB (1999) Health effects and bioavailability of dietary flavonols. *Free Radical Research*, **31**, S75–80.

Homocysteine Studies Collaboration (2002) Homocysteine and risk of ischemic heart disease and stroke: a meta-analysis. *Journal of the American Medical Association*, **288**, 2015–22.

Homocysteine-Lowering Trialists' Collaboration (2005) Dose-dependent effects of folic acid on plasma homocysteine concentrations. A meta-analysis of the randomised trials. *American Journal of Clinical Nutrition*, **82**, 806–12.

Hooper L, Thompson R, Harrison R, *et al.* (2006) Risks and benefits of omega-3 fats for mortality, cardiovascular disease, and cancer: systematic review. *British Medical Journal*, **332**, 752–60.

Hooper MM, Stellato TA, Hallowell PT, *et al.* (2007) Musculoskeletal findings in obese subjects before and after weight loss following bariatric surgery. *International Journal of Obesity*, **31**, 114–20.

Hope AK and Down EC (1986) Dietary fibre and fluid in the control of constipation in a nursing home population. *Medical Journal of Australia*, **144**, 306–7.

Hopkins MJ, Sharp R and Macfarlane GT (2001) Age and disease related changes in intestinal bacterial populations assessed by cell culture, 16S rRNA abundance, and community cellular fatty acid profiles. *Gut*, **48**, 198–205.

Hori O, Yan SD, Ogawa S, *et al.* (1996) The receptor for advanced glycation end-products has a central role in mediating the effects of advanced glycation end-products on the development of vascular disease in diabetes mellitus. *Nephrology Dialysis Transplantation*, **11 (Suppl 5)**, 13–16.

House of Lords (2005) *Ageing: Scientific Aspects. Report from the Science and Technology Committee.* London, Stationery Office.

Hsing AW, Hansson LE, McLaughlin JK, *et al.* (1993) Pernicious anemia and subsequent cancer. A population-based cohort study. *Cancer*, **71**, 745–50.

Hu F (2003) Plant-based foods and prevention of cardiovascular disease: an overview. *American Journal of Clinical Nutrition*, **78**, 544S–51S.

Hu F (2005) Protein, body weight and cardiovascular health. *American Journal of Clinical Nutrition*, **82**, 242S–7S.

Hu F and Stampfer M (1999) Nut consumption and risk of coronary heart disease: a review of epidemiologic evidence. *Current Atherosclerosis Reports*, **1**, 204–9.

Hu F, Bronner L, Willett W, *et al.* (2002) Fish and omega-3 fatty acid intake and risk of coronary heart disease in women. *The Journal of the American Medical Association*, **10**, 1815–21.

Hu F, Manson J and Willett W (2001) Types of dietary fat and risk of coronary heart disease: a critical review. *Journal of the American College of Nutrition*, **20**, 5–19.

Hu F, Rimm E, Stampfer M, *et al.* (2000) Prospective study of major dietary patterns and risk of coronary heart disease in men. *American Journal of Clinical Nutrition*, **72**, 912–21.

Hu F, Stampfer MJ, Colditz GA, *et al.* (2000) Physical activity and risk of stroke in women. *Journal of the American Medical Association*, **11**, 1784–5.

Hu FB, Stampfer MJ, Rimm EB, *et al.* (1999) A prospective study of egg consumption and risk of cardiovascular disease in men and women. *Journal of the American Medical Association*, **281**, 1387–94.

Hu FB, Willett WC, Li T, *et al.* (2004) Adiposity as compared with physical activity in predicting mortality among women. *New England Journal of Medicine*, **351**, 2694–703.

Hu Y, Martin J, Le Leu R and Young GP (2002) The colonic response to genotoxic carcinogens in the rat: regulation by dietary fibre. *Carcinogenesis*, **23**, 1131–7.

Huang Y, Macera CA, Blair SN, *et al.* (1998) Physical fitness, physical activity, and functional limitation in adults aged 40 and older. *Medicine & Science in Sports & Exercise*, **30**, 1430–5.

Hughes V, Frontera W, Roubenoff R, *et al.* (2002) Longitudinal changes in body composition in older men and women: role of body weight change and physical activity. *American Journal of Clinical Nutrition*, **76**, 473–81.

Hughes V, Frontera W, Wood M, *et al.* (2001) Longitudinal muscle strength changes in older adults: influence of muscle mass, physical activity, and health. *The Journals of Gerontology, Series A, Biological Sciences and Medical Sciences*, **56**, B209–17.

Hull M, Eistetter J, Fiebich BL and Bauer J (1999) Glutamate but not interleukin-6 influences the phosphorylation of tau in primary rat hippocampal neurons. *Neuroscience Letters*, **261**, 33–6.

Hulse G, Lautenschlager N, Tait R and Almeida O (2005) Dementia associated with alcohol and other drug use. *International Psychogeriatrics*, **17 (Suppl 1)**, S109–27.

Hulsey TK, O'Neill JA, Neblett WR and Meng HC (1980) Experimental wound healing in essential fatty acid deficiency. *Journal of Pediatric Surgery*, **15**, 505–8.

Hung CY, Perkins EH and Yang WK (1975) Age-related refractoriness of PHA-induced lymphocyte transformation. II. 125-I-PHA binding to spleen cells from young and old mice. *Mechanisms of Ageing & Development*, **4**, 103–12.

Hung HC, Willett W, Ascherio A, *et al.* (2003) Tooth loss and dietary intake. *Journal of the American Dental Association*, **134**, 1185–92.

Hunt D, Young P, Simes J, *et al.* (2001) Benefits of pravastatin on cardiovascular events and mortality in older patients with coronary heart disease are equal to or exceed those seen in younger patients: results from the LIPID trial. *Annals of Internal Medicine*, **134**, 931–40.

Hunt RJ, Eldredge JB and Beck JD (1989) Effect of residence in a fluoridated community on the incidence of coronal and root caries in an older adult population. *Journal of Public Health Dentistry*, **49**, 138–41.

Huppert F, Pinto E, Morgan K and Brayne C (2003) Survival in a population sample is predicted by proportions of lymphocyte subsets. *Mechanisms of Ageing & Development*, **124**, 449–51.

Hurson M, Regan M, Kirk S, *et al.* (1995) Metabolic effects of arginine in a healthy elderly population. *Journal of Parenteral and Enteral Nutrition*, **19**, 227–30.

Hurwitz A, Brady DA, Schaal SE, *et al.* (1997) Gastric acidity in older adults. *Journal of the American Medical Association*, **278**, 659–62.

Husebye E, Hellstrom PM, Sundler F, *et al.* (2001) Influence of microbial species on small intestinal myoelectric activity and transit in germ-free rats. *American Journal of Physiology – Gastrointestinal and Liver Physiology*, **280**, G368–80.

Huxley R, Barzi F and Woodward M (2006) Excess risk of fatal coronary heart disease associated with diabetes in men and women: meta-analysis of 37 prospective cohort studies. *British Medical Journal*, **332**, 73–8.

Hypponen E and Power C (2007) Hypovitaminosis D in British adults at age 45 y: nationwide cohort study of dietary and lifestyle predictors. *American Journal of Clinical Nutrition*, **85**, 860–8.

Ibs K-H and Rink L (2004) Zinc. In: *Diet and Human Immune Function*. Ed. D. A. Hughes, L. G. Darlington and A. Bendich. Totawa, NJ, Humana Press.

Ikata J, Wakatsuki T, Oishi Y, *et al.* (2000) Leukocyte counts and concentrations of soluble adhesion molecules as predictors of coronary atherosclerosis. *Coronary Artery Disease*, **11**, 445–9.

International ARM Epidemiological Study Group (1995) An international classification and grading system for age-related maculopathy and age-related macular degeneration. *Survey of Ophthalmology*, **39**, 367–74.

Intersalt Cooperative Research Group (1988) Intersalt: an international study of electrolyte excretion and blood pressure. Results for 24 hour urinary sodium and potassium excretion. *British Medical Journal*, **297**, 319–28.

Ipsos MORI (2006) *Public Consultation into Ageing: Research into Public Attitudes towards BBSRC and MRC-funded Research on Ageing*. http://www.bbsrc.ac.uk/society/dialogue/attitude/ageing_mori_sri.pdf. Ipsos MORI.

Ishihara L and Brayne C (2005) A systematic review of nutritional risk factors of Parkinson's disease. *Nutrition Research Reviews*, **18**, 259–82.

Ishikawa H, Akedo I, Otani T, *et al.* (2005) Randomized trial of dietary fiber and *Lactobacillus* casei administration for prevention of colorectal tumors. *International Journal of Cancer*, **116**, 762–7.

Isidori AM, Strollo F, More M, *et al.* (2000) Leptin and aging: correlation with endocrine changes in male and female healthy adult populations of different body-weights. *Journal of Clinical Endocrinology & Metabolism*, **85**, 1954–62.

Iso H, Sato S, Umemura U, *et al.* (2002) Linoleic acid, other fatty acids, and the risk of stroke. *Stroke*, **33**, 2086–93.

Iso H, Stampfer M, Manson J, *et al.* (2001) Prospective study of fat and protein intake and risk of intraparenchymal hemorrhage in women. *Circulation*, **103**, 856–63.

Issa AM, Mojica WA, Morton SC, *et al.* (2006) The efficacy of omega-3 fatty acids on cognitive function in aging and dementia: a systematic review. *Dementia & Geriatric Cognitive Disorders*, **21**, 88–96.

Issa JP (2003) Age-related epigenetic changes and the immune system. *Clinical Immunology*, **109**, 103–8.

Issa JP, Ahuja N, Toyota M, *et al.* (2001) Accelerated age-related CpG island methylation in ulcerative colitis. *Cancer Research*, **61**, 3573–7.

Issa JP, Ottaviano YL, Celano P, *et al.* (1994) Methylation of the oestrogen receptor CpG island links ageing and neoplasia in human colon. *Nature Genetics*, **7**, 536–40.

Issemann I and Green S (1990) Activation of a member of the steroid hormone receptor superfamily by peroxisome proliferators. *Nature*, **347**, 645–50.

Italian-American Cataract Study Group (1991) Risk factors for age-related cortical, nuclear, and posterior subcapsular cataracts. *American Journal of Epidemiology*, **133**, 541–53.

Jackson GR, Owsley C and Curcio CA (2002) Photoreceptor degeneration and dysfunction in aging and age-related maculopathy. *Ageing Research Reviews*, **1**, 381–96.

Jacobs D, Meyer K, Kushi L and Folsom A (1998) Whole grain intake may reduce the risk of ischemic heart disease death in postmenopausal women: the Iowa Women's Health Study. *American Journal of Nutrition*, **68**, 248–57.

Jacobs D, Meyer K, Kushi L and Folsom A (1999) Is whole grain intake associated with reduced total and cause-specific death rates in older women? The Iowa Women's Health Study. *American Journal of Public Health*, **89**, 322–9.

Jacobzone S (1999) *Ageing and Care for the Frail Elderly Persons: An Overview of International Perspectives*. OECD Labour Market and Social Policy – Occasional Papers, No. 38. Paris, OECD.

Jacques PF and Chylack LT, Jr. (1991) Epidemiologic evidence of a role for the antioxidant vitamins and carotenoids in cataract prevention. *American Journal of Clinical Nutrition*, **53**, 352S–5S.

Jacques PF, Chylack LT, Jr., Hankinson SE, *et al.* (2001) Long-term nutrient intake and early age-related nuclear lens opacities. *Archives of Ophthalmology*, **119**, 1009–19.

Jacques PF, Chylack LT, Jr., McGandy RB and Hartz SC (1988) Antioxidant status in persons with and without senile cataract. *Archives of Ophthalmology*, **106**, 337–40.

Jacques PF, Moeller SM, Hankinson SE, *et al.* (2003) Weight status, abdominal adiposity, diabetes, and early age-related lens opacities. *American Journal of Clinical Nutrition*, **78**, 400–5.

Jacques PF, Taylor A, Moeller S, *et al.* (2005) Long-term nutrient intake and 5-year change in nuclear lens opacities. *Archives of Ophthalmology*, **123**, 517–26.

Janciauskiene S, Moraga F and Lindgren S (2001) C-terminal fragment of alpha1-antitrypsin activates human monocytes to a pro-inflammatory state through interactions with the CD36 scavenger receptor and LDL receptor. *Atherosclerosis*, **158**, 41–51.

Janssen I, Baumgartner R, Ross R, *et al.* (2004) Skeletal muscle cutpoints associated with elevated physical disability risk in older men and women. *American Journal of Epidemiology*, **159**, 413–21.

Janssen I, Shepard D, Katzmarzyk P and Roubenoff R (2004) The healthcare costs of sarcopenia in the United States. *Journal of the American Geriatric Society*, **52**, 80–5.

Jarvis M (1993) Does caffeine enhance intake above absolute levels of cognitive performance? *Psychopharmacology*, **110**, 45–52.

Jehle S, Zanetti A, Hulter HN *et al.* (2006) Partial neutralization of the acidogenic Western diet with potassium citrate increases bone mass in postmenopausal women with osteopenia. *Journal of the American Society of Nephrology*, **17**, 3213–22.

Jenab M, Ferrari P, Slimani N, *et al.* (2004) Association of nut and seed intake with colorectal cancer risk in the European Prospective Investigation into Cancer and Nutrition. *Cancer Epidemiology, Biomarkers & Prevention*, **13**, 1595–603.

Jenab M, Riboli E, Cleveland RJ, *et al.* (2007) Serum C-peptide, IGFBP-1 and IGFBP-2 and risk of colon and rectal cancers in the European Prospective Investigation into Cancer and Nutrition. *International Journal of Cancer*, **121**, 368–76.

Jenab M, Riboli E, Ferrari P, *et al.* (2006a) Plasma and dietary carotenoid, retinol and tocopherol levels and the risk of gastric adenocarcinomas in the European prospective investigation into cancer and nutrition. *British Journal of Cancer*, **95**, 406–15.

Jenab M, Riboli E, Ferrari P, *et al.* (2006b) Plasma and dietary vitamin C levels and risk of gastric cancer in the European Prospective Investigation into Cancer and Nutrition (EPIC-EURGAST). *Carcinogenesis*, **27**, 2250–7.

Jenkins D, Kendall C, Faulkner D, *et al.* (2002) A dietary portfolio approach to cholesterol reduction: combined effects of plant sterols, vegetable proteins, and viscous fibers in hypercholesterolemia. *Metabolism*, **51**, 1596–604.

Jenkins D, Popovich D, Kendall C *et al.* (1997) Effect of a diet high in vegetables, fruit, and nuts on serum lipids. *Metabolism*, **46**, 530–7.

Jenkins G (2002) Molecular mechanisms of skin ageing. *Mechanisms of Ageing & Development*, **123**, 801–10.

Jiang H and Chess L (2004) An integrated view of suppressor T cell subsets in immunoregulation. *Journal of Clinical Investigation*, **114**, 1198–208.

John J, Ziebland S, Yudkin P, *et al.* (2002) Effects of fruit and vegetable consumption on plasma antioxidant concentrations and blood pressure: a randomised controlled trial. *Lancet*, **359**, 1969–74.

Johnell O (2003) Non-nutritional risk factors for bone fragility. In: *Nutritional Aspects of Bone Health*. Ed. S. A. New and J. P. Bonjour. Cambridge, Royal Society of Chemistry.

Johnson-Kozlow M, Kritz-Silverstein D, Barrett-Connor E and Morton D (2002) Coffee consumption and cognitive function among older adults. *American Journal of Epidemiology*, **156**, 842–50.

Johnston KL, Clifford MN and Morgan LM (2003) Coffee acutely modifies gastrointestinal hormone secretion and glucose tolerance in humans: glycemic effects of chlorogenic acid and caffeine. *American Journal of Clinical Nutrition*, **78**, 728–33.

Jonas CR, McCullough ML, Teras LR, *et al.* (2003) Dietary glycemic index, glycemic load, and risk of incident breast cancer in postmenopausal women. *Cancer Epidemiology, Biomarkers & Prevention*, **12**, 573–7.

Jones C, Beaupre L, Johnston D and Suarez-Almazor M (2005) Total joint arthroplasties: current concepts of patient outcomes after surgery. *Clinics in Geriatric Medicine*, **21**, 527–41.

Jones C, Dewar B and Donaldson C (2005) Recipe for Life: Helping Older People to Eat Well. www.qmuc.ac.uk/opa/Pb/Recipe%20for%20Liife%20research%20report2.pdf.

Jones DP, Mody VC, Jr., Carlson JL, *et al.* (2002) Redox analysis of human plasma allows separation of pro-oxidant events of aging from decline in antioxidant defenses. *Free Radical Biology & Medicine*, **33**, 1290–300.

Jones G, White C, Nguyen T, *et al.* (1995) Cigarette smoking and vertebral body deformity. *Journal of the American Medical Association*, **274**, 1834–5.

Jones P, MacDougall D, Ntanios F and Vanstone C (1997) Dietary phytosterols as cholesterol-lowering agents in humans. *Canadian Journal of Physiology and Pharmacology*, **75**, 217–27.

Jonsson B, Ringsberg K, Josefsson PO, *et al.* (1992) Effects of physical training on bone mineral content and muscle strength in women: a cross-sectional study. *Bone*, **13**, 191–5.

Jordan K, Sawyer S, Coakley P, *et al.* (2004) The use of conventional and complementary treatments for knee osteoarthritis in the community. *Rheumatology*, **43**, 381–4.

Joshipura K, Ascherio A, Manson J, *et al.* (1999) Fruit and vegetable intake in relation to risk of ischemic stroke. *Journal of the American Medical Association*, **282**, 1233–9.

Joshipura KJ, Willett WC and Douglass CW (1996) The impact of edentulousness on food and nutrient intake.

Journal of the American Dental Association, **127**, 459–67.

Jubrias S, Odderson I, Esselman P and Conley K (1997) Decline in isokinetic force with age: muscle cross-sectional area and specific force. *Pflugers Archive: European Journal of Physiology*, **434**, 246–53.

Juni P, Reichenbach S and Dieppe P (2006) Osteoarthritis: rational approach to treating the individual. Best practice & research. *Clinical Rheumatology*, **20**, 721–40.

Kaaks R, Tuyns AJ, Haelterman M and Riboli E (1998) Nutrient intake patterns and gastric cancer risk: a case-control study in Belgium. *International Journal of Cancer*, **78**, 415–20.

Kado D, Karlamangla A, Huang M, *et al.* (2005) Homocysteine versus the vitamin folate, B6, and B12 as predictors of cognitive function and decline in older high-functioning adults: MacArthur Studies of Successful Aging. *American Journal of Medicine*, **118**, 161–7.

Kagan HM and Li W (2003) Lysyl oxidase: properties, specificity, and biological roles inside and outside of the cell. *Journal of Cellular Biochemistry*, **88**, 660–72.

Kalviainen N, Salovaara H and Tuorila H (2002) Sensory attributes and preference mapping for muesli oat flakes. *Journal of Food Science*, **67**, 455–60.

Kang GH, Lee HJ, *et al.* (2003) Aberrant CpG island hypermethylation of chronic gastritis, in relation to aging, gender, intestinal metaplasia, and chronic inflammation. *American Journal of Pathology*, **163**, 1551–6.

Kang JH, Ascherio A and Grodstein F (2005) Fruit and vegetable consumption and cognitive decline in aging women. *Annals of Neurology*, **57**, 713–20.

Kang JH, Pasquale LR, Rosner BA, *et al.* (2003) Prospective study of cigarette smoking and the risk of primary open-angle glaucoma. *Archives of Ophthalmology*, **121**, 1762–8.

Kang JH, Pasquale LR, Willett W, *et al.* (2003) Antioxidant intake and primary open-angle glaucoma: a prospective study. *American Journal of Epidemiology*, **158**, 337–46.

Kang JH, Pasquale LR, Willett WC, *et al.* (2004) Dietary fat consumption and primary open-angle glaucoma. *American Journal of Clinical Nutrition*, **79**, 755–64.

Kang S, Chung JH, Lee JH, *et al.* (2003) Topical N-acetyl cysteine and genistein prevent ultraviolet-light-induced signaling that leads to photoaging in human skin in vivo. *Journal of Investigative Dermatology*, **120**, 835–41.

Kang S, Fisher GJ and Voorhees JJ (2001) Photoaging: pathogenesis, prevention, and treatment. *Clinics in Geriatric Medicine*, **17**, 643–59.

Kannel W (2002) Coronary heart disease risk factors in the elderly. *American Journal of Geriatric Cardiology*, **11**, 101–7.

Kannel W, Wolf P, Castelli W and D'Agostino R (1987) Fibrinogen and risk of cardiovascular disease. *Journal of the American Medical Association*, **258**, 1183–6.

Kappeler L, Gourdji D, Zizzari P, *et al.* (2003) Age-associated changes in hypothalamic and pituitary neuroendocrine gene expression in the rat. *Journal of Neuroendocrinology*, **15**, 592–601.

Karin M and Greten FR (2005) NF-kappaB: linking inflammation and immunity to cancer development and progression. *Nature Reviews Immunology*, **5**, 749–59.

Karlsson C, Lindell K, Ottosson M, *et al.* (1998) Human adipose tissue expresses angiotensinogen and enzymes required for its conversion to angiotensin II. *Journal of Clinical Endocrinology & Metabolism*, **83**, 3925–9.

Karpe F (2005) Lipid-related factors. In: *Cardiovascular Disease: Diet, Nutrition and Emerging Risk Factors*. Ed. S. Stanner. Oxford, Blackwell Publishing: 50–62.

Karthikeyan K and Thappa DM (2002) Pellagra and skin. *International Journal of Dermatology*, **41**, 476–81.

Katan M (1998) Effect of low-fat diets on plasma high-density lipoprotein concentrations. *American Journal of Clinical Nutrition*, **67**, 573S–6S.

Katan M, Grundy S and Willett W (1997) Should a low-fat, high carbohydrate diet be recommended for everyone? Beyond low-fat diets. *New England Journal of Medicine*, **337**, 563–6.

Katelaris PH, Seow F, Lin BP, *et al.* (1993) Effect of age, *Helicobacter pylori* infection, and gastritis with atrophy on serum gastrin and gastric acid secretion in healthy men. *Gut*, **34**, 1032–7.

Katiyar S (2007) UV-induced immune suppression and photocarcinogenesis: chemoprevention by dietary botanical agents. *Cancer Letters*. Epub ahead of print.

Katiyar SK (2003) Skin photoprotection by green tea: antioxidant and immunomodulatory effects. *Current Drug Targets – Immune Endocrine & Metabolic Disorders*, **3**, 234–42.

Katiyar SK, Afaq F, Perez A and Mukhtar H (2001) Green tea polyphenol (−)-epigallocatechin-3-gallate treatment of human skin inhibits ultraviolet radiation-induced oxidative stress. *Carcinogenesis*, **22**, 287–94.

Katiyar SK, Korman NJ, Mukhtar H and Agarwal R (1997) Protective effects of silymarin against photocarcinogenesis in a mouse skin model. *Journal of the National Cancer Institute*, **89**, 556–66.

Katiyar SK, Perez A and Mukhtar H (2000) Green tea polyphenol treatment to human skin prevents formation of ultraviolet light B-induced pyrimidine dimers in DNA. *Clinical Cancer Research*, **6**, 3864–9.

Kato I, Dnistrian AM, Schwartz M, *et al.* (1999) Serum folate, homocysteine and colorectal cancer risk in women: a nested case-control study. *British Journal of Cancer*, **79**, 1917–22.

Katznelson L, Finkelstein JS, Schoenfeld DA, *et al.* (1996) Increase in bone density and lean body mass during testosterone administration in men with acquired hypogonadism. *Journal of Clinical Endocrinology & Metabolism*, **81**, 4358–65.

Kaur P (2006) Interfollicular epidermal stem cells: identification, challenges, potential. *Journal of Investigative Dermatology*, **126**, 1450–8.

Keaney JF, Jr., Larson MG, Vasan RS, *et al.* (2003) Obesity and systemic oxidative stress: clinical correlates of oxidative stress in the Framingham Study. *Arteriosclerosis, Thrombosis & Vascular Biology*, **23**, 434–9.

Keen RW, Hart DJ, Arden NK, *et al.* (1999) Family history of appendicular fracture and risk of osteoporosis: a population-based study. *Osteoporosis International*, **10**, 161–6.

Keil U (2000) Coronary artery disease: the role of lipids, hypertension and smoking. *Basic Research in Cardiology*, **95 (Suppl 1)**, I52–8.

Keinan-Boker L, van Der Schouw YT, Grobbee DE and Peeters PHM (2004) Dietary phytoestrogens and breast cancer risk. *American Journal of Clinical Nutrition*, **79**, 282–8.

Kellgren J and Moore R (1952) Generalised osteoarthritis and Heberden's nodes. *British Medical Journal*, **1**, 181–7.

Kelly CP, Pothoulakis C and LaMont JT (1994) Clostridium difficile colitis. *New England Journal of Medicine*, **330**, 257–62.

Kelly F, Sinclair AJ, Mann NJ, *et al.* (2001) A stearic acid-rich diet improves thrombogenic and atherogenic risk factor profiles in healthy males. *European Journal of Clinical Nutrition*, **55**, 88–96.

Kelly M, Steele JG, Nuttal N, *et al.* (2000) *Adult Dental Health Survey, Oral Health in the United Kingdom 1998.* London, Stationery Office.

Kelly P, Feakins R, Domizio P, *et al.* (2004) Paneth cell granule depletion in the human small intestine under infective and nutritional stress. *Clinical & Experimental Immunology*, **135**, 303–9.

Kelly S, Frost G, Whittaker V and Summerbell C (2004) Low glycaemic index diets for coronary heart disease. *Cochrane Database of Systematic Reviews*, CD004467.

Kelly SP, Thornton J, Lyratzopoulos G, *et al.* (2004) Smoking and blindness. *British Medical Journal*, **328**, 537–8.

Kemp FW, DeCandia J, Li W, *et al.* (2002) Relationships between immunity and dietary and serum antioxidants, B vitamins, and homocysteine in elderly men and women. *Nutrition Research*, **22**, 45–53.

Kempen JH, Mitchell P, Lee KE, *et al.* (2004) The prevalence of refractive errors among adults in the United States, Western Europe, and Australia. *Archives of Ophthalmology*, **122**, 495–505.

Kempen JH, O'Colmain BJ, Leske MC, *et al.* (2004) The prevalence of diabetic retinopathy among adults in the United States. *Archives of Ophthalmology*, **122**, 552–63.

Kendrick Z, Scafidi K and Lowenthal D (1994) Metabolic and nutritional considerations for exercising older adults. *Comprehensive Therapy*, **20**, 558–69.

Kenyon C, Chang J, Gensch E, *et al.* (1993) A C. elegans mutant that lives twice as long as wild type. *Nature*, **366**, 461–4.

Key T, Appleby P, Barnes I, *et al.* (2002) Endogenous sex hormones and breast cancer in postmenopausal women: reanalysis of nine prospective studies. *Journal of the National Cancer Institute*, **94**, 606–16.

Key TJ, Allen N, Appleby P, *et al.* (2004a) Fruits and vegetables and prostate cancer: no association among 1104 cases in a prospective study of 130544 men in the European Prospective Investigation into Cancer and Nutrition (EPIC). *International Journal of Cancer*, **109**, 119–24.

Key TJ, Schatzkin A, Willett WC, *et al.* (2004b) Diet, nutrition and the prevention of cancer. *Public Health Nutrition*, **7**, 187–200.

Khachik F, Spangler CJ, Smith JC, Jr., *et al.* (1997) Identification, quantification, and relative concentrations of carotenoids and their metabolites in human milk and serum. *Analytical Chemistry*, **69**, 1873–81.

Khader Y, Albashaireh Z and Alomari M (2004) Periodontal diseases and the risk of coronary heart and cerebrovascular diseases: a meta-analysis. *Journal of Periodontology*, **75**, 1046–53.

Khalil DA, Lucas EA, Juma S, *et al.* (2002) Soy protein supplementation increases serum insulin-like growth factor-I in young and old men but does not affect markers of bone metabolism. *Journal of Nutrition*, **132**, 2605–8.

Khaw K-T (1997) Healthy aging. *British Medical Journal*, **315**, 1090–6.

Kidd B, Photiou A and Inglis J (2004) The role of inflammatory mediators on nicioception and pain in arthritis. *Novartis Foundation Symposium*, **260**, 122–38.

Kiecolt-Glaser JK, Preacher KJ, MacCallum RC, *et al.* (2003) Chronic stress and age-related increases in the proinflammatory cytokine IL-6. *Proceedings of the National Academy of Sciences of the United States of America*, **100**, 9090–5.

Kilhovd BK, Berg TJ, Birkeland KI, *et al.* (1999) Serum levels of advanced glycation end products are increased in patients with type 2 diabetes and coronary heart disease. *Diabetes Care*, **22**, 1543–8.

Kim HJ, Camilleri M, McKinzie S, *et al.* (2003) A randomized controlled trial of a probiotic, VSL#3, on gut transit and symptoms in diarrhoea-predominant irritable bowel syndrome. *Alimentary Pharmacology & Therapeutics*, **17**, 895–904.

Kim HJ, Vazquez Roque MI, Camilleri M, *et al.* (2005) A randomized controlled trial of a probiotic combination VSL# 3 and placebo in irritable bowel syndrome with bloating. *Neurogastroenterology & Motility*, **17**, 687–96.

Kim J, Hwang JS, Cho YK, *et al.* (2001) Protective effects of (−)-epigallocatechin-3-gallate on UVA- and UVB-induced skin damage. *Skin Pharmacology & Applied Skin Physiology*, **14**, 11–19.

Kim JZ, Wang Z, Heymsfield S, *et al.* (2002) Total-body skeletal muscle mass: estimation by a new dual-energy X-ray absorptiometry method. *American Journal of Clinical Nutrition*, **76**, 378–83.

Kim S-H, Kaminker P and Campisi J (2002) Telomeres, aging and cancer: in search of a happy ending. *Oncogene*, **21**, 503–11.

Kim S-Y, Kim S-J, Lee J-Y, *et al.* (2004) Protective effects of dietary soy isoflavones against UV-induced skin-aging in hairless mouse model. *Journal of the American College of Nutrition*, **23**, 157–62.

Kimball SR and Jefferson LS (2006) Signaling pathways and molecular mechanisms through which branched-chain amino acids mediate translational control of protein synthesis. *Journal of Nutrition*, **136**, 227S–31S.

Kimura KD, Tissenbaum HA, Liu Y and Ruvkun G (1997) daf-2, an insulin receptor-like gene that regulates longevity and diapause in Caenorhabditis elegans. *Science*, **277**, 942–6.

Kino T, De Martino MU, Charmandari E, *et al.* (2003) Tissue glucocorticoid resistance/hypersensitivity syndromes. *Journal of Steroid Biochemistry & Molecular Biology*, **85**, 457–67.

Kirk SJ, Hurson M, Regan MC, *et al.* (1993) Arginine stimulates wound healing and immune function in elderly human beings. *Surgery*, **114**, 155–60.

Kirkwood TB (1977) Evolution of ageing. *Nature*, **270**, 301–4.

Kirkwood TB (1997) The origins of human ageing. *Philosophical Transactions of the Royal Society of London – Series B: Biological Sciences*, **352**, 1765–72.

Kirkwood TB and Cremer T (1982) Cytogerontology since 1881: a reappraisal of August Weismann and a review of modern progress. *Human Genetics*, **60**, 101–21.

Kirkwood TB and Holliday R (1979) The evolution of ageing and longevity. *Proceedings of the Royal Society of London – Series B: Biological Sciences*, **205**, 531–46.

Kirkwood TB and Rose MR (1991) Evolution of senescence: late survival sacrificed for reproduction. *Philosophical Transactions of the Royal Society of London – Series B: Biological Sciences*, **332**, 15–24.

Kirkwood TBL (2005) Understanding the odd science of aging. *Cell*, **120**, 437–47.

Kirkwood TBL (2006) Nutrition for a longer life. BNF Annual Lecture 2005. *Nutrition Bulletin*, **31(2)**, 88–92.

Kirkwood TBL, Boys RJ, Gillespie CS, *et al.* (2003) Towards an e-biology of ageing: integrating theory and data. *Nature Reviews Molecular Cell Biology*, **4**, 243–9.

Kissileff HR, Pi-Sunyer FX, Thornton J and Smith GP (1981) C-terminal octapeptide of cholecystokinin decreases food intake in man. *American Journal of Clinical Nutrition*, **34**, 154–60.

Kivipelto M, Ngandu T, Laatikainen T, *et al.* (2006) Risk score for the prediction of dementia risk in 20 years among middle aged people: a longitudinal, population-based study. *Lancet Neurology*, **5**, 735–41.

Kjaer M (2004) Role of extracellular matrix in adaptation of tendon and skeletal muscle to mechanical loading. *Physiological Reviews*, **84**, 649–98.

Kleessen B, Sykura B, Zunft HJ and Blaut M (1997) Effects of inulin and lactose on fecal microflora, microbial activity, and bowel habit in elderly constipated persons. *American Journal of Clinical Nutrition*, **65**, 1397–402.

Klein R, Davis MD, Magli Y, *et al.* (1991) The Wisconsin Age Related Maculopathy Grading System. *Ophthalmology*, **98**, 1128–34.

Klein R, Klein BE and Linton KL (1992) Prevalence of age-related maculopathy. The Beaver Dam Eye Study. *Ophthalmology*, **99**, 933–43.

Klein RE, Klein BE, Jensen SC and Meuer SM (1997) The five-year incidence and progression of age-related maculopathy. *Ophthalmology*, **104**, 7–21.

Klurfeld DM, Weber MM and Kritchevsky D (1987) Inhibition of chemically induced mammary and colon tumor promotion by caloric restriction in rats fed increased dietary fat. *Cancer Research*, **47**, 2759–62.

Knapen MH, Schurgers LJ and Vermeer C (2007) Vitamin K2 supplementation improves hip bone geometry and bone strength indices in postmenopausal women. *Osteoporosis International*, **18**, 963–72.

Knekt P, Heliovaara M, Rissanen A, *et al.* (1992) Serum antioxidant vitamins and risk of cataract. *British Medical Journal*, **305**, 1392–4.

Knoops K, de Groot L, Kromhout D, *et al.* (2004) Mediterranean diet, lifestyle, and 10-year mortality in elderly European men and women. *Journal of the American Medical Association*, **292**, 1433–9.

Knowler WC, Barrett-Connor E, Fowler SE, *et al.* (2002) Reduction in the incidence of type 2 diabetes with lifestyle intervention or metformin. *New England Journal of Medicine*, **346**, 393–403.

Kohl HW (2001) Physical activity and cardiovascular disease: evidence for a dose response. *Medicine and Science in Sports and Exercise*, **33**, S472–83.

Kohrt W, Snead D, Slatopolsky E and Birge SJ (1995) Additive effects of weight-bearing exercise and estrogen on bone mineral density in older women. *Journal of Bone & Mineral Research*, **10**, 1303–11.

Kohrt WM, Bloomfield SA, Little KD, *et al.* (2004) Physical activity and bone health. *Medicine and Science in Sports and Exercise*, **36**, 1985–96.

Kohyama K, Mioche L and Bourdiol P (2003) Influence of age and dental status on chewing behaviour studied by EMG recordings during consumption of various food samples. *Gerodontology*, **20**, 15–23.

Komuves LG, Hanley K, Lefebvre AM, *et al.* (2000) Stimulation of PPARalpha promotes epidermal keratinocyte differentiation in vivo. *Journal of Investigative Dermatology*, **115**, 353–60.

Konsman JP, Parnet P and Dantzer R (2002) Cytokine-induced sickness behaviour: mechanisms and implications. *Trends in Neurosciences*, **25**, 154–9.

Kop WJ, Gottdiener JS, Tangen CM, *et al.* (2002) Inflammation and coagulation factors in persons >65 years of age with symptoms of depression but without evidence of myocardial ischemia. *American Journal of Cardiology*, **89**, 419–24.

Köpke W and Krutmann J (2008) Protection from sunburn with beta-carotene – a meta-analysis. *Photochemistry and Photobiology*, **84**, 284–8.

Kornman KS (2006) Interleukin 1 genetics, inflammatory mechanisms, and nutrigenetic opportunities to modulate diseases of aging. *American Journal of Clinical Nutrition*, **83**, 475S–83S.

Kot TV and Pettit-Young NA (1992) Lactulose in the management of constipation: a current review. *Annals of Pharmacotherapy*, **26**, 1277–82.

Kotsopoulos D, Dalais FS, Liang YL, *et al.* (2000) The effects of soy protein containing phytoestrogens on menopausal symptoms in postmenopausal women. *Climacteric*, **3**, 161–7.

Kouris-Blazos A, Gnardellis C, Walqvist M, *et al.* (1999) Are the advantages of the Mediterranean diet transferable to other populations? A cohort study in Melbourne, Australia. *British Journal of Nutrition*, **82**, 57–61.

Koushik A, Hunter DJ, Spiegelman D, *et al.* (2005) Fruits and vegetables and ovarian cancer risk in a pooled analysis of 12 cohort studies. *Cancer Epidemiology, Biomarkers & Prevention*, **14**, 2160–7.

Kovalenko S, Kopsidas G, Kelso J and Linnane A (1997) Deltoid human muscle mtDNA is extensively rearranged in old age subjects. *Biochemical and Biophysical Research Communications*, **232**, 147–52.

Kowald A and Kirkwood TB (2000) Accumulation of defective mitochondria through delayed degradation of damaged organelles and its possible role in the ageing of post-mitotic and dividing cells. *Journal of Theoretical Biology*, **202**, 145–60.

Krall E, Hayes C and Garcia R (1998) How dentition status and masticatory function affect nutrient intake. *Journal of the American Dental Association*, **129**, 1261–9.

Krall EA and Dawson-Hughes B (1993) Heritable and life-style determinants of bone mineral density. *Journal of Bone & Mineral Research*, **8**, 1–9.

Kraus V, Huebner J, Stabler T, *et al.* (2004) Ascorbic acid increases the severity of spontaneous knee osteoarthritis in the guinea pig model. *Arthritis & Rheumatism*, **50**, 1822–31.

Krebs EE, Ensrud KE, MacDonald R and Wilt TJ (2004) Phytoestrogens for treatment of menopausal symptoms: a systematic review. *Obstetrics & Gynecology*, **104**, 824–36.

Krebs HA (1972) The Pasteur effect and relation between respiration and fermentation. In: *Essays in Biochemistry*. Ed. P. N. Campbell and F. Dickens. London, Academic Press. **8**, 1–34.

Kreijkamp-Kaspers S, Kok L, Bots M, *et al.* (2005) Randomized controlled trial of the effects of soy protein containing isoflavones on vascular function in postmenopausal women. *American Journal of Clinical Nutrition*, **81**, 189–95.

Kreijkamp-Kaspers S, Kok L, Grobbee DE, *et al.* (2004) Effect of soy protein containing isoflavones on cognitive function, bone mineral density, and plasma lipids in postmenopausal women: a randomized controlled trial. *Journal of the American Medical Association*, **292**, 65–74.

Kremer JM, Jubiz W, Michalek A, *et al.* (1987) Fish-oil fatty acid supplementation in active rheumatoid arthritis. A double-blinded, controlled, crossover study. *Annals of Internal Medicine*, **106**, 497–503.

Kris-Etherton P, Zhao G, Binkoski A, *et al.* (2001) The effects of nuts on coronary heart disease risk. *Nutrition Reviews*, **59**, 103–11.

Krishnan KJ, Harbottle A and Birch-Machin MA (2004) The use of a 3895 bp mitochondrial DNA deletion as a marker for sunlight exposure in human skin. *Journal of Investigative Dermatology*, **123**, 1020–4.

Kriska AM, Sandler RB, Cauley JA, *et al.* (1988) The assessment of historical physical activity and its relation to adult bone parameters. *American Journal of Epidemiology*, **127**, 1053–63.

Kritchevsky S, Cesari M and Pahor M (2005) Inflammatory markers and cardiovascular health in older adults. *Cardiovascular Research*, **66**, 265–75.

Kubaszek A, Pihlajamaki J, Punnonen K, *et al.* (2003) The C-174G promoter polymorphism of the IL-6 gene affects energy expenditure and insulin sensitivity. *Diabetes*, **52**, 558–61.

Kubo K, Kanehisa H, Azuma K, *et al.* (2003) Muscle architectural characteristics in young and elderly men and women. *International Journal of Sports Medicine*, **24**, 125–30.

Kuh D, Bassey J, Hardy R, *et al.* (2002) Birth weight, childhood size, and muscle strength in adult life: evidence from a birth cohort study. *American Journal of Epidemiology*, **156**, 627–33.

Kuiper GG, Carlsson B, Grandien K, *et al.* (1997) Comparison of the ligand binding specificity and transcript tissue distribution of estrogen receptors alpha and beta. *Endocrinology*, **138**, 863–70.

Kuiper GG, Lemmen JG, Carlsson B, *et al.* (1998) Interaction of estrogenic chemicals and phytoestrogens with estrogen receptor beta. *Endocrinology*, **139**, 4252–63.

Kuipers EJ, Uyterlinde AM, Pena AS, *et al.* (1995) Long-term sequelae of *Helicobacter pylori* gastritis. *Lancet*, **345**, 1525–8.

Kuller L, Shemanski L, Psaty B, *et al.* (1995) Subclinical disease as an independent risk factor for cardiovascular disease. *Circulation*, **92**, 720–6.

Kuper H, Marmot M and Hemingway H (2002) Systematic review of prospective cohort studies of psychosocial factors in the etiology and prognosis of coronary heart disease. *Seminars in Vascular Medicine*, **2**, 267–314.

Kyle U, Unger P, Dupertuis Y, *et al.* (2002) Body composition in 995 acutely ill or chronically ill patients at hospital admission: a controlled population study. *Journal of the American Dietetic Association*, **102**, 944–55.

La Croix AZ, Lipson S, Miles TP and White L (1989) Prospective study of pneumonia hospitalization and mortality of US older people: the role of chronic conditions, health behaviors and nutritional status. *Public Health Reports*, **104**, 350–60.

Laaksonen D, Nyyssonen K, Niskanen L, *et al.* (2005) Prediction of cardiovascular mortality in middle-aged men by dietary and serum linoleic and polyunsaturated fatty acids. *Archives of Internal Medicine*, **165**, 193–9.

Lagergren J (2005) Adenocarcinoma of oesophagus: what exactly is the size of the problem and who is at risk? *Gut*, **54 (Suppl 1)**, 11–15.

Lagergren J, Bergstrom R and Nyren O (1999) Association between body mass and adenocarcinoma of the esophagus and gastric cardia. *Annals of Internal Medicine*, **130**, 883–90.

Lahmann PH, Friedenreich C, Schuit AJ, *et al.* (2007) Physical activity and breast cancer risk: the European Prospective Investigation into Cancer and Nutrition. *Cancer Epidemiology, Biomarkers & Prevention*, **16**, 36–42.

Lahmann PH, Hoffmann K, Allen N, *et al.* (2004) Body size and breast cancer risk: findings from the European Prospective Investigation into Cancer and Nutrition (EPIC). *International Journal of Cancer*, **111**, 762–71.

Lahmann PH, Schulz M, Hoffmann K, *et al.* (2005) Long-term weight change and breast cancer risk: the European Prospective Investigation into Cancer and Nutrition (EPIC). *British Journal of Cancer*, **93**, 582–9.

Lakatta E (2002) Age-associated cardiovascular changes in health: impact on cardiovascular disease in older persons. *Heart Failure Reviews*, **7**, 29–49.

Lakka TA, Laaksonen DE, Lakka HM, *et al.* (2003) Sedentary lifestyle, poor cardiorespiratory fitness, and the metabolic syndrome. *Medicine and Science in Sports and Exercise*, **35**, 1279–86.

Lakshmi AV (1998) Riboflavin metabolism – relevance to human nutrition. *Indian Journal of Medical Research*, **108**, 182–90.

LaMonte MJ, Barlow CE, Jurca R, *et al.* (2005) Cardiorespiratory fitness is inversely associated with the incidence of metabolic syndrome: a prospective study of men and women. *Circulation*, **112**, 505–12.

Lampe JW (1999) Health effects of vegetables and fruit: assessing mechanisms of action in human experimental studies. *American Journal of Clinical Nutrition*, **70**, 475S–90S.

Landi S, Moreno V, Gioia-Patricola L, *et al.* (2003) Association of common polymorphisms in inflammatory genes interleukin (IL)6, IL8, tumor necrosis factor alpha, NFKB1, and peroxisome proliferator-activated receptor gamma with colorectal cancer. *Cancer Research*, **63**, 3560–6.

Lands WE (1992) Biochemistry and physiology of n-3 fatty acids. *FASEB Journal*, **6**, 2530–6.

Lang A and Lozano A (1998) Parkinson's disease. First of two parts. *New England Journal of Medicine*, **339**, 1044–53.

Lange KHW, Andersen JL, Beyer N, *et al.* (2002) GH administration changes myosin heavy chain isoforms in skeletal muscle but does not augment muscle strength or hypertrophy, either alone or combined with resistance exercise training in healthy elderly men. *Journal of Clinical Endocrinology & Metabolism*, **87**, 513–23.

Lange Skovgaard GR, Jensen AS and Sigler ML (2006) Effect of a novel dietary supplement on skin aging in postmenopausal women. *European Journal of Clinical Nutrition*, **60**, 1201–6.

Lanham-New S (2007) The balance of bone health: tipping the scales in favour of potassium-rich, bicarbonate-rich foods. *Journal of Nutrition*, **138**, 172S–7S.

Lanham-New SA (2006) Fruit and vegetables: the unexpected natural answer to the question of osteoporosis prevention? *American Journal of Clinical Nutrition*, **83**, 1254–5.

Lansdown AB (1996) Zinc in the healing wound. *Lancet*, **347**, 706–7.

Lansdown AB (2001) Iron: a cosmetic ingredient but an essential nutrient for healthy skin. *International Journal of Cosmetic Science*, **23**, 129–37.

Lansdown AB, Sampson B and Rowe A (1999) Sequential changes in trace metal, metallothionein and calmodulin concentrations in healing skin wounds. *Journal of Anatomy*, **195**, 375–86.

Lansdown ABG (2004a) Nutrition 1: a vital consideration in the management of skin wounds. *British Journal of Nursing*, **13**, S22–8.

Lansdown ABG (2004b) Nutrition 2: a vital consideration in the management of skin wounds. *British Journal of Nursing*, **13**, 1199–210.

Larsen ER, Mosekilde L and Foldspang A (2004) Vitamin D and calcium supplementation prevents osteoporotic fractures in elderly community dwelling residents: a pragmatic population-based 3-year intervention study. *Journal of Bone & Mineral Research*, **19**, 370–8.

Larsen L, Jespersen J and Marckmann P (1999) Are olive oil diets antithrombotic? Diets enriched with olive, rapeseed or sunflower oil affect postprandial factor VII differently. *American Journal of Clinical Nutrition*, **70**, 976–82.

Larsen PL, Albert PS and Riddle DL (1995) Genes that regulate both development and longevity in *Caenorhabditis elegans*. *Genetics*, **139**, 1567–83.

Larson E, Wang L, Bowen J, *et al.* (2006) Exercise is associated with reduced risk for incident dementia among persons 65 years of age and older. *Annals of Internal Medicine*, **144**, 73–81.

Larsson L, Grimby G and Karlsson J (1979) Muscle strength and speed of movement in relation to age and muscle morphology. *Journal of Applied Physiology*, **46**, 451–6.

Lassus A, Jeskanen L, Happonen HP and Santalahti J (1991) Imedeen for the treatment of degenerated skin in females. *Journal of International Medical Research*, **19**, 147–52.

Lau E, Donnan S, Barker DJ and Cooper C (1988) Physical activity and calcium intake in fracture of the proximal femur in Hong Kong. *British Medical Journal*, **297**, 1441–3.

Laugier R, Bernard JP, Berthezene P and Dupuy P (1991) Changes in pancreatic exocrine secretion with age: pancreatic exocrine secretion does decrease in the elderly. *Digestion*, **50**, 202–11.

Laurberg P, Pedersen KM, Hreidarsson A, *et al.* (1998) Iodine intake and the pattern of thyroid disorders: a comparative epidemiological study of thyroid abnormalities in the elderly in Iceland and in Jutland, Denmark. *Journal of Clinical Endocrinology & Metabolism*, **83**, 765–9.

Lautenschlager N and Almeida O (2006) Physical activity and cognition in old age. *Current Opinion in Psychiatry*, **19**, 190–3.

Law C, Shiell A, Newsome C, *et al.* (2002) Fetal, infant, and childhood growth and adult blood pressure: a longitudinal study from birth to 22 years of age. *Circulation*, **105**, 1088–92.

Law M (2000) Plant sterol and stanol margarines and health. *British Medical Journal*, **320**, 861–4.

Lawlor D, Ebrahim S and Davey Smith G (2004) The metabolic syndrome and coronary heart disease in older women: findings from the British Women's Heart and Health Study. *Diabetic Medicine*, **21**, 906–13.

Lawrence J, Bremner J and Bier F (1966) Osteoarthritis: prevalence in the population and relationship between symptoms and x-ray changes. *Annals of the Rheumatic Diseases*, **25**, 1–24.

Layman D, Boileau R, Erickson D, *et al.* (2003) A reduced ratio of dietary carbohydrate to protein improves body composition and blood lipid profiles during weight loss in adult women. *Journal of Nutrition*, **J133**, 411–7.

Lee CD, Blair SN and Jackson AS (1999) Cardiorespiratory fitness, body composition, and all-cause and cardiovascular disease mortality in men. *American Journal of Clinical Nutrition*, **69**, 373–80.

Lee CK, Klopp RG, Weindruch R and Prolla TA (1999) Gene expression profile of aging and its retardation by caloric restriction. *Science*, **285**, 1390–3.

Lee CK, Weindruch R and Prolla TA (2000) Gene-expression profile of the ageing brain in mice. *Nature Genetics*, **25**, 294–7.

Lee IM (2003) Physical activity and cancer prevention – data from epidemiologic studies. *Medicine & Science in Sports & Exercise*, **35**, 1823–7.

Lee SA, Kang D, Shim KN, *et al.* (2003) Effect of diet and *Helicobacter pylori* infection to the risk of early gastric cancer. *Journal of Epidemiology*, **13**, 162–8.

Lenchik L, Vatti S and Register TC (2004) Interpretation of bone mineral density as it relates to bone health and fracture risk. In: *Nutrition and Bone Health*. Ed. M. F. Holick and B. Dawson-Hughes. New Jersey, Humana Press: 63–84.

Lengauer C, Kinzler KW and Vogelstein B (1997) DNA methylation and genetic instability in colorectal cancer cells. *Proceedings of the National Academy of Sciences of the United States of America*, **94**, 2545–50.

Lengyel CO, Zello GA, Smith JT and Whiting SJ (2003) Evaluation of menu and food service practices of long-term care facilities of a health district in Canada. *Journal of Nutrition for the Elderly*, **22**, 29–42.

Leonhardt JM and Heymann WR (2002) Thyroid disease and the skin. *Dermatologic Clinics*, **20**, 473–81.

Leske MC, Chylack LT, Jr., He Q, *et al.* (1998) Antioxidant vitamins and nuclear opacities: the longitudinal study of cataract. *Ophthalmology*, **105**, 831–6.

Leske MC, Chylack LT, Jr. and Wu SY (1991) The Lens Opacities Case-Control Study. Risk factors for cataract. *Archives of Ophthalmology*, **109**, 244–51.

Leske MC, Connell AM, Wu SY, *et al.* (1995) Risk factors for open-angle glaucoma. The Barbados Eye Study. *Archives of Ophthalmology*, **113**, 918–24.

Leske MC, Wu SY, Hennis A, *et al.* (2005) Hyperglycemia, blood pressure, and the 9-year incidence of diabetic retinopathy: the Barbados Eye Studies. *Ophthalmology*, **112**, 799–805.

Leske MC, Wu SY, Hyman L, *et al.* (1995) Biochemical factors in the lens opacities. Case-control study. The Lens Opacities Case-Control Study Group. *Archives of Ophthalmology*, **113**, 1113–19.

Lesourd B (1999) Immune response during disease and recovery in the elderly. *Proceedings of the Nutrition Society*, **58**, 85–98.

Lesourd B and Mazari L (1999) Nutrition and immunity in the elderly. *Proceedings of the Nutrition Society*, **58**, 685–95.

Lesourd B, Decarli B and Dirren H (1996) Longitudinal changes in iron and protein status of elderly Europeans. SENECA Investigators. *European Journal of Clinical Nutrition*, **50 (Suppl 2)**, S16–24.

Lesourd BM, Mazari L and Ferry M (1998) The role of nutrition in immunity in the aged. *Nutrition Reviews*, **56**, S113–25.

Levenson SM and Demetriou AA (1992) Metabolic factors. In: *Wound Healing: Biochemical and Clinical Aspects.* Ed. I. K. Cohen, R. Diegelmann and W. J. Lindblad. Philadelphia, WB Saunders: 248–73.

Levi F, Randimbison L, Lucchini F, *et al.* (2001) Epidemiology of adenocarcinoma and squamous cell carcinoma of the oesophagus. *European Journal of Cancer Prevention*, **10**, 91–6.

Levine M, Rumsey SC, Daruwala R, *et al.* (1999) Criteria and recommendations for vitamin C intake. *Journal of the American Medical Association*, **281**, 1415–23.

Lewerin C, Matousek M, Steen G, *et al.* (2005) Significant correlations of plasma homocysteine and serum methylmalonic acid with movement and cognitive performance in elderly subjects but no improvement from short-term vitamin therapy: a placebo-controlled randomized study. *American Journal of Clinical Nutrition*, **81**, 1155–62.

Lewis S, Burmeister S and Brazier J (2005a) Effect of the prebiotic oligofructose on relapse of Clostridium difficile-associated diarrhea: a randomized, controlled study. *Clinical Gastroenterology & Hepatology*, **3**, 442–8.

Lewis S, Burmeister S, Cohen S, *et al.* (2005b) Failure of dietary oligofructose to prevent antibiotic-associated diarrhoea. *Alimentary Pharmacology & Therapeutics*, **21**, 469–77.

Lewis SE, Goldspink DF, Phillips JG, *et al.* (1985) The effects of aging and chronic dietary restriction on whole body growth and protein turnover in the rat. *Experimental Gerontology*, **20**, 253–63.

Lexell J, Downham D and Sjostrom M (1986) Distribution of different fibre types in human skeletal muscles. Fibre type arrangement in m. vastus lateralis from three groups of healthy men between 15 and 83 years. *Journal of the Neurological Sciences*, **72**, 211–22.

Ley SJ, Horwath CC and Stewart JM (1999) Attention is needed to the high prevalence of vitamin D deficiency in our older population. *New Zealand Medical Journal*, **112**, 471–2.

Li G-Z, Eller MS, Firoozabadi R and Gilchrest BA (2003) Evidence that exposure of the telomere 3' overhang sequence induces senescence. *Proceedings of the National Academy of Sciences of the United States of America*, **100**, 527–31.

Licinio J and Wong ML (1999) The role of inflammatory mediators in the biology of major depression: central nervous system cytokines modulate the biological substrate of depressive symptoms, regulate stress-responsive systems, and contribute to neurotoxicity and neuroprotection. *Molecular Psychiatry*, **4**, 317–27.

Lim K, Rogers J, Shepstone L and Dieppe P (1995) The evolutionary origins of osteoarthritis. *Journal of Rheumatology*, **22**, 2132–4.

Lin F-H, Lin J-Y, Gupta RD, *et al.* (2005) Ferulic acid stabilizes a solution of vitamins C and E and doubles its photoprotection of skin. *Journal of Investigative Dermatology*, **125**, 826–32.

Lin J-Y, Selim MA, Shea CR, *et al.* (2003) UV photoprotection by combination topical antioxidants vitamin C and vitamin E. *Journal of the American Academy of Dermatology*, **48**, 866–74.

Lin PH, Ginty F, Appel LJ, *et al.* (2003) The DASH diet and sodium reduction improve markers of bone turnover and calcium metabolism in adults. *Journal of Nutrition*, **133**, 3130–6.

Lindenbaum J, Healton E, Savage D, *et al.* (1988) Neuropsychiatric disorders caused by cobalamin deficiency in the absence of anemia or macrocytosis. *New England Journal of Medicine*, **318**, 1720–8.

Lindle R, Metter E, Lynch N, *et al.* (1997) Age and gender comparisons of muscle strength in 654 women and men aged 20–93 yr. *Journal of Applied Physiology*, **83**, 1581–7.

Lindstrom J, Ilanne-Parikka P, Peltonen M, *et al.* (2006) Sustained reduction in the incidence of type 2 diabetes by lifestyle intervention: follow-up of the Finnish Diabetes Prevention Study. *Lancet*, **368**, 1673–9.

Lineback DR (2005) Role of diet in blood glucose response and related health outcomes: summary of a meeting. *Nutrition Reviews*, **63**, 126–31.

Linnane A, Marzuki S, Ozawa T and Tanaka M (1989) Mitochondrial DNA mutations as an important contributor to ageing and degenerative diseases. *Lancet*, **1**, 642–5.

Lio D, Candore G, Crivello A, *et al.* (2004) Opposite effects of interleukin 10 common gene polymorphisms in cardiovascular diseases and in successful ageing: genetic background of male centenarians is protective against coronary heart disease. *Journal of Medical Genetics*, **41**, 790–4.

Lio D, D'Anna C, Scola L, *et al.* (1999) Interleukin-5 production by mononuclear cells from aged individuals: implication for autoimmunity. *Mechanisms of Ageing & Development*, **106**, 297–304.

Lio D, Scola L, Crivello A, *et al.* (2002a) Gender-specific association between -1082 IL-10 promoter polymorphism and longevity. *Genes & Immunity*, **3**, 30–3.

Lio D, Scola L, Crivello A, *et al.* (2002b) Allele frequencies of +874T→A single nucleotide polymorphism at the first intron of interferon-gamma gene in a group of Italian centenarians. *Experimental Gerontology*, **37**, 315–19.

Little RD, Carulli JP, Del Mastro RG, *et al.* (2002) A mutation in the LDL receptor-related protein 5 gene results in the autosomal dominant high-bone-mass trait. *American Journal of Human Genetics*, **70**, 11–19.

Liu PT, Stenger S, Li H, *et al.* (2006) Toll-like receptor triggering of a vitamin D-mediated human antimicrobial response. *Science*, **311**, 1770–3.

Liu PY, Swerdloff RS and Veldhuis JD (2004) Clinical review 171: the rationale, efficacy and safety of androgen therapy in older men: future research and current practice recommendations. *Journal of Clinical Endocrinology & Metabolism*, **89**, 4789–96.

Liu S, Manson J, Stampfer M, *et al.* (2000) Whole grain consumption and risk of ischemic stroke in women: a prospective study. *Journal of the American Medical Association*, **284**, 1534–40.

Liu S, Stampfer M, Hu F, *et al.* (1999) Whole grain consumption and risk of coronary heart disease: results from the Nurses' Health Study. *American Journal of Clinical Nutrition*, **70**, 412–19.

Liu S, West R, Randell E, *et al.* (2004) A comprehensive evaluation of food fortification with folic acid for primary prevention of neural tube defects. *Biomed Central Pregnancy and Childbirth*, **4**, 20.

Liu YL, Yakar S, Otero-Corchon V, *et al.* (2002) Ghrelin gene expression is age-dependent and influenced by gender and the level of circulating IGF-1. *Molecular & Cellular Endocrinology*, **189**, 97–103.

Liu Y-Z, Liu Y-J, Recker RR and Deng H-W (2003) Molecular studies of identification of genes for osteoporosis: the 2002 update. *Journal of Endocrinology*, **177**, 147–96.

Lloyd T, Schaeffer JM, Walker MA and Demers LM (1991) Urinary hormonal concentrations and spinal bone densities of premenopausal vegetarian and non-vegetarian women. *American Journal of Clinical Nutrition*, **54**, 1005–10.

Loeser R and Shakoor N (2003) Ageing or osteoarthritis: which is the problem? *Rheumatic Diseases Clinics of North America*, **29**, 653–74.

Lohman T, Going S, Pamenter R, *et al.* (1995) Effects of resistance training on regional and total bone mineral density in premenopausal women: a randomized prospective study. *Journal of Bone & Mineral Research*, **10**, 1015–24.

Lohwasser C, Neureiter D, Weigle B, *et al.* (2006) The receptor for advanced glycation end products is highly expressed in the skin and upregulated by advanced glycation end products and tumor necrosis factor-alpha. *Journal of Investigative Dermatology*, **126**, 291–9.

Longcope C, Feldman HA, McKinlay JB and Araujo AB (2000) Diet and sex hormone-binding globulin. *Journal of Clinical Endocrinology & Metabolism*, **85**, 293–6.

Lonn E, Yusuf S, Arnold M, *et al.* (2006) Homocysteine lowering with folic acid and B vitamins in vascular disease. *New England Journal of Medicine*, **354**, 1567–77.

Looker A, Cogswell M and Gunter E (2002) Iron deficiency – United States, 1999–2000. *MMWR*, **51**, 897–9.

Lopez-Segura F, Velasco F, Lopez-Miranda J, *et al.* (1996) Monounsaturated fatty acid-enriched diet decreases plasma plasminogen activator inhibitor type 1. *Arteriosclerosis, Thrombosis and Vascular Biology*, **16**, 82–8.

Louard R, Fryburg D, Gelfand R and Barrett E (1992) Insulin sensitivity of protein and glucose metabolism in human forearm skeletal muscle. *Journal of Clinical Investigation*, **90**, 2348–54.

Louis M, Poortmans JR, Francaux M, *et al.* (2003a) Creatine supplementation has no effect on human muscle protein turnover at rest in the postabsorptive or fed states. *American Journal of Physiology – Endocrinology & Metabolism*, **284**, E764–70.

Louis M, Poortmans JR, Francaux M, *et al.* (2003b) No effect of creatine supplementation on human myofibrillar and sarcoplasmic protein synthesis after resistance exercise. *American Journal of Physiology – Endocrinology & Metabolism*, **285**, E1089–94.

Lovegrove J, Clohessy A, Milon H and Williams C (2000) Modest doses of beta-glucan do not reduce concentrations of potentially atherogenic lipoproteins. *American Journal of Clinical Nutrition*, **72**, 49–55.

Low Y-L, Taylor JI, Grace PB, *et al.* (2005) Phytoestrogen exposure correlation with plasma estradiol in postmenopausal women in European Prospective Investigation of Cancer and Nutrition – Norfolk may involve diet-gene interactions. *Cancer Epidemiology, Biomarkers & Prevention*, **14**, 213–20.

Lu CT, Yen YY, Ho CS, *et al.* (1996) A case-control study of oral cancer in Changhua County, Taiwan. *Journal of Oral Pathology & Medicine*, **25**, 245–8.

Lubree HG, Rege SS, Bhat DS, *et al.* (2002) Body fat and cardiovascular risk factors in Indian men in three geographical locations. *Food & Nutrition Bulletin*, **23**, 146–9.

Lukanova A and Kaaks R (2005) Endogenous hormones and ovarian cancer: epidemiology and current hypotheses. *Cancer Epidemiology, Biomarkers & Prevention*, **14**, 98–107.

Lukaski H (2000) Magnesium, zinc, and chromium nutriture and physical activity. *American Journal of Clinical Nutrition*, **72**, 585S–93S.

Lundman P, Eriksson MJ, Silveira A, *et al.* (2003) Relation of hypertriglyceridemia to plasma concentrations of biochemical markers of inflammation and endothelial activation (C-reactive protein, interleukin-6, soluble adhesion molecules, von Willebrand factor, and endothelin-1). *American Journal of Cardiology*, **91**, 1128–31.

Lunn J and Buttriss J (2007) Carbohydrates and dietary fibre. *Nutrition Bulletin*, **32**, 21–64.

Lunn J and Theobald H (2006) The health effects of dietary unsaturated fatty acids. *Nutrition Bulletin*, **31**, 178–224.

Lyle BJ, Mares-Perlman JA, Klein BE, *et al.* (1999a) Antioxidant intake and risk of incident age-related nuclear cataracts in the Beaver Dam Eye Study. *American Journal of Epidemiology*, **149**, 801–9.

Lyle BJ, Mares-Perlman JA, Klein BE, *et al.* (1999b) Serum carotenoids and tocopherols and incidence of age-related nuclear cataract. *American Journal of Clinical Nutrition*, **69**, 272–7.

Macdonald HM, Black AJ, Sandison R, *et al.* (2006) Two year double blind randomized controlled trial in postmenopausal women shows no gain in BMD with potassium citrate treatment. *Journal of Bone & Mineral Research*, **21 (Suppl 1)**, S15.

Macdonald HM, New SA, Golden MHN, *et al.* (2004) Nutritional associations with bone loss during the menopausal transition: evidence of a beneficial effect of calcium, alcohol, and fruit and vegetable nutrients and of a detrimental effect of fatty acids. *American Journal of Clinical Nutrition*, **79**, 155–65.

MacGregor G and He F (2002) Effect of modest salt reduction on blood pressure: a meta-analysis of randomized trials. Implications for public health. *Journal of Human Hypertension*, **16**, 761–70.

MacIntosh CG, Morley JE, Wishart J, *et al.* (2001) Effect of exogenous cholecystokinin (CCK)-8 on food intake and plasma CCK, leptin, and insulin concentrations in older and young adults: evidence for increased CCK activity as a cause of the anorexia of aging. *Journal of Clinical Endocrinology & Metabolism*, **86**, 5830–7.

Madsen JL and Graff J (2004) Effects of ageing on gastrointestinal motor function. *Age & Ageing*, **33**, 154–9.

Maggio D, Barabani M, Pierandrei M, *et al.* (2003) Marked decrease in plasma antioxidants in aged osteoporotic women: results of a cross-sectional study. *Journal of Clinical Endocrinology & Metabolism*, **88**, 1523–7.

Mallbris L, Edstrom DW, Sundblad L, *et al.* (2005) UVB upregulates the antimicrobial protein hCAP18 mRNA in human skin. *Journal of Investigative Dermatology*, **125**, 1072–4.

Malnutrition Advisory Group (2003) *A Guide to the 'Malnutrition Universal Screening Tool' ('MUST') for Adults*. Redditch, BAPEN.

Mandal A, Abernathy T, Nelluri S and Stitzel V (1995) Is quinine effective and safe in leg cramps? *Journal of Clinical Pharmacology*, **35**, 588–93.

Mangelsdorf DJ, Thummel C, Beato M, *et al.* (1995) The nuclear receptor superfamily: the second decade. *Cell*, **83**, 835–9.

Mangelsdorf DJ, Umesono K and Evans RM (1994) The retinoid receptors. In: *The Retinoids: Biology, Chemistry and Medicine*. Ed. M. B. Sporn, A. B. Roberts and D. S. Goodman. New York, Raven: 319–50.

Mangione CM, Berry S, Spritzer K, *et al.* (1998) Identifying the content area for the 51-item National Eye Institute Visual Function Questionnaire: results from focus groups with visually impaired persons. *Archives of Ophthalmology*, **116**, 227–33.

Manini TM, Everhart JE, Patel KV, *et al.* (2006) Daily activity energy expenditure and mortality among older adults. *Journal of the American Medical Association*, **296**, 171–9.

Mann G (1975) Letter: bone mineral content of North Alaskan Eskimos. *American Journal of Clinical Nutrition*, **28**, 566–7.

Mannisto S, Smith-Warner SA, Spiegelman D, *et al.* (2004) Dietary carotenoids and risk of lung cancer in a pooled analysis of seven cohort studies. *Cancer Epidemiology, Biomarkers & Prevention*, **13**, 40–8.

Manson J, Greenland P, LaCroix A, *et al.* (2002) Walking compared with vigorous exercise for the prevention of cardiovascular events in women. *New England Journal of Medicine*, **347**, 716–25.

Manson J, Hu F, Rich-Edwards J, *et al.* (1999) A prospective study of walking as compared with vigorous exercise in the prevention of CHD in women. *New England Journal of Medicine*, **26**, 650–8.

Man-Son-Hing M, Wells G and Lau A (1998) Quinine for nocturnal leg cramps: a meta-analysis including unpublished data. *Journal of General Internal Medicine*, **13**, 600–6.

Marcell T (2003) Sarcopenia: causes, consequences, and preventions. *The Journals of Gerontology, Series A, Biological Sciences and Medical Sciences*, **58**, M911–16.

Marculescu R, Endler G, Schillinger M, *et al.* (2002) Interleukin-1 receptor antagonist genotype is associated with coronary atherosclerosis in patients with type 2 diabetes. *Diabetes*, **51**, 3582–5.

Mares-Perlman JA, Brady WE, Klein BE, *et al.* (1995) Serum carotenoids and tocopherols and severity of nuclear and cortical opacities. *Investigative Ophthalmology and Visual Science*, **36**, 276–88.

Mares-Perlman JA, Brady WE, Klein R, *et al.* (1995a) Dietary fat and age-related maculopathy. *Archives of Ophthalmology*, **113**, 743–8.

Mares-Perlman JA, Brady WE, Klein R, *et al.* (1995b) Serum antioxidants and age-related macular degeneration in a population-based case-control study. *Archives of Ophthalmology*, **113**, 1518–23.

Mares-Perlman JA, Fisher AI, Klein R, *et al.* (2001) Lutein and zeaxanthin in the diet and serum and their relation to age-related maculopathy in the third national health and nutrition examination survey. *American Journal of Epidemiology*, **153**, 424–32.

Mares-Perlman JA, Klein BE, Klein R and Ritter LL (1994) Relation between lens opacities and vitamin and mineral supplement use. *Ophthalmology*, **101**, 315–25.

Mares-Perlman JA, Klein R, Klein BE, *et al.* (1996) Association of zinc and antioxidant nutrients with age-related maculopathy. *Archives of Ophthalmology*, **114**, 991–7.

Mares-Perlman JA, Lyle BJ, Klein R, *et al.* (2000) Vitamin supplement use and incident cataracts in a population-based study. *Archives of Ophthalmology*, **118**, 1556–63.

Marfella R, Esposito K, Giunta R, *et al.* (2000) Circulating adhesion molecules in humans: role of hyperglycemia and hyperinsulinemia. *Circulation*, **101**, 2247–51.

Marmot M, Elliot P, Shipley M, *et al.* (1994) Alcohol and blood pressure: the INTERSALT study. *British Medical Journal*, **308**, 1263–7.

Marotta F, Barreto R, Tajiri H, *et al.* (2004) The aging/precancerous gastric mucosa: a pilot nutraceutical trial. *Annals of the New York Academy of Sciences*, **1019**, 195–9.

Marshall J, Lopez T, Shetterly S, *et al.* (1999) Indicators of nutritional risk in rural elderly Hispanic and non-Hispanic white population: San Luis Valley Health and Aging Study. *Journal of the American Dietetic Association*, **99**, 315–22.

Martin GM, Austad SN and Johnson TE (1996) Genetic analysis of ageing: role of oxidative damage and environmental stresses. *Nature Genetics*, **13**, 25–34.

Martin K, Potten CS, Roberts SA and Kirkwood TB (1998) Altered stem cell regeneration in irradiated intestinal crypts of senescent mice. *Journal of Cell Science*, **111**, 2297–303.

Martin R (1998) The role of nutrition and diet in rheumatoid arthritis. *Proceedings of the Nutrition Society*, **57**, 231–4.

Martinez DE (1998) Mortality patterns suggest lack of senescence in hydra. *Experimental Gerontology*, **33**, 217–25.

Mascarucci P, Taub D, Saccani S, *et al.* (2001) Age-related changes in cytokine production by leukocytes in rhesus monkeys. *Aging – Clinical & Experimental Research*, **13**, 85–94.

Masoro EJ (1995) Dietary restriction. *Experimental Gerontology*, **30**, 291–8.

Massague J (2000) How cells read TGF-beta signals. *Nature Reviews Molecular Cell Biology*, **1**, 169–78.

Massey L and Whiting S (2003) Excess dietary protein and bone health. In: *Nutritional Aspects of Bone Health*. Ed. S. A. New and J. P. Bonjour. Cambridge, Royal Society of Chemistry: 213–28.

Mathers JC (2002) Pulses and carcinogenesis: potential for the prevention of colon, breast and other cancers. *British Journal of Nutrition*, **88 (Suppl 3)**, S273–9.

Mathers JC (2003) Nutrients and apoptosis. In: *Molecular Nutrition*. Ed. J. Zemplini and H. Daniel. Wallingford, CAB International: 73–89.

Mathers JC, Kennard J and James OF (1993) Gastrointestinal responses to oats consumption in young adult and elderly rats: digestion, large bowel fermentation and crypt cell proliferation rates. *British Journal of Nutrition*, **70**, 567–84.

Mathews-Roth MM, Pathak MA, Parrish J, *et al.* (1972) A clinical trial of the effects of oral beta-carotene on the responses of human skin to solar radiation. *Journal of Investigative Dermatology*, **59**, 349–53.

Matkovic V, Goel PK, Badenhop-Stevens NE, *et al.* (2005) Calcium supplementation and bone mineral density in females from childhood to young adulthood: a randomized controlled trial. *American Journal of Clinical Nutrition*, **81**, 175–88.

Matkovic V, Jelic T, Wardlaw GM, *et al.* (1994) Timing of peak bone mass in Caucasian females and its implication for the prevention of osteoporosis. Inference from a cross-sectional model. *Journal of Clinical Investigation*, **93**, 799–808.

Mattes R (2002) The chemical senses and nutrition in aging: challenging old assumptions. *Journal of the American Dietetic Association*, **102**, 192–6.

Mattes-Kulig DA and Henkin RI (1985) Energy and nutrient consumption of patients with dysgeusia. *Journal of the American Dietetic Association*, **85**, 822–6.

Matthews DR, Stratton IM, Aldington SJ, *et al.* (2004) Risks of progression of retinopathy and vision loss related to tight blood pressure control in type 2 diabetes mellitus: UKPDS 69. *Archives of Ophthalmology*, **122**, 1631–40.

Matthews F and Brayne C (2005) Medical Research Council Cognitive Function and Ageing Study Investigators. *PLoS Med*, **2**, 193.

Mattison JA, Lane MA, Roth GS and Ingram DK (2003) Calorie restriction in rhesus monkeys. *Experimental Gerontology*, **38**, 35–46.

May P, Barber A, D'Olimpio J, *et al.* (2002) Reversal of cancer-related wasting using oral supplementation with a combination of beta-hydroxy-beta-methylbutyrate, arginine, and glutamine. *American Journal of Surgery*, **183**, 471–9.

Mayberry JF (2001) Epidemiology and demographics of achalasia. *Gastrointestinal Endoscopy Clinics of North America*, **11**, 235–48.

Mayer H, Bollag W, Hanni R and Ruegg R (1978) Retinoids, a new class of compounds with prophylactic and therapeutic activities in oncology and dermatology. *Experientia*, **34**, 1105–19.

Mayer-Davis EJ, D'Agostino R, Jr, Karter AJ, *et al.* (1998) Intensity and amount of physical activity in relation to insulin sensitivity: the Insulin Resistance

Atherosclerosis Study. *Journal of the American Medical Association*, **279**, 669–74.

Mayer-Davis EJ, Bell RA, Reboussin BA, *et al.* (1998) Antioxidant nutrient intake and diabetic retinopathy: the San Luis Valley Diabetes Study. *Ophthalmology*, **105**, 2264–70.

Mayes JS and Watson GH (2004) Direct effects of sex steroid hormones on adipose tissues and obesity. *Obesity Reviews*, **5**, 197–216.

Mayne ST, Risch HA, Dubrow R, *et al.* (2001) Nutrient intake and risk of subtypes of esophageal and gastric cancer. *Cancer Epidemiology, Biomarkers & Prevention*, **10**, 1055–62.

Mazess RB and Mather W (1974) Bone mineral content of North Alaskan Eskimos. *American Journal of Clinical Nutrition*, **27**, 916–25.

Mazess RB and Mather WE (1975a) Bone mineral content in Canadian Eskimos. *Human Biology*, **47**, 44–63.

Mazess RB and Mather WE (1975b) Letter: bone mineral content of North Alaskan Eskimos. *American Journal of Clinical Nutrition*, **28**, 567.

McAlindon T and Biggee B (2005) Nutritional factors and osteoarthritis: recent developments. *Current Opinion in Rheumatology*, **17**, 647–52.

McAlindon TE, Jacques P, Zhang Y, *et al.* (1996) Do antioxidant micronutrients protect against the development and progression of knee osteoarthritis? *Arthritis & Rheumatism*, **39**, 648–56.

McArdle F, Rhodes LE, Parslew R, *et al.* (2002) UVR-induced oxidative stress in human skin in vivo: effects of oral vitamin C supplementation. *Free Radical Biology & Medicine*, **33**, 1355–62.

McCabe B (2004) Prevention of food–drug interactions with special emphasis on older adults. *Current Opinions in Clinical Nutrition and Metabolic Care*, **7**, 21–36.

McCarty CA and Taylor HR (2002) A review of the epidemiologic evidence linking ultraviolet radiation and cataracts. *Developments in Ophthalmology*, **35**, 21–31.

McCay CM, Crowell MF and Maynard LA (1935) The effect of retarded growth upon the length of the lifespan and upon the ultimate body size. *Journal of Nutrition*, **10**, 63–79.

McCully K (1969) Vascular pathology of homocysteinemia: implications for the pathogenesis of arteriosclerosis. *American Journal of Pathology*, **56**, 111–28.

McFarland LV (1993) Diarrhea acquired in the hospital. *Gastroenterology Clinics of North America*, **22**, 563–77.

McFarland LV (1998) Epidemiology, risk factors and treatments for antibiotic-associated diarrhea. *Digestive Diseases*, **16**, 292–307.

McFarland LV (2006) Meta-analysis of probiotics for the prevention of antibiotic associated diarrhea and the treatment of Clostridium difficile disease. *American Journal of Gastroenterology*, **101**, 812–22.

McGrath JA, Eady RAJ and Pope FM (2004) Anatomy and organization of human skin. *Rook's Textbook of Dermatology*. Ed. T. Burns, S. Breathnach, N. Cox and C. Griffiths. Oxford, Blackwell.

McLean RR, Jacques PF, Selhub J, *et al.* (2004) Homocysteine as a predictive factor for hip fracture in older persons. *New England Journal of Medicine*, **350**, 2042–9.

McMahon J, Green T, Skeaff M, *et al.* (2006) A controlled trial of homocysteine-lowering on cognitive performance in older people. *New England Journal of Medicine*, **354**, 2764–72.

McMurray DN (1984) Cell-mediated immunity in nutritional deficiency. *Progress in Food & Nutrition Science*, **8**, 193–228.

McMurray DN, Loomis SA, Casazza LJ, Rey H and Miranda R (1981) Development of impaired cell-mediated immunity in mild and moderate malnutrition. *American Journal of Clinical Nutrition*, **34**, 68–77.

McNamara D (2000) Dietary cholesterol and atherosclerosis. *Biochimica Biophysica Acta*, **1529**, 310–20.

McNeil JJ, Robman L, Tikellis G, *et al.* (2004) Vitamin E supplementation and cataract: randomized controlled trial. *Ophthalmology*, **111**, 75–84.

McPherson K, Marsh T and Brown M (2007) *Foresight: Tackling Obesities: Future Choices – Modelling Future Trends in Obesity & Their Impact on Health*, 2nd edition. Government Office for Science. http://www.foresight.gov.uk/Obesity/14.pdf.

McTiernan A, Tworoger SS, Rajan KB, *et al.* (2004) Effect of exercise on serum androgens in postmenopausal women: a 12-month randomized clinical trial. *Cancer Epidemiology, Biomarkers & Prevention*, **13**, 1099–105.

Meance S, Turchet P, Raimondi A, *et al.* (1999) Effect of a milk fermented by Bifidobacterium SP DN-173010 (BIO) on the oro-fecal transit time in elderly. *Gut*, **45 (Suppl 5)**, A327.

Medawar PB (1952) *An Unsolved Problem of Biology*. London, Lewis.

Melhus H (2003) Vitamin A and fracture risk. In: *Nutritional Aspects of Bone Health*. Ed. S. A. New and J. P. Bonjour. Cambridge, Royal Society of Chemistry: 369–402.

Melov S, Ravenscroft J, Malik S, *et al.* (2000) Extension of life-span with superoxide dismutase/catalase mimetics. *Science*, **289**, 1567–9.

Melton LI, Khosla S, Crowson C, *et al.* (2000) Epidemiology of sarcopenia. *Journal of the American Geriatric Society*, **48**, 625–30.

Melton LJ (1995) How many women have osteoporosis now? *Journal of Bone & Mineral Research*, **10**, 175–7.

Meneilly GS, Ryan AS, Minaker KL and Elahi D (1998) The effect of age and glycemic level on the response of the beta-cell to glucose-dependent insulinotropic polypeptide and peripheral tissue sensitivity to endogenously released insulin. *Journal of Clinical Endocrinology & Metabolism*, **83**, 2925–32.

Meneilly GS, Ryan AS, Veldhuis JD and Elahi D (1997) Increased disorderliness of basal insulin release, attenuated insulin secretory burst mass, and reduced ultradian rhythmicity of insulin secretion in older individuals. *Journal of Clinical Endocrinology & Metabolism*, **82**, 4088–93.

Meneilly GS, Veldhuis JD and Elahi D (1999) Disruption of the pulsatile and entropic modes of insulin release during an unvarying glucose stimulus in elderly individuals. *Journal of Clinical Endocrinology & Metabolism*, **84**, 1938–43.

Menkes A, Mazel S, Redmond RA, *et al.* (1993) Strength training increases regional bone mineral density and bone remodeling in middle-aged and older men. *Journal of Applied Physiology*, **74**, 2478–84.

Mensink G, Ziese T and Kok F (1999) Benefits of leisure-time physical activity on the cardiovascular risk profile at older age. *International Journal of Epidemiology*, **28**, 659–66.

Mensink R, Zock P, Kester A and Katan M (2003) Effects of dietary fatty acids and carbohydrates on the ratio of serum total to HDL cholesterol and on serum lipids and apolipoproteins: a meta-analysis of 60 controlled trials. *American Journal of Clinical Nutrition*, **77**, 1146–55.

Meshkinpour H, Selod S, Movahedi H, *et al.* (1998) Effects of regular exercise in management of chronic idiopathic constipation. *Digestive Diseases & Sciences*, **43**, 2379–83.

Messier SP, Loeser RF, Miller GD, *et al.* (2004) Exercise and dietary weight loss in overweight and obese older adults with knee osteoarthritis: the Arthritis, Diet, and Activity Promotion Trial. *Arthritis & Rheumatism*, **50**, 1501–10.

Mestheneos E and Triantafillou J (1999) *Background Report on Greece*. Athens, Sextant.

Meurman J, Sanz M and Janket S (2004) Oral health, atherosclerosis, and cardiovascular disease. *Critical Reviews in Oral Biology and Medicine*, **15**, 403–13.

Meydani SN, Han SN and Hamer DH (2004) Vitamin E and respiratory infection in the elderly. *Annals of the New York Academy of Sciences*, **1031**, 214–22.

Meydani SN, Meydani M, Blumberg JB, *et al.* (1997) Vitamin E supplementation and *in vivo* immune response in healthy elderly subjects. A randomized controlled trial. *Journal of the American Medical Association*, **277**, 1380–6.

Meydani SN, Ribaya-Mercado JD, Russell RM, *et al.* (1991) Vitamin B-6 deficiency impairs interleukin 2 production and lymphocyte proliferation in elderly adults. *American Journal of Clinical Nutrition*, **53**, 1275–80.

Meydani SN, Wu D, Santos MS and Hayek MG (1995) Antioxidants and immune response in aged persons: overview of present evidence. *American Journal of Clinical Nutrition*, **62**, 1462S–76S.

Meyer CH and Sekundo W (2005) Nutritional supplementation to prevent cataract formation. *Developments in Ophthalmology*, **38**, 103–19.

Meyer HE, Smedshaug GB, Kvaavik E, *et al.* (2002) Can vitamin D supplementation reduce the risk of fracture in the elderly? A randomized controlled trial. *Journal of Bone & Mineral Research*, **17**, 709–15.

Meyer KA, Kushi LH, Jacobs DR, Jr., *et al.* (2000) Carbohydrates, dietary fiber, and incident type 2 diabetes in older women. *American Journal of Clinical Nutrition*, **71**, 921–30.

Meyer NA, Muller MJ and Herndon DN (1994) Nutrient support of the healing wound. *New Horizons*, **2**, 202–14.

Michaelsson K, Lithell H, Vessby B and Melhus H (2003) Serum retinol levels and the risk of fracture. *New England Journal of Medicine*, **348**, 287–94.

Michalik L and Wahli W (2006) Involvement of PPAR nuclear receptors in tissue injury and wound repair. *Journal of Clinical Investigation*, **116**, 598–606.

Michetti P, Dorta G, Wiesel PH, *et al.* (1999) Effect of whey-based culture supernatant of Lactobacillus acidophilus (johnsonii) La1 on *Helicobacter pylori* infection in humans. *Digestion*, **60**, 203–9.

Miettinen T, Alfthan G, Huttunen J, *et al.* (1983) Serum selenium concentration related to myocardial infarction and fatty acid content of serum lipids. *British Medical Journal*, **287**, 517–19.

Miettinen T, Naukkarinen V and Huttunen J (1982) Fatty-acid composition of serum lipids predicts myocardial infarction. *British Medical Journal*, **285**, 993–6.

Miettinen T, Pyörälä K, Olsson A, *et al.* (1997) Cholesterol-lowering therapy in women and elderly patients with myocardial infarction or angina pectoris findings from the Scandinavian Simvastatin Survival Study (4S). *Circulation*, **96**, 4211–18.

Miles EA, Thies F, Wallace FA, *et al.* (2001) Influence of age and dietary fish oil on plasma soluble adhesion molecule concentrations. *Clinical Science*, **100**, 91–100.

Miles L (2007a) Physical activity and the prevention of cancer: a review of recent findings. *Nutrition Bulletin*, **32**, 250–82.

Miles L (2007b) Physical activity and health. *Nutrition Bulletin*, **32**, 314–63.

Millen AE, Gruber M, Klein R, *et al.* (2003) Relations of serum ascorbic acid and alpha-tocopherol to diabetic retinopathy in the Third National Health and Nutrition Examination Survey. *American Journal of Epidemiology*, **158**, 225–33.

Miller G and Bruckdorfer KR (2005) The haemostatic system: coagulation, platelets and fibrinolysis. In: *Cardiovascular Disease: Diet, Nutrition and Emerging Risk Factors*. Ed. S Stanner. Oxford, Blackwell Publishing: 100–27.

Miller GD, Nicklas BJ, Davis C, *et al.* (2006) Intensive weight loss program improves physical function in older obese adults with knee osteoarthritis. *Obesity*, **14**, 1219–30.

Miller GE, Stetler CA, Carney RM, *et al.* (2002) Clinical depression and inflammatory risk markers for coronary heart disease. *American Journal of Cardiology*, **90**, 1279–83.

Miller RA (1998) Aging and immune function. In: *Fundamental Immunology*. Ed. W. E. Paul. Philadelphia, Lippincott, Williams and Wilkins: 947–66.

Miller RA and Stutman O (1981) Decline, in aging mice, of the anti-2,4,6-trinitrophenyl (TNP) cytotoxic T cell response attributable to loss of Lyt-2-, interleukin 2-producing helper cell function. *European Journal of Immunology*, **11**, 751–6.

Mills J and Signore C (2004) Neural tube defect rates before and after food fortification with folic acid. *Birth Defects Research. Part A, Clinical & Molecular Teratology*, **70**, 844–5.

Mills SJ, Ashworth JJ, Gilliver SC, *et al.* (2005) The sex steroid precursor DHEA accelerates cutaneous wound healing via the estrogen receptors. *Journal of Investigative Dermatology*, **125**, 1053–62.

Millward D (2000) Postprandial protein utilization: implications for clinical nutrition. *Nestle Nutrition Workshop Series. Clinical and Performance Programme*, **3**, 135–52.

Millward D and Jackson A (2004) Protein/energy ratios of current diets in developed and developing countries compared with a safe protein/energy ratio: implications for recommended protein and amino acid intake. *Public Health Nutrition*, **7**, 387–405.

Milne AC, Potter J and Avenell A (2005) Protein and energy supplementation in elderly people at risk from malnutrition. *Cochrane Database of Systematic Reviews*, CD003288.

Minihane A, Khan S, Leigh-Firbank E, *et al.* (2000) ApoE polymorphism and fish oil supplementation in subjects with an atherogenic lipoprotein phenotype. *Arteriosclerosis, Thrombosis and Vascular Biology*, **20**, 1990–7.

Ministry of Agriculture FaF (1997) *National Food Survey. Annual Report on Food Expenditure, Consumption and Nutrient Food Consumption and Expenditure Intakes.* London, Stationery Office.

Ministry of Health (2002) *Health of Older People in New Zealand. A Statistical Reference.* Wellington, Ministry of Health.

Mioche L, Bourdiol P, Monier S, *et al.* (2004) Changes in jaw muscles activity with age: effects on food bolus properties. *Physiology & Behavior*, **82**, 621–7.

Mitchell P, Smith W, Cumming RG, *et al.* (2003) Nutritional factors in the development of age-related eye disease. *Asia Pacific Journal of Clinical Nutrition*, **12 (Suppl)**, S5.

Mitsiopoulos N, Baumgartner R, Heymsfield S, *et al.* (1998) Cadaver validation of skeletal muscle measurement by magnetic resonance imaging and computerized tomography. *Journal of Applied Physiology*, **85**, 115–22.

Mitsuoka T (1992) Intestinal flora and aging. *Nutrition Reviews*, **50**, 438–46.

Mittendorfer B, Andersen JL, Plomgaard P, *et al.* (2005) Protein synthesis rates in human muscles: neither anatomical location nor fibre-type composition are major determinants. *Journal of Physiology*, **563**, 203–11.

Mocchegiani E, Costarelli L, Giacconi R, *et al.* (2006) Nutrient–gene interaction in ageing and successful ageing. A single nutrient (zinc) and some target genes related to inflammatory/immune response. *Mechanisms of Ageing & Development*, **127**, 517–25.

Moeller SM, Blumberg JB and Jacques PF (2000) The potential role of dietary xanthophylls in cataract and age-related macular degeneration. *Journal of the American College of Nutrition*, **19**, 522S–7S.

Moeller SM, Taylor A, Tucker KL, *et al.* (2004) Overall adherence to the dietary guidelines for Americans is associated with reduced prevalence of early age-related nuclear lens opacities in women. *Journal of Nutrition*, **134**, 1812–19.

Moffat SD, Zonderman AB, Metter EJ, *et al.* (2002) Longitudinal assessment of serum free testosterone concentration predicts memory performance and cognitive status in elderly men. *Journal of Clinical Endocrinology & Metabolism*, **87**, 5001–7.

Mohamed-Ali V and Coppack S (2005) Adipose tissue – derived factors. In: *Cardiovascular Disease: Diet, Nutrition and Emerging Risk Factors*. Ed. S. Stanner. Oxford, Blackwell Publishing: 160–76.

Mojet J, Heidema J and Christ-Hazelhof E (2003) Taste perception with age: generic or specific losses in suprathreshold intensities of five taste qualities? *Chemical Senses*, **28**, 397–413.

Mojet J, Heidema J and Christ-Hazelhof E (2004) Effect of concentration on taste–taste interactions in foods for elderly and young subjects. *Chemical Senses*, **29**, 671–81.

Molokhia MM and Portnoy B (1969) Neutron activation analysis of trace elements in skin. 3. Zinc in normal skin. *British Journal of Dermatology*, **81**, 759–62.

Montebugnoli L, Servidio D, Miaton R, *et al.* (2005) Periodontal health improves systemic inflammatory and haemostatic status in subjects with coronary heart disease. *Journal of Clinical Periodontology*, **32**, 188–92.

Mooradian AD, Reed RL, Osterweil D and Scuderi P (1991) Detectable serum levels of tumor necrosis factor alpha may predict early mortality in elderly institutionalized patients. *Journal of the American Geriatrics Society*, **39**, 891–4.

Moore C, Murphy M, Keast D, *et al.* (2004) Vitamin D intake in the United States. *Journal of the American Dietetic Association*, **104**, 980–3.

Moore LL, Bradlee ML, Singer MR, *et al.* (2004) BMI and waist circumference as predictors of lifetime colon cancer risk in Framingham Study adults. *International Journal of Obesity & Related Metabolic Disorders: Journal of the International Association for the Study of Obesity*, **28**, 559–67.

Morabito N, Crisafulli A, Vergara C, *et al.* (2002) Effects of genistein and hormone-replacement therapy on bone loss in early postmenopausal women: a randomized double-blind placebo-controlled study. *Journal of Bone & Mineral Research*, **17**, 1904–12.

Morelli V, Naquin C and Weaver V (2003) Alternative therapies for traditional disease states: osteoarthritis. *American Family Physician*, **67**, 339–44.

Morley JE (2001) Hormones, aging and endocrine disease in the elderly. In: 4th edition. *Endocrinology and Metabolism* Ed. P. Felig and L. A. Frohman. New York, McGraw-Hill: 1455–82.

Morris M, Evans D, Bienias J, *et al.* (2003) Dietary fats and the risk of incident Alzheimer disease. *Archives of Neurology*, **60**, 194–200.

Morris M, Evans D, Bienias J, *et al.* (2005) Dietary folate and vitamin B12 intake and cognitive decline among community-dwelling older persons. *Archives of Neurology*, **62**, 641–5.

Morris MC, Evans DA, Tangney CC, *et al.* (2006) Associations of vegetable and fruit consumption with age-related cognitive change. *Neurology*, **67**, 1370–6.

Morris MS, Jacques PF, Rosenberg IH and Selhub J (2007) Folate and vitamin B-12 status in relation to anemia, macrocytosis, and cognitive impairment in older Americans in the age of folic acid fortification. *American Journal of Clinical Nutrition*, **85**, 193–200.

Morse C, Thom J, Reeves N, *et al.* (2005) *In vivo* physiological cross-sectional area and specific force are reduced in the gastrocnemius of elderly men. *Journal of Applied Physiology*, **99**, 1050–5.

Mosmann TR and Sad S (1996) The expanding universe of T-cell subsets: Th1, Th2 and more. *Immunology Today*, **17**, 138–46.

Mosmann TR, Cherwinski H, Bond MW, *et al.* (1986) Two types of murine helper T cell clone. I. Definition according to profiles of lymphokine activities and secreted proteins. *Journal of Immunology*, **136**, 2348–57.

Mowlana F, Heath MR, Van der Bilt A and Van der Glas HW (1994) Assessment of chewing efficiency: a comparison of particle size distribution determined using optical scanning and sieving of almonds. *Journal of Oral Rehabilitation*, **21**, 545–51.

Moynihan PJ, Butler TJ, Thomason JM and Jepson NJ (2000) Nutrient intake in partially dentate patients: the effect of prosthetic rehabilitation. *Journal of Dentistry*, **28**, 557–63.

Moynihan PJ, Snow S, Jepson NJ and Butler TJ (1994) Intake of non-starch polysaccharide (dietary fibre) in edentulous and dentate persons: an observational study. *British Dental Journal*, **177**, 243–7.

Mozaffarian D, Katan M, Ascherio A, *et al.* (2006) Trans fatty acids and cardiovascular disease. *New England Journal of Medicine*, **354**, 1601–13.

Mozaffarieh M, Sacu S and Wedrich A (2003) The role of the carotenoids, lutein and xeaxanthein, in protecting against age-related macular degneration: a review based on controversial evidence. *Nutrition Journal*, **2**, 20.

Muiras ML, Muller M, Schachter F, *et al.* (1998) Increased poly(ADP-ribose) polymerase activity in lymphoblastoid cell lines from centenarians. *Journal of Molecular Medicine*, **76**, 346–54.

Muller M and Kersten S (2003) Nutrigenomics: goals and strategies. *Nature Reviews Genetics*, **4**, 315–22.

Muller-Hocker J (1989) Cytochrome-c-oxidase deficient cardiomyocytes in the human heart – an age-related phenomenon. A histochemical ultracytochemical study. *American Journal of Pathology*, **134**, 1167–73.

Muller-Hocker J, Seibel P, Schneiderbanger K and Kadenbach B (1993) Different in situ hybridization patterns of mitochondrial DNA in cytochrome c oxidase-deficient extraocular muscle fibres in the elderly. *Virchows Archiv – A, Pathological Anatomy & Histopathology*, **422**, 7–15.

Munger RG, Cerhan JR and Chiu BC (1999) Prospective study of dietary protein intake and risk of hip fracture in postmenopausal women. *American Journal of Clinical Nutrition*, **69**, 147–52.

Munro HN (1974) Report of a conference on protein and amino acid needs for growth and development. *American Journal of Clinical Nutrition*, **27**, 55–8.

Murgatroyd P, Goldberg G, Leahy F, *et al.* (1999) Effects of inactivity and diet composition on human energy balance. *International Journal of Obesity and Related Metabolic Disorders*, **23**, 1269–75.

Murphy CT, McCarroll SA, Bargmann CI, *et al.* (2003) Genes that act downstream of DAF-16 to influence the lifespan of Caenorhabditis elegans. *Nature*, **424**, 277–83.

Murphy TK, Calle EE, Rodriguez C, *et al.* (2000) Body mass index and colon cancer mortality in a large prospective study. *American Journal of Epidemiology*, **152**, 847–54.

Murray DR and Freeman GL (2003) Proinflammatory cytokines: predictors of a failing heart? *Circulation*, **107**, 1460–2.

Murray J and Lopez A (1996) *The Global Burden of Disease*. Geneva, World Heath Organization.

Myllykangas-Luosujarvi R, Aho K and Isomake H (2000) Mortality in rheumatoid arthritis. *Seminars in Arthritis & Rheumatism*, **72**, 42–8.

Mysliwska J, Bryl E, Foerster J and Mysliwski A (1998) Increase of interleukin 6 and decrease of interleukin 2 production during the ageing process are influenced by the health status. *Mechanisms of Ageing & Development*, **100**, 313–28.

Nagata C, Takatsuka N, Inaba S, *et al.* (1998) Association of diet and other lifestyle with onset of menopause in Japanese women. *Maturitas*, **29**, 105–13.

Nagata C, Takatsuka N, Kawakami N and Shimizu H (2000) Association of diet with the onset of menopause in Japanese women. *American Journal of Epidemiology*, **152**, 863–7.

Nappo F, Esposito K, Cioffi M, *et al.* (2002) Postprandial endothelial activation in healthy subjects and in type 2 diabetic patients: role of fat and carbohydrate meals. *Journal of the American College of Cardiology*, **39**, 1145–50.

Närhi TO, Meurman JH, Ainamo A, *et al.* (1992) Association between salivary flow rate and the use of systemic medication among 76-, 81-, and 86-year-old inhabitants in Helsinki, Finland. *Journal of Dental Research*, **71**, 1875–80.

Narici MV, Maganaris CN, Reeves ND and Capodaglio P (2003) Effect of aging on human muscle architecture. *Journal of Applied Physiology*, **95**, 2229–34.

Naru E, Suzuki T, Moriyama M, *et al.* (2005) Functional changes induced by chronic UVA irradiation to cultured human dermal fibroblasts. *British Journal of Dermatology*, **153 (Suppl 2)**, 6–12.

National Academy of Sciences (2002) *Dietary Reference Intakes for Energy, Carbohydrate, Fiber, Fat, Fatty Acids, Cholesterol, Protein, and Amino Acids*. Washington, National Academies Press.

National Academy of Sciences (2004) *Dietary Reference Intakes for Water, Potassium, Sodium, Chloride, and Sulfate*. Washington DC, National Academies Press.

National Center for Health Statistics (2005) Data Warehouse on Trends in Health and Aging. http://www.cdc.gov/nchs/agingact.htm. Accessed 5 January 2005.

National Institute for Health and Clinical Excellence (2007) MI: Secondary Prevention in Primary and Secondary Care for Patients Following a Myocardial Infarction. www.nice.org.uk.

National Institute for Health and Clinical Excellence (2008) Osteoarthritis: National Clinical Guidelines for Care and Management in Adults. www.nice.org.uk/nicemedia/pdf/CG059FullGuideline.pdf.

National Institutes of Health, Lung and Blood Institute (1998) Clinical Guidelines on Identification, Evaluation, and Treatment of Overweight and Obesity in Adults. The Evidence Report. www.nhlbi.nih.gov.

National Osteoporosis Society. What is Osteoporosis? www.nos.org.uk/osteo.asp. Accessed 24 January 2006.

National Statistics (2004) *National Travel Survey 2004*. London, Department of Transport.

National Statistics Online (2004) Older People. www.statistics.gov.uk. Accessed 19 May 2004.

Nawaz A, Mohammed I, Ahsan K, *et al.* (1998) Clostridium difficile colitis associated with treatment of *Helicobacter pylori* infection. *American Journal of Gastroenterology*, **93**, 1175–6.

Naylor J and Young J (1994) A general population survey of rest cramps. *Age & Ageing*, **23**, 418–20.

Neer RM, Arnaud CD, Zanchetta JR, *et al.* (2001) Effect of parathyroid hormone (1–34) on fractures and bone mineral density in postmenopausal women with osteoporosis. *New England Journal of Medicine*, **344**, 1434–41.

Nelson HD, Humphrey LL, Nygren P, *et al.* (2002) Postmenopausal hormone replacement therapy: scientific review. *Journal of the American Medical Association*, **288**, 872–81.

Nelson M, Erens B, Bates B, Church S and Boshier T (2007) *Low Income Diet and Nutrition Survey*. London, Stationery Office.

Neuropathology Group. Medical Research Council Cognitive Function and Aging Study (2001) Pathological correlates of late-onset dementia in a multicentre, community-based population in England and Wales. Neuropathology Group of the Medical Research Council Cognitive Function and Ageing Study (MRC CFAS). *Lancet*, **357**, 169–75.

Neve J (1996) Selenium as a risk factor for cardiovascular diseases. *Journal of Cardiovascular Risk*, **3**, 42–7.

Nevitt M, Xu L, Zhang Y, *et al.* (2000) Chinese in Beijing have a very low prevalence of hip OA compared to US Caucasians. *Arthritis & Rheumatism*, **43**, S171.

New SA (2004) Do vegetarians have a normal bone mass? *Osteoporosis International*, **15**, 679–88.

New SA, Bolton-Smith C, Grubb DA and Reid DM (1997) Nutritional influences on bone mineral density: a cross-sectional study in premenopausal women. *American Journal of Clinical Nutrition*, **65**, 1831–9.

Newton JP, Yemm R, Abel RW and Menhinick S (1993) Changes in human jaw muscles with age and dental state. *Gerodontology*, **10**, 16–22.

Ng K, Woo J, Kwan M, *et al.* (2004) Effect of age and disease on taste perception. *Journal of Pain and Symptom Management*, **28**, 28–34.

Ngandu T, Helkala E, Soininen H, *et al.* (2006) Alcohol drinking and cognitive functions: findings from the Cardiovascular Risk Factors Aging and Dementia (CAIDE) Study. *Dementia & Geriatric Cognitive Disorders*, **23**, 140–9.

Nicoll JA, Mrak RE, Graham DI, *et al.* (2000) Association of interleukin-1 gene polymorphisms with Alzheimer's disease. *Annals of Neurology*, **47**, 365–8.

Niedzielin K, Kordecki H and Birkenfeld B (2001) A controlled, double-blind, randomized study on the efficacy of Lactobacillus plantarum 299V in patients with irritable bowel syndrome. *European Journal of Gastroenterology & Hepatology*, **13**, 1143–7.

Nikander E, Metsa-Heikkila M, Ylikorkala O and Tiitinen A (2004) Effects of phytoestrogens on bone turnover in postmenopausal women with a history of breast cancer. *Journal of Clinical Endocrinology & Metabolism*, **89**, 1207–12.

Nilsson B-O, Ernerudh J, Johansson B, *et al.* (2003) Morbidity does not influence the T-cell immune risk phenotype in the elderly: findings in the Swedish NONA Immune Study using sample selection protocols. *Mechanisms of Ageing & Development*, **124**, 469–76.

Ning Y, Xu J-F, Li Y, *et al.* (2003) Telomere length and the expression of natural telomeric genes in human fibroblasts. *Human Molecular Genetics*, **12**, 1329–36.

Niu XT, Cushin B, Reisner A, *et al.* (1987) Effect of dietary supplementation with vitamin A on arterial healing in rats. *Journal of Surgical Research*, **42**, 61–5.

Niv E, Naftali T, Hallak R and Vaisman N (2005) The efficacy of Lactobacillus reuteri ATCC 55730 in the treatment of patients with irritable bowel syndrome – a double-blind, placebo-controlled, randomized study. *Clinical Nutrition*, **24**, 925–31.

Njemini R, Abeele MV, Demanet C, *et al.* (2002) Age-related decrease in the inducibility of heat-shock protein 70 in human peripheral blood mononuclear cells. *Journal of Clinical Immunology*, **22**, 195–205.

Nobaek S, Johansson ML, Molin G, *et al.* (2000) Alteration of intestinal microflora is associated with reduction in abdominal bloating and pain in patients with irritable bowel syndrome. *American Journal of Gastroenterology*, **95**, 1231–8.

Noel P, Williams JJ, Unutzer J, *et al.* (2004) Depression and comorbid illness in elderly primary care patients: impact on multiple domains of health status and well-being. *Annals of Family Medicine* **2**, 555–62.

Noguchi T, Tsujisaki M, Imai K, *et al.* (1998) Relationship among risk factors of atherosclerosis, leukocyte count, and soluble intercellular adhesion molecule-1. *Internal Medicine*, **37**, 123–6.

Norat T, Bingham S, Ferrari P, *et al.* (2005) Meat, fish, and colorectal cancer risk: the European Prospective Investigation into cancer and nutrition. *Journal of the National Cancer Institute*, **97**, 906–16.

Nordgaard I, Mortensen PB and Langkilde AM (1995) Small intestinal malabsorption and colonic fermentation of resistant starch and resistant peptides to short-chain fatty acids. *Nutrition*, **11**, 129–37.

Nordin BE, Need AG, Morris HA and Horowitz M (1993) The nature and significance of the relationship between urinary sodium and urinary calcium in women. *Journal of Nutrition*, **123**, 1615–22.

Nordin BEC, Need AG, Morris HA, *et al.* (2004) Effect of age on calcium absorption in postmenopausal women. *American Journal of Clinical Nutrition*, **80**, 998–1002.

Nordin S, Razani LJ, Markison S and Murphy CJ (2003) Age-associated increases in intensity discrimination for taste. *Experimental Aging Research*, **29**, 371–81.

Nowjack-Raymer RE and Sheiham A (2003) Association of edentulism and diet and nutrition in US adults. *Journal of Dental Research*, **82**, 123–6.

Nugent AP (2004) The metabolic syndrome. *Nutrition Bulletin*, **29**, 36–43.

Nugent AP (2005) Health properties of resistant starch. *Nutrition Bulletin*, **30**, 27–54.

Nusselder W, Looman C and Mackenbach J (2005) Non-disease factors affected trajectories of disability in a prospective study. *Journal of Clinical Epidemiology*, **58**, 484–94.

Nuttall SL, Martin U, Sinclair AJ and Kendall MJ (1998) Glutathione: in sickness and in health. *Lancet*, **351**, 645–6.

Nygaard E and Sanchez J (1982) Intramuscular variation of fiber types in the brachial biceps and the lateral vastus muscles of elderly men: how representative is a small biopsy sample? *The Anatomy Record*, **203**, 451–9.

O'Brien PMS, Wheeler T and Barker DJP (1999) *Fetal Programming: Influences on Development and Disease in Later Life.* London, Royal College of Obstetricians and Gynaecologists.

O'Neill T (2007) Assessment of risk. In: *Managing Osteoporosis.* Ed. S. A. Lanham-New, T. O'Neill, R. Morris, D. Skeleton and A. Sutcliffe. Oxford, Clinical Publishing: 117–33.

Oberg S, Wenner J, Johansson J, *et al.* (2005) Barrett esophagus: risk factors for progression to dysplasia and adenocarcinoma. *Annals of Surgery*, **242**, 49–54.

Obermayer-Pietsch BM, Bonelli CM, Walter DE, *et al.* (2004) Genetic predisposition for adult lactose intolerance and relation to diet, bone density, and bone fractures. *Journal of Bone & Mineral Research*, **19**, 42–7.

Oderberg G (2004) Characterisation of joint pain in human OA. *Novartis Foundation Symposium*, **260**, 105–15.

Oeppen J and Vaupel JW (2002) Demography. Broken limits to life expectancy. *Science*, **296**, 1029–31.

Office of Deputy Prime Minister (2006) A Sure Start to Later Life – Ending Inequalities for Older People, 2007. archive.cabinetoffice.gov.uk/seu/downloaddoc7b5f.pdf?id=797.

Office for National Statistics (2001) National Statistics Online. Census 2001: CD supplement to the National report for England and Wales and key statistics for local authorities in England and Wales. London, ONS. www.statistics.gov.uk/census2001/access_results.asp.

Office for National Statistics (2002) *Census 2001.* London, Stationery Office.

Ohata H, Kitauchi S, Yoshimura N, *et al.* (2004) Progression of chronic atrophic gastritis associated with *Helicobacter pylori* infection increases risk of gastric cancer. *International Journal of Cancer*, **109**, 138–43.

Ohkusu K, Du J, Isobe KI, *et al.* (1997) Protein kinase C alpha-mediated chronic signal transduction for immunosenescence. *Journal of Immunology*, **159**, 2082–4.

Oldfield EC, 3rd (2004) Clostridium difficile-associated diarrhea: risk factors, diagnostic methods, and treatment. *Reviews in Gastroenterological Disorders*, **4**, 186–95.

Oliva MS and Taylor H (2005) Ultraviolet radiation and the eye. *International Ophthalmology Clinics*, **45**, 1–17.

Olivieri F, Antonicelli R, Cardelli M, *et al.* (2006) Genetic polymorphisms of inflammatory cytokines and myocardial infarction in the elderly. *Mechanisms of Ageing & Development*, **127**, 552–9.

Olsen S, Aagaard P, Kadi F, *et al.* (2006) Creatine supplementation augments the increase in satellite cell and myonuclei number in human skeletal muscle induced by strength training. *Journal of Physiology*, **573(Pt 2)**, 525–34.

Olsson J, Wikby A, Johansson B, *et al.* (2000) Age-related change in peripheral blood T-lymphocyte subpopulations and cytomegalovirus infection in the very old: the Swedish longitudinal OCTO immune study. *Mechanisms of Ageing & Development*, **121**, 187–201.

Omenn G, Goodman G, Thornquist M, *et al.* (1996) Risk factors for lung cancer and for intervention effects in CARET, the Beta-Carotene and Retinol Efficacy Trial. *Journal of the National Cancer Institute*, **88**, 1550–9.

Ono T, Hori K, Ikebe K, *et al.* (2003) Factors influencing eating ability of old inpatients in a rehabilitation hospital in Japan. *Gerodontology*, **20**, 24–31.

Oommen AM, Griffin JB, Sarath G and Zempleni J (2005) Roles for nutrients in epigenetic events. *Journal of Nutritional Biochemistry*, **16**, 74–7.

Ophir G, Amariglio N, Jacob-Hirsch J, *et al.* (2005) Apolipoprotein E4 enhances brain inflammation by modulation of the NF-kappaB signaling cascade. *Neurobiology of Disease*, **20**, 709–18.

Ordovas J (1999) The genetics of serum lipid responsiveness to dietary interventions. *Proceedings of the Nutrition Society*, **58**, 171–87.

Orengo IF, Black HS, Kettler AH and Wolf JE, Jr. (1989) Influence of dietary menhaden oil upon carcinogenesis and various cutaneous responses to ultraviolet radiation. *Photochemistry & Photobiology*, **49**, 71–7.

Orlander J, Kiessling K and Larsson L (1979) Skeletal muscle metabolism, morphology and function in sedentary smokers and nonsmokers. *Acta Physiologica Scandinavica*, **107**, 39–46.

Orrhage K, Sjostedt S and Nord CE (2000) Effect of supplements with lactic acid bacteria and oligofructose on the intestinal microflora during administration of cefpodoxime proxetil. *Journal of Antimicrobial Chemotherapy*, **46**, 603–12.

Ortega R, Mena M, Faci M, *et al.* (2001) Vitamin status in different groups of the Spanish population: a meta-analysis of national studies performed between 1990 and 1999. *Public Health Nutrition*, **4**, 1325–9.

Osler W (1892) The Principles and Practice of Medicine. *(Reprinted by The Classics of Medicine, Division of Gryphon Editions Ltd. Birmingham Alabama 1978.)* New York, Appleton.

Osmond C, Barker D, Winter P, *et al.* (1993) Early growth and death from cardiovascular disease in women. *British Medical Journal*, **307**, 1519–24.

Osteoporosis Prevention, Diagnosis, and Therapy. NIH Consensus Statement Online 2000 March 27–29; **17**(1): 1–36. consensus.nih.gov/2000/2000Osteoporosis111html. htm. Accessed 24 January 2006.

Ouwehand AC, Lagstrom H, Suomalainen T and Salminen S (2002) Effect of probiotics on constipation, fecal azoreductase activity and fecal mucin content in the elderly. *Annals of Nutrition & Metabolism*, **46**, 159–62.

Ouyang Q, Cicek G, Westendorp RG, *et al.* (2000) Reduced IFN-gamma production in elderly people following in vitro stimulation with influenza vaccine and endotoxin. *Mechanisms of Ageing & Development*, **121**, 131–7.

Ouyang Q, Wagner WM, Wikby A, *et al.* (2003) Large numbers of dysfunctional CD8+ T lymphocytes bearing receptors for a single dominant CMV epitope in the very old. *Journal of Clinical Immunology*, **23**, 247–57.

Ozawa T (1998) Mitochondrial DNA mutations and age. *Annals of the New York Academy of Sciences*, **854**, 128–54.

Ozcan U, Cao Q, Yilmaz E, *et al.* (2004) Endoplasmic reticulum stress links obesity, insulin action, and type 2 diabetes. *Science*, **306**, 457–61.

Pacht ER, DeMichele SJ, Nelson JL, *et al.* (2003) Enteral nutrition with eicosapentaenoic acid, gamma-linolenic acid, and antioxidants reduces alveolar inflammatory mediators and protein influx in patients with acute respiratory distress syndrome. *Critical Care Medicine*, **31**, 491–500.

Packer L and Valacchi G (2002) Antioxidants and the response of skin to oxidative stress: vitamin E as a key indicator. *Skin Pharmacology & Applied Skin Physiology*, **15**, 282–90.

Padyukov L, Camilla S, Patrik S, *et al.* (2004) A gene–environment interaction between smoking and shared epitope genes in HLA-DR provides a high risk of seropositive rheumatoid arthritis. *Arthritis & Rheumatism*, **50**, 3085–92.

Paganelli R, Quinti I, Fagiolo U, *et al.* (1992) Changes in circulating B cells and immunoglobulin classes and subclasses in a healthy aged population. *Clinical & Experimental Immunology*, **90**, 351–4.

Paganini-Hill A, Chao A, Ross RK and Henderson BE (1991) Exercise and other factors in the prevention of hip fracture: the Leisure World study. *Epidemiology*, **2**, 16–25.

Pageon H and Asselineau D (2005) An *in vitro* approach to the chronological aging of skin by glycation of the collagen: the biological effect of glycation on the reconstructed skin model. *Annals of the New York Academy of Sciences*, **1043**, 529–32.

Painter NS (1985) The cause of diverticular disease of the colon, its symptoms and its complications. Review and hypothesis. *Journal of the Royal College of Surgeons of Edinburgh*, **30**, 118–22.

Pallast EG, Schouten EG, de Waart FG, *et al.* (1999) Effect of 50- and 100-mg vitamin E supplements on cellular immune function in noninstitutionalized elderly persons. *American Journal of Clinical Nutrition*, **69**, 1273–81.

Palmer RM, Wilson RF, Hasan AS and Scott DA (2005) Mechanisms of action of environmental factors – tobacco smoking. *Journal of Clinical Periodontology*, **32 (Suppl 6)**, 180–95.

Pan XR, Li GW, Hu YH, *et al.* (1997) Effects of diet and exercise in preventing NIDDM in people with impaired glucose tolerance. The Da Qing IGT and Diabetes Study. *Diabetes Care*, **20**, 537–44.

Paolisso G, Di Maro G, Galzerano D, *et al.* (1994) Pharmacological doses of vitamin E and insulin action in elderly subjects. *American Journal of Clinical Nutrition*, **59**, 1291–6.

Papassotiropoulos A, Bagli M, Jessen F, *et al.* (1999) A genetic variation of the inflammatory cytokine interleukin-6 delays the initial onset and reduces the risk for sporadic Alzheimer's disease. *Annals of Neurology*, **45**, 666–8.

Parfitt A (1990) Osteomalacia and related disorders. In: *Metabolic bone disease and clinically related disorders.* Ed. L. Avioli and S. Krane. Philadelphia, WB Saunders: 329–96.

Parish S, Collins R, Peto R, *et al.* (1995) Cigarette smoking, tar yields, and non-fatal myocardial infarction: 14000 cases and 32000 controls in the United Kingdom. *British Medical Journal*, **311**, 471–7.

Park Y, Hunter DJ, Spiegelman D, *et al.* (2005) Dietary fiber intake and risk of colorectal cancer: a pooled analysis of prospective cohort studies. *Journal of the American Medical Association*, **294**, 2849–57.

Parker B, Noakes M, Luscombe N and Clifton P (2002) Effect of a high-protein, high-monounsaturated fat weight loss diet on glycemic control and lipid levels in type 2 diabetes. *Diabetes Care*, **25**, 425–30.

Parker BA and Chapman IM (2004) Food intake and ageing – the role of the gut. *Mechanisms of Ageing & Development*, **125**, 859–66.

Parkes TL, Elia AJ, Dickinson D, *et al.* (1998) Extension of Drosophila lifespan by overexpression of human SOD1 in motorneurons. *Nature Genetics*, **19**, 171–4.

Parle JV, Franklyn JA, Cross KW, *et al.* (1991) Prevalence and follow-up of abnormal thyrotrophin (TSH) concentrations in the elderly in the United Kingdom. *Clinical Endocrinology*, **34**, 77–83.

Pasquali R and Gambineri A (2006) Polycystic ovary syndrome: a multifaceted disease from adolescence to adult age. *Annals of the New York Academy of Sciences*, **1092**, 158–74.

Pathmakanthan S, Meance S and Edwards CA (2000) Probiotics: a review of human studies to date and methodological approaches. *Microbial Ecology in Health & Disease*, **12 (Suppl 2)**, 10–30.

Paulionis L, Kane S-L and Meckling KA (2005) Vitamin status and cognitive function in a long-term care population. *BMC Geriatrics*, **5**, 16.

Pawelec G and Solana R (1997) Immunosenescence. *Immunology Today*, **18**, 514–16.

Pawelec G, Adibzadeh M, Pohla H and Schaudt K (1995) Immunosenescence: ageing of the immune system. *Immunology Today*, **16**, 420–2.

Pawelec G, Adibzadeh M, Solana R and Beckman I (1997) The T cell in the ageing individual. *Mechanisms of Ageing & Development*, **93**, 35–45.

Pawelec G, Akbar A, Caruso C, *et al.* (2005) Human immunosenescence: is it infectious? *Immunological Reviews*, **205**, 257–68.

Pawelec G, Barnett Y, Forsey R, *et al.* (2002) T cells and aging. *Frontiers in Bioscience*, **7**, d1056–183.

Pawelec G, Mariani E, Bradley B and Solana R (2000) Longevity in vitro of human CD4+ T helper cell clones derived from young donors and elderly donors, or from progenitor cells: age-associated differences in cell surface molecule expression and cytokine secretion. *Biogerontology*, **1**, 247–54.

Payne S (2004) Gender influences on men's health. *The Journal of The Royal Society for the Promotion of Health*, **124**, 206–7.

Pearson S, Young A, Macaluso A, *et al.* (2002) Muscle function in elite master weightlifters. *Medicine and Science in Sports and Exercise*, **34**, 1199–206.

Pechere-Bertschi A and Burnier M (2004) Female sex hormones, salt, and blood pressure regulation. *American Journal of Hypertension*, **17**, 994–1001.

Pedersen WA, Wan R and Mattson MP (2001) Impact of aging on stress-responsive neuroendocrine systems. *Mechanisms of Ageing & Development*, **122**, 963–83.

Pelletier G and Ren L (2004) Localization of sex steroid receptors in human skin. *Histology & Histopathology*, **19**, 629–36.

Penn ND, Purkins L, Kelleher J, *et al.* (1991) The effect of dietary supplementation with vitamins A, C and E on cell-mediated immune function in elderly long-stay patients: a randomized controlled trial. *Age & Ageing*, **20**, 169–74.

Pepersack T, Fuss M, Otero J, *et al.* (1992) Longitudinal study of bone metabolism after ethanol withdrawal in alcoholic patients. *Journal of Bone & Mineral Research*, **7**, 383–7.

Pera P, Bucca C, Borro R, *et al.* (2002) Influence of mastication on gastric emptying. *Journal of Dental Research*, **81**, 179–81.

Percheron G, Hogrel J-Y, Denot-Ledunois S, *et al.* (2003) Effect of 1-year oral administration of dehydroepiandrosterone to 60- to 80-year-old individuals on muscle function and cross-sectional area: a double-blind placebo-controlled trial. *Archives of Internal Medicine*, **163**, 720–7.

Perl D and Brody AR (1980) Alzheimer's disease: X-ray spectrometric evidence of aluminum accumulation in neurofibrillary tangle-bearing neurons. *Science*, **208**, 297–9.

Persson PG, Bernell O, Leijonmarck CE, *et al.* (1996) Survival and cause-specific mortality in inflammatory bowel disease: a population-based cohort study. *Gastroenterology*, **110**, 1339–45.

Peters R, Beckett N, Forette F, *et al.* (2008) Incident dementia and blood pressure lowering in the Hypertension in the Very Elderly Trial cognitive function assessment (HYVET-COG): a double-blind, placebo controlled trial. *Lancet Neurology*, **7**, 683–9.

Petersen DN, Tkalcevic GT, Koza-Taylor PH, *et al.* (1998) Identification of estrogen receptor beta2, a functional variant of estrogen receptor beta expressed in normal rat tissues. *Endocrinology*, **139**, 1082–92.

Petersen K, Befroy D, Dufour S, *et al.* (2003) Mitochondrial dysfunction in the elderly: possible role in insulin resistance. *Science*, **300**, 1140–2.

Peterson PK, Chao CC, Carson P, *et al.* (1994) Levels of tumor necrosis factor alpha, interleukin 6, interleukin 10, and transforming growth factor beta are normal in the serum of the healthy elderly. *Clinical Infectious Diseases*, **19**, 1158–9.

Petersson I (1996) Occurrence of osteoarthritis of the peripheral joints in European populations. *Annals of the Rheumatic Diseases*, **55**, 659–61.

Petti S and Scully C (2005) Oral cancer: the association between nation-based alcohol-drinking profiles and oral cancer mortality. *Oral Oncology*, **41**, 828–34.

Pfeifer M, Begerow B, Minne HW, *et al.* (2001) Vitamin D status, trunk muscle strength, body sway, falls, and fractures among 237 postmenopausal women with osteoporosis. *Exp Clin Endocrinol Diabetes*, **109**, 87–92.

Pfeiffer C, Caudill S, Gunter E, *et al.* (2005) Biochemical indicators of B vitamin status in the US Population after folic acid fortification: results form the National Health and Nutrition Examination Survey 1999–2000. *American Journal of Clinical Nutrition*, **82**, 442–50.

Phelan JP and Austad SN (1989) Natural selection, dietary restriction, and extended longevity. *Growth, Development, & Aging*, **53**, 4–6.

Philpott MP and Kealey T (1991) Metabolic studies on isolated hair follicles: hair follicles engage in aerobic glycolysis and do not demonstrate the glucose fatty acid cycle. *Journal of Investigative Dermatology*, **96**, 875–9.

Philpott MP, Green MR and Kealey T (1990) Human hair growth *in vitro*. *Journal of Cell Science*, **97**, 463–71.

Picavet H and Schouten J (2003) Musculoskeletal pain in the Netherlands: prevalence, consequences and risk groups. *Pain*, **102**, 167–78.

Pietinen P, Malila N, Virtanen M, *et al.* (1999) Diet and risk of colorectal cancer in a cohort of Finnish men. *Cancer Causes & Control*, **10**, 387–96.

Pietinen P, Rimm E, Korhonen P, *et al.* (1996) Intake of dietary fibre and risk of coronary heart disease in a cohort of Finnish men. The Alpha-tocopherol, Beta-carotene Cancer Prevention Study. *Circulation*, **94**, 2720–7.

Pilotto A (2004) Aging and upper gastrointestinal disorders. *Best Practice & Research: Clinical Gastroenterology*, **18 (Suppl)**, 73–81.

Pilotto A, Franceschi M and Di Mario F (2000) *Helicobacter pylori*-associated peptic ulcer disease in elderly patients. *Clinical Geriatrics*, **8**, 49–58.

Pilotto A, Franceschi M, Di Mario F, *et al.* (1998) The long-term clinical outcome of elderly patients with *Helicobacter pylori*-associated peptic ulcer disease. *Gerontology*, **44**, 153–8.

Pinnell SR (1985) Regulation of collagen biosynthesis by ascorbic acid: a review. *Yale Journal of Biology & Medicine*, **58**, 553–9.

Pirich C, Mullner M and Sinzinger H (2000) Prevalence and relevance of thyroid dysfunction in 1922 cholesterol screening participants. *Journal of Clinical Epidemiology*, **53**, 623–9.

Pischon T, Lahmann PH, Boeing H, *et al.* (2006) Body size and risk of colon and rectal cancer in the European Prospective Investigation Into Cancer and Nutrition (EPIC). *Journal of the National Cancer Institute*, **98**, 920–31.

Pittas AG, Lau J, Hu FB and Dawson-Hughes B (2007) The role of vitamin D and calcium in type 2 diabetes. A systematic review and meta-analysis. *Journal of Clinical Endocrinology and Metabolism*, **92**, 2017–29.

Place RJ and Simmang CL (2002) Diverticular disease. *Best Practice & Research: Clinical Gastroenterology*, **16**, 135–48.

Pocock NA, Eisman JA, Gwinn TH, *et al.* (1989) Mechanical load and the skeleton: the interaction of regional muscle strength, physical fitness and weight with bone mass. *Journal of Bone & Mineral Research*, **4**, 441–8.

Podas T, Eaden J, Mayberry M and Mayberry J (1998) Achalasia: a critical review of epidemiological studies. *American Journal of Gastroenterology*, **93**, 2345–7.

Poehlman E, Toth MJ, Fishman PS, *et al.* (1995) Sarcopenia in aging humans: the impact of menopause and disease. *The Journals of Gerontology, Series A, Biological Sciences and Medical Sciences*, **50**, 73–7.

Policy Research Institute on Ageing and Ethnicity (2004) Minority Elderly Health and Social Care in Europe. www.priae.org.

Pols M, Peeters P, Twisk J, *et al.* (1997) Physical activity and cardiovascular disease risk profile in women. *American Journal of Epidemiology*, **146**, 322–8.

Ponnappan U (1998) Regulation of transcription factor NF kappa B in immune senescence. *Frontiers in Bioscience*, **3**, d152–68.

Popkin BM, Armstrong LE, Bray GM, *et al.* (2006) A new proposed guidance system for beverage consumption in the United States. *American Journal of Clinical Nutrition*, **83**, 529–42.

Poppitt S, Keogh G, Mulvey T, *et al.* (2002) Lipid-lowering effects of a modified butterfat: a controlled intervention trial in healthy men. *European Journal of Clinical Nutrition*, **56**, 64–71.

Porthouse J, Cockayne S, King C, *et al.* (2005) Randomised controlled trial of calcium and supplementation with cholecalciferol (vitamin D3) for prevention of fractures in primary care. *British Medical Journal*, **330**, 1003–6.

Potter J (2003) Bowel care in older people. *Clinical Medicine*, **3**, 48–51.

Potter JD (1999) Colorectal cancer: molecules and populations. *Journal of the National Cancer Institute*, **91**, 916–32.

Potter JD and McMichael AJ (1986) Diet and cancer of the colon and rectum: a case-control study. *Journal of the National Cancer Institute*, **76**, 557–69.

Potter JD, Slattery ML, Bostick RM and Gapstur SM (1993) Colon cancer: a review of the epidemiology. *Epidemiologic Reviews*, **15**, 499–545.

Pottern LM, Morris LE, Blot WJ, *et al.* (1981) Esophageal cancer among black men in Washington, DC. I. Alcohol, tobacco, and other risk factors. *Journal of the National Cancer Institute*, **67**, 777–83.

Poynter ME and Daynes RA (1998) Peroxisome proliferator-activated receptor alpha activation modulates cellular redox status, represses nuclear factor-kappaB signaling, and reduces inflammatory cytokine production in aging. *Journal of Biological Chemistry*, **273**, 32833–41.

Prasad R, Lakshmi AV and Bamji MS (1983) Impaired collagen maturity in vitamins B2 and B6 deficiency – probable molecular basis of skin lesions. *Biochemical Medicine*, **30**, 333–41.

Prentice A and Jebb S (2003) Fast foods, energy density and obesity: a possible mechanistic link. *Obesity Reviews*, **4**, 187–94.

Prentice RL, Caan B, Chlebowski RT, *et al.* (2006) Low-fat dietary pattern and risk of invasive breast cancer: the Women's Health Initiative Randomized Controlled Dietary Modification Trial. *Journal of the American Medical Association*, **295**, 629–42.

Preshaw PM, Heasman L, Stacey F, *et al.* (2005) The effect of quitting smoking on chronic periodontitis. *Journal of Clinical Periodontology*, **32**, 869–79.

Price G, Uauy R, Breeze E, *et al.* (2006) Weight, shape and mortality risk in older people: elevated waist hip ratio rather than high BMI is associated with greater risk of death. *American Journal of Clinical Nutrition*, **84**, 449–60.

Proctor D, O'Brien P, Atkinson E and Nair K (1999) Comparison of techniques to estimate total body skeletal muscle mass in people of different age groups. *American Journal of Physiology – Endocrinology and Metabolism*, **277**, E489–95.

Promislow DE (1994) DNA repair and the evolution of longevity: a critical analysis. *Journal of Theoretical Biology*, **170**, 291–300.

Prospective Studies Collaboration (1995) Cholesterol, diastolic blood pressure, and stroke: 13,000 strokes in 450,000 people in 45 prospective cohorts. *Lancet*, **346**, 1647–53.

Prospective Studies Collaboration (2002) Age-specific relevance of usual blood pressure to vascular mortality: a meta-analysis of individual data for one million adults in 61 prospective studies. *Lancet*, **360**, 1903–13.

Provinciali M, Montenovo A, Di Stefano G, *et al.* (1998) Effect of zinc or zinc plus arginine supplementation on antibody titre and lymphocyte subsets after influenza vaccination in elderly subjects: a randomized controlled trial. *Age & Ageing*, **27**, 715–22.

Pryer J, Cook A and Shetty P (2001) Identification of groups who report similar patterns of diet among a representative national sample of British adults aged 65 years of age or more. *Public Health Nutrition*, **4**, 787–95.

Prynne CJ, Mishra GD, O'Connell MA, *et al.* (2006) Fruit and vegetable intakes and bone mineral status: a cross sectional study in 5 age and sex cohorts. *American Journal of Clinical Nutrition*, **83**, 1420–8.

Pupe A, Moison R, De Haes P, *et al.* (2002) Eicosapentaenoic acid, a *n*-3 polyunsaturated fatty acid differentially modulates TNF-alpha, IL-1alpha, IL-6 and PGE2 expression in UVB-irradiated human keratinocytes. *Journal of Investigative Dermatology*, **118**, 692–8.

Purba MB, Kouris-Blazos A, Wattanapenpaiboon N, *et al.* (2001) Skin wrinkling: can food make a difference? *Journal of the American College of Nutrition*, **20**, 71–80.

Pusateri DJ, Roth WT, Ross JK and Shultz TD (1990) Dietary and hormonal evaluation of men at different risks for prostate cancer: plasma and faecal hormone–nutrient interrelationships. *American Journal of Clinical Nutrition*, **51**, 371–7.

Quan T, He T, Voorhees JJ and Fisher GJ (2005) Ultraviolet irradiation induces Smad7 via induction of transcription factor AP-1 in human skin fibroblasts. *Journal of Biological Chemistry*, **280**, 8079–85.

Rafferty K and Heaney RP (2008) Nutrient effects on the calcium economy: emphasizing the potassium controversy. *Journal of Nutrition*, **138**, 166S–171S.

Rafter J, Bennett M, Caderni G, *et al.* (2007) Dietary synbiotics reduce cancer risk factors in polypectomized and colon cancer patients. *American Journal of Clinical Nutrition*, **85**, 488–96.

Raisz LG (2004a) Bone physiology, bone cells, modeling, remodeling. *Nutrition and Bone Health*. Ed. M. F. Holick and B. Dawson-Hughes. Totowa, NJ, Humana Press: 43–62.

Raisz LG (2004b) Homocysteine and osteoporotic fractures – culprit or bystander? *New England Journal of Medicine*, **350**, 2089–90.

Rajala SA, Salminen SJ, Seppanen JH and Vapaatalo H (1988) Treatment of chronic constipation with lactitol sweetened yogurt supplemented with guar gum and wheat bran in elderly hospital in-patients. *Comprehensive Gerontology Section A, Clinical & Laboratory Sciences*, **2**, 83–6.

Ralston SH (2003) Genetic determinants of susceptibility to osteoporosis. *Current Opinion in Pharmacology*, **3**, 286–90.

Ralston SH (2007) Genetics of osteoporosis. *Proceedings of the Nutrition Society*, **66**, 158–65.

Rantanen T, Masaki K, Foley D, *et al.* (1998) Grip strength changes over 27 yr in Japanese-American men. *Journal of Applied Physiology*, **85**, 2047–53.

Rapuri PB, Gallagher JC, Balhorn KE and Ryschon KL (2000) Alcohol intake and bone metabolism in elderly women. *American Journal of Clinical Nutrition*, **72**, 1206–13.

Rasmussen U, Krustrup P, Kjaer M and Rasmussen H (2003) Experimental evidence against the mitochondrial theory of aging. A study of isolated human skeletal muscle mitochondria. *Experimental Gerontology*, **38**, 877–86.

Ravelli A, van der Meulen J, Michels R, *et al.* (1998) Glucose tolerance in adults after prenatal exposure to famine. *Lancet*, **351**, 173–7.

Ray AJ, Turner R, Nikaido O, *et al.* (2000) The spectrum of mitochondrial DNA deletions is a ubiquitous marker of ultraviolet radiation exposure in human skin. *Journal of Investigative Dermatology*, **115**, 674–9.

Ray S, Rana P, Rajput M and Haleem MA (2007) Nutrition management of stroke: from current evidence to conjecture. *Nutrition Bulletin*, **32**, 145–53.

Rayman M, Thompson A, Warren-Perry M, *et al.* (2006) Impact of selenium on mood and quality of life: a randomized, controlled trial. *Biological Psychiatry*, **59**, 147–54.

Read NW, Welch IM, Austen CJ, *et al.* (1986) Swallowing food without chewing; a simple way to reduce postprandial glycaemia. *British Journal of Nutrition*, **55**, 43–7.

Rebrin I, Kamzalov S and Sohal RS (2003) Effects of age and caloric restriction on glutathione redox state in mice. *Free Radical Biology & Medicine*, **35**, 626–35.

Recker RR, Davies KM, Hinders SM, *et al.* (1992) Bone gain in young adult women. *Journal of the American Medical Association*, **268**, 2403–8.

Reddy BS and Rivenson A (1993) Inhibitory effect of Bifidobacterium longum on colon, mammary, and liver carcinogenesis induced by 2-amino-3-methylimidazo [4,5-f]quinoline, a food mutagen. *Cancer Research*, **53**, 3914–18.

Reddy VN (1990) Glutathione and its function in the lens – an overview. *Experimental Eye Research*, **50**, 771–8.

Redmond E, Sitzmann J and Cahill P (2000) Potential mechanisms for cardiovascular protective effect of ethanol. *Acta Pharmacologica Sinica*, **21**, 385–90.

Reed JA, Anderson JJ, Tylavsky FA and Gallagher PN, Jr. (1994) Comparative changes in radial-bone density of elderly female lacto-ovo-vegetarians and omnivores. *American Journal of Clinical Nutrition*, **59**, 1197S–202S.

Reed MJ, Penn PE, Li Y, *et al.* (1996) Enhanced cell proliferation and biosynthesis mediate improved wound repair in refed, caloric-restricted mice. *Mechanisms of Ageing & Development*, **89**, 21–43.

Rees D, Miles EA, Banerjee T, *et al.* (2006) Dose-related effects of eicosapentaenoic acid on innate immune function in healthy humans: a comparison of young and older men. *American Journal of Clinical Nutrition*, **83**, 331–42.

Reginster J, Deroisy R, Rovati L, *et al.* (2001) Long-term effects of glucosamine sulphate on osteoarthritis progression: a randomised, placebo-controlled clinical trial. *Lancet*, **357**, 251–6.

Reichenbach S, Sterchi R, Scherer M, *et al.* (2007) Meta-analysis: chondroitin for osteoarthritis of the knee or hip. *Annals of Internal Medicine*, **146**, 580–90.

Reidy A, Minassian DC, Vafidis G, *et al.* (1998) Prevalence of serious eye disease and visual impairment in a north London population: population based, cross-sectional study. *British Medical Journal*, **316**, 1643–6.

Reilly DM, Ferdinando D, Johnston C, *et al.* (1997) The epidermal nerve fibre network: characterization of nerve fibres in human skin by confocal microscopy and assessment of racial variations. *British Journal of Dermatology*, **137**, 163–70.

Reilly J, Lord A, Bunker V, *et al.* (1993) Energy balance in healthy elderly women. *British Journal of Nutrition*, **69**, 21–7.

Reilly JJ, Jackson DM, Montgomery C, *et al.* (2004) Total energy expenditure and physical activity in young Scottish children: mixed longitudinal study. *Lancet*, **363**, 211–12.

Remarque E and Pawelec G (1998) T-cell immunosenescence and its clinical relevance in man. *Reviews in Clinical Gerontology*, **8**, 5–14.

Remarque EJ, Bollen EL, Weverling-Rijnsburger AW, *et al.* (2001) Patients with Alzheimer's disease display a pro-inflammatory phenotype. *Experimental Gerontology*, **36**, 171–6.

Remer T, Pietrzik K and Manz F (1998) Short-term impact of a lactovegetarian diet on adrenocortical activity and adrenal androgens. *Journal of Clinical Endocrinology & Metabolism*, **83**, 2132–7.

Renehan AG, Zwahlen M, Minder C, *et al.* (2004) Insulin-like growth factor (IGF)-I, IGF binding protein-3, and cancer risk: systematic review and meta-regression analysis. *Lancet*, **363**, 1346–53.

Rennie M (2001) Control of muscle protein synthesis as a result of contractile activity and amino acid availability: implications for protein requirements. *International Journal of Sport Nutrition and Exercise Metabolism*, **11**, S170–6.

Rennie M and Millward D (1983) 3-Methylhistidine excretion and the urinary 3-methylhistidine/creatinine ratio are poor indicators of skeletal muscle protein breakdown. *Clinical Science (Lond)*, **65**, 217–25.

Rennie M and Tipton K (2000) Protein and amino acid metabolism during and after exercise and the effects of nutrition. *Annual Review of Nutrition*, **20**, 457–83.

Rennie MJ (2003) Claims for the anabolic effects of growth hormone: a case of the emperor's new clothes? *British Journal of Sports Medicine*, **37**, 100–5.

Resnick NM (1996) An 89-year-old woman with urinary incontinence. *Journal of the American Medical Association*, **276**, 1832–40.

Reuben DB, Cheh AI, Harris TB, *et al.* (2002) Peripheral blood markers of inflammation predict mortality and functional decline in high-functioning community-dwelling older persons. *Journal of the American Geriatrics Society*, **50**, 638–44.

Reul JM, Labeur MS, Wiegers GJ and Linthorst AC (1998) Altered neuroimmunoendocrine communication during a condition of chronically increased brain corticotropin-releasing hormone drive. *Annals of the New York Academy of Sciences*, **840**, 444–55.

Rhodes LE, Durham BH, Fraser WD and Friedmann PS (1995) Dietary fish oil reduces basal and ultraviolet B-generated PGE2 levels in skin and increases the threshold to provocation of polymorphic light eruption. *Journal of Investigative Dermatology*, **105**, 532–5.

Rhodes LE, O'Farrell S, Jackson MJ and Friedmann PS (1994) Dietary fish-oil supplementation in humans reduces UVB-erythemal sensitivity but increases epidermal lipid peroxidation. *Journal of Investigative Dermatology*, **103**, 151–4.

Rhodes LE, Shahbakhti H, Azurdia RM, *et al.* (2003) Effect of eicosapentaenoic acid, an omega-3 polyunsaturated fatty acid, on UVR-related cancer risk in humans. An assessment of early genotoxic markers. *Carcinogenesis*, **24**, 919–25.

Ricci TA, Heymsfield SB, *et al.* (2001) Moderate energy restriction increases bone resorption in obese postmenopausal women. *American Journal of Clinical Nutrition*, **73**, 347–52.

Richard MJ and Roussel AM (1999) Micronutrients and ageing: intakes and requirements. *Proceedings of the Nutrition Society*, **58**, 573–8.

Richardson D (2000) The grain, the whole-grain and nothing but the grain: the science behind the whole-grain and the reduced risk of heart disease and cancer. *Nutrition Bulletin*, **25**, 353–60.

Richelle M, Sabatier M, Steiling H and Williamson G (2006) Skin bioavailability of dietary vitamin E, carotenoids, polyphenols, vitamin C, zinc and selenium. *British Journal of Nutrition*, **96**, 227–38.

Ridker P (2001) Role of inflammatory biomarkers in prediction of coronary heart disease. *Lancet*, **358**, 946–8.

Rigamonti AE, Pincelli AI, Corra B, *et al.* (2002) Plasma ghrelin concentrations in elderly subjects: comparison with anorexic and obese patients. *Journal of Endocrinology*, **175**, R1–5.

Rimm E, Ascherio A, Giovannucci E, *et al.* (1996) Vegetable, fruit and cereal fiber intake and risk of coronary heart disease among men. *Journal of the American Medical Association*, **275**, 447–51.

Rinaldi S, Peeters PHM, Berrino F, *et al.* (2006) IGF-1, IGFBP-3 and breast cancer risk in women: The European Prospective Investigation into Cancer and Nutrition (EPIC). *Endocrine-Related Cancer*, **13**, 593–605.

Ringsdorf WM, Jr. and Cheraskin E (1982) Vitamin C and human wound healing. *Oral Surgery, Oral Medicine, Oral Pathology*, **53**, 231–6.

Ringstad J and Fonnebo V (1987) The Tromso Heart Study: serum selenium in a low-risk population for cardiovascular disease and cancer and matched controls. *Annals of Clinical Research*, **19**, 351–4.

Ritchie CS (2002) Oral health, taste, and olfaction. *Clinics in Geriatric Medicine*, **18**, 709–17.

Ritz P (2001) Factors affecting energy and macronutrient requirements in elderly people. *Public Health Nutrition*, **4**, 561–8.

Rivas M, Garay R, Escanero J, *et al.* (2002) Soy milk lowers blood pressure in men and women with mild to moderate essential hypertension. *Journal of Nutrition*, **132**, 1900–2.

Rizzoli R, Ammann P, Pierson RN, Jr., *et al.* (2003) Effects of dietary protein insufficiency on the skeleton. In: *Nutritional Aspects of Bone Health*. Ed. S. A. New and J. P. Bonjour. Cambridge, Royal Society of Chemistry: 193–212.

Roberfroid M (1993) Dietary fiber, inulin, and oligofructose: a review comparing their physiological effects. *Critical Reviews in Food Science & Nutrition*, **33**, 103–48.

Roberts S, Young V, Fuss P, *et al.* (1992) What are the dietary needs of elderly adults? *International Journal of Obesity*, **16**, 969–76.

Robertson G, Meshkinpour H, Vandenberg K, *et al.* (1993) Effects of exercise on total and segmental colon transit. *Journal of Clinical Gastroenterology*, **16**, 300–3.

Robertson MD, Livesey G, Morgan LM, *et al.* (1999) The influence of the colon on postprandial glucagon-like peptide 1 (7–36) amide concentration in man. *Journal of Endocrinology*, **161**, 25–31.

Roche H, Zampelas A, Jackson K, *et al.* (1998) The effect of test meal monounsaturated fatty acid: saturated fatty acid ratio on postprandial lipid metabolism. *British Journal of Nutrition*, **79**, 419–24.

Roe DA (1986) Current etiologies and cutaneous signs of vitamin deficiencies. In: *Nutrition and the Skin. Contemporary Issues in Clinical Nutrition*. Ed. D. A. Roe. New York, Alan R Liss Inc: 81–98.

Roe DA (1991) Riboflavin deficiency: mucocutaneous signs of acute and chronic deficiency. *Seminars in Dermatology*, **10**, 293–5.

Rogers D, Toder E and Jones L (2000) *Economic Consequences of an Aging Population*. Washington, Urban Institute.

Rogers I, Emmett P, Gunnell D, *et al.* (2006) Milk as a food for growth? The insulin-like growth factors link. *Public Health Nutrition*, **9**, 359–68.

Rogers J and Dieppe P (2003) The paleopathology of osteoarthritis. In: *Osteoarthritis*. Ed. K. Brandt, M. Doherty and S. Lohmander. Oxford, Oxford University Press: 59–66.

Rogers P (2007) Caffeine, mood and mental performance in everyday life. *Nutrition Bulletin*, **32 (Suppl 1)**, 84–9.

Rohde LE, Hennekens CH and Ridker PM (1999) Cross-sectional study of soluble intercellular adhesion molecule-1 and cardiovascular risk factors in apparently healthy men. *Arteriosclerosis, Thrombosis & Vascular Biology*, **19**, 1595–9.

Roininen K, Fillion L, Kilcast D and Lahteenmaki L (2004) Exploring difficult textural properties of fruit and vegetables for the elderly in Finland and the United Kingdom. *Food Quality and Preference*, **15**, 517–30.

Rondeau V (2002) A review of epidemiologic studies on aluminum and silica in relation to Alzheimer's disease and associated disorders. *Reviews on Environmental Health*, **17**, 107–21.

Roos TC, Jugert FK, Merk HF and Bickers DR (1998) Retinoid metabolism in the skin. *Pharmacological Reviews*, **50**, 315–33.

Rooyackers O, Adey D, Ades P and Nair K (1996) Effect of age on in vivo rates of mitochondrial protein synthesis in human skeletal muscle. *Proceedings of the National Academy of Sciences of the United States of America*, **93**, 15364–9.

Rosen CJ (1999) Serum insulin-like growth factors and insulin-like growth factor-binding proteins: clinical implications. *Clinical Chemistry*, **45**, 1384–90.

Rosen CJ (2004) Nutrition and bone health in the elderly. In: *Nutrition and Bone Health*. Ed. M. F. Holick and B. Dawson-Hughes. Totawa, NJ, Humana Press.

Rosen ED and Spiegelman BM (2001) PPARgamma: a nuclear regulator of metabolism, differentiation, and cell growth. *Journal of Biological Chemistry*, **276**, 37731–4.

Rosen P, Nawroth PP, King G, *et al.* (2001) The role of oxidative stress in the onset and progression of diabetes and its complications: a summary of a Congress Series sponsored by UNESCO-MCBN, the American Diabetes Association and the German Diabetes Society. *Diabetes/Metabolism Research and Reviews*, **17**, 189–212.

Rosenberg I (1997) Sarcopenia: origins and clinical relevance. *Journal of Nutrition*, **127**, 990S–1S.

Ross J, Belding H and Paegel B (1947) The development and progression of subacute combined degeneration of the spinal cord in patients with pernicious anemia treated with synthetic pteroylglutamic (folic) acid. *Blood*, **68**, 3.

Rossouw JE, Anderson GL, Prentice RL, *et al.* (2002) Risks and benefits of estrogen plus progestin in healthy postmenopausal women: principal results from the women's health initiative randomized controlled trial. *Journal of the American Medical Association*, **288**, 321–33.

Roth GS, Lane MA, Ingram DK, *et al.* (2002) Biomarkers of caloric restriction may predict longevity in humans. *Science*, **297**, 811.

Roth S, Ferrel LR and Hurley B (2000) Strength training for the prevention and treatment of sarcopenia. *The Journal of Nutrition, Health and Aging*, **4**, 143–55.

Rothwell P, Coull A, Silver L, *et al.* (2005) Population-based study of event-rate, incidence, case fatality, and mortality for all acute vascular events in all arterial territories (Oxford Vascular Study). *Lancet*, **366**, 1773–83.

Roubenoff R, Harris TB, Abad LW, *et al.* (1998) Monocyte cytokine production in an elderly population: effect of age and inflammation. *Journals of Gerontology Series A – Biological Sciences & Medical Sciences*, **53**, M20–6.

Rouhiainen P, Rouhiainen H and Salonen JT (1996) Association between low plasma vitamin E concentration and progression of early cortical lens opacities. *American Journal of Epidemiology*, **144**, 496–500.

Rowland IR and Gangolli SD (1999) Role of gastrointestinal flora in the metabolic and toxicological activities of xenobiotics. In: *General and Applied Toxicology*. Ed. B. Ballantyne, T. C. Marrs and T. Syverson. London, Macmillan: 561–76.

Rowland IR, Rumney CJ, Coutts JT and Lievense LC (1998) Effect of Bifidobacterium longum and inulin on gut bacterial metabolism and carcinogen-induced aberrant crypt foci in rats. *Carcinogenesis*, **19**, 281–5.

Royal College of Physicians (2000) *Osteoporosis Clinical Guidelines for Prevention and Treatment*. London, Royal College of Physicians.

Rubiano F, Nunez C and Heymsfield S (2000) A comparison of body composition techniques. *Annals of the New York Academy of Sciences*, **904**, 335–8.

Rush EC, Patel M, Plank LD and Ferguson LR (2002) Kiwi fruit promotes laxation in the elderly. *Asia Pacific Journal of Clinical Nutrition*, **11**, 164–8.

Russell SJ and Kahn CR (2007) Endocrine regulation of ageing. *Nature Reviews Molecular Cell Biology*, **8**, 681–91.

Ruston D, Hoare J, Henderson L, *et al.* (2004) *The National Diet and Nutrition Survey: Adults aged 19 to 64 Years. Volume 4: Nutritional Status (Anthropometry and Blood Analytes), Blood Pressure and Physical Activity*. London, Stationery Office.

Sacks FM, Lichtenstein A, Van Horn L, *et al.* (2006) Soy protein, isoflavones, and cardiovascular health. *Circulation*, **113**, 1034–44.

Sacks F, Svetkey L, Vollmer W, *et al.* (2001) Effects on blood pressure of reduced dietary sodium and the Dietary Approaches to Stop Hypertension (DASH) diet. *New England Journal of Medicine*, **344**, 3–10.

Sadeghi HM, Schnelle JF, Thoma JK, *et al.* (1999) Phenotypic and functional characteristics of circulating monocytes of elderly persons. *Experimental Gerontology*, **34**, 959–70.

Safer JD, Crawford TM and Holick MF (2005) Topical thyroid hormone accelerates wound healing in mice. *Endocrinology*, **146**, 4425–30.

Sahyoun N, Jacques P, Zhang X, *et al.* (2006) Whole grain intake is inversely associated with the metabolic syndrome and mortality in older adults. *American Journal of Clinical Nutrition*, **83**, 124–31.

Sahyoun N, Lin C-H and Krall E (2003) Nutritional status of the older adult is associated with dentition status. *Journal of the American Dietetic Association*, **103**, 61–6.

Sakamoto I, Igarashi M, Kimura K, *et al.* (2001) Suppressive effect of Lactobacillus gasseri OLL 2716 (LG21) on *Helicobacter pylori* infection in humans. *Journal of Antimicrobial Chemotherapy*, **47**, 709–10.

Salmeron J, Ascherio A, Rimm EB, *et al.* (1997a) Dietary fiber, glycemic load, and risk of NIDDM in men. *Diabetes Care*, **20**, 545–50.

Salmeron J, Manson JE, Stampfer MJ, *et al.* (1997b) Dietary fiber, glycemic load, and risk of non-insulin-dependent diabetes mellitus in women. *Journal of the American Medical Association*, **277**, 472–7.

Salminen E, Heikkila S, Poussa T, *et al.* (2002) Female patients tend to alter their diet following the diagnosis of rheumatoid arthritis and breast cancer. *Preventive Medicine*, **34**, 529–35.

Salonen J, Alfthan G, Huttunen J, *et al.* (1982) Association between cardiovascular death and myocardial infarction and serum selenium in a matched-pair longitudinal study. *Lancet*, **2**, 175–9.

Salvini S, Hennekens C, Morris J, *et al.* (1995) Plasma levels of the antioxidant selenium and risk of myocardial infarction among U.S. physicians. *American Journal of Cardiology*, **76**, 1218–21.

Sambrook P (2005) Vitamin D and fractures: quo vadis? *Lancet*, **365**, 1599–600.

San Giovanni JP and Chew EY (2005) The role of omega-3 long-chain polyunsaturated fatty acids in health and disease of the retina. *Progress in Retinal and Eye Research*, **24**, 87–138.

San Millan JL, Corton M, Villuendas G, *et al.* (2004) Association of the polycystic ovary syndrome with genomic variants related to insulin resistance, type 2 diabetes mellitus, and obesity. *Journal of Clinical Endocrinology & Metabolism*, **89**, 2640–6.

Sanders T (2003) High- versus low-fat diets in human diseases. *Current Opinion in Clinical Nutrition and Metabolic Care*, **6**, 151–5.

Sanders TA, Haines AP, Wormald R, *et al.* (1993) Essential fatty acids, plasma cholesterol, and fat-soluble vitamins in subjects with age-related maculopathy and matched control subjects. *American Journal of Clinical Nutrition*, **57**, 428–33.

Santhanam U, Green MR, Feinberg C and Weinkauf R (2005) A new cosmetic antiageing ingredient for improvement of photoaged skin. *Journal of the American Academy of Dermatology*, **52 (Suppl)**, P83.

Santos MS, Meydani SN, Leka L, *et al.* (1996) Natural killer cell activity in elderly men is enhanced by beta-carotene supplementation. *American Journal of Clinical Nutrition*, **64**, 772–7.

Sardana K and Sehgal VN (2003) Retinoids: fascinating up-and-coming scenario. *Journal of Dermatology*, **30**, 355–80.

Saris W (2005) DiOGenes: an integrated multidisciplinary approach to the obesity problem in Europe. *Nutrition Bulletin*, **30**, 188–93.

Saris W, Astrup A, Prentice A, *et al.* (2000) Randomized controlled trial of changes in dietary carbohydrate/fat ratio and simple vs complex carbohydrates on body weight and blood lipids: the CARMEN study. The carbohydrate ratio management in European national diets. *International Journal of Obesity*, **24**, 1310–18.

Sarma U, Brunner E, Evans J and Wormald R (1994) Nutrition and the epidemiology of cataract and age-related maculopathy. *European Journal of Clinical Nutrition*, **48**, 1–8.

Sarzi-Puttini P, Cimmino M, Scarpa R, *et al.* (2005) Osteo-arthritis: an overview of the disease and its treatment strategies. *Seminars in Arthritis & Rheumatism*, **35**, 1–10.

Sato K, Kawakami N, Ohtsu T, *et al.* (2004) Broccoli consumption and chronic atrophic gastritis among Japanese males: an epidemiological investigation. *Acta Medica Okayama*, **58**, 127–33.

Sator P-G, Schmidt JB, Rabe T and Zouboulis CC (2004) Skin aging and sex hormones in women – clinical perspectives for intervention by hormone replacement therapy. *Experimental Dermatology*, **13 (Suppl 4)**, 36–40.

Sattar N and Ferns G (2005) Endothelial dysfunction. *Cardiovascular Disease: Diet, Nutrition and Emerging Risk Factors*. Ed. S. Stanner. Oxford, Blackwell: 63–77.

Saurwein-Teissl M, Schonitzer D and Grubeck-Loebenstein B (1998) Dendritic cell responsiveness to stimulation with influenza vaccine is unimpaired in old age. *Experimental Gerontology*, **33**, 625–31.

Sawin CT (2001) Endocrinology of aging. In: *Endocrinology and Metabolism*. Ed. A. Pinchera. Maidenhead, McGraw-Hill: 575–80.

Sawin CT, Castelli WP, Hershman JM, *et al.* (1985) The aging thyroid. Thyroid deficiency in the Framingham Study. *Archives of Internal Medicine*, **145**, 1386–8.

Sayer A, Poole J, Cox V, *et al.* (2003) Weight from birth to 53 years: a longitudinal study of the influence on clinical hand osteoarthritis. *Arthritis & Rheumatism*, **48**, 1030–3.

Sayer A, Syddall H, Dennison E, *et al.* (2004) Birth weight, weight at 1 y of age, and body composition in older men: findings from the Hertfordshire Cohort Study. *American Journal of Clinical Nutrition*, **80**, 199–203.

Sayer A, Syddall H, Gilbody H, *et al.* (2004) Does sarcopenia originate in early life? Findings from the Hertfordshire cohort study. *The Journals of Gerontology, Series A, Biological Sciences and Medical Sciences*, **59**, M930–4.

Scarmeas N, Stern Y, Tang M, *et al.* (2006) Mediterranean diet and risk of Alzheimer's disease. *Annals of Neurology*, **59**, 912–21.

Schatzkin A, Lanza E, Corle D, *et al.* (2000) Lack of effect of a low-fat, high-fiber diet on the recurrence of colorectal adenomas. Polyp Prevention Trial Study Group. *New England Journal of Medicine*, **342**, 1149–55.

Schaumberg DA, Glynn RJ, Christen WG, *et al.* (2000) Relations of body fat distribution and height with cataract in men. *American Journal of Clinical Nutrition*, **72**, 1495–502.

Scheen AJ, Sturis J, Polonsky KS and Van Cauter E (1996) Alterations in the ultradian oscillations of insulin secretion and plasma glucose in aging. *Diabetologia*, **39**, 564–72.

Schenker S (2003) Undernutrition in the UK. *Nutrition Bulletin*, **28**, 87–120.

Scheppach W (1994) Effects of short chain fatty acids on gut morphology and function. *Gut*, **35**, S35–8.

Schiekofer S, Andrassy M, Chen J, *et al.* (2003) Acute hyperglycemia causes intracellular formation of CML and activation of ras, p42/44 MAPK, and nuclear factor kappaB in PBMCs. *Diabetes*, **52**, 621–33.

Schiffman S and Graham B (2000) Taste and smell perception affect appetite and immunity in the elderly. *European Journal of Clinical Nutrition*, **50 (Suppl 3)**, S54–S63.

Schiffman S, Gatlin L, Frey A, *et al.* (1994) Taste perception of bitter compounds in young and elderly persons: relation to lipophilicity of bitter compounds. *Neurobiology of Aging*, **15**, 743–50.

Schiffman SS and Warwick ZS (1993) Effect of flavor enhancement of foods for the elderly on nutritional status: food intake, biochemical indices, and anthropometric measures. *Physiology & Behavior*, **53**, 395–402.

Scholfield WN (1985) Predicting basal metabolic rate, new standards and review of previous work. *Human Nutrition: Clinical Nutrition*, **39C (Suppl 1)**: 5–41.

Scholz J and Woolf CJ (2002) Can we conquer pain? *Nature Neuroscience*, **5 Suppl**, 1062–7.

Schonhoff SE, Giel-Moloney M and Leiter AB (2004) Minireview: development and differentiation of gut endocrine cells. *Endocrinology*, **145**, 2639–44.

Schottenfeld D (1984) Epidemiology of cancer of the esophagus. *Seminars in Oncology*, **11**, 92–100.

Schrauwen-Hinderling V, van Loon L, Koopman R, *et al.* (2003) Intramyocellular lipid content is increased after exercise in nonexercising human skeletal muscle. *Journal of Applied Physiology*, **95**, 2328–32.

Schroll K, Carbajal A, Decarli B, *et al.* (1996) Food patterns of elderly Europeans. *European Journal of Clinical Nutrition*, **50 (Suppl 2)**, S86–S100.

Schroll M, Bjomsbo-Scroll K, Ferrt N and Livingstone M (1996) Health and physical performances of elderly Europeans. *European Journal of Clinical Nutrition*, **50 (Suppl 2)**, S105–11.

Schroll M, Ferry M, Lund-Larsen K and Enzi G (1991) Assessment of health: self-perceived health, chronic disease, use of medicine. *European Journal of Clinical Nutrition*, **45 (Suppl 3)**, 169–82.

Schurch MA, Rizzoli R, Slosman D, *et al.* (1998) Protein supplements increase serum insulin-like growth factor-I levels and attenuate proximal femur bone loss in patients with recent hip fracture. A randomized, double-blind, placebo-controlled trial. *Annals of Internal Medicine,* **128**, 801–9.

Schwartz AG and Pashko LL (1994) Role of adrenocortical steroids in mediating cancer-preventive and age-retarding effects of food restriction in laboratory rodents. *Journal of Gerontology,* **49**, B37–41.

Scientific Advisory Committee on Nutrition (2003) *Salt and Health.* London, Stationery Office.

Scientific Advisory Committee on Nutrition (2004) *Advice on Fish Consumption: Benefits and Risks.* London, TSO.

Scientific Advisory Committee on Nutrition (2005a) *Review of Dietary Advice on Vitamin A.* London, Stationery Office.

Scientific Advisory Committee on Nutrition (2005b) The nutritional health of the population. Draft report (SACN/05/13), Scientific Advisory Committee on Nutrition: www.sacn.gov.uk/pdfs/sacn_05_13.pdf.

Scientific Advisory Committee on Nutrition (2006) *Folate and Disease Prevention.* Report 20. London, Stationery Office.

Scientific Advisory Committee on Nutrition (2007a) The Nutritional Health of the Population SACN/07/14. www.sacn.gov.uk.

Scientific Advisory Committee on Nutrition (2007b) National Diet and Nutrition Survey: Adults 19–64 Years Further Analysis SACN/07/13. www.sacn.gov.uk.

Scientific Advisory Committee on Nutrition (2007c) *Update on Vitamin D. Position Statement by the Scientific Advisory Committee on Nutrition.* London, Stationery Office.

Scientific Advisory Committee on Nutrition (2007d) *The Nutrition Wellbeing of the UK Population – Synthesis Paper* SACN/07/15. www.sacn.gov.uk.

Scientific Advisory Committee on Nutrition (2007e) *Update on Trans Fatty Acids and Health: Position Statement by the Scientific Advisory Committee on Nutrition.* London, Stationery Office.

Scientific Advisory Committee on Nutrition and COT (Committee on Toxicity of Chemicals in Food, Consumer Products and the Environment) (2004) *Advice on Fish Consumption: Benefits and Risks.* London, Stationery Office.

Scott I and Green MR (2005) The human periorbital wrinkle. In: *Textbook of Cosmetic Dermatology.* Ed. R. Baran and H. I. Maibach. London, Taylor & Francis: 277–82.

Scott JA and King GL (2004) Oxidative stress and antioxidant treatment in diabetes. *Annals of the New York Academy of Science,* **1031**, 204–13.

Scuteri A, Najjar SS, Morrell CH and Lakatta EG (2005) The metabolic syndrome in older individuals: prevalence and prediction of cardiovascular events: The Cardiovascular Health Study. *Diabetes Care,* **28**, 882–7.

Scuteri A, Najjar S, Muller D, *et al.* (2004) Metabolic syndrome amplifies the age-associated increases in vascular thickness and stiffness. *Journal of the American College of Cardiology,* **43**, 1388–95.

Seal EC, Metz J, Flicker L and Melny J (2002) A randomized, double-blind, placebo-controlled study of oral vitamin B12 supplementation in older patients with subnormal or borderline serum vitamin B12 concentrations. *Journal of American Geriatric Society,* **50**, 146–51.

Sebastian A, Harris ST, Ottaway JH, *et al.* (1994) Improved mineral balance and skeletal metabolism in postmenopausal women treated with potassium bicarbonate. *New England Journal of Medicine,* **330**, 1776–81.

Seddon JM, Ajani UA, Sperduto RD, *et al.* (1994) Dietary carotenoids, vitamins A, C, and E, and advanced age-related macular degeneration. Eye Disease Case-Control Study Group. *Journal of the American Medical Association,* **272**, 1413–20.

Seddon JM, Christen WG, Manson JE, *et al.* (1994) The use of vitamin supplements and the risk of cataract among US male physicians. *American Journal of Public Health,* **84**, 788–92.

Seddon JM, Cote J, Davis N and Rosner B (2003) Progression of age-related macular degeneration: association with body mass index, waist circumference, and waist:hip ratio. *Archives of Ophthalmology,* **121**, 785–92.

Seddon JM, Rosner B, Sperduto RD, *et al.* (2001) Dietary fat and risk for advanced age-related macular degeneration. *Archives of Ophthalmology,* **119**, 1191–9.

Seeman TE, Singer B, Wilkinson CW and McEwen B (2001) Gender differences in age-related changes in HPA axis reactivity. *Psychoneuroendocrinology,* **26**, 225–40.

Segger D and Schonlau F (2004) Supplementation with Evelle improves skin smoothness and elasticity in a double-blind, placebo-controlled study with 62 women. *Journal of Dermatological Treatment,* **15**, 222–6.

Sehl M and Yates F (2001) Kinetics of human aging: I. Rates of senescence between ages 30 and 70 years in healthy people. *The Journals of Gerontology, Series A, Biological Sciences and Medical Sciences,* **56**, V.

Seinost G, Wimmer G, Skerget M, *et al.* (2005) Periodontal treatment improves endothelial dysfunction in patients with severe periodontitis. *American Heart Journal,* **149**, 1050–4.

Sell C (2003) Caloric restriction and insulin-like growth factors in aging and cancer. *Hormone & Metabolic Research,* **35**, 705–11.

Sellmeyer DE, Schloetter M and Sebastian A (2002) Potassium citrate prevents increased urine calcium excretion and bone resorption induced by a high sodium chloride diet. *Journal of Clinical Endocrinology & Metabolism*, **87**, 2008–12.

Sellmeyer DE, Stone KL, Sebastian A and Cummings SR (2001) A high ratio of dietary animal to vegetable protein increases the rate of bone loss and the risk of fracture in postmenopausal women. Study of Osteoporotic Fractures Research Group. *American Journal of Clinical Nutrition*, **73**, 118–22.

Selvaag E, Bohmer T and Benkestock K (2002) Reduced serum concentrations of riboflavin and ascorbic acid, and blood thiamine pyrophosphate and pyridoxal-5-phosphate in geriatric patients with and without pressure sores. *Journal of Nutrition, Health & Aging*, **6**, 75–7.

Seo YR, Kelley MR and Smith ML (2002) Selenomethionine regulation of p53 by a ref1-dependent redox mechanism. *Proceedings of the National Academy of Sciences of the United States of America*, **99**, 14548–53.

Seshadri S, Beiser A, Selhub J, *et al.* (2002) Plasma homocysteine as a risk factor for dementia and Alzheimer's disease. *New England Journal of Medicine*, **346**, 476–83.

Shaban H and Richter C (2002) A2E and blue light in the retina: the paradigm of age-related macular degeneration. *Biological Chemistry*, **383**, 537–45.

Shah MG and Maibach HI (2001) Estrogen and skin. An overview. *American Journal of Clinical Dermatology*, **2**, 143–50.

Shaheen NJ (2005) Advances in Barrett's esophagus and esophageal adenocarcinoma. *Gastroenterology*, **128**, 1554–66.

Shang F, Lu M, Dudek E, Reddan J and Taylor A (2003) Vitamin C and vitamin E restore the resistance of GSH-depleted lens cells to H2O2. *Free Radical Biology and Medicine*, **34**, 521–30.

Shanley DP and Kirkwood TB (2000) Calorie restriction and aging: a life-history analysis. *Evolution*, **54**, 740–50.

Shapses S and Cifuentes M (2003) Weight reduction and bone health. In: *Nutritional Aspects of Bone Health*. Ed. S. A. New and J. P. Bonjour. Cambridge, Royal Society of Chemistry: 589–608.

Sharkey J, Branch L, Giuliani C, *et al.* (2004) Nutrient intake and BMI as predictors of severity of ADL disability over 1 year in homebound elders. *Journal of Nutrition and Healthy Aging*, **8**, 131–9.

Shaw DI, Hall WL and Williams CM (2005) Metabolic syndrome: what is it and what are the implications? *Proceedings of the Nutrition Society*, **64**, 349–57.

Shea B, Wells G, Cranney A, *et al.* (2004) Calcium supplementation on bone loss in postmenopausal women. *Cochrane Database of Systematic Reviews*, CD004526.

Shearer GM (1997) Th1/Th2 changes in aging. *Mechanisms of Ageing & Development*, **94**, 1–5.

Shearer MJ, Bach A and Kohlmeier M (1996) Chemistry, nutritional sources, tissue distribution and metabolism of vitamin K with special reference to bone health. *Journal of Nutrition*, **126**, 1181S–6S.

Shearer MJ, Cockrayne R, Adamson J, *et al.* (2007) Vitamin K and bone health. *Archives of Internal Medicine*, **167**, 94–5.

Sheiham A, Steele JG, Marcenes W, *et al.* (2001a) The relationship among dental status, nutrient intake, and nutritional status in older people. *Journal of Dental Research*, **80**, 408–13.

Sheiham A, Steele JG, Marcenes W, *et al.* (2001b) Prevalence of impacts of dental and oral disorders and their effects on eating among older people; a national survey in Great Britain. *Community Dentistry & Oral Epidemiology*, **29**, 195–203.

SHEP Cooperative Research Group (1991) Prevention of stroke by antihypertensive drug treatment in older persons with isolated systolic hypertension. *Journal of the American Medical Association*, **265**, 3255–64.

Shepherd J, Blauw G, Murphy M, *et al.* (2002) Pravastatin in elderly individuals at risk of vascular disease (PROSPER): a randomised controlled trial. *Lancet*, **360**, 623–30.

Sherlock M and Toogood AA (2007) Aging and the growth hormone/insulin like growth factor-I axis. *Pituitary*, **10**, 189–203.

Shih GL, Brensinger C, Katzka DA and Metz DC (2003) Influence of age and gender on gastric acid secretion as estimated by integrated acidity in patients referred for 24-hour ambulatory pH monitoring. *American Journal of Gastroenterology*, **98**, 1713–18.

Shimamoto C, Hirata I, Hiraike Y, *et al.* (2002) Evaluation of gastric motor activity in the elderly by electrogastrography and the (13)C-acetate breath test. *Gerontology*, **48**, 381–6.

Short K, Vittone J, Bigelow M, *et al.* (2004) Age and aerobic exercise training effects on whole body and muscle protein metabolism. *American Journal of Physiology – Endocrinology & Metabolism*, **286**, E92–101.

Shuman C (1953) Nocturnal cramps in diabetes mellitus; clinical and physiological correlations. *The American Journal of the Medical Sciences*, **225**, 54–60.

Sijben JWC and Calder PC (2007) Differential immunomodulation with long-chain n-3 PUFA in health and chronic disease. *Proceedings of the Nutrition Society*, **66**, 237–59.

Siler U, Barella L, Spitzer V, *et al.* (2004) Lycopene and vitamin E interfere with autocrine/paracrine loops in the Dunning prostate cancer model. *FASEB Journal*, **18**, 1019–21.

Silman A and Pearson J (2002) Epidemiology and genetics of rheumatoid arthritis. *Arthritis Research*, **4 (Suppl 3)**, S265–72.

Simmons SF and Schnelle JF (2004) Effects of an exercise and scheduled-toileting intervention on appetite and constipation in nursing home residents. *Journal of Nutrition, Health & Aging*, **8**, 116–21.

Simon JA and Hudes ES (1999) Serum ascorbic acid and other correlates of self-reported cataract among older Americans. *Journal of Clinical Epidemiology*, **52**, 1207–11.

Simoneau JA and Bouchard C (1995) Genetic determinism of fiber type proportion in human skeletal muscle. *FASEB Journal*, **9**, 1091–5.

Simons D, Brailsford SR, Kidd EAM and Beighton D (2002) The effect of medicated chewing gums on oral health in frail older people: a 1-year clinical trial. *Journal of the American Geriatrics Society*, **50**, 1348–53.

Simons L, Simons J, Friedlander Y and McCallum J (2001) Cholesterol and other lipids predict coronary heart disease and ischaemic stroke in the elderly, but only in those below 70 years. *Atherosclerosis*, **159**, 201–8.

Simopoulos AP (1991) Omega-3 fatty acids in health and disease and in growth and development. *American Journal of Clinical Nutrition*, **54**, 438–63.

Singh R, Rastogi V, Rastogi S, *et al.* (1996) Effect of diet and moderate exercise on central obesity and associated disturbances, myocardial infarction and mortality in patients with and without coronary artery disease. *Journal of the American College of Nutrition*, **15**, 592–601.

Sirtori C, Tremoli E, Gatti E, *et al.* (1986) Controlled evaluation of fat intake in the Mediterranean diet: comparative activities of olive oil and corn oil on plasma lipids and platelets in high-risk patients. *American Journal of Clinical Nutrition*, **44**, 635–42.

Siscovick D, Schwartz, SM, Corey L, *et al.* (2000) Chlamydia pneumoniae, herpes simplex virus type 1, and cytomegalovirus and incident myocardial infarction and coronary heart disease death in older adults: the Cardiovascular Health Study. *Circulation*, **102**, 2335–40.

Slattery ML, Potter JD, Coates A, *et al.* (1997) Plant foods and colon cancer: an assessment of specific foods and their related nutrients (United States). *Cancer Causes & Control*, **8**, 575–90.

Slemenda C, Brandt K, Heilman D, *et al.* (1997) Quadriceps weakness and osteoarthritis of the knee. *Annals of Internal Medicine*, **127**, 97–104.

Slemenda CW, Miller JZ, Hui SL, *et al.* (1991) Role of physical activity in the development of skeletal mass in children. *Journal of Bone & Mineral Research*, **6**, 1227–33.

Slominski A, Wortsman J, Luger T, *et al.* (2000) Corticotropin releasing hormone and proopiomelanocortin involvement in the cutaneous response to stress. *Physiological Reviews*, **80**, 979–1020.

Smith AN, Drummond E and Eastwood MA (1981) The effect of coarse and fine Canadian red spring wheat and French soft wheat bran on colonic motility in patients with diverticular disease. *American Journal of Clinical Nutrition*, **34**, 2460–3.

Smith H, Anderson F, Raphael H, *et al.* (2007) Effect of annual intramuscular vitamin D on fracture risk in elderly men and women – a population-based, randomized, double-blind, placebo-controlled trial. *Rheumatology*, **46**, 1852–7.

Smith K and Rennie MJ (1996) The measurement of tissue protein turnover. *Baillieres Clinical Endocrinology & Metabolism*, **10**, 469–95.

Smith W, Mitchell P and Leeder SR (2000) Dietary fat and fish intake and age-related maculopathy. *Archives of Ophthalmology*, **118**, 401–4.

Smith W, Mitchell P, Leeder SR and Wang JJ (1998) Plasma fibrinogen levels, other cardiovascular risk factors, and age-related maculopathy: the Blue Mountains Eye Study. *Archives of Ophthalmology*, **116**, 583–7.

Smith W, Mitchell P and Rochester C (1997) Serum beta carotene, alpha tocopherol, and age-related maculopathy: the Blue Mountains Eye Study. *American Journal of Ophthalmology*, **124**, 838–40.

Smith W, Mitchell P, Webb K and Leeder SR (1999) Dietary antioxidants and age-related maculopathy: the Blue Mountains Eye Study. *Ophthalmology*, **106**, 761–7.

Smith-Warner SA, Spiegelman D, Yaun S-S, *et al.* (2003) Fruits, vegetables and lung cancer: a pooled analysis of cohort studies. *International Journal of Cancer*, **107**, 1001–11.

Snow-Harter C, Bouxsein ML, Lewis BT, *et al.* (1992) Effects of resistance and endurance exercise on bone mineral status of young women: a randomized exercise intervention trial. *Journal of Bone & Mineral Research*, **7**, 761–9.

Snow-Marcus H and Mikuls T (2005) Rheumatoid arthritis and cardiovascular disease. *Current Opinion in Rheumatology*, **17**, 234–41.

Soeken K, Lee W, Bausell R, *et al.* (2002) Safety and efficacy of S-adenosylmethionine for osteoarthritis. *Journal of Family Practice*, **51**, 425–30.

Solana R and Mariani E (2000) NK and NK/T cells in human senescence. *Vaccine*, **18**, 1613–20.

Solana R and Pawelec G (1998) Molecular and cellular basis of immunosenescence. *Mechanisms of Ageing & Development*, **102**, 115–29.

Solana R, Alonso MC and Pena J (1999) Natural killer cells in healthy aging. *Experimental Gerontology*, **34**, 435–43.

Sommer BR, Hoff AL and Costa M (2003) Folic acid supplementation in dementia: a preliminary report.

Journal of Geriatric Psychiatry and Neurology, **16**, 156–9.

Sontag S and Wanner J (1988) The cause of leg cramps and knee pains: an hypothesis and effective treatment. *Medical Hypotheses*, **25**, 35–41.

Spangenburg E and Booth F (2003) Molecular regulation of individual skeletal muscle fibre types. *Acta Physiologica Scandinavica*, **178**, 413–24.

Sparrow JR, Nakanishi K and Parish CA (2000) The lipofuscin fluorophore A2E mediates blue light-induced damage to retinal pigmented epithelial cells. *Investigative Ophthalmology and Visual Science*, **41**, 1981–9.

Spencer NF, Norton SD, Harrison LL, *et al.* (1996) Dysregulation of IL-10 production with aging: possible linkage to the age-associated decline in DHEA and its sulfated derivative. *Experimental Gerontology*, **31**, 393–408.

Spencer RC (1998) Clinical impact and associated costs of Clostridium difficile-associated disease. *Journal of Antimicrobial Chemotherapy*, **41 (Suppl C)**, 5–12.

Sperduto RD, Hu TS, Milton RC, *et al.* (1993) The Linxian cataract studies. Two nutrition intervention trials. *Archives of Ophthalmology*, **111**, 1246–53.

Spranger J, Kroke A, Mohlig M, *et al.* (2003) Inflammatory cytokines and the risk to develop type 2 diabetes: results of the prospective population-based European Prospective Investigation into Cancer and Nutrition (EPIC)-Potsdam Study. *Diabetes*, **52**, 812–17.

Sprenger MJ, Mulder PG, Beyer WE, *et al.* (1993) Impact of influenza on mortality in relation to age and underlying disease, 1967–1989. *International Journal of Epidemiology*, **22**, 334–40.

Sproston K and Mindell J (2006) Health Survey for England 2004: Volume 1: The Health of Minority Ethnic Groups. www.ic.nhs.uk/pubs.

Sproston K and Primatesta P (2004) *Health Survey for England 2003. Volume 2: Risk Factors for Cardiovascular Disease*. London, Stationery Office.

Sprott RL (1997) Diet and calorie restriction. *Experimental Gerontology*, **32**, 205–14.

Sreebny LM and Schwartz SS (1997) A reference guide to drugs and dry mouth, 2nd edition. *Gerodontology*, **14**, 33–47.

Staessen J, Fagard R, Thijs L, *et al.* (1997) Randomised double-blind comparison of placebo and active treatment for older patients with isolated systolic hypertension. *Lancet*, **350**, 757–64.

Staessen J, Wang J, Thijs L and Fagard R (1999) Overview of the outcome trials in older patients with isolated systolic hypertension. *Journal of Human Hypertension*, **13**, 859–63.

Stahl W and Sies H (1997) Antioxidant defense: vitamins E and C and carotenoids. *Diabetes*, **46 (Suppl 2)**, S14–18.

Stahl W, Heinrich U, Jungmann H, *et al.* (1998) Increased dermal carotenoid levels assessed by noninvasive reflection spectrophotometry correlate with serum levels in women ingesting Betatene. *Journal of Nutrition*, **128**, 903–7.

Stahl W, Heinrich U, Wiseman S, *et al.* (2001) Dietary tomato paste protects against ultraviolet light-induced erythema in humans. *Journal of Nutrition*, **131**, 1449–51.

Stamm JW, Banting DW and Imrey PB (1990) Adult root caries survey of two similar communities with contrasting natural water fluoride levels. *Journal of the American Dental Association*, **120**, 143–9.

Stammers T, Sibbald B and Freeling P (1992) Efficacy of cod liver oil as an adjunct to non-steroidal anti-inflammatory drug treatment in the management of osteoarthritis in general practice. *Annals of the Rheumatic Diseases*, **51**, 128–9.

Stamp L, James M and Cleland L (2005) Diet and rheumatoid arthritis: a review of the literature. *Seminars in Arthritis and Rheumatism*, **35**, 77–94.

Stanner S (2005) *Cardiovascular Disease: Diet, Nutrition and Emerging Risk Factors. The Report of the British Nutrition Foundation Task Force*. Oxford, Blackwell Publishing.

Stanner S (2007) Does adding milk remove the benefits of your daily cuppa? *Nutrition Bulletin*, **32**, 101–3.

Stanner S, Kelly C, Hughes J and Buttriss J (2004) A review of the epidemiological evidence for the 'antioxidant hypothesis'. *Public Health Nutrition*, **7**, 407–22.

Steele J, Sheiham A, Marcenes W and Walls A (1998) *National Diet and Nutrition Survey: People Aged 65 years and over. Volume 2: Report of the Oral Health Survey*. London, HMSO.

Steele J, Sheiham A, Marcenes W and Walls A (1998) *National Diet and Nutrition Survey: People Aged 65 Years and Over. Volume 2: Report of the Oral Health Survey*. London, HMSO.

Steele JG, Sheiham A, Fay N and Walls AW (2001) Clinical and behavioural risk indicators for root caries in older people. *Gerodontology*, **18**, 95–101.

Stern D, Yan SD, Yan SF and Schmidt AM (2002) Receptor for advanced glycation endproducts: a multiligand receptor magnifying cell stress in diverse pathologic settings. *Advanced Drug Delivery Reviews*, **54**, 1615–25.

Sternbach H (1998) Age-associated testosterone decline in men: clinical issues for psychiatry. *American Journal of Psychiatry*, **155**, 1310–18.

Stitt AW (2005) The maillard reaction in eye diseases. *Annals of the New York Academy of Science*, **1043**, 582–97.

Stokowski RP, Pant PV, Dadd T, *et al.* (2007) A genome-wide association study of skin pigmentation in a South Asian population. *American Journal of Human Genetics*, **81**, 1119–32.

Stott DJ, MacIntosh G, Lowe GD, *et al.* (2005) Randomized controlled trial of homocysteine-lowering vitamin treatment in elderly patients with vascular disease. *American Journal of Clinical Nutrition*, **82**, 1320–6.

Stratton IM, Kohner EM, Aldington SJ, *et al.* (2001) UKPDS 50: risk factors for incidence and progression of retinopathy in Type II diabetes over 6 years from diagnosis. *Diabetologia*, **44**, 156–63.

Stratton RJ, King CL, Stroud MA, Jackson AA and Elia M (2006) 'Malnutrition Universal Screening Tool' predicts mortality and length of hospital stay in acutely ill elderly. *British Journal of Nutrition*, **95**, 325–30.

Straub RH, Konecna L, Hrach S, *et al.* (1998) Serum dehydroepiandrosterone (DHEA) and DHEA sulfate are negatively correlated with serum interleukin-6 (IL-6), and DHEA inhibits IL-6 secretion from mononuclear cells in man in vitro: possible link between endocrinosenescence and immunosenescence. *Journal of Clinical Endocrinology & Metabolism*, **83**, 2012–17.

Straub RH, Miller LE, Scholmerich J and Zietz B (2000) Cytokines and hormones as possible links between endocrinosenescence and immunosenescence. *Journal of Neuroimmunology*, **109**, 10–15.

Strickland FM and Kripke ML (1997) Immune response associated with nonmelanoma skin cancer. *Clinics in Plastic Surgery*, **24**, 637–47.

Stucker M, Altmeyer P, Struk A, *et al.* (2000) The transepidermal oxygen flux from the environment is in balance with the capillary oxygen supply. *Journal of Investigative Dermatology*, **114**, 533–40.

Sturm K, MacIntosh CG, Parker BA, *et al.* (2003) Appetite, food intake, and plasma concentrations of cholecystokinin, ghrelin, and other gastrointestinal hormones in undernourished older women and well-nourished young and older women. *Journal of Clinical Endocrinology & Metabolism*, **88**, 3747–55.

Su L, Bui M, Kardinaal A, *et al.* (1998) Differences between plasma and adipose tissue biomarkers of carotenoids and tocopherols. *Cancer Epidemiology, Biomarkers & Prevention*, **7**, 1043–8.

Su LJ and Arab L (2001) Nutritional status of folate and colon cancer risk: evidence from NHANES I epidemiologic follow-up study. *Annals of Epidemiology*, **11**, 65–72.

Suau A, Bonnet R, Sutren M, *et al.* (1999) Direct analysis of genes encoding 16S rRNA from complex communities reveals many novel molecular species within the human gut. *Applied & Environmental Microbiology*, **65**, 4799–807.

Sugimoto M, Yamashita R and Ueda M (2006) Telomere length of the skin in association with chronological aging and photoaging. *Journal of Dermatological Science*, **43**, 43–7.

Summers LKM, Fielding BA, Bradshaw HA, *et al.* (2002) Substituting dietary saturated fat with polyunsaturated fat changes abdominal fat distribution and improves insulin sensitivity. *Diabetologia*, **45**, 369–77.

Synder PJ, Peachey H, Berlin JA, *et al.* (2000) Effects of testosterone replacement in hypogonadal men. *Journal of Clinical Endocrinology & Metabolism*, **85**, 2670–7.

Szulc P, Duboeuf F, Marchand F and Delmas P (2004) Hormonal and lifestyle determinants of appendicular skeletal muscle mass in men: the MINOS study. *American Journal of Clinical Nutrition*, **80**, 496–503.

Tahir M, Foley B, Pate G, *et al.* (2005) Impact of vitamin E and C supplementation on serum adhesion molecules in chronic degenerative aortic stenosis: a randomized controlled trial. *American Heart Journal*, **150**, 302–6.

Takahashi K (1961) Statistical study on caries incidence in the first molar in relation to the amount of sugar consumption. *Bulletin of the Tokyo Dental College*, **2**, 44–57.

Talbott MC, Miller LT and Kerkvliet NI (1987) Pyridoxine supplementation: effect on lymphocyte responses in elderly persons. *American Journal of Clinical Nutrition*, **46**, 659–64.

Talley NJ, Jones M, Nuyts G and Dubois D (2003) Risk factors for chronic constipation based on a general practice sample. *American Journal of Gastroenterology*, **98**, 1107–11.

Tallon D, Chard J and Dieppe P (2000) Relation between the agendas of the research community and the research consumer. *Lancet*, **355**, 2037–40.

Tanasescu M, Cho E, Manson JE and Hu FB (2004) Dietary fat and cholesterol and the risk of cardiovascular disease among women with type 2 diabetes. *American Journal of Clinical Nutrition*, **79**, 999–1005.

Tarazona R, DelaRosa O, Alonso C, *et al.* (2000) Increased expression of NK cell markers on T lymphocytes in aging and chronic activation of the immune system reflects the accumulation of effector/senescent T cells. *Mechanisms of Ageing & Development*, **121**, 77–88.

Tavani A and La Vecchia C (1999) Beta-carotene and risk of coronary heart disease. A review of observational and intervention studies. *Biomedicine & Pharmacotherapy*, **53**, 409–16.

Taylor A and Hobbs M (2001) Assessment of nutritional influences on risk for cataract. *Nutrition*, **17**, 845–57.

Taylor A, Jacques PF, Chylack LT, Jr., *et al.* (2002) Long-term intake of vitamins and carotenoids and odds of early age-related cortical and posterior subcapsular lens opacities. *American Journal of Clinical Nutrition*, **75**, 540–9.

Taylor AH, Cable NT, Faulkner G, *et al.* (2004) Physical activity and older adults: a review of health benefits and the effectiveness of interventions. *Journal of Sports Sciences*, **22**, 703–25.

Taylor B, Tofler G, Carey H, *et al.* (2006) Full-mouth tooth extraction lowers systemic inflammatory and thrombotic markers of cardiovascular risk. *Journal of Dental Research*, **85**, 74–8.

Taylor HR (1999) Epidemiology of age-related cataract. *Eye*, **13 (Pt 3b)**, 445–8.

Taylor HR, Tikellis G, Robman LD, *et al.* (2002) Vitamin E supplementation and macular degeneration: randomised controlled trial. *British Medical Journal*, **325**, 11.

Taylor HR, West S, Munoz B, *et al.* (1992) The long-term effects of visible light on the eye. *Archives of Ophthalmology*, **110**, 99–104.

Taylor RW, Barron MJ, Borthwick GM, *et al.* (2003) Mitochondrial DNA mutations in human colonic crypt stem cells. *Journal of Clinical Investigation*, **112**, 1351–60.

Tchernof A, Calles-Escandon J, Sites CK and Poehlman ET (1998) Menopause, central body fatness, and insulin resistance: effects of hormone-replacement therapy. *Coronary Artery Disease*, **9**, 503–11.

Teede HJ, Dalais FS, Kotsopoulos D, *et al.* (2001) Dietary soy has both beneficial and potentially adverse cardiovascular effects: a placebo-controlled study in men and postmenopausal women. *Journal of Clinical Endocrinology and Metabolism*, **86**, 3053–60.

Teikari JM, Laatikainen L, Virtamo J, *et al.* (1998) Six-year supplementation with alpha-tocopherol and beta-carotene and age-related maculopathy. *Acta Ophthalmologica Scandinavica*, **76**, 224–9.

Teikari JM, Rautalahti M, Haukka J, *et al.* (1998) Incidence of cataract operations in Finnish male smokers unaffected by alpha tocopherol or beta carotene supplements. *Journal of Epidemiology and Community Health*, **52**, 468–72.

Tepaske R, Velthuis H, Oudemans-van Straaten HM, *et al.* (2001) Effect of preoperative oral immune-enhancing nutritional supplement on patients at high risk of infection after cardiac surgery: a randomised placebo-controlled trial. *Lancet*, **358**, 696–701.

ter Riet G, Kessels AG and Knipschild PG (1995) Randomized clinical trial of ascorbic acid in the treatment of pressure ulcers. *Journal of Clinical Epidemiology*, **48**, 1453–60.

Terry P, Giovannucci E, Michels KB, *et al.* (2001) Fruit, vegetables, dietary fiber, and risk of colorectal cancer. *Journal of the National Cancer Institute*, **93**, 525–33.

Terry P, Lagergren J, Hansen H, *et al.* (2001) Fruit and vegetable consumption in the prevention of oesophageal and cardia cancers. *European Journal of Cancer Prevention*, **10**, 365–9.

Terry P, Lagergren J, Ye W, *et al.* (2000) Antioxidants and cancers of the esophagus and gastric cardia. *International Journal of Cancer*, **87**, 750–4.

Terry P, Lagergren J, Ye W, *et al.* (2001) Inverse association between intake of cereal fiber and risk of gastric cardia cancer. *Gastroenterology*, **120**, 387–91.

Terry P, Nyren O and Yuen J (1998) Protective effect of fruits and vegetables on stomach cancer in a cohort of Swedish twins. *International Journal of Cancer*, **76**, 35–7.

Tesar R, Notelovitz M, Shim E, *et al.* (1992) Axial and peripheral bone density and nutrient intakes of postmenopausal vegetarian and omnivorous women. *American Journal of Clinical Nutrition*, **56**, 699–704.

Teuri U and Korpela R (1998) Galacto-oligosaccharides relieve constipation in elderly people. *Annals of Nutrition & Metabolism*, **42**, 319–27.

Thearle M and Brillantes AMB (2005) Unique characteristics of the geriatric diabetic population and the role for therapeutic strategies that enhance glucagon-like peptide-1 activity. *Current Opinion in Clinical Nutrition & Metabolic Care*, **8**, 9–16.

Thiele JJ, Hsieh SN and Ekanayake-Mudiyanselage S (2005) Vitamin E: critical review of its current use in cosmetic and clinical dermatology. *Dermatologic Surgery*, **31**, 805–13.

Thies F, Nebe-von-Caron G, Powell JR, *et al.* (2001) Dietary supplementation with gamma-linolenic acid or fish oil decreases T lymphocyte proliferation in healthy older humans. *Journal of Nutrition*, **131**, 1918–27.

Thoman ML and Weigle WO (1989) The cellular and subcellular bases of immunosenescence. *Advances in Immunology*, **46**, 221–61.

Thompson D, Williams C, McGregor SJ, *et al.* (2001) Prolonged vitamin C supplementation and recovery from demanding exercise. *International Journal of Sport Nutrition & Exercise Metabolism*, **11**, 466–81.

Thompson P, Clarkson P and Karas R (2003) Statin-associated myopathy. *Journal of the American Medical Association*, **289**, 1681–90.

Toole J, Malinow M, Chambless L, *et al.* (2004) Lowering homocysteine in patients with ischemic stroke to prevent recurrent stroke, myocardial infarction, and death: the Vitamin Intervention for Stroke Prevention (VISP) randomized controlled trial. *Journal of the American Medical Association*, **291**, 565–75.

Torgerson DJ, Iglesias C and Reid DM (2001) *Economics of Osteoporosis*. London, Key Advance Series.

Tortorella C, Piazzolla G, Spaccavento F, *et al.* (1999) Age-related effects of oxidative metabolism and cyclic AMP signaling on neutrophil apoptosis. *Mechanisms of Ageing & Development*, **110**, 195–205.

Tower J (2000) Transgenic methods for increasing Drosophila life span. *Mechanisms of Ageing & Development*, **118**, 1–14.

Townsend DM, Tew KD and Tapiero H (2003) The importance of glutathione in human disease. *Biomedicine & Pharmacotherapy*, **57**, 145–55.

Trautwein E, Duchateau G, Lin Y, *et al.* (2003) Proposed mechanisms of cholesterol-lowering action of plant sterols. *European Journal of Lipid Science and Technology*, **105**, 171–85.

Trayhurn P (2005) The biology of obesity. *Proceedings of the Nutrition Society*, **64**, 31–8.

Trichopoulou A, Costacou T, Bamia C and Trichopoulos D (2003) Adherence to a Mediterranean diet and survival in a Greek population. *New England Journal of Medicine*, **348**, 2599–608.

Trichopoulou A, Kouris-Blazos A, Walqvist M, *et al.* (1995) Diet and overall survival in elderly people. *British Medical Journal*, **311**, 1457–60.

Trichopoulou A, Orfanos P, Norat T, *et al.* (2005) Modified Mediterranean diet and survival: EPIC-elderly prospective cohort study. *British Medical Journal*, **330**, 991–7.

Tricon S, Burdge G, Williams C, *et al.* (2005) The effects of conjugated linoleic acid on human health-related outcomes. *Proceedings of the Nutrition Society*, **64**, 171–82.

Trifunovic A, Wredenberg A, Falkenberg M, *et al.* (2004) Premature ageing in mice expressing defective mitochondrial DNA polymerase. *Nature*, **429**, 417–23.

Trivedi DP, Doll R and Khaw KT (2003) Effect of four monthly oral vitamin D3 (cholecalciferol) supplementation on fractures and mortality in men and women living in the community: randomised double blind controlled trial. *British Medical Journal*, **326**, 469–74.

Trounce I, Byrne E and Marzuki S (1989) Decline in skeletal muscle mitochondrial respiratory chain function: possible factor in ageing. *Lancet*, **1**, 637–9.

Trumbo PR and Ellwood KC (2006) Lutein and zeaxanthin intakes and risk of age-related macular degeneration and cataracts: an evaluation using the Food and Drug Administration's evidence-based review system for health claims. *American Journal of Clinical Nutrition*, **84**, 971–4.

Truswell A (2002) Cereal grains and coronary heart disease. *European Journal of Clinical Nutrition*, **56**, 1–14.

Tselepis AD and John Chapman M (2002) Inflammation, bioactive lipids and atherosclerosis: potential roles of a lipoprotein-associated phospholipase A2, platelet activating factor-acetylhydrolase. *Atherosclerosis Supplements*, **3**, 57–68.

Tsugane S (2005) Salt, salted food intake, and risk of gastric cancer: epidemiologic evidence. *Cancer Science*, **96**, 1–6.

Tucker KL, Hannan MT, Chen H, *et al.* (1999) Potassium, magnesium, and fruit and vegetable intakes are associated with greater bone mineral density in elderly men and women. *American Journal of Clinical Nutrition*, **69**, 727–36.

Tuohy KM, Kolida S, Lustenberger AM and Gibson GR (2001) The prebiotic effects of biscuits containing partially hydrolysed guar gum and fructo-oligosaccharides – a human volunteer study. *British Journal of Nutrition*, **86**, 341–8.

Tuomilehto J, Lindstrom J, Eriksson JG, *et al.* (2001) Prevention of type 2 diabetes mellitus by changes in lifestyle among subjects with impaired glucose tolerance. *New England Journal of Medicine*, **344**, 1343–50.

Turnbull W, Leeds A and Edwards G (1990) Effect of mycoprotein on blood lipids. *American Journal of Clinical Nutrition*, **52**, 646–50.

Turnbull W, Leeds A and Edwards D (1992) Mycoprotein reduces blood lipids in free-living subjects. *American Journal of Clinical Nutrition*, **55**, 415–19.

Turner NC and Clapham JC (1998) Insulin resistance, impaired glucose tolerance and non-insulin-dependent diabetes, pathologic mechanisms and treatment: current status and therapeutic possibilities. *Progress in Drug Research*, **51**, 33–94.

Tuyns AJ (1983) Oesophageal cancer in non-smoking drinkers and in non-drinking smokers. *International Journal of Cancer*, **32**, 443–4.

Tylavsky FA, Anderson JJ, Talmage RV and Taft TN (1992) Are calcium intakes and physical activity patterns during adolescence related to radial bone mass of white college-age females? *Osteoporosis International*, **2**, 232–40.

Tylavsky FA, Holliday K, Danish R, *et al.* (2004) Fruit and vegetable intakes are an independent predictor of bone size in early pubertal children. *American Journal of Clinical Nutrition*, **79**, 311–17.

Tyler H (1970) Neurologic disorders seen in the uremic patient. *Archives of Internal Medicine*, **126**, 781–6.

Uauy R, Aro A, Clarke R, *et al.* (2008) *WHO Scientific Update on Trans Fatty Acids: Summary and Conclusions.* Geneva, WHO.

Urban RJ, Bodenburg YH, Gilkison C, *et al.* (1995) Testosterone administration to elderly men increases skeletal muscle strength and protein synthesis. *American Journal of Physiology*, **269**, E820–6.

Utian WH (2005) Psychosocial and socioeconomic burden of vasomotor symptoms in menopause: a comprehensive review. *Health & Quality of Life Outcomes*, **3**, 47.

Valachovicova M, Krajcovicova-Kudlackova M, Blazicek P and Babinska K (2006) No evidence of insulin resistance in normal weight vegetarians. A case control study. *European Journal of Nutrition*, **45**, 52–4.

Valdes AM, Andrew T, Gardner JP, *et al.* (2005) Obesity, cigarette smoking, and telomere length in women. *Lancet*, **366**, 662–4.

Valenti G (2002) Adrenopause: an imbalance between dehydroepiandrosterone (DHEA) and cortisol secretion. *Journal of Endocrinological Investigation*, **25**, 29–35.

Valero MP, Fletcher AE, De Stavola BL, *et al.* (2002) Vitamin C is associated with reduced risk of cataract in a Mediterranean population. *Journal of Nutrition*, **132**, 1299–306.

Vallee BL (1956) Metabolic role of zinc: report of Council of Foods and Nutrition. *Journal of the American Medical Association*, **162**, 1053.

van Dam RM and Hu FB (2005) Coffee consumption and risk of type 2 diabetes: a systematic review. *Journal of the American Medical Association*, **294**, 97–104.

Van Den Biggelaar AHJ, De Craen AJM, Gussekloo J, *et al.* (2004) Inflammation underlying cardiovascular mortality is a late consequence of evolutionary programming. *FASEB Journal*, **18**, 1022–4.

van den Heuvel EG, Muys T, van Dokkum W and Schaafsma G (1999) Oligofructose stimulates calcium absorption in adolescents. *American Journal of Clinical Nutrition*, **69**, 544–8.

van den Heuvel EG, Schoterman MH and Muijs T (2000) Transgalactooligosaccharides stimulate calcium absorption in postmenopausal women. *Journal of Nutrition*, **130**, 2938–42.

van der Bilt A, van der Glas HW, Mowlana F *et al.* (1993) A comparison between sieving and optical scanning for the determination of particle size distributions obtained by mastication in man. *Archives of Oral Biology*, **38**, 159–62.

van Gils CH, Peeters PHM, Bueno-de-Mesquita HB, *et al.* (2005) Consumption of vegetables and fruits and risk of breast cancer. *Journal of the American Medical Association*, **293**, 183–93.

van Leeuwen R (2003) Age related macular disease. Studies on incidence, risk factors and prognosis. *Ophthalmology*. Rotterdam, The Netherlands, Erasmus University.

van Leeuwen R, Klaver CC, Vingerling JR, *et al.* (2003) Epidemiology of age-related maculopathy: a review. *European Journal of Epidemiology*, **18**, 845–54.

van Leeuwen R, Klaver CCW, Vingerling JR, *et al.* (2003) The risk and natural course of age-related maculopathy. *Archives of Ophthalmology*, **121**, 519–26.

van Meurs JBJ, Dhonukshe-Rutten RAM, Pluijm SMF, *et al.* (2004) Homocysteine levels and the risk of osteoporotic fracture. *New England Journal of Medicine*, **350**, 2033–41.

van Ommen B and Stierum R (2002) Nutrigenomics: exploiting systems biology in the nutrition and health arena. *Current Opinion in Biotechnology*, **13**, 517–21.

van Saase J, van Romunde L, Cats A, *et al.* (1989) Epidemiology of osteoarthritis: Zoetermeer survey. Comparison of radiological osteoarthritis in a Dutch population with that in 10 other populations. *Annals of the Rheumatic Diseases*, **48**, 271–80.

van Soest EM, Dieleman JP, Siersema PD, *et al.* (2005) Increasing incidence of Barrett's oesophagus in the general population. *Gut*, **54**, 1062–6.

VandenLangenberg GM, Mares-Perlman JA, Klein R, *et al.* (1998) Associations between antioxidant and zinc intake and the 5-year incidence of early age-related maculopathy in the Beaver Dam Eye Study. *American Journal of Epidemiology*, **148**, 204–14.

Vander AJ, Sherman JH and Luciano DS (1990) *Human Physiology: The Mechanisms of Body Function*. New York, McGraw-Hill.

Vanek C and Connor WE (2007) Do *n*-3 fatty acids prevent osteoporosis? *American Journal of Clinical Nutrition*, **85**, 647–8.

Varani J, Perone P, Fligiel SEG, *et al.* (2002) Inhibition of type I procollagen production in photodamage: correlation between presence of high molecular weight collagen fragments and reduced procollagen synthesis. *Journal of Investigative Dermatology*, **119**, 122–9.

Varani J, Spearman D, Perone P, *et al.* (2001) Inhibition of type I procollagen synthesis by damaged collagen in photoaged skin and by collagenase-degraded collagen in vitro. *American Journal of Pathology*, **158**, 931–42.

Varani J, Warner RL, Gharaee-Kermani M, *et al.* (2000) Vitamin A antagonizes decreased cell growth and elevated collagen-degrading matrix metalloproteinases and stimulates collagen accumulation in naturally aged human skin. *Journal of Investigative Dermatology*, **114**, 480–6.

Varma SD (1987) Ascorbic acid and the eye with special reference to the lens. *Annals of the New York Academy of Science*, **498**, 280–306.

Vasan RS, Sullivan LM, Roubenoff R, *et al.* (2003) Inflammatory markers and risk of heart failure in elderly subjects without prior myocardial infarction: the Framingham Heart Study. *Circulation*, **107**, 1486–91.

Vassilakopoulos T, Karatza M-H, Katsaounou P, *et al.* (2003) Antioxidants attenuate the plasma cytokine response to exercise in humans. *Journal of Applied Physiology*, **94**, 1025–32.

Vayalil PK, Elmets CA and Katiyar SK (2003) Treatment of green tea polyphenols in hydrophilic cream prevents UVB-induced oxidation of lipids and proteins, depletion of antioxidant enzymes and phosphorylation of MAPK proteins in SKH-1 hairless mouse skin. *Carcinogenesis*, **24**, 927–36.

Vazquez H, Mazure R, Gonzalez D, *et al.* (2000) Risk of fractures in celiac disease patients: A cross-sectional, case-control study. *American Journal of Gastroenterology*, **95**, 183–9.

Vehkalahti MM and Paunio IK (1988) Occurrence of root caries in relation to dental health behavior. *Journal of Dental Research*, **67**, 911–14.

Vellas B, Balas D, Moreau J, *et al.* (1998) Exocrine pancreatic secretion in the elderly. *International Journal of Pancreatology*, **3**, 497–502.

Verdier-Sevrain S, Bonte F and Gilchrest B (2006) Biology of estrogens in skin: implications for skin aging. *Experimental Dermatology*, **15**, 83–94.

Vermeer S, van Dijk E, Koudstaal P, *et al.* (2002) Homocysteine, silent brain infarcts, and white matter lesions: The Rotterdam Scan Study. *Annals of Neurology*, **51**, 285–90.

Verthelyi D (2001) Sex hormones as immunomodulators in health and disease. *International Immunopharmacology*, **1**, 983–93.

Vessby B, Unsitupa M, Hermansen K, *et al.* (2001) Substituting dietary saturated for monounsaturated fat impairs insulin sensitivity in healthy men and women: The KANWU Study. *Diabetologia*, **44**, 312–19.

Vestergaard P and Mosekilde L (2002) Fractures in patients with hyperthyroidism and hypothyroidism: a nationwide follow-up study in 16,249 patients. *Thyroid*, **12**, 411–19.

Vico L, Collet P, Guignandon A, *et al.* (2000) Effects of long-term microgravity exposure on cancellous and cortical weight-bearing bones of cosmonauts. *Lancet*, **355**, 1607–11.

Vieth R, Bischoff-Ferrari H, Boucher BJ, *et al.* (2007) The urgent need to recommend an intake of vitamin D that is effective. *American Journal of Clinical Nutrition*, **85**, 649–50.

Villareal DT and Holloszy JO (2006) DHEA enhances effects of weight training on muscle mass and strength in elderly women and men. *American Journal of Physiology – Endocrinology & Metabolism*, **291**, E1003–8.

Vingerling JR, Dielemans I, Hofman A, *et al.* (1995) The prevalence of age-related maculopathy in the Rotterdam Study. *Ophthalmology*, **102**, 205–10.

Virtamo J, Valkeila E, Alfthan G, *et al.* (1985) Serum selenium and the risk of coronary heart disease and stroke. *American Journal of Epidemiology*, **122**, 276–82.

Visscher T, Seidell J, Molarius A, *et al.* (2001) A comparison of body mass index, waist–hip ratio and waist circumference as predictors of all-cause mortality among the elderly: the Rotterdam study. *International Journal of Obesity and Related Metabolic Disorders*, **25**, 1730–5.

Visser M, Deeg DJH, Lips P and Longitudinal Aging Study Amsterdam (2003) Low vitamin D and high parathyroid hormone levels as determinants of loss of muscle strength and muscle mass (sarcopenia): the Longitudinal Aging Study Amsterdam. *Journal of Clinical Endocrinology & Metabolism*, **88**, 5766–72.

Visser M, Pahor M, Taaffe D, *et al.* (2002) Relationship of interleukin-6 and tumor necrosis factor-alpha with muscle mass and muscle strength in elderly men and women: the Health ABC Study. *The Journals of Gerontology, Series A, Biological Sciences and Medical Sciences*, **57**, M326–32.

Visser M, Pahor M, Tylavsky F, *et al.* (2003) One- and two-year change in body composition as measured by DXA in a population-based cohort of older men and women. *Journal of Applied Physiology*, **94**, 2368–74.

Vitale S, West S, Hallfrisch J, *et al.* (1993) Plasma antioxidants and risk of cortical and nuclear cataract. *Epidemiology*, **4**, 195–203.

Voedingsnormen (2001) *Energie, Eiwitten, Vetten en Verteerbare Koolhydraten*. Den Haag, Gezondheidsraad.

Volkert D, Kreuel K, Heseker H and Stehle P (2004) Energy and nutrient intake of young-, old, old-old and very old elderly in Germany. *European Journal of Clinical Nutrition*, **58**, 1190–2000.

Volpato S, Guralnik JM, Ferrucci L, *et al.* (2001) Cardiovascular disease, interleukin-6, and risk of mortality in older women: the women's health and aging study. *Circulation*, **103**, 947–53.

Volpi E, Mittendorfer B, Rasmussen B and Wolfe R (2000) The response of muscle protein anabolism to combined hyperaminoacidemia and glucose-induced hyperinsulinemia is impaired in the elderly. *Journal of Clinical Endocrinology and Metabolism*, **85**, 4481–90.

Volpi E, Sheffield-Moore M, Rasmussen B and Wolfe R (2001) Basal muscle amino acid kinetics and protein synthesis in healthy young and older men. *Journal of the American Medical Association*, **286**, 1206–12.

vom Saal FS, Quadagno DM, Even MD, *et al.* (1990) Paradoxical effects of maternal stress on fetal steroids and postnatal reproductive traits in female mice from different intrauterine positions. *Biology of Reproduction*, **43**, 751–61.

von Zglinicki T (2002) Oxidative stress shortens telomeres. *Trends in Biochemical Sciences*, **27**, 339–44.

von Zglinicki T, Burkle A and Kirkwood TB (2001) Stress, DNA damage and ageing – an integrative approach. *Experimental Gerontology*, **36**, 1049–62.

von Zglinicki T, Serra V, Lorenz M, *et al.* (2000) Short telomeres in patients with vascular dementia: an indicator of low antioxidative capacity and a possible risk factor? *Laboratory Investigation*, **80**, 1739–47.

Vyas A, Greenhalgh A, Cade J, *et al.* (2003) Nutrient intakes of an adult Pakistani, European and African-Caribbean community in inner city Britain. *Journal of Human Nutrition and Dietetics*, **16**, 327–37.

Wahle K, Lindsay D and Bourne L (2005) Plant and plant-derived lipids. In: *Plants: Diet and Health*. Ed. G. Goldberg. Oxford, Blackwell: 183–208.

Wahlqvist M and Saviage G (2000) Interventions aimed at dietary and lifestyle changes to promote healthy aging. *European Journal of Clinical Nutrition*, **54 (Suppl 3)**, S148–56.

Wainwright LJ, Barrett KE and Jenkins G (2006) Chronic stress and its role in skin ageing. *Journal of Investigative Dermatology*, **126**, 1678.

Wainwright LJ, Middleton PG and Rees JL (1995) Changes in mean telomere length in basal cell carcinomas of the skin. *Genes, Chromosomes & Cancer*, **12**, 45–9.

Wald DS, Wald NJ, Morris JK and Law M (2006) Folic acid, homocysteine, and cardiovascular disease: judging causality in the face of inconclusive trial evidence. *British Medical Journal*, **333**, 1114–17.

Wald N and Law M (2003) A strategy to reduce cardiovascular disease by more than 80%. *British Medical Journal*, **326**, 1419–24.

Wallace DC (1992) Mitochondrial genetics: a paradigm for aging and degenerative diseases? *Science*, **256**, 628–32.

Wallis JL, Lipski PS, Mathers JC, *et al.* (1993) Duodenal brush-border mucosal glucose transport and enzyme activities in aging man and effect of bacterial contamination of the small intestine. *Digestive Diseases & Sciences*, **38**, 403–9.

Walston J, McBurnie MA, Newman A, *et al.* (2002) Frailty and activation of the inflammation and coagulation systems with and without clinical comorbidities: results from the Cardiovascular Health Study. *Archives of Internal Medicine*, **162**, 2333–41.

Wang B, Jenkins JR and Trayhurn P (2005) Expression and secretion of inflammation-related adipokines by human adipocytes differentiated in culture: integrated response to TNF-alpha. *American Journal of Physiology – Endocrinology & Metabolism*, **288**, E731–40.

Wang C, Harris W, Chung M, *et al.* (2006) n-3 Fatty acids from fish or fish-oil supplements, but not alpha-linolenic acid, benefit cardiovascular disease outcomes in primary- and secondary-prevention studies: a systematic review. *American Journal of Clinical Nutrition*, **84**, 5–17.

Wang J, Chi DS, Kalin GB, *et al.* (2002) *Helicobacter pylori* infection and oncogene expressions in gastric carcinoma and its precursor lesions. *Digestive Diseases & Sciences*, **47**, 107–13.

Wang JJ, Foran S, Smith W and Mitchell P (2003) Risk of age-related macular degeneration in eyes with macular drusen or hyperpigmentation. *Archives of Ophthalmology*, **121**, 658–63.

Wang L, Larson EB, Bowen JD and van Belle G (2006) Performance-based physical function and future dementia in older people. *Archives of Internal Medicine*, **166**, 1115–20.

Wang N, Wu H and Fan Z (2002) Primary angle closure glaucoma in Chinese and Western populations. *Chinese Medical Journal*, **115**, 1706–15.

Wang X, Qin X, Demirtash H, *et al.* (2007) Efficacy of folic acid supplementation in stroke prevention: a meta-analysis. *Lancet*, **369**, 1876–82.

Wang ZY, Agarwal R, Bickers DR and Mukhtar H (1991) Protection against ultraviolet B radiation-induced photocarcinogenesis in hairless mice by green tea polyphenols. *Carcinogenesis*, **12**, 1527–30.

Wanless D (2004) *Securing Good Health for the Whole Population*. London, HMSO.

Wannamethee S and Shaper A (2002) Physical activity and cardiovascular disease. *Seminars in Vascular Medicine*, **2**, 257–65.

Wannamethee S, Shaper A and Walker M (1998) Changes in physical activity, mortality, and incidence of coronary heart disease in older men. *Lancet*, **351**, 1603–8.

Ward WF and Shibatani T (1994) Calorie-modulation of protein turnover. *Modulation of Aging Processes by Dietary Restriction*. Ed. B. P. Yu. Boca Raton, FL, CRC Press Inc: 121–42.

Warholm O, Skaar S, Hedman E and Molmen H (2003) The effects of a standardized herbal remedy made from a subtype of rosa canina in patients with osteoarthritis. *Current Therapeutic Research, Clinical & Experimental*, **64**, 21–31.

Warnakulasuriya S (2004) Smokeless tobacco and oral cancer. *Oral Diseases*, **10**, 1–4.

Watanabe Y, Ozasa K, Higashi A, *et al.* (1997) *Helicobacter pylori* infection and atrophic gastritis. A case-control study in a rural town of Japan. *Journal of Clinical Gastroenterology*, **25**, 391–4.

Watson RR, Prabhala RH, Plezia PM and Alberts DS (1991) Effect of beta-carotene on lymphocyte subpopulations in elderly humans: evidence for a dose–response relationship. *American Journal of Clinical Nutrition*, **53**, 90–4.

Watt I and Doherty M (2003) Plain radiographic features of osteoarthritis. In: *Osteoarthritis*. Ed. K. Brandt, M. Doherty and S. Lohmander. Oxford, Oxford University Press: 211–25.

Weaver JD, Huang MH, Albert M, *et al.* (2002) Interleukin-6 and risk of cognitive decline: MacArthur studies of successful aging. *Neurology*, **59**, 371–8.

Weaver W, Litwin PE, Martin JS, *et al.* (1991) Effect of age on use of thrombolytic therapy and mortality in acute myocardial infarction. The MITI Project Group. *Journal of the American College of Cardiology*, **18**, 657–62.

Weber G, Heilborn JD, Chamorro Jimenez CI, *et al.* (2005) Vitamin D induces the antimicrobial protein hCAP18 in human skin. *Journal of Investigative Dermatology*, **124**, 1080–2.

Wefers H and Sies H (1988) The protection by ascorbate and glutathione against microsomal lipid peroxidation is dependent on vitamin E. *European Journal of Biochemistry*, **174**, 353–7.

Wei H, Saladi R, Lu Y, *et al.* (2003) Isoflavone genistein: photoprotection and clinical implications in dermatology. *Journal of Nutrition*, **133**, 3811S–19S.

Wei Q, Shen H, Wang LE, *et al.* (2003) Association between low dietary folate intake and suboptimal cellular DNA repair capacity. *Cancer Epidemiology, Biomarkers & Prevention*, **12**, 963–9.

Weindruch R and Sohal RS (1997) Caloric intake and aging. *New England Journal of Medicine*, **337**, 986–94.

Weindruch R and Walford RL (1982) Dietary restriction in mice beginning at 1 year of age: effect on life-span and spontaneous cancer incidence. *Science*, **215**, 1415–18.

Weindruch R and Walford RL (1988) *The Retardation of Aging and Disease by Dietary Restriction.* Springfield, IL, Charles C. Thomas.

Weiss JM, Huang W-Y, Rinaldi S, *et al.* (2007) IGF-1 and IGFBP-3: risk of prostate cancer among men in the Prostate, Lung, Colorectal and Ovarian Cancer Screening Trial. *International Journal of Cancer*, **121**, 2267–73.

Weiss LA, Barrett-Connor E and von Mühlen D (2005) Ratio of *n*-6 to *n*-3 fatty acids and bone mineral density in older adults: the Rancho Bernardo Study. *American Journal of Clinical Nutrition*, **81**, 934–8.

Weksler ME (1981) The senescence of the immune system. *Hospital Practice (Office Edition)*, **16**, 53–64.

Welle S, Thornton C and Statt M (1995) Myofibrillar protein synthesis in young and old human subjects after three months of resistance training. *American Journal of Physiology*, **268**, E422–7.

Wellinghausen N, Martin M and Rink L (1997) Zinc inhibits interleukin-1-dependent T cell stimulation. *European Journal of Immunology*, **27**, 2529–35.

Wendt T, Bucciarelli L, Qu W, *et al.* (2002) Receptor for advanced glycation endproducts (RAGE) and vascular inflammation: insights into the pathogenesis of macrovascular complications in diabetes. *Current Atherosclerosis Reports*, **4**, 228–37.

Werninghaus K, Meydani M, Bhawan J, *et al.* (1994) Evaluation of the photoprotective effect of oral vitamin E supplementation. *Archives of Dermatology*, **130**, 1257–61.

Wespes E and Schulman CC (2002) Male andropause: myth, reality, and treatment. *International Journal of Impotence Research*, **14 (Suppl 1)**, S93–8.

West S, Vitale S, Hallfrisch J, *et al.* (1994) Are antioxidants or supplements protective for age-related macular degeneration? *Archives of Ophthalmology*, **112**, 222–7.

Westergaard M, Henningsen J, Svendsen ML, *et al.* (2001) Modulation of keratinocyte gene expression and differentiation by PPAR-selective ligands and tetradecylthio-
acetic acid. *Journal of Investigative Dermatology*, **116**, 702–12.

Weyand CM, Brandes JC, Schmidt D, *et al.* (1998) Functional properties of CD4+ CD28− T cells in the aging immune system. *Mechanisms of Ageing & Development*, **102**, 131–47.

Wharton B and Bishop N (2003) Rickets. *Lancet*, **362**, 1389–400.

Whelton HP, Holland TJ and O'Mullane DM (1993) The prevalence of root surface caries amongst Irish adults. *Gerodontology*, **10**, 72–5.

Whelton P, Appel L, Espeland M, *et al.* (1998) Sodium reduction and weight loss in the treatment of hypertension in older persons: a randomized controlled trial of nonpharmacologic interventions in the elderly (TONE). TONE Collaborative Research Group. *Journal of the American Medical Association*, **279**, 839–46.

Whitehead WE, Drinkwater D, Cheskin LJ, *et al.* (1989) Constipation in the elderly living at home. Definition, prevalence, and relationship to lifestyle and health status. *Journal of the American Geriatrics Society*, **37**, 423–9.

Whorwell PJ, Altringer L, Morel J, *et al.* (2006) Efficacy of an encapsulated probiotic Bifidobacterium infantis 35624 in women with irritable bowel syndrome. *American Journal of Gastroenterology*, **101**, 1581–90.

Wigler I, Grotto I, Caspi D and Yaron M (2003) The effects of Zintona EC (a ginger extract) on symptomatic osteoarthritis. *Osteoarthritis and Cartilage*, **11**, 783–9.

Wikby A, Ferguson F, Forsey R, *et al.* (2005) An immune risk phenotype, cognitive impairment, and survival in very late life: impact of allostatic load in Swedish octogenarian and nonagenarian humans. *Journals of Gerontology Series A – Biological Sciences & Medical Sciences*, **60**, 556–65.

Wikby A, Johansson B, Olsson J, *et al.* (2002) Expansions of peripheral blood CD8 T-lymphocyte subpopulations and an association with cytomegalovirus seropositivity in the elderly: the Swedish NONA immune study. *Experimental Gerontology*, **37**, 445–53.

Wikby A, Maxson P, Olsson J, *et al.* (1998) Changes in CD8 and CD4 lymphocyte subsets, T cell proliferation responses and non-survival in the very old: the Swedish longitudinal OCTO-immune study. *Mechanisms of Ageing & Development*, **102**, 187–98.

Wild S and McKeigue P (1997) Cross sectional analysis of mortality by country of birth in England and Wales, 1970–92. *British Medical Journal*, **314**, 705–10.

Wilkerson W and Sane D (2002) Aging and thrombosis. *Seminars in Thrombosis & Hemostasis*, **28**, 555–68.

Wilkins CH, Sheline YI, Roe CM, Birge SJ and Morris JC (2006) Vitamin D deficiency is associated with low mood and worse cognitive performance in older adults. *American Journal of Geriatric Psychiatry*, **14**, 1032–40.

Willett W (2002) Dietary fat plays a major role in obesity: no. *Obesity Reviews*, **3**, 59–68.

Willett W, Manson J and Liu S (2002) Glycemic index, glycemic load, and risk of type 2 diabetes. *American Journal of Clinical Nutrition*, **76**, 274S–80S.

Williams C (2003) Chips with everything? Nutritional genomics and the application of diet in disease prevention. *Nutrition Bulletin*, **28**, 139–46.

Williams G (1957) Pleiotropy, natural selection and the evolution of senescence. *Evolution*, **11**, 398–411.

Williams JZ and Barbul A (2003) Nutrition and wound healing. *Surgical Clinics of North America*, **83**, 571–96.

Williams L (2002) Assessing patients' nutritional needs in the wound-healing process. *Journal of Wound Care*, **11**, 225–8.

Williams M, Fleg J, Ades P, *et al.* (2002) Secondary prevention of coronary heart disease in the elderly (with emphasis on patients 75 years of age). An American Heart Association Scientific Statement From the Council on Clinical Cardiology Subcommittee on Exercise, Cardiac Rehabilitation, and Prevention. *Circulation*, **105**, 1735–43.

Williams ME and Pannill FC, 3rd (1982) Urinary incontinence in the elderly: physiology, pathophysiology, diagnosis, and treatment. *Annals of Internal Medicine*, **97**, 895–907.

Williams PT and Wood PD (2006) The effects of changing exercise levels on weight and age-related weight gain. *International Journal of Obesity*, **30**, 543–51.

Williams R, Philpott MP and Kealey T (1993) Metabolism of freshly isolated human hair follicles capable of hair elongation: a glutaminolytic, aerobic glycolytic tissue. *Journal of Investigative Dermatology*, **100**, 834–40.

Wilson S, Parle JV, Roberts LM, *et al.* (2006) Prevalence of subclinical thyroid dysfunction and its relation to socioeconomic deprivation in the elderly: a community-based cross-sectional survey. *Journal of Clinical Endocrinology & Metabolism*, **91**, 4809–16.

Winkler BS, Boulton ME, Gottsch JD and Sternberg P (1999) Oxidative damage and age-related macular degeneration. *Molecular Vision*, **5**, 32.

Winzell MS, Nogueiras R, Dieguez C and Ahren B (2004) Dual action of adiponectin on insulin secretion in insulin-resistant mice. *Biochemical & Biophysical Research Communications*, **321**, 154–60.

Wittert G, Chapman I, Haren M, *et al.* (2003) Oral testosterone supplementation increases muscle and decreases fat mass in healthy elderly males with low-normal gonadal status. *The Journals of Gerontology, Series A, Biological Sciences and Medical Sciences*, **58**, 618–25.

Wlaschek M, Ma W, Jansen-Durr P and Scharffetter-Kochanek K (2003) Photoaging as a consequence of natural and therapeutic ultraviolet irradiation – studies on PUVA-induced senescence-like growth arrest of human dermal fibroblasts. *Experimental Gerontology*, **38**, 1265–70.

Wojtaszewski JFP, Nielsen JN and Richter EA (2002) Invited review: effect of acute exercise on insulin signaling and action in humans. *Journal of Applied Physiology*, **93**, 384–92.

Wolbach SB and Howe PR (1978) Nutrition classics. *The Journal of Experimental Medicine*, **42**, 753–77, 1925.

Wolf C, Steiner A and Honigsmann H (1988) Do oral carotenoids protect human skin against ultraviolet erythema, psoralen phototoxicity, and ultraviolet-induced DNA damage? *Journal of Investigative Dermatology*, **90**, 55–7.

Wolk A (2004) The growth hormone and insulin-like growth factor I axis, and cancer. *Lancet*, **363**, 1336–7.

Wolters M, Strohle A and Hahn A (2004) Cobalamin: a critical vitamin in the elderly. *Preventive Medicine*, **39**, 1256–66.

Wong ML, Wee S, Pin CH, *et al.* (1999) Sociodemographic and lifestyle factors associated with constipation in an elderly Asian community. *American Journal of Gastroenterology*, **94**, 1283–91.

Woodmansey EJ, McMurdo MET, Macfarlane GT and Macfarlane S (2004) Comparison of compositions and metabolic activities of fecal microbiotas in young adults and in antibiotic-treated and non-antibiotic-treated elderly subjects. *Applied & Environmental Microbiology*, **70**, 6113–22.

Woodward M and Turnstall-Pedoe H (1999) Coffee and tea consumption in the Scottish Heart Health Study: conflicting relations with coronary risk factors, coronary disease amd all cause mortality. *Journal of Epidemiology and Community Health*, **53**, 481–7.

World Cancer Research Fund/American Institute for Cancer Research (1997) *Food, Nutrition and the Prevention of Cancer: A Global Perspective*. Washington, DC, American Institute for Cancer Research.

World Cancer Research Fund/American Institute for Cancer Research (2007) *Food, Nutrition, Physical Activity, and the Prevention of Cancer: a Global Perspective*. Washington, DC, AICR.

World Health Organization (1994) *Study Group on Assessment of Fracture Risk and its Application to Screening and Postmenopausal Osteoporosis*. Report of a WHO Study Group. Technical Report series No. 84. Geneva, WHO.

World Health Organization (1996) *Guidelines Series for Healthy Ageing 1 – The Heidelberg Guidelines for Promoting Physical Activity among Older People*. Geneva, WHO.

World Health Organization (2001) *Men, Ageing and Health*. Geneva, WHO.

World Health Organization (2002a) *Active Ageing. A Policy Framework*. Geneva, WHO.

World Health Organization (2002b) *Keep Fit for Life. Meeting the Nutritional Needs of Older People.* Geneva, WHO.

World Health Organization (2003a) WHO Technical Report Series 916 Joint WHO/FAO Expert Consultation on Diet, Nutrition and the Prevention of Chronic Diseases. Geneva, WHO. www.who.int/dietphysicalactivity/publications/trs916/en/gsfao_global.pdf.

World Health Organization (2003b) *World Health Report 2003 – Shaping the Future.* Geneva, WHO.

World Health Organization (2004a) *Atlas of Heart Disease and Stroke.* Geneva, WHO.

World Health Organization (2004b) *Global Strategy on Diet and Physical Activity.* Geneva, WHO.

World Health Organization (2005) *The SuRF Report 2: Surveillance of Chronic Disease Risk Factors.* Geneva, WHO.

World Health Organization Regional Office for Africa. Ageing and Health. www.afro.who.int/ageingandhealth/epidemiology.html. Accessed December 2007.

World Health Organization Regional Office for the Western Pacific Region. Regional Office for the Western Pacific Region. Statistical Tables. www.who.int/about/regions/wpro/en/index.html. Accessed December 2007.

World Health Organization Statistics. www3.who.int/whois/mort. Accessed 5 November 2004.

Worwag M, Classen HG and Schumacher E (1999) Prevalence of magnesium and zinc deficiencies in nursing home residents in Germany. *Magnesium Research*, **12**, 181–9.

Woudstra T and Thomson ABR (2002) Nutrient absorption and intestinal adaptation with ageing. *Best Practice & Research: Clinical Gastroenterology*, **16**, 1–15.

Wouters-Wesseling W, Vos AP, Van Hal M, *et al.* (2005) The effect of supplementation with an enriched drink on indices of immune function in frail elderly. *Journal of Nutrition, Health & Aging*, **9**, 281–6.

Wright S (1991) Essential fatty acids and the skin. *British Journal of Dermatology*, **125**, 503–15.

Wu AH, Wan P and Bernstein L (2001) A multiethnic population-based study of smoking, alcohol and body size and risk of adenocarcinomas of the stomach and esophagus (United States). *Cancer Causes & Control*, **12**, 721–32.

Wu SY and Leske MC (1997) Associations with intraocular pressure in the Barbados Eye Study. *Archives of Ophthalmology*, **115**, 1572–6.

Xu HE, Lambert MH, Montana VG, *et al.* (1999) Molecular recognition of fatty acids by peroxisome proliferator-activated receptors. *Molecular Cell*, **3**, 397–403.

Xu Q, Schett G, Perschinka H, *et al.* (2000) Serum soluble heat shock protein 60 is elevated in subjects with atherosclerosis in a general population. *Circulation*, **102**, 14–20.

Xu Y, Voorhees JJ and Fisher GJ (2006) Epidermal growth factor receptor is a critical mediator of ultraviolet B irradiation-induced signal transduction in immortalized human keratinocyte HaCaT cells. *American Journal of Pathology*, **169**, 823–30.

Yamazaki S, Machii K, Tsuyuki S, *et al.* (1985) Immunological responses to monoassociated Bifidobacterium longum and their relation to prevention of bacterial invasion. *Immunology*, **56**, 43–50.

Yaqoob P and Calder PC (2003) N-3 polyunsaturated fatty acids and inflammation in the arterial wall. *European Journal of Medical Research*, **8**, 337–54.

Yaqoob P and Ferns G (2005) Inflammation-related factors. In: *Cardiovascular Disease: Diet, Nutrition and Emerging Risk Factors.* Ed. S. Stanner. Oxford, Blackwell Publishing: 128–46.

Yaqoob P, Knapper JA, Webb DH, *et al.* (1998) Effect of olive oil on immune function in middle aged men. *American Journal of Clinical Nutrition*, **67**, 129–35.

Ye W and Nyren O (2003) Risk of cancers of the oesophagus and stomach by histology or subsite in patients hospitalised for pernicious anaemia. *Gut*, **52**, 938–41.

Yeh CK, Johnson DA and Dodds MW (1998) Impact of aging on human salivary gland function: a community-based study. *Aging (Milano)*, **10**, 421–8.

Yochum L, Kushi L, Meyer K and Folsom A (1999) Dietary flavonoid intake and risk of cardiovascular disease in postmenopausal women. *American Journal of Epidemiology*, **149**, 943–9.

Yoshikawa T (1997) Perspective: aging and infectious diseases: past, present, and future. *Journal of Infectious Diseases*, **176**, 1053–7.

Young DG, Skibinski G, Mason JI and James K (1999) The influence of age and gender on serum dehydroepiandrosterone sulphate (DHEA-S), IL-6, IL-6 soluble receptor (IL-6 sR) and transforming growth factor beta 1 (TGF-beta1) levels in normal healthy blood donors. *Clinical & Experimental Immunology*, **117**, 476–81.

Yu BP (1994) How diet influences the aging process of the rat. *Proceedings of the Society for Experimental Biology & Medicine*, **205**, 97–105.

Yu MC, Garabrant DH, Peters JM and Mack TM (1988) Tobacco, alcohol, diet, occupation, and carcinoma of the esophagus. *Cancer Research*, **48**, 3843–8.

Yudkin J (2003) Adipose tissue, insulin action and vascular disease: inflammatory signals. *International Journal of Obesity*, **27**, S25–8.

Yudkin J, Eringa E and Stehouwer C (2005) 'Vasocrine' signalling from perivascular fat: a mechanism linking insulin resistance to vascular disease. *Lancet*, **365**, 1817–20.

Yudkin JS, Kumari M, Humphries SE and Mohamed-Ali V (2000) Inflammation, obesity, stress and coronary heart disease: is interleukin-6 the link? *Atherosclerosis*, **148**, 209–14.

Yurkstas A and Emerson W (1964) Dietary selections of persons with natural and artificial teeth. *Journal of Prosthetic Dentistry*, **14**, 695–7.

Yven C, Bonnet L, Cormier D, *et al.* (2006) Impaired mastication modifies the dynamics of bolus formation. *European Journal of Oral Sciences*, **114**, 184–90.

Zain RB, Ikeda N, Gupta PC, Gupta PC, *et al.* (1999) Oral mucosal lesions associated with betel quid, areca nut and tobacco chewing habits: consensus from a workshop held in Kuala Lumpur, Malaysia, November 25–27, 1996. *Journal of Oral Pathology & Medicine*, **28**, 1–4.

Zamboni M, Zoico E, Scartezzini T, *et al.* (2003) Body composition changes in stable-weight elderly subjects: the effect of sex. *Aging Clinical and Experimental Research*, **15**, 321–7.

Zampelas A, Peel A, Gould B, *et al.* (1994) Polyunsaturated fatty acids of the *n*-6 and *n*-3 series: effects of low-fat dietary treatment with and without fish oil supplementation. *European Journal of Clinical Nutrition*, **48**, 842–8.

Zaninotto P, Wardle H, Stamatakis E, Mindell J and Head J (2006) *Forecasting Obesity to 2010. Report Prepared for Department of Health.* London, Department of Health.

Zarbin MA (2004) Current concepts in the pathogenesis of age-related macular degeneration. *Archives of Ophthalmology*, **122**, 598–614.

Zava DT and Duwe G (1997) Estrogenic and antiproliferative properties of genistein and other flavonoids in human breast cancer cells in vitro. *Nutrition & Cancer*, **27**, 31–40.

Zetterberg A and Engstrom W (1981) Glutamine and the regulation of DNA replication and cell multiplication in fibroblasts. *Journal of Cellular Physiology*, **108**, 365–73.

Zhang HM, Wakisaka N, Maeda O and Yamamoto T (1997) Vitamin C inhibits the growth of a bacterial risk factor for gastric carcinoma: *Helicobacter pylori*. *Cancer*, **80**, 1897–903.

Zhang W, Doherty M, Bardin T, *et al.* (2006) EULAR evidence-based recommendations for gout. Part II: Management. Report of a task force of the EULAR Standing Committee for International Clinical Studies Including Therapeutics (ESCISIT). *Annals of the Rheumatic Diseases*, **65**, 1312–24.

Zhang X, Shu X-O, Li H, *et al.* (2005) Prospective cohort study of soy food consumption and risk of bone fracture among postmenopausal women. *Archives of Internal Medicine*, **165**, 1890–5.

Zhang Y, Hannan MT, Chaisson CE, *et al.* (2000) Bone mineral density and risk of incident and progressive radiographic knee osteoarthritis in women: the Framingham Study. *Journal of Rheumatology*, **27**, 1032–7.

Zhou T, Edwards CK, 3rd and Mountz JD (1995) Prevention of age-related T cell apoptosis defect in CD2-fas-transgenic mice. *Journal of Experimental Medicine*, **182**, 129–37.

Ziccardi P, Nappo F, Giugliano G, *et al.* (2002) Reduction of inflammatory cytokine concentrations and improvement of endothelial functions in obese women after weight loss over one year. *Circulation*, **105**, 804–9.

Zock PL (2001) Dietary fats and cancer. *Current Opinion in Lipidology*, **12**, 5–10.

Zouboulis CC (2001a) Retinoids – which dermatological indications will benefit in the near future? *Skin Pharmacology & Applied Skin Physiology*, **14**, 303–15.

Zouboulis CC (2001b) Is acne vulgaris a genuine inflammatory disease? *Dermatology*, **203**, 277–9.

Index